NEONATAL NURSING

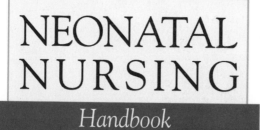

Handbook

NEONATAL NURSING

Handbook

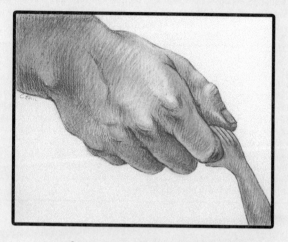

Carole Kenner, DNS, RNC, FAAN
Associate Dean for Academic Advancement
Professor, Clinical Nursing
University of Illinois at Chicago
Chicago, Illinois

Judy Wright Lott, DSN, RNC, NNP
Dean and Associate Professor
Louise Herrington School of Nursing
Baylor University
Dallas, Texas

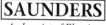

SAUNDERS
An Imprint of Elsevier

SAUNDERS

An Imprint of Elsevier

11830 Westline Industrial Drive
St. Louis, Missouri 63146

NOTICE

Nursing is an ever-changing field. Standard safety precautions must be followed, but as new research and clinical experience broaden our knowledge, changes in treatment and drug therapy may become necessary or appropriate. Readers are advised to check the most current product information provided by the manufacturer of each drug to be administered to verify the recommended dose, the method and duration of administration, and contraindications. It is the responsibility of the licensed prescriber, relying on experience and knowledge of the patient, to determine dosages and the best treatment for each individual patient. Neither the publisher nor the author assumes any liability for any injury and/or damage to persons or property arising from this publication.

ISBN-13: 978-0-7216-0023-9
ISBN-10: 0-7216-0023-9

Executive Editor: Michael S. Ledbetter
Developmental Editor: Amanda Sunderman Politte
Publishing Services Manager: Catherine Albright Jackson
Project Manager: Celeste Clingan
Design Coordinator: Teresa Breckwoldt
Cover Art: Claire Hirn

Printed in USA

Last digit is the print number: 9   8   7   6   5   4   3   2

Healthcare delivery has changed dramatically in the last decade. Decisions are made quickly and with more thought toward cost and efficiency. Health professionals need reference materials that provide "at a glance" answers. This handbook will serve that purpose.

The content addresses the most common neonatal nursing problems. Its format is brief with charts and illustrations to assist in its use in a clinical situation. For students the algorithms and decision-trees provide a visual overview of the material. Where possible, care maps, protocols, and charts are included that have been used in institutions and critiqued by multidisciplinary committees. These can be adapted for your institution's use based on the population that you serve.

As you use this material please give us feedback—what you liked, did not like, what should be included in future editions, and what should be revised. You can reach us through the Elsevier website at www.elsevierhealth.com.

Carole Kenner, DNS, RNC, FAAN
Judy Wright Lott, DSN, RNC, NNP

Acknowledgments

We wish to acknowledge the help of several institutions and individuals who assisted in the development of this book. Leslie Altimier, MSN, RN, Nurse Manager, Neonatal Services TriHealth, Cincinnati, Ohio who spearheaded the writing of a Competency Based Orientation Program along with policies and procedures for the Neonatal Intensive Care Unit (NICU). This material was published by the National Association of Neonatal Nurses (NANN), Glenview, Ill. We are grateful that NANN had the vision to make this material commercially available. Catherine Theorell, MSN, RNC, NNP, Neonatal Nurse Practitioner, University of Illinois Medical Center, Chicago, Ill., willingly shared policies and procedures that were written for the NICU and Intermediate Care Nursery (ICN). Karen Trebel, an undergraduate nursing student at University of Illinois at Chicago College of Nursing helped gather guidelines.

Deborah Harris, RN, Neonatal Nurse Practitioner, Waikato Hospital, Hamiton, New Zealand, brought the international perspective to this book. She willingly shared resources and added a depth to the content that would otherwise have been missing. Her contribution reminds us that neonatal nursing care is global.

Some of the materials in this book were adapted from Kenner C and Lott JW (2003). *Comprehensive neonatal nursing: a physiologic perspective*, ed 3, St Louis: WB Saunders. We wish to thank the following authors in that book whose materials have been quoted in this handbook: Susan Blackburn, Nancy Shaw, Stephanie Durfor, Michelle Ratcliffe, Karen Sweetwyne-Thomas, Marlene Walden, and Linda Franck.

There are many people who worked on the production of this book. Jan Zasada, The In Bin, Inc, Johnsburg, Ill., spent hours editing the manuscript and getting copyright permissions. We could not have produced this book without her support. We also want to thank the people behind the scenes at Elsevier who believed in the project and then helped us bring it to fruition, Amanda Politte and Michael Ledbetter. Thank you, too, to the many neonatal nurses from around the world who willingly told us what they needed in practice.

Carole Kenner, DNS, RNC, FAAN
Judy Wright Lott, DSN, RNC, NNP

and

Deborah Harris, RN

Contents

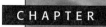

PRENATAL, INTRAPARTAL, AND POSTPARTAL RED FLAGS

New neonatal nurses frequently are in the position to observe maternal or perinatal conditions that lead to a high-risk delivery or a sick neonate. Some of these signs or **red flags** can be used to help identify a potential abnormal condition, develop the differential diagnoses, and plan nursing care.

PHYSICAL ABUSE DURING PREGNANCY*

Reports of physical abuse during pregnancy are on the increase. These signs should serve as red flags during assessment:
1. Unexplained bruises or repeated trips to the emergency room for potential miscarriage (usually caused by punches to the stomach)
2. Withdrawn behavior
3. Refusal to discuss home situation—or at least gives few details
4. When the woman is asked about potential abuse, gives false reassurances that everything is fine or appears to fear discussing the topic

Assess the family situation, and if possible find out as much as you can about the people who live in the household. Consider the characteristics of a potential batterer.

Characteristics of a Potential Batterer*
- Low self-esteem
- Commonly experiences problems with abandonment, loss, helplessness, dependency, insecurity, intimacy
- Inadequate verbal skills, especially difficulty expressing feelings
- Deficits in assertiveness
- Frequently diagnosed as having personality disorders
- Low frustration tolerance (loses temper easily)
- Higher incidence of growing up in an abusive or violent home
- Denies, minimizes, blames, and lies about own actions
- Violence is consistent with his view of himself and the world; it is an acceptable way of dealing with everyday life
- Unable to empathize with others
- Rigidity in male and female behaviors (gender-role stereotypes)

---

*From Lowdermilk DL, et al. (2000). Maternity & women's health care, ed 7, St Louis: Mosby, p. 227.

- Often perceives self as "special" and deserves special attention for being the provider, protector
- Substance abuse problems common
- Displays an unusual amount of jealousy (e.g., expects partner to spend all her time with him or to keep him informed of her whereabouts)

   Table 1-1 gives additional myths and facts about batterers.

   Box 1-1 gives indicators of nutritional risk in pregnancy.

SUBSTANCE ABUSE

Alcohol consumption and other substance abuse are significant health problems. The CAGE questionnaire can be a quick assessment for problem drinking. During pregnancy the TACE (Tolerance, Annoyance, Cut-Down, and Eye-Opener) questionnaire may be more appropriate because it replaces the G that stands for guilt with T for tolerance and seems to remove some of the guilt.

   Agents crossing the placenta can also lead to TORCH (toxoplasmosis, other agents, rubella, cytomegalovirus, herpes simplex) infection in newborns (Table 1-2).

ASTHMA AND PREGNANCY

Since adult-onset asthma is on the rise, more pregnant women are treated for this condition. The medications used have implications for the neonate (Table 1-3).

Box 1-1

Indicators of Nutritional Risk in Pregnancy

Recent pregnancies: three within 2 years
Poor fetal outcome in a previous pregnancy
Obesity
Poor diet habits with resistance to change
Use of tobacco, alcohol, or drugs
Weight at conception, under or over normal weight
Problems with weight gain
Weight gain of less than 1 kg/mo after the first trimester
Weight gain of more than 1 kg/wk after the first trimester
Medical pregnancy
Hemoglobin and/or hematocrit values

From Lowdermilk DL, et al. (2000). Maternity & women's health care, ed 7, St Louis: Mosby, p. 363.

Table **1-1**	Myths and Facts About Battering
Myths	**Facts**
Battering occurs in a small percentage of the population.	One fifth to one third of all women experience battering by an intimate partner.
Being pregnant protects the woman from battering.	From 25% to 45% of all women who are battered are battered during pregnancy. Battering frequently begins or escalates in frequency and intensity during pregnancy. Pregnancy may be the result of forced sex or the man's control of contraception.
Battering occurs only in "problem" or lower-class families.	Domestic violence can occur in any family. Although lower-class families have a higher reported incidence of battering (Gelles, 1993), it also occurs in middle- and upper-income families. Incidence is not really known because of the tendency of middle- and upper-income families to hide their battering.
Battered women like to be beaten and deliberately provoke the attack. They are masochistic.	Women are terrified of their assailants and go to great lengths to avoid a confrontation. In some cases the woman may provoke her partner to release tension that, if left unchecked, might lead to a more severe beating and possible death.
Only men with psychologic problems abuse women.	Many batterers are successful professionals, including politicians, ministers, physicians, and lawyers. In fact, research indicates that only a small number of abusers have psychologic problems.
Only people who come from abusive families end up in abusive relationships.	Most battered women report that their partners were the first person to beat them.

Continued

| Table **1-1** | Myths and Facts About Battering—cont'd |

Myths	**Facts**
Alcohol abuse and drug abuse cause battering.	Although alcohol may be involved in abusive incidents, it is not the cause. Many batterers use alcohol as an excuse to batter and shift the blame to the alcohol.
Women would leave the relationship if the abuse were really that bad.	Those women who stay in the relationship do so out of fear and financial dependence. Shelters have long waiting lists.
Batterers and battered women cannot change.	Counseling can effectively help resocialize both batterers and battered women.

From Campbell J, et al. (1995). The influence of abuse on pregnancy intention. Women's health issues, 5(4), 214-223; Campbell J, Landenburger K (1995). Violence against women. In Fogel C, Woods N, editors. Women's health care. Thousand Oaks, Calif: Sage; Gelles R, Loseke D, editors. (1993). Current controversies on family violence. Newbury Park, Calif: Sage; Lowdermilk DL, et al. (2000). Maternity & women's health care, ed 7, St Louis: Mosby, p. 232.

SICKLE CELL ANEMIA

With advances in care, women with sickle cell anemia can become pregnant and deliver healthy infants (Table 1-4). Knowledge of the care of pregnant women with sickle cell anemia and the implications for the neonate allows the neonatal nurse to provide improved care for the newborn.

REVIEW OF OBSTETRIC AND PERINATAL HISTORY*

1. Routine prenatal care
   a. Last menstrual period
   b. Estimated date of conception (by dates and ultrasound)
   c. Onset of prenatal care
2. Previous pregnancies
   a. Number
   b. Outcome of each
   c. Previous prenatal, intrapartal, neonatal complications

---

*From D'Harlingue AE, Durand DJ (2001). Recognition, stabilization, and transport of the high-risk newborn. In Klaus MH, Fanaroff AA, editors. Care of the high-risk neonate, ed 5, Philadelphia: WB Saunders, p. 66.

Table 1-2	Maternal Infection: TORCH		
Infection	Maternal Effects	Fetal Effects	Counseling: Prevention, Identification, and Management
Toxoplasmosis (protozoa)	Acute infection similar to influenza, lymph-adenopathy Woman immune after first episode (except in immunocompromised patients)	With maternal acute infection, parasitemia Less likely to occur with maternal chronic infection Miscarriage likely with acute infection early in pregnancy	Use good hand-washing technique. Avoid eating raw meat and exposure to litter used by infected cats; if cats in house, have *Toxoplasma* titer checked. If titer is rising during early pregnancy, abortion may be considered an option.
Other Hepatitis A (infectious hepatitis) virus	Miscarriage, cause of liver failure during pregnancy Fever, malaise, nausea, and abdominal discomfort	Exposure during first trimester: fetal anom-alies, fetal or neonatal hepatitis, preterm birth, intrauterine fetal death	Usually spread by droplet or hand contact, especially by culinary workers; gamma-globulin can be given as prophylaxis for hepatitis

Continued

Table 1-2	Maternal Infection: TORCH—cont'd		
Infection	**Maternal Effects**	**Fetal Effects**	**Counseling: Prevention, Identification, and Management**
Hepatitis B (serum hepatitis) virus	May be transmitted sexually; symptoms variable—fever, rash, arthralgia, depressed appetite, dyspepsia, abdominal pain, generalized aching, malaise, weakness, jaundice, tender and enlarged liver	Infection occurs during birth Maternal vaccination during pregnancy should present no risk for fetus (however, data are not available)	Generally passed by contaminated needles, syringes, or blood transfusions; also can be transmitted orally or by coitus (but incubation period is longer); hepatitis B immune globulin can be given prophylactically after exposure Hepatitis B vaccine recommended for populations at risk: women from Asia, Pacific Islands, Indochina, Haiti, South Africa, Alaska (women of Eskimo descent); other women at risk include health care providers, users of IV drugs, those sexually active with multiple partners or single partner with multiple risks

Rubella (3-day German measles) virus	Rash, fever, mild symptoms; suboccipital lymph nodes may be swollen; some photophobia Occasionally arthritis or encephalitis Miscarriage	Incidence of congenital anomalies—first month 50%, second month 25%, third month 10%, fourth month 4% Exposure during first 2 mo—malformations of heart, eyes, ears, or brain; abnormal dermatoglyphics Exposure after fourth month—systemic infection, hepatosplenomegaly, intrauterine growth restriction, rash	Vaccination of pregnant women contraindicated; pregnancy should be prevented for 3 mo after vaccination; pregnant women, nonreactive to hemagglutinin-inhibition antigen or can be safely vaccinated after birth
Cytomegalovirus (CMV) (a herpesvirus)	Respiratory or sexually transmitted asymptomatic illness or mononucleosis-like syndrome, may have cervical discharge No immunity develops	Fetal death or severe, generalized disease—hemolytic anemia and jaundice, hydrocephaly or microcephaly, pneumonitis, hepatosplenomegaly, deafness	Virus may be reactivated and cause disease in utero or during birth in subsequent pregnancies; fetal infection may occur during passage through infected birth canal; disease is commonly progressive through infancy and childhood

Continued

Table 1-2	Maternal Infection: TORCH—cont'd		
Infection	Maternal Effects	Fetal Effects	Counseling: Prevention, Identification, and Management
Herpes genitalis (herpes simplex virus, type 2 [HSV-2])	Primary blisters, rash, fever, malaise, nausea, headache; pregnancy risks included miscarriage, preterm labor, stillbirths	Transplacental infection is rare; congenital effects include skin lesions and scarring, intrauterine growth retardation (IUGR), mental retardation, microcephaly	Risk of transmission greatest during vaginal birth if woman has active lesions Acyclovir not recommended in pregnancy; treat symptomatically

From Lowdermilk DL, et al. (2000). Maternity & women's health care, ed 7, St Louis: Mosby, pp. 171-172.

Table **1-3**		Medications Used in Pregnancy by Clients with Asthma
Stage/Condition of Pregnancy	**Preferred Medication**	**Medication(s) to Avoid (Rationale)**
Labor	Continue asthma medications	
Induction	Oxytocin	Prostaglandins (may cause bronchoconstriction or bronchospasm)
Pain relief	Fentanyl	Morphine and Demerol (release histamine)
	Epidural anesthesia	Beta-agonist if client is already taking one for her asthma (may cause respiratory distress)
		Nonsteroidal antiinflammatory drugs (NSAIDs; may exacerbate asthma)
Postpartal hemorrhage	Oxytocin	Methylergonovine and 15-methyl prostaglandin $F_{2\alpha}$ (may worsen asthma)

From Lowdermilk, DL, et al. (2000). Maternity & women's health, ed 7, St Louis: Mosby, p. 904. Data from Mabie W (1996). Asthmas in pregnancy. Clinical obstetrics and gynecology, 39(1), 56-69.

3. Maternal laboratory studies
   a. Blood type and Rh
   b. Antibody screen
   c. Rapid plasma reagin
   d. Hepatitis B surface antigen
   e. Rubella immunity
   f. Human immunodeficiency virus antibody
   g. Alpha-fetoprotein
   h. Results of cultures or antibody titers
4. Maternal illnesses and infections
   a. Diabetes
   b. Hypertension
   c. Thyroid disease
   d. Seizure disorder
   e. Sexually transmitted infections (gonorrhea, syphilis, *Chlamydia*, herpes)
5. Pregnancy-related conditions
   a. Pregnancy-induced hypertension
   b. Chorioamnionitis
   c. Premature labor (use of tocolytics)

Table 1-4	Sickle Cell Anemia: Potential Problems, Prevention, and Maintenance
Potential Problem	**Prevention and Maintenance**
1. Inadequate oxygen to meet needs of labor and prevent sickling	1. a. Monitor Hb level and HCT to maintain Hb at 8% and HCT at 20% b. Have typed and cross-matched blood available c. Assist with transfusions d. Administer oxygen continuously during labor
2. Infection: UTI, pyelonephritis, pneumonia	2. a. Continue actions as under no. 1 b. Maintain adequate hydration c. Administer antibiotics as ordered d. Maintain strict asepsis e. Encourage frequent voiding to keep bladder empty
3. Sequestration crisis caused by need for and destruction of RBCs	3. Administer folic acid supplement (1 mg/day) to decrease erythropoietic demands and reduce probability of capillary stasis
4. Crisis caused by hypoxia, hypotension, acidosis, dehydration, exertion, sudden cooling, low-grade fever	4. a. Continue actions as under no. 1 b. Avoid supine hypotension c. Maintain adequate hydration d. Maintain comfortable room temperature: use warm blanket or cool cloths as needed e. Assist with analgesia and anesthesia
5. Pseudotoxemia (hypertension, proteinuria, no large weight gain); often accompanying bone pain crisis	5. a. If true PIH occurs, care is the same as for PIH b. Monitor blood pressure and urine
6. Thromboembolism (from increased blood viscosity)	6. a. Monitor for positive Homans' sign b. Initiate bed rest if Homans' sign is positive or if not reddened, warm areas, or lump appears in the calf

Table **1-4**	Sickle Cell Anemia: Potential Problems, Prevention, and Maintenance—cont'd
Potential Problem	**Prevention and Maintenance**
6. Thrombo-embolism—cont'd	c. Maintain adequate hydration d. Administer heparin as ordered e. Apply warm compresses f. Apply antiembolism stockings
7. Congestive heart failure	7. a. Assess pulse, respiratory rate b. Place in semirecumbent position; lateral position for labor c. Auscultate for crackles in the lungs frequently d. Administer oxygen and medication (e.g., digitalis, antibiotics, diuretics, analgesics) e. Use regional analgesia for pain relief in labor
8. Pulmonary infarction (hemoptysis, cough, temperature to 38.9° C, friction rub)	8. Assess for this possible complication to facilitate early diagnosis
9. Postpartal hemorrhage (resulting from heparin therapy)	9. Administer ordered oxytocin medication

From Lowdermilk DL, et al. (2000). Maternity & women's health care, ed 7, St Louis: Mosby, p. 902.
Hb, Hemoglobin; HCT, hematocrit; UTI, urinary tract infection; RBC, red blood cell; PIH, pregnancy-induced hypertension.

6. Maternal medications and drug use
   a. Steroids
   b. Tocolytics
   c. Antibiotics
   d. Sedatives
   e. Analgesics
   f. Anesthetics
   g. Tobacco
   h. Alcohol
   i. Marijuana
   j. Cocaine
   k. Amphetamines
   l. Heroin or methadone
   m. Phencyclidine (PCP)

7. Fetal laboratory studies
   a. Amniotic fluid lung studies
   b. Fetal chromosome results
   c. Amniotic fluid delta 450 to assess fetal bilirubin
   d. Cordocentesis labs (complete blood count, platelet count)
   e. Scalp pH
8. Fetal status
   a. Singleton, twins, and so on
   b. Ultrasound findings (weight, gestation age anomalies, intrauterine growth restriction)
   c. Amniotic fluid (polyhydramnios, oligohydramnios, meconium staining)
9. Time of rupture of membranes
10. Cord injuries or prolapse
    a. Results of fetal heart rate monitoring
    b. Maternal bleeding (Figure 1-1); placenta previa (Figure 1-2), abruptio placentae (Figure 1-3)
11. Delivery
    a. Method of delivery: vaginal or cesarean (indication)
    b. Instrumentation at delivery: forceps, vacuum
    c. Presentation (Figures 1-4 to 1-6) and position
    d. Prolonged second stage
    e. Shoulder dystocia
    f. Cord complications: nuchal cord true knot, laceration, avulsion
12. Social factors
    a. Maternal support system
    b. History of family violence, neglect, or abuse
    c. Previous children in foster care
    d. Stable living situation, homelessness
    e. History of depression, psychosis

Figure 1-7 shows the fetal head entering the pelvis, including various diameters; and Figure 1-8 shows decelerations from various causes. Table 1-5 lists maternal medical conditions and their potential effects on the newborn. Table 1-6 gives maternal medications and toxins with their potential effects on the newborn.

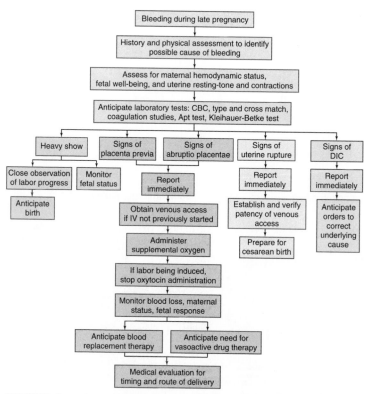

FIGURE **1-1**
Bleeding during late pregnancy. CBC, Complete blood count; *IV*, intravenous. (From Lowdermilk DL, et al. [2000]. *Maternity & women's health care*, ed 7, St Louis: Mosby, p. 850.)

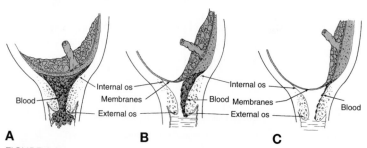

FIGURE **1-2**
Types of placenta previa after onset of labor. **A,** Complete, or total. **B,** Incomplete, or partial. **C,** Marginal, or low lying. (From Lowdermilk DL, et al. [2000]. *Maternity & women's health care*, ed 7, St Louis: Mosby, p. 850.)

Abruptio placentae (premature separation)

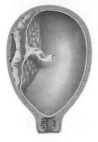
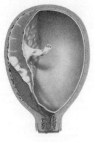
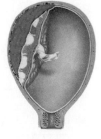

Partial separation
(concealed hemorrhage)

Partial separation
(apparent hemorrhage)

Complete separation
(concealed hemorrhage)

FIGURE **1-3**
Abruptio placentae. Premature separation of normally implanted placenta.
(From Lowdermilk DL, et al. [2000]. *Maternity & women's health care*, ed 7, St
Louis: Mosby, p. 855.)

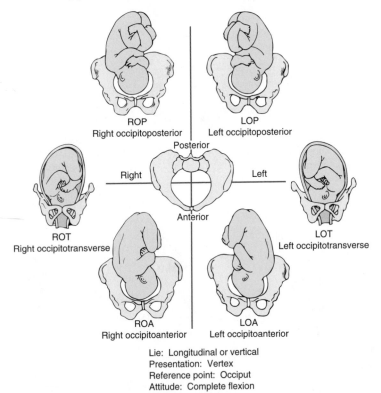

ROP
Right occipitoposterior

LOP
Left occipitoposterior

Posterior

Right

Left

Anterior

ROT
Right occipitotransverse

LOT
Left occipitotransverse

ROA
Right occipitoanterior

LOA
Left occipitoanterior

Lie: Longitudinal or vertical
Presentation: Vertex
Reference point: Occiput
Attitude: Complete flexion

FIGURE **1-4**
Examples of fetal vertex (occiput) presentations in relation to front, back, or
side of maternal pelvis. (From Lowdermilk DL, et al. [2000]. *Maternity &
women's health care*, ed 7, St Louis: Mosby, p. 446.)

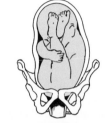

A

Frank breech

Lie: Longitudinal or vertical
Presentation: Breech (incomplete)
Presenting part: Sacrum
Attitude: Flexion, except for
legs at knees

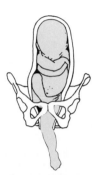

B

Single footling breech

Lie: Longitudinal or vertical
Presentation: Breech (incomplete)
Presenting part: Sacrum
Attitude: Flexion, except for one
leg extended at hip and knee

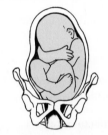

C

Complete breech

Lie: Longitudinal or vertical
Presentation: Breech (sacrum
and feet presenting)
Presenting part: Sacrum (with feet)
Attitude: General flexion

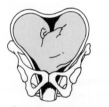

D

Shoulder presentation

Lie: Transverse or horizontal
Presentation: Shoulder
Presenting part: Scapula
Attitude: Flexion

FIGURE **1-5**

Fetal presentations. **A** to **C,** Breech (sacral) presentation. **D,** Shoulder presentation. (From Lowdermilk DL, et al. [2000]. *Maternity & women's health care*, ed 7, St Louis: Mosby, p. 447.)

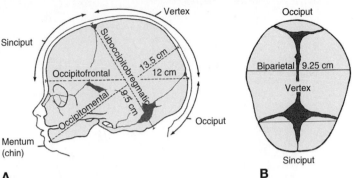

FIGURE **1-6**

Diameters of the fetal head at term. **A,** Cephalic presentations: occiput, vertex, and sinciput; and cephalic diameters: suboccipitobregmatic, occipitofrontal, and occipitomental. **B,** Biparietal diameter. (From Lowdermilk DL, et al. [2000]. *Maternity & women's health care,* ed 7, St Louis: Mosby, p. 448.)

EFFECTS OF PRENATAL STEROIDS ON THE PREMATURE NEWBORN*

- Increased tissue and alveolar surfactant
- Maturational effects on the lung: structural and biochemical
- Possible maturational effects on brain, gastrointestinal tract, and other organs
- Decreased mortality rate
- Decreased incidence and severity of respiratory distress syndrome
- Decreased incidence of necrotizing enterocolitis
- Decreased incidence of intraventricular hemorrhage
- Decreased incidence of significant patent ductus arteriosus
- Decreased length of stay and costs of hospitalizations

CLINICOPATHOLOGIC CORRELATION†

1. **Preterm labor**
   a. Acute chorioamnionitis
   b. Abruption (acute or chronic)
   c. Chronic uteroplacental underperfusion
   d. Idiopathic chronic uterine inflammation

---

*From D'Harlingue AE, Durand DJ (2001). Recognition, stabilization, and transport of the high-risk newborn. In Klaus MH, Fanaroff AA, editors. Care of the high-risk neonate, ed 5, Philadelphia: WB Saunders, p. 73.
†From Redline R (2002). Placental pathology. In Fanaroff AA, Martin RJ, editors. Neonatal-perinatal medicine: diseases of the fetus and infant, ed 7, St Louis: Mosby, p. 399.

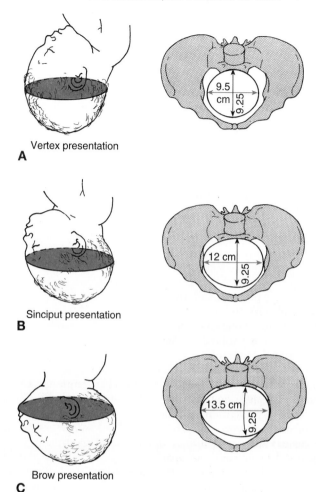

Vertex presentation

A

Sinciput presentation

B

Brow presentation

C

FIGURE **1-7**
Head entering pelvis. Biparietal diameter is indicated with shading (9.25
cm). **A,** Suboccipitobregmatic diameter: complete flexion of head on chest
so that smallest diameter enters. **B,** Occipitofrontal diameter: moderate
extension (military attitude) so that large diameter enters. **C,** Occipitomental diameter: marked extension (deflection) so that largest diameter,
which is too large to permit head to enter pelvis, is presenting. (From
Lowdermilk DL, et al. [2000]. *Maternity & women's health care*, ed 7, St Louis:
Mosby, p. 448.)

2. **Intrauterine growth retardation (restriction)**
   a. Chronic uteroplacental underperfusion
   b. Villitis of unknown etiology
   c. Abruption (chronic)
   d. Fetal thrombotic vasculopathy
   e. Perivillous fibrin
3. **Intrauterine fetal demise**
   a. Large placenta with delayed villous maturation
   b. Massive fetomaternal hemorrhage (intervillous)
   c. Thrombi
   d. Hydrops fetalis (any cause)
   e. Multiple placental lesions
4. **Neonatal encephalopathy**
   a. Abruption (acute)
   b. Umbilical cord accident (Figure 1-9)
   c. Rupture of fetal vessels
5. **Cerebral palsy (preterm)**
   a. Severe villous edema
   b. Chorionic vessel thrombi
   c. Multiple placental lesions
6. **Cerebral palsy (term)**
   a. Fetal thrombotic vasculopathy
   b. Severe fetal chorioamnionitis
   c. Abruption (chronic)
   d. Multiple placental lesions

The U.S. Centers for Disease Control and Prevention (CDC) recommend that physicians and hospitals follow these GBS (group B streptococcus) prevention strategies*:

• All pregnant women should be screened at 35-37 weeks' gestation for vaginal and rectal GBS colonization. At the time of labor or rupture of membranes, intrapartum chemoprophylaxis should be given to all pregnant women identified as GBS carriers. Colonization during a previous pregnancy is not an indication for intrapartum prophylaxis in subsequent deliveries. Screening to detect GBS colonization in each pregnancy will determine the need for prophylaxis in that pregnancy.

• Women with GBS isolated from the urine in any concentration (e.g., 10^3) during their current pregnancy should receive intrapartum chemoprophylaxis because such women usually are heavily colonized with GBS and are at increased risk of delivering an infant with early-onset GBS disease. Labels on urine specimens from prenatal patients should clearly state the patient's pregnancy status to assist laboratory processing and reporting of results. Prenatal culture-based screening at 35-37 weeks' gestation is not necessary for women with GBS bacteriuria. Women with sympto-

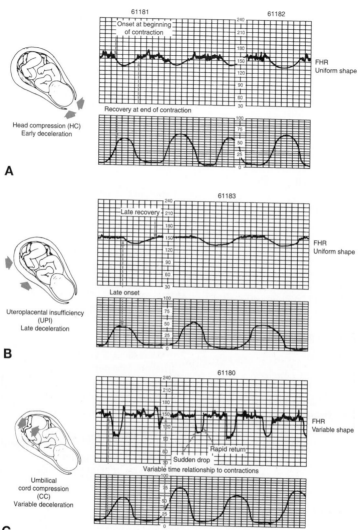

FIGURE 1-8

A, Early decelerations caused by head compression. **B,** Late decelerations caused by uteroplacental insufficiency. **C,** Variable decelerations caused by cord compression. (From Tucker S [2000]. *Pocket guide to fetal monitoring and assessment*, ed 4, St Louis: Mosby. In Lowdermilk DL, et al. [2000]. *Maternity & women's health care*, ed 7, St Louis: Mosby, p. 497.)

Table **1-5**	Maternal Medical Conditions and the Newborn
Maternal Condition	**Potential Effects on the Fetus or Newborn**
Endocrine, Metabolic	
Diabetes mellitus*	Hypoglycemia, macrosomia, hyperbilirubinemia, polycythemia, increased risk for birth defects, birth trauma, small left colon syndrome, cardiomyopathy, and respiratory distress syndrome
Hypoparathyroidism	Fetal hypocalcemia, neonatal hyperparathyroidism
Hyperparathyroidism	Neonatal hypocalcemia and hypoparathyroidism
Graves' disease	Fetal and neonatal hyperthyroidism, intrauterine growth restriction, prematurity
Obesity	Macrosomia, birth trauma
Phenylketonuria (untreated pregnancies)	Mental retardation, microcephaly, congenital heart disease
Cardiopulmonary	
Asthma	Increased rates of prematurity, toxemia, and perinatal loss
Congenital heart disease	Effects of cardiovascular drugs
Pregnancy-induced hypertension	Premature delivery caused by uncontrolled hypertension or eclampsia
	Uteroplacental insufficiency, abruptio placentae, fetal loss, growth retardation (restriction), thrombocytopenia, neutropenia
Hematologic	
Severe anemia (hemoglobin <6 mg/dl)	Impaired oxygen delivery, fetal loss
Iron deficiency anemia	Reduced iron stores, lower mental and developmental scores in follow-up
Idiopathic thrombocytopenic purpura	Thrombocytopenia, central nervous system (CNS) hemorrhage
Fetal platelet antigen sensitization	Thrombocytopenia, CNS hemorrhage
Rh or ABO sensitization	Jaundice, anemia, hydrops fetalis

Table 1-5	Maternal Medical Conditions and the Newborn—cont'd
Maternal Condition	**Potential Effects on the Fetus or Newborn**
Hematologic—cont'd	
Sickle cell anemia	Increased prematurity and intrauterine growth retardation (restriction)
Infectious	
Chorioamnionitis	Increased risk for neonatal sepsis, prematurity
Gonorrhea	Ophthalmia neonatorum
Hepatitis A	Perinatal transmission
Hepatitis B	Perinatal transmission, chronic hepatitis, hepatic carcinoma
Herpes simplex	Encephalitis, disseminated herpes (risk for neonatal disease is much higher with primary than recurrent maternal infection)
Human immunodeficiency virus	25% risk of infectious transmission, lower with zidovudine use
Syphilis	Congenital syphilis, growth restriction
Tuberculosis	Perinatal and postnatal transmission
Inflammatory, Immunologic	
Systemic lupus erythematosus	Fetal death, spontaneous abortions, heart block, neonatal lupus, thrombocytopenia, neutropenia, hemolytic anemia
Inflammatory bowel disease	Increase in prematurity, fetal loss, and growth restriction
Renal, Urologic	
Urinary tract infection	Prematurity, intrauterine growth restriction
Chronic renal failure	Prematurity, intrauterine growth restriction
Transplant recipients	Prematurity, intrauterine growth restriction, possible effects of maternal immunosuppressive therapy and mineral disorders

From D'Harlingue AE, Durand DJ (2001). Recognition, stabilization, and transport of the high-risk newborn. In Klaus MH, Fanaroff AA, editors. Care of the high-risk neonate, ed 5, Philadelphia: WB Saunders, p. 67.
From the Human Genome Project there are now indications that there are genetic defects in some maternal diabetes cases that lead to neural tube defects in offspring. This linkage is just beginning to be explored in 2002.

Table **1-6**	Maternal Medications and Toxins: Possible Effects on the Fetus and Newborn
Medication	**Effect on Fetus and Newborn**
Analgesics and Antiinflammatories	
Acetaminophen	Generally safe except with maternal overdose
Aspirin	Hemorrhage, premature closure of ductus arteriosus, pulmonary artery hypertension (effects not seen at ≤100 mg/day)
Opiates	Neonatal abstinence syndrome with chronic use
Ibuprofen	Reduced amniotic fluid volume when used in tocolysis; risk for premature ductus arteriosus closure and pulmonary hypertension
Indomethacin	Closure of fetal ductus arteriosus and pulmonary artery hypertension
Meperidine	Respiratory depression peaks 2-3 hr after maternal dose
Propoxyphene	Drug withdrawal reported
Anesthetics	
General anesthesia	Respiratory depression of infant at delivery with prolonged anesthesia just before delivery
Lidocaine	High serum levels cause central nervous system (CNS) depression; accidental direct injection into the fetal head causes seizures
Antibiotics	
Aminoglycosides	Ototoxicity reported after use of kanamycin and streptomycin
Cephalosporins	Some drugs in this group displace bilirubin from albumin binding sites
Isoniazid	Risk for folate deficiency
Metronidazole	Potential teratogen and carcinogen but not proven in humans
Penicillins	Generally no adverse effect
Tetracyclines	Yellow-brown staining of infant's teeth (when given at >5 months' gestation); stillbirth and prematurity caused by maternal hepatotoxicity
Sulfonamides	Some drugs in this group displace bilirubin from albumin; can cause kernicterus
Trimethoprim	Folate antagonism
Vancomycin	Potential for ototoxicity
Anticonvulsants	
Carbamazepine	Neural tube defects; midfacial hypoplasia

Table **1-6**	Maternal Medications and Toxins: Possible Effects on the Fetus and Newborn—cont'd
Medication	**Effect on Fetus and Newborn**

Anticonvulsants—cont'd

Phenobarbital	Withdrawal symptoms, hemorrhagic disease; midfacial hypoplasia
Phenytoin	Hemorrhagic disease; fetal hydantoin syndrome; growth and mental deficiency, midfacial hypoplasia, hypoplasia of distal phalanges
Trimethadione	Fetal trimethadione syndrome: growth and mental deficiency, abnormal facies (including synophrys with up-slanting eyebrows), cleft lip and palate, cardiac and genital anomalies
Valproic acid	Neural tube defects, midfacial hypoplasia

Anticoagulants

Warfarin (Coumadin)	Warfarin embryopathy; stippled epiphyses, growth and mental deficiencies, seizures, hypoplastic nose, eye defects, CNS anomalies including Dandy-Walker syndrome
Heparin	No direct adverse effects on the fetus

Antineoplastics

Aminopterin	Cleft palate, hydrocephalus, meningomyelocele, growth retardation
Cyclophosphamide	Growth retardation, cardiovascular and digital anomalies
Methotrexate	Absent digits, CNS malformation

Antithyroid Drugs

Iodide-containing drugs	Hypothyroidism
Methimazole	Hypothyroidism, cutis aplasia
Potassium iodide	Hypothyroidism and goiter, especially with long-term use
Propylthiouracil	Hypothyroidism
Iodine-131	Hypothyroidism, partial to complete ablation of thyroid gland

Antivirals

Acyclovir	*No* adverse effects reported; reserved for life-threatening maternal illness
Ribavirin	Teratogenic and embryo-lethal in animals

Continued

Table **1-6**	Maternal Medications and Toxins: Possible Effects on the Fetus and Newborn—cont'd
Medication	**Effect on Fetus and Newborn**
Antivirals—cont'd	
Zidovudine	Potential for fetal bone marrow suppression; combined maternal and neonatal treatment reduces perinatal transmission of human immunodeficiency virus
Cardiovascular Drugs and Antihypertensives	
Angiotensin-converting enzyme inhibitors	Fetal hypocalvaria, oligohydramnios and fetal compression, oliguria, renal failure
Beta-blockers (propranolol)	Neonatal bradycardia, hypoglycemia
Calcium channel blockers	If maternal hypotension occurs, this could affect placental blood flow
Diazoxide	Hyperglycemia; decreased placental perfusion with maternal hypotension
Digoxin	Fetal toxicity with maternal overdose
Hydralazine	If maternal hypotension occurs, this could affect placental blood flow
Methyldopa	Mild, clinically insignificant decrease in neonatal blood pressure
Diruetics	
Furosemide	Increases fetal urinary sodium and potassium levels
Thiazides	Thrombocytopenia, hypoglycemia, hyponatremia, hypokalemia
Hormones and Related Drugs	
Androgenics (danazol)	Masculinization of female fetuses
Corticosteroids	Cleft palate in animals but not humans
Diethylstilbestrol (DES)	DES daughters: vaginal adenosis, genital tract anomalies, increased incidence of clear cell adenocarcinoma, increased rate of premature delivery in future pregnancies; DES sons: possible increase in genitourinary anomalies
Estrogens, progestins	Risk for virilization of female fetuses reported with progestins; small, if any, risk for other anomalies
Insulin	No apparent direct adverse effects, uncertain risk of maternal hypoglycemia

Table 1-6	Maternal Medications and Toxins: Possible Effects on the Fetus and Newborn—cont'd
Medication	**Effect on Fetus and Newborn**
Hormones and Related Drugs–cont'd	
Tamoxifen	Animal studies suggest potential for DES-like effect
Sedatives, Tranquilizers, and Psychiatric Drugs	
Barbiturates	Risk for hemorrhage and drug withdrawal
Benzodiaze-pines	Drug withdrawal; cleft lip/palate in animals but not humans
Fluoxetine	No obvious effect on neurodevelopment
Lithium	Ebstein's anomaly, diabetes insipidus, thyroid depression, cardiovascular dysfunction
Thalidomide	Limb deficiency, cardiac defects, ear malformations
Tricyclic antidepressants	No obvious effect on neurodevelopment; nortriptyline: neonatal urinary retention; imipramine: neonatal withdrawal
Social and Illicit Drugs	
Alcohol	Fetal alcohol syndrome
Amphetamines	Withdrawal, prematurity, decreased birth weight and head circumference, cerebral injury
Cocaine	Decreased birth weight, microcephaly, prematurity, abruptio placentae, decreased placental blood flow, stillbirth, cerebral hemorrhage; possible teratogen: genitourinary, cardiac, facial, limb
Heroin	Increased incidence of low birth weight and small for gestational age, drug withdrawal, postnatal growth and behavioral disturbances; increased incidence of respiratory distress syndrome
Marijuana	Elevated blood carboxyhemoglobin; possible cause of shorter gestation, dysfunctional labor, intrauterine growth restriction, and anomalies
Methadone	Increased birth weight compared with heroin, drug withdrawal (worse than with heroin alone)
Phencyclidine (PCP)	Irritability, jitteriness, hypertonia, poor feeding

Continued

Table 1-6	Maternal Medications and Toxins: Possible Effects on the Fetus and Newborn—cont'd
Medication	**Effect on Fetus and Newborn**
Social and Illicit Drugs–cont'd	
Tobacco smoking	Elevated blood carboxyhemoglobin; decreases birth weight by 175-250 g, increased prematurity rate, increased premature rupture of membranes, placental abruption and previa, increased fetal death, cleft lip
Tocolytics	
Magnesium sulfate	Respiratory depression, hypotonia, bone demineralization with prolonged (weeks) use for tocolysis
Ritodrine	Neonatal hypoglycemia
Terbutaline	Neonatal hypoglycemia
Vitamins and Related Drugs	
A (preformed, not carotene)	Excessive doses ($\geq$50,000 IU/day) may be teratogenic
Acitretin (activated form of etretinate)	See Etritinate
D	Megadoses may cause hypercalcemia, craniosynostosis
Etretinate	Limb deficiency, neural tube defect; ear, cardiac, and CNS anomalies
Folate deficiency	Neural tube defects
Isotretinoin (13-*cis*-retinoic acid)	Ear, cardiac, CNS, and thymic anomalies
Mendione (vitamin K_3)	Hyperbilirubinemia, kernicterus
Phytonadione (vitamin K_1)	No adverse effects
Miscellaneous	
Anticholinergics	Neonatal meconium ileus
Antiemetic	Doxylamine succinate and/or dicyclomine HCl with pyridoxine reported to be teratogens, but bulk of evidence is clearly negative
Aspartame	Contains phenylalanine; potential risk to fetus of a mother with phenylketonuria
Chorionic villus sampling (CVS)	Limb deficiency with early CVS

Table 1-6	Maternal Medications and Toxins: Possible Effects on the Fetus and Newborn—cont'd
Medication	**Effect on Fetus and Newborn**
Irradiation	Adverse effects primarily associated with therapeutic not diagnostic doses and are dose dependent: fetal death, microcephaly, growth retardation
Lead	Decreased IQ (dose related)
Methylene blue	Hemolytic anemia, hyperbilirubinemia, methemoglobinemia; intraamniotic injection in early pregnancy associated with intestinal atresia
Methylmercury	CNS injury, neurodevelopmental abnormalities, microcephaly
Misoprostol	Moebius sequence
Oral hypoglycemics	Neonatal hypoglycemia
Polychlorinate biphenyls	Cola skin coloration, minor skeletal anomalies, neurodevelopmental deficits

From D'Harlingue AE, Durand DJ (2001). Recognition, stabilization, and transport of the high-risk newborn. (p. 69). In Klaus MH, Fanaroff AA, editors. Care of the high-risk neonate, ed 5, Philadelphia: WB Saunders.

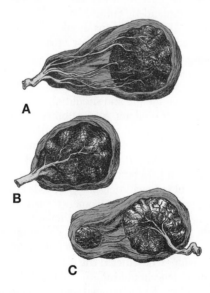

FIGURE **1-9**
Cord insertion and placental variations. **A,** Velamentous insertion of cord. **B,** Battledore placenta. **C,** Placenta succenturiate. (From Lowdermilk DL, et al. [2000]. *Maternity & women's health care*, ed 7, St Louis: Mosby, p. 857.)

matic or asymptomatic GBS urinary tract infection detected during pregnancy should be treated according to current standards of care for urinary tract infection during pregnancy.

- Women who have previously given birth to an infant with invasive GBS disease should receive intrapartum chemoprophylaxis; prenatal culture-based screening is not necessary for these women.
- If the result of GBS culture is not known at the onset of labor, intrapartum chemoprophylaxis should be administered to women with any of the following risk factors: gestation <37 weeks, duration of membrane rupture ≥18 hours, or a temperature of ≥100.4° F (≥38.0° C). Women with known negative results from vaginal and rectal GBS screening cultures within 5 weeks of delivery do not require prophylaxis to prevent GBS disease even if any of the intrapartum risk factors develop.
- Women with threatened preterm (<37 weeks' gestation) delivery should be assessed for need for intrapartum prophylaxis to prevent perinatal GBS disease. An algorithm for management of women with threatened preterm delivery is provided. Other management approaches, developed by individual physicians or institutions, may be appropriate.
- Culture techniques that maximize the likelihood of GBS recovery are required for prenatal screening. Collection of specimens for culture may be conducted in the outpatient clinic setting by either the patient, with appropriate instruction, or health-care provider. This involves swabbing the lower vagina and rectum (i.e., through the anal sphincter). Because lower vaginal as opposed to cervical cultures are recommended, cultures should not be collected by speculum examination. Specimens should be placed in a nonnutritive transport medium (e.g., Amies or Stuart's without charcoal). Specimen labels should clearly identify that specimens are for group B streptococcal culture. If susceptibility testing is ordered for penicillin-allergic women, specimen labels should also identify the patient as penicillin allergic and should specify that if GBS is isolated, it should be tested for susceptibility to clindamycin and erythromycin. Specimens should be inoculated into a selective broth medium (examples of appropriate commercially available media include Trans-Vag Broth supplemented with 5% defibrinated sheep blood or LIM broth), incubated overnight, and subcultured onto solid blood agar medium. Methods of testing prenatal isolates from penicillin-allergic women for susceptibility to clindamycin and erythromycin are outlined. Laboratories should report culture results (positive and negative) and susceptibility testing results to the anticipated site of delivery (when known) and to the health-care provider who ordered the test.
- Health-care providers should inform women of their GBS screening test result and the recommended interventions. In the absence of GBS urinary tract infection, antimicrobial agents should not be

used before the intrapartum period to treat GBS colonization. Such treatment is not effective in eliminating carriage or preventing neonatal disease and may cause adverse consequences.

- GBS-colonized women who have a planned cesarean delivery performed before rupture of membranes and onset of labor are at low risk for having an infant with early-onset GBS disease. These women should not routinely receive intrapartum chemoprophylaxis for perinatal GBS disease prevention.

- For intrapartum chemoprophylaxis, the following regimen is recommended for women without penicillin allergy: penicillin G, 5 million units intravenously initial dose, then 2.5 million units intravenously every 4 hours until delivery. Because of its narrow spectrum of activity, penicillin is the preferred agent. An alternative regimen is ampicillin, 2 g intravenously initial dose, then 1 g intravenously every 4 hours until delivery.

- Intrapartum chemoprophylaxis for penicillin-allergic women takes into account increasing resistance to clindamycin and erythromycin among GBS isolates. During prenatal care, history of penicillin allergy should be assessed to determine whether a patient is at high risk for anaphylaxis, i.e., has a history of immediate hyper-sensitivity reactions to penicillin (e.g., anaphylaxis, angioedema, or urticaria) or history of asthma or other conditions that would make anaphylaxis more dangerous. Women who are not at high risk for anaphylaxis should be given cefazolin, 2 g intravenously initial dose, then 1 g intravenously every 8 hours until delivery. For women at high risk for anaphylaxis, clindamycin and erythromycin susceptibility testing, if available, should be performed on isolates obtained during GBS prenatal carriage screening. Women with clindamycin- and erythromycin-susceptible isolates should be given either clindamycin, 900 mg intravenously every 8 hours until delivery; OR erythromycin, 500 mg intravenously every 6 hours until delivery. If susceptibility testing is not possible, susceptibility results are not known, or isolates are resistant to erythromycin or clindamycin, the following regimen can be used for women with immediate penicillin hypersensitivity: vancomycin, 1 g intravenously every 12 hours until delivery.

- Routine use of antimicrobial prophylaxis for newborns whose mothers received intrapartum chemoprophylaxis for GBS infection is not recommended. However, therapeutic use of these agents is appropriate for infants with clinically suspected sepsis. An updated algorithm for management of infants born to mothers who received intrapartum chemoprophylaxis for GBS infection is provided. This revised algorithm is not an exclusive approach to management; variation that incorporates individual circumstances or institutional preferences may be appropriate.

- Local and state public health agencies, in conjunction with appropriate groups of hospitals, are encouraged to establish surveillance for early-onset GBS disease and to take other steps to promote perinatal GBS disease prevention and education to reduce the incidence of early-onset GBS disease in their states. Efforts to monitor the emergence of perinatal infections caused by other organisms are also encouraged.

Before full implementation of this strategy can be expected in all health-care settings, all members of the health-care team will need to improve protocols for isolation and reporting of GBS culture results, to improve information management to ensure communication of screening results, and to educate medical and nursing staff responsible for prenatal and intrapartum care. Within institutions, such efforts may take several months.

Even with ideal implementation, cases of early-onset GBS disease will continue to occur. Tools to help promote prevention and educate parents of infants with early-onset GBS disease are available at *http://www.cdc.gov/groupbstrep. Additional tools available to assist with prevention implementation are available at http://www.acog.org, http://sales.acog.com, http://www.aap.org and http://www.health.state.mn.us/divs/dpc/ades/invbact/strepb.htm Multiple copies of educational materials published by CDC are available at the Public Health Foundation, 1220 L St., NW Suite 350, Washington, DC 20005, telephone 877-252-1200, or online at http://www.phf.org.*

Table 1-7 gives milestones in human fetal development.

PSYCHOSOCIAL ASSESSMENT*

1. **Language**
   a. Identify the primary language spoken in the home.
   b. Assess whether there are any language barriers to receiving support.
2. **Community resources and access to care**
   a. Identify primary and secondary means of transportation.
   b. Identify community agencies family currently uses for health care and support.
   c. Assess cultural and psychosocial barriers to receiving care.
3. **Social support**
   a. Determine the people living with the pregnant woman.
   b. Identify who assists with household chores.
   c. Identify who assists with child care and parenting activities.
   d. Identify who the pregnant woman turns to for problems or during a crisis.

From Lowdermilk DL, et al. (2000). Maternity & women's health care, ed 7, St Louis: Mosby, p. 45.

Table 1-7	Milestones in Human Development Before Birth Since Last Menstrual Period (LMP)	
4 Weeks	**8 Weeks**	**12 Weeks**
External Appearance		
Body flexed, C-shaped; arm and leg buds present; head at right angles to body	Body fairly well formed; nose flat, eyes far apart; digits well formed; head elevating; tail almost disappeared; eyes, ears, nose, and mouth recognizable	Nails appearing, resembling a human, head erect but disproportionately large, skin pink, delicate
Crown-to-Rump Measurement, Weight		
	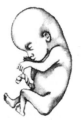	
0.4-0.5 cm, 0.4 g	2.5-3 cm, 2 g	6-9 cm, 19 g
Gastrointestinal System		
Stomach at midline and fusiform, conspicuous liver, esophagus short, intestine a short tube	Intestinal villi developing, small intestines coiling within umbilical cord; palatal folds present, liver very large	Bile secreted, palatal fusion complete, intestines withdrawn from cord and assume characteristic positions
Musculoskeletal System		
All somites present	First indication of ossification—occiput, mandible, and humerus; embryo capable of some movement, definitive muscles of trunk, limbs, and head well represented	Some bones well outlined, ossification spreading, upper cervical to lower sacral arches and bodies ossify; smooth muscle layers indicated in hollow viscera

Continued

Table 1-7	Milestones in Human Development Before Birth Since LMP—cont'd		
4 Weeks	**8 Weeks**	**12 Weeks**	

Circulatory System

4 Weeks	8 Weeks	12 Weeks
Heart developing; double chambers visible, beginning to beat; aortic arch and major veins completed	Main blood vessels assume final plan, enucleated red cells predominate in blood; heartbeat detectable with sonography	Blood forming in marrow; heart beat audible by Doppler

Respiratory System

4 Weeks	8 Weeks	12 Weeks
Primary lung buds appear	Pleural and pericardial cavities forming, branching bronchioles, nostrils closed by epithelial plugs	Lungs acquiring definite shape, vocal cords appear

Renal System

4 Weeks	8 Weeks	12 Weeks
Rudimentary ureteral buds appear	Earliest secretory tubules differentiating, bladder-urethra separates from rectum	Kidney able to secrete urine, bladder expands as a sac

Nervous System

4 Weeks	8 Weeks	12 Weeks
Well-marked midbrain flexure, no hindbrain or cervical flexures, neural groove closed	Cerebral cortex begins to acquire typical cells; differentiation of cerebral cortex, meninges, ventricular foramina, cerebrospinal fluid circulation; spinal cord extends entire length of spine	Brain structural configuration roughly complete, cord showing cervical and lumbar enlargements, fourth ventricle foramina developed, sucking present

Table 1-7	Milestones in Human Development Before Birth Since LMP—cont'd	
4 Weeks	**8 Weeks**	**12 Weeks**
Sensory Organs		
Eye and ear appearing as optic vessel and otocyst	Primordial choroids plexuses develop, ventricles large relative to cortex, development progressing, eyes converging rapidly, internal ear developing	Earliest taste buds indicated, characteristic organization of eye attained
Genital System		
Genital ridge appearing (fifth week)	Testes and ovaries distinguishable, external genitals sexless but beginning to differentiate	Sex recognizable, internal and external sex organs specific

From Wong D, Perry S (1998). *Maternal child nursing care.* St Louis: Mosby.

4. **Interpersonal relationship**
   a. Identify the way decisions are made in the family.
   b. Identify the family's perception of the need for home care.
   c. Identify roles of adults in caring for family members.
5. **Caregiver**
   a. Identify the primary caregiver for the home care treatments.
   b. Identify other caregivers and their roles.
   c. Assess the caregiver's knowledge of treatments and the care process.
   d. Identify potential strain from the caregiver role.
   e. Identify the level of satisfaction with the caregiver role.
6. **Stress and coping**
   a. Identify what the woman perceives as lifestyle changes and their impact on her and her family.
   b. Identify the changes she and her family have made to adjust to her health condition and home health care treatments.

EMERGENCY

*Amniotic Fluid Embolism**

Signs

Respiratory distress
- Restlessness
- Dyspnea
- Cyanosis
- Pulmonary edema
- Respiratory arrest

Circulatory collapse
- Hypotension
- Tachycardia
- Shock
- Cardiac arrest

Hemorrhage
- Coagulation failure: bleeding from incisions, venipuncture sites, trauma (lacerations), petechiae, ecchymoses, purpura
- Uterine atony

Interventions

Oxygenation
- Administer oxygen by face mask (8 to 10 L/min) or resuscitation bag delivering 100% oxygen.
- Prepare for intubation and mechanical ventilation.
- Initiate or assist with cardiopulmonary resuscitation. Tilt pregnant woman 30 degrees to side to displace uterus.

Maintain cardiac output and replace fluid losses
- Position woman on her side.
- Administer intravenous (IV) fluids.
- Administer blood: packed cells, fresh frozen plasma.
- Insert indwelling catheter, and measure hourly urine output.

Correct coagulation failure
- Monitor fetal and maternal status.
- Prepare for emergency birth once woman's condition is stabilized.
- Provide emotional support to woman, her partner, and family.

The neonatal nurse does not generally provide care to the mother but does need knowledge of pertinent antenatal, intrapartal, and postpartal history that will potentially affect the neonate's health. Assessment is the key feature of the nursing process when considering perinatal **red flags.** If abuse is suspected, however, it may be the neonatal nurse who has the opportunity to identify the problem and

---

*From Lowdermilk DL, et al. (2000). Maternity & women's health care, ed 7, St Louis: Mosby, p. 1017.

make the appropriate referral to social services, security in some cases, and law enforcement authorities. Steps for reporting such cases are dictated by institutional policies and state law. Refer to these sources for more information.

BIBLIOGRAPHY

Ahrari M, et al. (2002). Factors associated with successful pregnancy outcomes in upper Egypt: a positive deviance inquiry. *Food nutrition bulletin*, 23(1), 83-88.

Bartal M (2001). Health effects of tobacco use and exposure. *Monaldi archives of chest disease*, 56(6), 545-554.

Beck LF, et al. (2002). Prevalence of selected maternal behaviors and experiences, Pregnancy Risk Assessment Monitoring System (PRAMS), 1999. MMWR *(morbidity & mortality weekly report) CDC surveillance summary*, 51(2), 1-27.

Cifuentes J, et al. (2002). Mortality in low birth weight infants according to level of neonatal care at hospital of birth. *Pediatrics*, 109(5), 745-751.

Lessaris KJ, et al. (2002). Effects of changing health care financial policy on very low birth weight neonatal outcomes. *Southern medical journal*, 95(4), 426-430.

Murphy CC, et al. (2001). Abuse: a risk factor for low birth weight? A systematic review and meta-analysis. *Canadian medical association journal*, 164(11), 1567-1572.

Pittini R, et al. (2002). Risk factors for early death among extremely low-birth-weight infants. *American journal of obstetrics & gynecology*, 186(4), 796-802.

Quinlivan JA, Evans SF (2001). A prospective cohort study of the impact of domestic violence on young teenage pregnancy outcomes. *Journal of pediatric & adolescent gynecology*, 14(1), 17-23.

Shumway J, et al. (1999). Preterm labor, placental abruption, and premature rupture of membranes in relation to maternal violence or verbal abuse. *Journal of maternal & fetal medicine*, 8(3), 76-80.

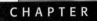

RESUSCITATION AND STABILIZATION

The transition from intrauterine to extrauterine existence requires many complex changes and adaptations by the newborn. For the majority of newborns, the transition from intrauterine to extrauterine life is smooth and uneventful. However, some newborns may experience difficulty in the transition because of various reasons. Careful assessment, skillful care, and timely intervention by the health care team can improve outcomes. Neonatal nurse practitioners (NNPs) or other skilled neonatal nurses are frequently present to facilitate successful transition or to intervene when necessary. Successful identification of distress and appropriate intervention are associated with an improved hospital course. Successful resuscitation, whether in the delivery situation or in the nursery, is systematic and focuses on the basics: airway, breathing, and circulation (ABC). The American Heart Association publishes guidelines for neonatal resuscitation (Kattwinkel, 2000). This chapter contains a guideline for resuscitation in the delivery room, offered for adaptation to your unit. There is also a guideline for emergency equipment that is suggested for neonatal intensive care units (NICUs).

APGAR SCORES

Apgar scores (Table 2-1) assigned at delivery by an objective observer may be used to indicate the stability of the neonate. The validity of these scores for long-term consequence prognostication is under debate. These scores continue to be used as a guideline for resuscitation and stabilization.

UNIVERSITY OF ILLINOIS MEDICAL CENTER AT CHICAGO CLINICAL CARE GUIDELINE

Subject: Guidelines for Neonatal Resuscitation Team at Delivery*

Objectives
- To anticipate the need for neonatal resuscitation based on maternal, antepartal, intrapartal, fetal/neonatal risk factors. Those fac-

*From University of Illinois Medical Center at Chicago Women's and Children's Nursing Services. Used with permission by Dharmapuri Vidyasagar, MD; Catherine Theorell, RNC, MSN, NNP; Beena Peters, RN, MS.

Table 2-1	Apgar Scores		
	0 (heart rate absent)	**1 (heart rate slow [<100])**	**2 (heart rate >100)**
Respiratory rate	Absent	Slow, weak cry	Good cry
Tone	Flaccid	Some flexion of extremities	Well flexed
Irritability	No response	Grimace	Cry
Color	Blue, pale	Body pink, extremities blue	Completely pink

From Lowdermilk DL, et al. (2000). Maternity & women's health care, ed 7, St Louis: Mosby.

tors defined as *at risk* and *high risk* require the presence of the neonatal resuscitation team whereas those factors defined as *low risk* do not require notification of the neonatal team and may be appropriately managed by the delivery room staff. In addition, for *high-risk* infants, a neonatal intensive care nurse will accompany the resuscitation team.

- To provide ongoing communication between the obstetric and neonatal staff to ensure that adequate personnel and necessary equipment are available for all deliveries.

Definitions
For the purpose of this guideline, the following definitions apply:

Low Risk—*neonate managed by delivery room staff*

Factors that, when present, constitute a low risk of neonatal compromise. These factors include the following:

1. Uncomplicated pregnancies including delivery of twins at term gestation in vertex/vertex lie
2. Women receiving penicillin/ampicillin only for group B strep prophylaxis
3. Maternal methadone
4. Nitrous anesthesia

At Risk—*neonate managed by neonatal resuscitation team*

Maternal, antepartal, intrapartal, and fetal/neonatal risk factors that necessitate that the neonatal resuscitation team be present at delivery:

1. Low or mid forceps or vacuum extraction
2. Prolapsed cord
3. Cesarean delivery
4. Nonreassuring fetal heart rate tracing
5. Maternal magnesium or meperidine/morphine administration (if administered within 4 hours before delivery)

6. Poorly controlled maternal diabetes
7. Uncertain dates/lack of prenatal care
8. Preeclampsia
9. Chorioamnionitis
10. Isoimmunization
11. Abruption or significant antepartum hemorrhage
12. History of active substance abuse
13. Abnormal fetal lie or presentation
14. Suspected intrauterine growth restriction (IUGR)
15. Suspected fetal anomalies
16. Immature pulmonary indices
17. Term twins (vertex/nonvertex) and higher-order multiple births

Neonatal resuscitation team may be called at any time at the discretion of the delivery room staff.

High Risk—neonate managed by neonatal resuscitation team accompanied by NICU nurse

Maternal, antepartal, intrapartal, and fetal/neonatal risk factors that, when present, may result in a neonate requiring more skilled resuscitation after delivery:

1. Any meconium in amniotic fluid
2. Gestational age less than 35 weeks
3. Severe fetal distress as seen with:
   a. Cord prolapse
   b. Shoulder dystocia
   c. Abruption or significant antepartum hemorrhage
   d. Known or suspected fetal anomalies
   e. Immature pulmonary indices
   f. Term twins (vertex/nonvertex) and higher-order multiples

Neonatal Resuscitation—Interventions required that ensure the safe and healthy transition from the intrauterine environment to extrauterine life. The scope of interventions is broad and may include drying, stimulation, and providing warmth to the newborn or may extend to full cardiopulmonary support including intubation, ventilation, cardiac compressions, and pharmacologic intervention.

Neonatal Resuscitation Program (NRP)—The neonatal resuscitation education program endorsed by the American Academy of Pediatrics and the American Heart Association.

Position Statements

• The philosophy of the Obstetric and Neonatal staff at UIC is that the best care for the healthy newborn is to keep the baby with the mother as much as possible. Thus, immediately after the delivery of a healthy baby, the baby may be placed directly on the maternal abdomen where the initial newborn evaluation may be done.

- The delivery of a healthy newborn, in whom there are no identified risk factors, is a normal process and routinely requires drying, stimulation, and the provision of warmth after birth. Healthy newborns shall be kept with their mothers as their condition dictates.
- For every low-risk delivery at least one person skilled in initiating resuscitation should be present and dedicated to the care of the newborn. This individual shall be responsible for the initial assessment, care, and assignment of Apgar scores. A second individual to assist in the resuscitation should be readily available if needed.
- If, during or after the delivery of a low-risk infant, risk factors become apparent or further resuscitative measures are required, this nurse or designee shall notify the neonatal resuscitation team and assist in the resuscitative efforts.
- The neonatal resuscitation team shall be notified in a timely manner before, and be present at, all at-risk and high-risk deliveries and at the discretion of the obstetric (OB), family medicine, midwifery, or OB nursing staff.
- The individuals responsible for neonatal resuscitation will consist of a trained and experienced multidisciplinary team of physicians and nurses who are certified in the neonatal resuscitation program (NRP). For at-risk deliveries the resuscitation team shall always include a neonatologist, neonatal fellow, or neonatal nurse practitioner along with the senior resident. For high-risk deliveries a neonatal intensive care nurse will accompany the neonatal resuscitation team.
- On some occasions the neonatal resuscitation team will be notified of an at-risk delivery but may only be needed to visually assess the baby. For example, a baby whose mother received fentanyl 1 hour before birth who is vigorous by the time the cord is clamped should be left on the maternal abdomen and assessed by a member of the neonatal resuscitation team.
- Delivery room attendance by the neonatal resuscitation team does **NOT** imply that the infant is admitted to the observation nursery or neonatal intensive care unit unless warranted by the infant's condition.

Procedure

1. Maternal, antepartal, intrapartal, and fetal/neonatal risk factors are assessed for each pregnancy and labor.
2. At the beginning of each shift the charge nurse in labor and delivery (L&D) will give a verbal report of the census, risk factors, and progress of laboring women to the charge nurse in the NICU.
3. L&D updates will be conveyed to the NICU when there is one of the following:
   a. New admission to L&D
   b. Significant change in risk factors for any patient

4. The NICU shall keep an L&D progress report that describes the census, risk factors, and progress of patients in L&D.

5. The neonatal resuscitation team shall be notified of all *at-risk* deliveries or a fetus in distress as soon as feasible.

6. Notification of the neonatal team may be performed by the obstetrician, family medicine physician, midwife, or L&D nurse.

    a. Members of the neonatal resuscitation team will carry four identically programmed labor and delivery code pagers.

    b. Call the team by paging. If an NICU nurse is required, the room number followed by "911" should be entered.

    c. The neonatologists will carry one pager.

    d. The neonatal fellow or neonatal nurse practitioner will carry the second pager.

    e. The senior pediatric resident assigned to deliveries will carry the third pager.

    f. The NICU nurse assigned to first admission will carry the fourth pager and attend all high-risk deliveries. The second NICU admission nurse shall be available to assist in the resuscitation as needed. The code pager is passed on to the assigned nurse on next shift.

7. The resuscitation and pertinent information shall be documented on the delivery form and in the infant's medical record, as appropriate.

8. Neonates requiring some intervention after delivery need **NOT** be routinely admitted to the observation nursery. Infants requiring some intervention after delivery but in whom the transition to extrauterine life is now normal should stay with the mother. Infants should be admitted to the observation nursery or NICU only when the neonate's condition dictates.

9. A multidisciplinary team shall review all deliveries requiring neonatal resuscitation and the timing of the admissions to the observation nursery and NICU.

UNIVERSITY OF ILLINOIS MEDICAL CENTER AT CHICAGO CLINICAL CARE GUIDELINE

Subject: Emergency Equipment Checklist: NICU/ICN*

Objective

To ensure the adequate functioning and availability of equipment and medications necessary to effectively manage emergency situations in the NICU/ICN (intermediate care nursery).

---

*From University of Illinois Medical Center at Chicago Women's and Children's Nursing Services. Used with permission by Dharmapuri Vidyasagar, MD; Catherine Theorell, RNC, MSN, NNP; Beena Peters, RN, MS.

Definitions

Medication Box—A numbered, locked, self-contained storage box used as an additional supply of emergency medications.

Emergency Cart—A numbered, locked, self-contained cart stocked with emergency equipment, medications, and parenteral fluids required to resuscitate an infant.

Intubation Box—A numbered, locked, self-contained box that contains the emergency equipment required for infant intubation.

Defibrillator—An electrical device used for cardioversion.

Position Statements

- Equipment required for resuscitation of the newborn should be functional and readily available at all times.
- Security of the emergency equipment is maintained by monitoring the presence of numbered locks. ER (emergency) carts and medication boxes are locked when not in use.
- Emergency equipment is checked once per day by the nursing staff by verifying that the numbers on the locks have not been changed. Documentation of this inspection is performed using the emergency equipment checklist form.
- Every 30 days, pharmacy checks all crash carts and emergency drug boxes to confirm all items are present, intact, and functioning properly and have not reached the expiration date.
- Once an ER cart and medication box have been opened, pharmacy is responsible for taking it off the unit, restocking the used supplies, reapplying the numbered locks, and returning it to the unit.

Procedure

1. The ANI or charge nurse shall assign the duty of checking the emergency equipment (ER carts, medication boxes, defibrillator, intubation boxes) each day.
2. The nurse whose duty it is to check the emergency equipment shall be designated on the patient assignment sheets.
3. Emergency equipment must be checked daily.
4. The assigned RN should check emergency equipment early in the shift. If the assigned nurse is unable to check the equipment, the charge nurse may be notified.
5. The charge nurse is responsible to ensure that the emergency equipment has been checked. If the assigned RN is unable to complete the emergency equipment check, the charge nurse will reassign the duty.
6. The RN assigned to check the emergency equipment will ensure that the equipment is present and functional.
7. An RN who uses, or assists in the use of, equipment or medication from the emergency supplies will be responsible for ensuring that the used supplies are replaced.

8. A list of emergency equipment should be checked to ensure supplies needed are readily available.

9. The RN will contact the pharmacy to replace or restock the ER cart/medication box. The RN shall also ensure that a replacement ER cart(s) and medication box(es) is(are) available while the initial supplies are restocked. Pharmacy will ensure that any missing, nonfunctional, or outdated medications are replaced in the locked medication box(es) and locked ER cart(s).

10. The RN will replace/restock the intubation box(es) and ensure that any missing, outdated, or nonfunctional equipment is replaced. The RN will then sign and date the "Checked by" slip, place it inside the box, and secure the box with the appropriate lock.

11. The RN assigned to check the emergency equipment is responsible for completing a functional check of the defibrillator.
    a. The defibrillator monitor and base shall be plugged in when not in use. Battery charging light should be on.
    b. Check supply of electrocardiogram (ECG) paper. Insert new roll of paper as needed.
    c. Turn power on to both monitor and defibrillator base.
    d. Run an ECG strip to ensure that the stylus is working.
    e. Ensure that the monitor cables are in place, ECG gel is available, and pediatric paddles are present within the recessed storage area.
    f. Set joules to be delivered. Set the charge button.
    g. Ensure that the digital display correlates with the set joules.
    h. Press the internal discharge button. Observe for wave deflection on the oscilloscope.
    i. Turn off power to monitor and defibrillator base.
    j. The clinical engineering services (CES) shall be contracted should any problems or malfunction occur in the use or function of this device. CES checks the defibrillator every 6 months and replaces the batteries every 24 months.

12. The RN will document that the emergency equipment was checked by initialing the emergency equipment checklist form found on each ER cart.

13. The RN will document any follow-up actions taken to ensure that the emergency equipment is available and functional.

CARDIOVERSION AND DEFIBRILLATION IN THE NEONATE*

Definitions

Defibrillation is the untimed (asynchronous) depolarization of a critical mass of myocardial cells that allows a spontaneous organized beat to be initiated.

*From Altimier L, Brown B, Tedeschi L (2000). Tri-Health's manual of neonatal nursing policies, procedures, competencies, & clinical pathways, Glenview, Ill: National Association of Neonatal Nurses.

Cardioversion is a timed (synchronous) depolarization used in converting tachyarrhythmias so as to avoid the vulnerable period of cardiac cycle.

Indications for Use

1. Defibrillator (asynchronous mode):
   a. Ventricular fibrillation
   b. Ventricular tachycardia with cardiovascular collapse (when synchronized cardioversion may cause unacceptable delay)
2. Synchronized cardioversion; rhythms that are commonly cardioverted include the following:
   a. Atrial fibrillation or atrial flutter
   b. Paroxysmal atrial tachycardia (PAT) or junctional tachycardia
   c. Ventricular tachycardia

Contraindications

- Idiojunctional or idioventricular rhythms
- Second- or third-degree heart blocks
- Digitalis toxicity

Preparation and Diagnosis

- Obtain stat ECG, and have physician evaluate rhythm; or place recorder on monitors, obtain rhythm strip, and have physician evaluate.
- Plug patient monitor cable into monitor/defibrillator, obtain rhythm strip, and have physician evaluate.
- Consider all available methods of converting rhythm.

Defibrillation and Cardioversion Administration

Defibrillation and cardioversion can only be performed by physicians and nurses (under the direction of a physician present) who have been trained in the use of the monitor/defibrillator.

Safety Precautions

The safe use of the monitor/defibrillator must be an important concern of all using this equipment to avoid electrical hazards.

Electrode (Paddles) Interface

A low-impedance (-resistance) medium is recommended. Electrode gels, creams, and defibrillation pads only are recommended.

Electrode (Paddles) Position

Standard placement is one paddle on the upper right chest below the clavicle and the other to the left of the nipple in the anterior axillary line.

Energy Dosage

Available data in the pediatric age-group suggest a dose of 2 joules/(watt-seconds)/kg can be used initially. If defibrillation is not successful, dose should be doubled and repeated twice. If ventricular fibrillation persists, attention should be turned toward adequacy of ventilation, oxygenation, and the correction of acidosis before another defibrillation attempt is made. If rhythm initially converts and degenerates back into ventricular fibrillation, lidocaine or bretylium may raise the fibrillation threshold.

Defibrillation Sequence—if Ventricular Fibrillation

1. Continue cardiopulmonary resuscitation (CPR).
2. Apply conductive gel to paddles.
3. Turn on defibrillator power—nonsynchronous mode.
4. Select energy dosage—charge the unit.
5. Stop chest compressions, place paddles in the proper position on the chest.
6. Recheck rhythm on the monitor/defibrillator.
7. Clear area; yell "clear" making sure no one is touching patient or bedside.
8. Apply firm pressure to paddles while someone simultaneously depresses both discharge buttons.
9. Reassess ECG and pulse and vital signs:
   a. If ventricular fibrillation persists, repeat countershock using twice the energy.
   b. If organized rhythm has been established, check pulse and continue CPR methods as required.
   c. If ventricular fibrillation recurs, immediately repeat countershock using the same dose.

Synchronized Cardioversion Sequence

The sequence for synchronized cardioversion is the same as for defibrillation except for the following:
- Make sure patient cable is attached to defibrillator, or switch to paddles to monitor patient rhythm.
- Activate synchronizer circuit—sync mode lights and flashes with each QRS complex monitored.
- Discharge buttons must be pressed and held until the countershock is delivered and then released.
- If rhythm does not convert and cardioversion is to be repeated, push sync mode button again since the unit switches back to defibrillate mode automatically after each synchronous discharge.

Figure 2-1 gives an overview of resuscitation in the delivery room.

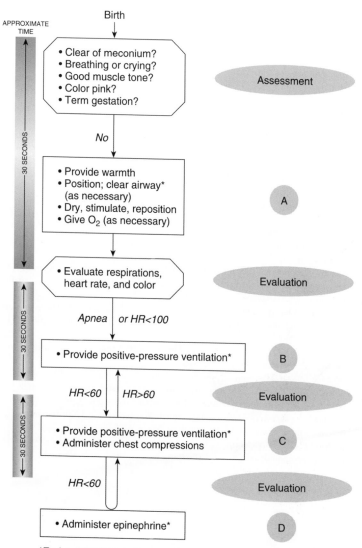

*Endotracheal intubation may be considered at several steps.

FIGURE **2-1**

Overview of resuscitation in the delivery room, basic diagram. (From Kattwinkel J [2000]. *Textbook of neonatal resuscitation,* ed 4, Dallas: American Heart Association. Used with permission of the American Academy of Pediatrics.)

BIBLIOGRAPHY

Brandon DH, Holditch-Davis D, Belyea M (2002). Preterm infants born at less than 31 weeks' gestation have improved growth in cycled light compared with continuous near darkness. *Journal of pediatrics*, 140(2), 192-199.

Carey BE, Trotter C (2000). Bronchopulmonary dysplasia. *Neonatal network*, 19(3), 45-49.

da Costa DE, Ghazal H, Al Khusaiby S (2002). Do Not Resuscitate orders and ethical decisions in a neonatal intensive care unit in a Muslim community. *Archives of disease in child fetal & neonatal education*, 86(2), F115-F119.

Finer NN, Rich W (2002). Neonatal resuscitation: toward improved performance. *Resuscitation*, 53(1), 47-51.

Furlong CM, Hamernick C (2000). Case study: listeriosis in the neonate. *Neonatal network*, 19(3), 53, 63.

Giannakopoulou C, et al. (2002). Comparative randomized study: administration of natural and synthetic surfactant to premature newborns with respiratory distress syndrome. *Pediatric international*, 44(2), 117-121.

Kattwinkel J (2000). *Textbook of neonatal resuscitation*, ed 4, Dallas: American Heart Association.

Leeman L, Leeman R (2002). Do all hospitals need cesarean delivery capability? An outcomes study of maternity care in a rural hospital without on-site cesarean capability. *Journal of family practice*, 51(2), 129-134.

Meininger D, Gerber J, Bremerich DH (2002). Neonatal assessment and resuscitation: current guidelines of the ICOR Pediatric Working Group. *Anaesthesist*, 51(1), 55-74; quiz 75, 77.

Miller SP, et al. (2002). Seizure-associated brain injury in term newborns with perinatal asphyxia. *Neurology*, 58(4), 542-548.

Moore CS (2000). Meconium aspiration syndrome. *Neonatal network*, 19(4), 41-44.

Wilder MA (2000). Ethical issues in the delivery room: resuscitation of extremely low birth weight infants. *Journal of perinatal & neonatal nursing*, 14(2), 44-57.

Wu TJ, Carlo WA (2002). Neonatal resuscitation guidelines 2000: framework for practice. *Journal of maternal & fetal medicine*, 11(1), 4-10.

Zaichkin J (2000). Introduction to the revised Neonatal Resuscitation Program guidelines: questions and answers to get you started. *Neonatal network*, 19(8), 49-54.

CHAPTER 3

NICU Admissions

Admission of an infant to either a level II or III nursery requires skill in assessment and implementation of a plan for stabilization. Nursing actions are the same whether the babies are born inside the hospital or transported in from another facility. The first step in the admission process is triage to determine the highest priority for this particular infant and family. This prioritization is set by the gestational age of the infant, prenatal history including intrapartal and delivery room care, and the stability of the infant at the time of admission.

Two guidelines for care are offered as examples of how to approach a new admission. Documentation of this process may be via paper or electronic charting or a combination. These guidelines give pointers as to the essential elements of documentation.

UNIVERSITY OF ILLINOIS MEDICAL CENTER AT CHICAGO CLINICAL CARE GUIDELINE

Subject: Admission to Neonatal Intensive Care Unit/Intermediate Care Nursery/Observation Nursery/Boarder Nursery*

Objectives

- To establish criteria for the admission or transfer of neonates to the neonatal intensive care unit (NICU), intermediate care nursery (ICN), observation nursery (OBS), and boarder nursery (BDN).
- To establish written guidelines for the process of triaging neonates when limited beds are available.
- To ensure appropriate equipment and supplies for neonatal admissions.
- To establish guidelines for the assessment of neonates admitted to the NICU, ICN, OBS, and BDN.

Definitions

For the purpose of this care guideline, the following definitions apply:

Neonatal Intensive Care Unit—A specialized intensive care unit designed to care for premature infants or critically ill, unstable infants with medical and/or surgical conditions.

*From University of Illinois Medical Center at Chicago Women's and Children's Nursing Services. Used with permission by Dharmapuri Vidyasagar, MD; Catherine Theorell, RNC, MSN, NNP; Beena Peters, RN, MS.

Intermediate Care Nursery—A specialized intermediate care unit designed to care for stable premature infants and/or infants convalescing from a variety of medical/surgical conditions.

Observational Nursery—A nursery designed to care for healthy infants whose mothers have been transferred out of the perinatal units (i.e., to the intensive care unit [ICU]) or have been discharged home or to another facility, or for healthy infants who are awaiting Department of Child and Family Services clearance.

Boarder Nursery—A nursery designed to care for healthy infants who are in need of hospitalization in an area away from the mother-baby unit and mothers who are unable to provide care.

Position Statements

- University of Illinois Medical Center at Chicago Women's and Children's Services strongly believes that all newborn infants should be cared for in partnership with their parents in a supportive, family-centered environment that promotes maternal and paternal infant care skills and integrates the newborn into the family. Healthy newborns are cared for on the mother-baby unit as part of a couplet residing within the mother's room.
- Healthy newborns whose mothers have been discharged or are hospitalized elsewhere other than the mother-baby unit may be transferred to the boarder nursery.
- For those newborns exhibiting symptoms of distress and admitted to any of the specialized nurseries, the staff encourages strong parental involvement in the care of their infant as appropriate for the condition.
- Newborns who are at risk for the development of problems related to antenatal or intrapartal conditions or are exhibiting transient, mild symptoms of distress after birth are admitted to the observation nursery for short-term surveillance/triage.
- Newborns exhibiting mild or moderate symptoms of illness or who are not feeding well may be admitted to the intermediate care nursery. In addition, neonates convalescing from medical and/or surgical conditions may be admitted to ICN in order to facilitate the transition of the parents and infant from hospital to home.
- Acutely ill newborns with complex diagnostic, medical, and/or surgical conditions will be admitted to the neonatal intensive care unit.

Procedures

A. Newborn recovery in labor and delivery
   1. After delivery, all newborns are immediately assessed as to their clinical condition.
   2. Newborns who are assessed to be healthy newborns shall remain in the same location as their mothers and be cared for

during the postdelivery recovery period by the same nurse. This may include providing simple screening procedures, such as testing blood glucose, complete blood count (CBC), blood culture, or other common laboratory indices.

3. All nurses caring for newborns will perform the appropriate identification procedure for the infant including placement of identification bands on the infant and the parent(s) and completion of the newborn footprint identification record.

4. All infants exhibiting signs of illness will be assessed by a physician, and if necessary, the physician will admit the infant to any of the specialized nurseries based on the infant's condition and the nursery's admission criteria. Infants may be admitted directly to OBS, NICU, or ICN from labor and delivery.

5. Neonates may be admitted to the boarder nursery from the labor and delivery only after a full admission assessment has been done and the baby fully stabilized after delivery.

B. Admission to *observation nursery*

1. Newborns at risk for or exhibiting mild symptoms of distress and in whom closer observation is required shall be admitted to the observation nursery for a period of time not to exceed 8 hours.

2. Admission criteria for *observation nursery* may include the evaluation of the following:

   a. Stable premature infants with a gestational age of 32 to 34 weeks to evaluate for apnea, feeding ability, and other consequences of prematurity

   b. Premature infants of 34 to 37 weeks who are exhibiting signs of physiologic instability

   c. Term or postterm infants experiencing transient, mild symptoms, such as mild tachypnea and grunting in whom the condition is not deteriorating

   d. Infants at risk for sepsis and requiring immediate treatment with intravenous (IV) antibiotics.

   e. Infants with initial abnormal blood glucose or hematocrit, who are asymptomatic but require monitoring or repeated testing

   f. Stable discordant twins

C. Admission criteria for *intermediate care nursery* may include the following:

1. Premature newborns <34 weeks' gestation requiring cardiorespiratory and oxygen saturation monitoring for apnea and bradycardia

2. Convalescent, very low–birth weight infants (>1100 g) with a postconceptual age of more than 28 weeks

3. Infants requiring gavage feeding and/or parenteral fluid administration

4. Infants with mild respiratory distress requiring oxygen b
   head hood or by nasal cannula
5. Infants who have hypoglycemia, need frequent monitorin
   for glucose, and/or require parenteral glucose infusions t
   maintain serum glucose levels within acceptable limits
6. Infants requiring a double volume exchange transfusion fo
   hyperbilirubinemia or a partial reduction exchange transfu
   sion for polycythemia
7. Infants requiring phototherapy
8. Infants exhibiting seizures with a potential for respirator
   arrest and requiring cardiorespiratory monitoring
9. Infants exhibiting symptoms of drug withdrawal requirin
   significant behavioral management
10. Stable infants with congenital anomalies requiring diagnos
    tic evaluation or therapeutic intervention
11. Mild bronchopulmonary dysplasia (BPD)
12. Mild apnea of prematurity

D. Admission criteria for the *neonatal intensive care unit* may includ
   all the above criteria as well as the following:

1. Preterm infants with a birth weight <1250 g and/or <2
   weeks' gestation
2. Infants exhibiting moderate to severe respiratory distress
   requiring assisted ventilation
3. Infants with suspected or proven congenital heart diseas
   requiring intensive cardiac monitoring and/or surgical inter
   vention
4. Infants requiring hemodynamic monitoring; arterial, umbil
   cal, or central lines
5. Infants with life-threatening congenital anomalies, such a
   trisomy 18, trisomy 13, or encephalocele
6. Infants requiring major surgical procedures with the poter
   tial for compromised respiratory or hemodynamic status pos
   operatively, such as diaphragmatic hernia, myelomeningocel
   gastroschises, omphalocele
7. Any infant in whom the physician has determined that ver
   close monitoring is needed (e.g., necrotizing enterocolit
   [NEC], sepsis)

E. Admission criteria for *boarder nursery*

1. Boarder nursery is not a point of admission; that is, the infar
   will have been admitted elsewhere in the hospital befor
   being transferred to the boarder nursery (i.e., from OB
   mother-baby unit, ICN, or NICU).
2. Admission criteria for *boarder nursery* may include any health
   newborn not requiring specialized care for whom their motl
   ers are unable to care for them because of the following:
   a. Maternal discharge or transfer to another unit

      b. Uncertain social status or pending Department of Child and Family Services investigation

F. Special conditions
1. In certain cases, mothers may be experiencing medical conditions that will temporarily prevent them from caring for their infant. Examples of mothers who are hospitalized in the maternal-child area but are unable to care for their newborns include the following:
    a. Maternal medical conditions, such as excessive bleeding
    b. Severe maternal hypertension requiring magnesium sulfate infusions
    c. Maternal absence from the unit for surgical procedures, such as a tubal ligation
2. In these cases, the mother-baby nurse will provide the required care for the baby, preferably in the room with the mother, but if necessary, in a separate room reserved for infants who cannot be cared for alongside their mother.

G. Neonates may be transferred to the care of their mother and of the mother-baby nurse from any of the specialized nurseries (NICU, ICN, OBS).

Standards

A. Admission of newly delivered infants into OBS, NICU, or ICN:
1. The registered nurse (RN) shall be responsible for the safe and efficient admission of newborns to the respective units.
2. Only RNs will be assigned to the admission of infants into OBS, NICU, or ICN and for transport duty. The exception may be when a hospitalized infant may be transferred from one unit to another because the infant requires a lower level of care.
3. The RN will ensure that the supplies needed for an admission are readily available.
4. The RN will ensure that the equipment and monitors needed for an admission are readily available and functional.
5. The RN will check the infant's identification band against the newborn identification sheet. If the information is correct, the sheet should be signed by the transferring RN and the receiving RN. If the information is not correct, the infant's and parental bands should be remade to reflect the correct information. For infants transferred from another institution, attach new infant and parental identification bands and complete a newborn identification sheet that corresponds to the correct information.
6. The RN will obtain the perinatal history from the labor and delivery staff or the referral hospital whenever possible.
7. The RN shall ensure that the appropriate pediatric resident, neonatal fellow/attending pediatrician, family practice physician,

or nurse practitioner is notified when the infant is admitted and/or with any change in the infant's condition.

8. The RN shall ensure that appropriate ancillary services are notified in a timely fashion.

B. Admission procedure of new infant to OBS, ICN, or NICU: on the neonate's arrival to the unit, the RN will do the following:

1. Weigh the neonate, as the condition allows.
2. Place the infant in the preheated radiant warmer, and secure temperature probe to the abdomen.
3. Administer oxygen therapy as ordered.
4. Obtain and record vital signs (temperature [T], heart rate [HR], respiratory rate [RR], blood pressure [BP] in all limbs).
5. Attach neonate to the appropriate monitoring equipment: temperature probes, cardiorespiratory and pulse oximeter monitors.
6. Ascertain that identification procedures are completed.
7. Perform a serum glucose check, and initiate IV infusion as ordered.
8. Complete a physical assessment of the infant, including length, head and chest circumference, and abdominal girth.
9. Obtain any admission labs as ordered.
10. If infant admitted to NICU, the nurse shall enter infant's name in the bedside monitoring station.

C. For NICU or ICN, the RN will further do the following:

1. Prepare for any additional procedures, and assist when necessary.
2. Ensure that the family is oriented to the parents' room, visiting guidelines, lactation consultation, and ancillary support services of the respective units.
3. Initiate and document a nursing plan of care.
4. Review the appropriateness of the infant's level of care.
   a. During daily rounds and at the weekly discharge planning conference, all neonates shall be evaluated to determine their readiness for transfer to one of the following:
      (1) Referral hospital
      (2) ICN
      (3) Mother-baby unit (if mother still hospitalized)
      (4) Boarder nursery

D. In the event that the demand for NICU beds exceeds the availability, bed space will be made available in the following ways:

1. Neonates who do not require NICU care shall be transferred to ICN, boarder nursery, mother-baby unit, or the referral hospital.
2. Neonates who require intensive care may be transferred to pediatric intensive care unit (PICU) if eligible as determined by patient size and PICU admission criteria.

3. If, despite these measures, space remains unavailable, the admission of neonates from referral hospitals will be triaged to another available NICU.

E. Documentation

1. In all nurseries, the admitting nurse will ensure that the newborn identification sheet and bands are properly completed.

2. The RN admitting the infant in labor and delivery will document the initial assessment in the newborn admission assessment.

3. The RN admitting infants in OBS, NICU, or ICN will use the NICU/ICN admission assessment to document initial findings.

4. After the initial stabilization is done, the RN will initiate the NICU/ICN flow sheet to document assessment and interventions on infants in OBS, NICU, or ICN.

5. For OBS patients, a note addressing the infant's presenting problem and summarizing the infant's course will be written and either resolved (if infant being transferred to the mother-baby unit) or continued (if being admitted to ICN or NICU) before transfer to another unit.

6. Infants who are admitted to boarder nursery from OBS, ICN, or NICU will have the newborn daily flow sheet initiated.

F. Clerical responsibilities

1. On admission to NICU, ICN, or OBS, the patient unit clerk will do the following:

a. Assemble clipboard to include admission database, nursing flow sheet, and master problem list.

b. Notify physician if authorization for admission form is not completed.

c. Send authorization for admission form to admitting office.

2. For infants admitted to NICU or ICN, the patient unit clerk will do the following:

a. Assemble brown chart with history and physical notes, physician order sheets, authorization for admission form, and consent for treatment form as needed.

b. Enter patient logbook.

c. Page physicians, respiratory therapist, and other personnel as needed.

d. Ensure patient's chart, lab slips, and clipboard are stamped with infant's Addressograph plate.

e. Assist in orienting family to signing into family logbook, the visiting guidelines, and hand-washing policies.

3. For all patients in NICU, ICN, OBS, and boarder nursery, the patient unit clerk will do the following:

a. Once per shift, verify that the infant's name and assigned bed space correspond with the actual location of the infant.

b. Transfer patients in the centralized medical record information system to correspond with any transfers to and from NICU, ICN, OBS, boarder, and mother-baby units.

NURSING RESPONSIBILITIES AND GENERAL ROUTINES*

Purpose

All patients admitted to the NICU/special care nursery (SCN) are treated in accordance with standards of care for nursing.

Patient Assignments

- The RN is responsible for total care of assigned patient load. The nursing process is utilized in assessing, planning, delegating, implementing, and evaluating care as identified in standards of care.
- The clinical team manager (CTM) takes a brief report on all patients at beginning of shift from previous-shift CTM.
- Assignments are posted at beginning of each shift. RNs take individual bedside reports on assigned patients at beginning of shift. The standards of care, clinical pathways, and Kardex primary/associate commitments, RN/PCA capabilities, and physical layout of the unit. Assignments should be rearranged by the CTM whenever necessary.
- RNs must be available to all rooms at all times to observe and monitor all infants.
- Lunches will be scheduled according to unit activity.
- RNs keep the CTM informed about major changes in patient condition and possible transfers.

Admission Assessment

All patients admitted to NICU/SCN should have a completed admission note and initial assessment sheet. The initial assessment is completed within 10 minutes and documented within 2 hours of admission. Infant reassessments/vital signs are an ongoing function of the RN and are documented as follows:

- At least every 4 hours (level III infants)
- Every 6 hours (level II infants)
- More often when deemed appropriate

All infants have standards of care/clinical pathway initiated on admission and completed within first 24 hours of admission. Standards of care are dynamic and updated as needed. Narrative documentation may be used for "pass throughs" in the NICU/SCN.

Charting

Charting is done on a daily nursing flow sheet (a 24-hour comprehensive outcome-focused documentation system). Initial assessment

*From Altimier L, Brown B, Tedeschi L (2000). Tri-Health's manual of neonatal nursing policies, procedures, competencies, & clinical pathways, Glenview, Ill: National Association of Neonatal Nurses.

is completed on each patient and documented on the "assessment sheet" of the nursing flow sheet. After completing the initial assessment, the RN focuses on actual patient outcomes.

Monitoring

1. Level II/III patients are continually monitored (unless otherwise ordered) with alarm systems functioning. Heart rate alarm limits should be set at 240 high limit + 90 low limit. These limits may be adjusted based on assessment of individual infant. Apnea alarms should be set at low limit of 5, with a 20-second delay. Pulse oximeter alarms should be set at low of 85 and high of 100. Alarm limits should be documented on nursing assessment.
2. Apply disposable electrodes according to package directions:
   a. Place chest leads above the nipple line on the **lateral** aspect of the chest.
   b. Place ground lead as far as possible from chest leads, usually on anterior aspect of thigh/abdomen.
3. Be responsible for seeing that monitor is utilized correctly and continuously on each patient (i.e., leads placed correctly, alarm assessed, monitor on).

Apnea/Bradycardia Episodes—Guidelines for Documentation

1. Apnea is defined as the cessation of respiratory airflow and/or respiratory movements for 20 seconds or longer.
2. The cardiorespiratory monitor should be set with a 20-second apnea delay.
3. When the monitor alarms, the infant should initially be evaluated for respiratory movements, color, and heart rate.
4. If the infant is apneic, appropriate stimulation should be initiated. If necessary, O_2 and positive pressure ventilation should be administered. Definitions of stimulation are as follows:
   a. Self: infant begins spontaneous respiration before any intervention occurs.
   b. Mild: infant responds immediately to minimal tactile stimulation.
   c. Moderate: infant requires tactile stimulation but responds within 5 seconds.
   d. Vigorous: infant requires extended tactile stimulation and responds after 5 seconds.
5. The duration of the episode should be from the time that the RN initially assesses the episode and be timed until the episode resolves.
6. Document episodes of apnea/bradycardia on apnea/bradycardia flow sheet.
7. When documenting, all entries should be dated and timed. Complete all columns, and use the color key to document infant's color.

Hemodynamic Monitoring

1. When using a transducer, calibrate to air on set-up and then once each shift and document.
2. Correlate transducer pressure with cuff pressure every shift.
3. Record BP on vital sign section of nursing flow sheet.

Vital Signs

1. Vital signs include temperature, BP, apical pulse, and respiratory rate and are taken as frequently as indicated by patient's condition. The assigned RN may increase or decrease the frequency of monitoring vital signs as deemed necessary but should notify the physician/certified nurse practitioner (CNP) of the action and rationale and document these. Frequency of vital signs depends on level of acuity:
   a. Level II/intubated infants: every 2 to 4 hours with BP at least every 4 hours
   b. Level II: every 3 to 6 hours with BP at least every 12 hours
2. Abnormal vital signs should be reported to the physician/CNP and reassessed.

I&O

1. *Intake:* Record hourly IV intake on IV section of nursing flow sheet. Record feeding intake on the feeding section of nursing flow sheet. Totals should be done every shift and then at 24 hours.
2. *Output*
   a. Level III infants or infants receiving IV fluid have all output measured if possible. Weigh diapers, and record urine output in nursing flow sheet. **Do not** weigh diapers of level II infants on oral (PO) feeds. Identify in output column by check mark (✓) that wet diaper was changed. Totals should be done every shift and then at 24 hours.
   b. Infants <1500 g should have a stool check daily or if any changes in clinical condition, stool pattern, stool character, abdominal distention, feeding difficulties developed or as ordered per physician/CNP.
   c. Infants >1500 g should have stool checks if symptoms occurred or as ordered. Nurses also have the discretion of doing stool checks if needed.
   d. Urine checks should be done as ordered.

Weighing

- All patients are weighed on admission and then daily on 1900-0700 shift, unless otherwise ordered by the physician/CNP. Time of weight should be documented on nursing flow sheet.
- Compare weights with previous weight, and document weight gain/loss on nursing flow sheet.

Medications

- Administer medications according to designated time on the medication administration record (MAR). A medication may be administered 1 hour before or 1 hour after designated time. If PO medication, such as NaCl or KCl, is missed with feeding, give in next feeding after reporting information to the physician.
- Keep all narcotics locked and checked every shift. Stock supply of emergency drugs is kept in resuscitation cart.

Newborn Eye Prophylaxis

Each newborn has erythromycin ophthalmic ointment (0.5%) instilled into each eye. Prophylaxis is given shortly after birth, with an acceptable delay of up to 1 hour, to facilitate initial maternal-infant bonding. This must be done before infant leaves delivery area. If not administered in labor and delivery area (L&D), it must be administered as soon as possible after admission to NICU.

- Carefully clean eyelids and surrounding area with a cotton ball.
- Gently open eyelid, place thin ribbon of ointment at least ½ inch (1 to 2 cm) along junction of bulbar and palpebral conjunction of lower lid. Try to cover whole lower conjunctival area. Carefully manipulate lids to ensure spread of ointment. Be careful not to touch eyelid or eyeball with tip of tube. Repeat same procedure for other eye. If eyes are fused, apply topically at eyelid junction. **Do not** force open.
- Discard tube after instillation.
- After 1 minute, gently wipe excess ointment from eyelids and surrounding tissue.
- Document administration of erythromycin ointment on the MAR.

Vitamin K Administration

- Should be given to all infants on admission
- Dose: <1000 g, 0.5 mg (0.25 cc); >1000 g, 1.0 mg (0.5 cc); intramuscularly (IM) only

Audits

Medication audits/chart audits are done every shift by two RNs at bedside during report.

Primary Care

Primary care is a goal. All babies should have a primary RN within 24 hours of admission.

Nursing Responsibilities in CPR Situations

All nurses will be certified in cardiopulmonary resuscitation (CPR)/neonatal resuscitation (NR) within first 12 months of employment. The first person to bedside is responsible for responding to immediate needs of patient. All drugs are given as ordered. Documentation should be completed on unit resuscitation sheet when available.

General Routines

1. Once cord is clamped, infant is no longer under obstetrician if pediatric staff members are in attendance.
2. All infants are initially placed under radiant warmer and are moved to an Isolette/open crib when stable according to thermoregulation procedure.
3. Isolette weaning may begin at RN's discretion when infant's temperature is stable on air temperature control and good weight gain is occurring.
4. Infants are transferred to a clean Isolette every month. Isolettes are dated with next schedule change date noted. Isolettes should be wiped down at bath time.
5. Bath and weight are routinely done according to Kardex days/times. To make optimum use of parent visitation, schedule times that accommodate parent visits. Baths are recommended two times per week.
6. Use alcohol with diaper change on umbilical cords without catheters until cord is off and area healed.
7. Method of feeding is determined by physician/CNP order, individualized to infant need.
   a. Collaboration with physician/CNP is necessary before initiating gavage feeding for a previously nipple-fed infant, as well as before initiating nipple feeding with the previously gavage-fed infant. Indwelling feeding tubes should be considered when planning care.
   b. Parents may feed infant at RN's discretion and in consideration of infant's capabilities.
   c. Level II/III infants must always be positioned prone or securely in side-lying position after a feed (on monitors). Boarder babies must be positioned securely in side-lying position or on back.
   d. Abdominal girth should be checked every shift on gavage-fed infants.
8. A glucose level should be obtained on admission to NICU/SCN and as ordered by physician/CNP. If glucose concentrations change or there is evidence of glucose instability, obtain a glucose level.
9. Take axillary temperature before giving bath. Take respiratory rate, pulse, BP before disturbing infant.
10. Discard used suction equipment between patients and as needed (prn). Write date/time on suction equipment when it is changed.

11. Check to be sure that infant is wearing two ID bracelets; verify infant identification. Also be sure bracelets are not too tight; if so, remove/replace with new ones. Be sure to include patient identification number. Document in nursing notes under safety check that infant has two ID bands.

12. Oral care is done every 2 hours with care for infants on ventilatory support, after orogastric feeds, every shift or prn.

13. Neonates are usually obligatory nose breathers—be sure both nares do not contain catheters or tubes (unless one is nasotracheal).

14. Infants may be in designated patient care rooms only.

15. Organize patient care and questions concerning the patient so that they may be clarified during rounds or as needed. The RN caring for the infant should be present for rounds on that patient.

16. Keep the patient care guidelines, Kardex, and clinical pathways current, and date additions or changes. Be certain nursing flow sheet is dated.

17. Head circumferences should be done every week (or as ordered) and documented.

Many units are implementing developmental care including how the infant is assessed. The following guideline incorporates this approach.

UNIVERSITY OF ILLINOIS MEDICAL CENTER AT CHICAGO CLINICAL CARE GUIDELINE

Subject: Assessment–Vital Sign Monitoring and Physical Assessment of Infants in the NICU/ICN*

Objectives

- To provide ongoing assessments at the clinically appropriate level.
- To provide hands-on assessment/intervention to the infant based on the infant's readiness and tolerance while providing safe and effective assessment of the infant's condition.

Definitions

Vital Signs—Heart rate, respiratory rate, oxygen saturation, skin temperature (taken by axillary route unless otherwise indicated), arterial blood pressure (central and/or peripheral), central venous pressure. Heart rate and breathing rate may be measured either mechanically or manually; temperature may be measured with thermometer or with continuous readout from the incubator. Arterial and venous blood pressures and oxygen saturation are only measured mechanically.

*From University of Illinois Medical Center at Chicago Women's and Children's Nursing Services. Used with permission by Dharmapuri Vidyasagar, MD; Catherine Theorell, RNC, MSN, NNP; Beena Peters, RN, MS.

Basic Monitor Vital Signs—Heart rate, respiratory rate, and oxygen saturation.

Complete Assessment—Thorough head-to-toe evaluation of the infant, consisting of checking skin integrity, neurologic integrity (daily head circumference, fontanels, behavioral state and reactivity, muscle tone and movement), circulatory system (heart rate, rhythm, point of maximal impulse [PMI], perfusion, peripheral pulses, overall skin color), respiratory (pattern, rate, effort, breath sounds), gastrointestinal (GI; softness, bowel sounds, abdominal girth), condition of the eyes.

Partial Assessment—Basic monitoring of vital signs, skin temperature, skin color and perfusion, behavioral state and activity, respiratory effort, breath sounds, GI (abdominal girth optional dependent on infant's status).

Hands-Off Assessment—Basic vital signs from monitor, skin color, behavioral state and activity, respiratory effort. **Note:** Even though this is a "hands-off" assessment, other practice guidelines state that peripheral IV sites must be assessed at least hourly and thus override this.

Pain Assessment—Standardized by using the Premature Infant Pain Profile (PIPP) and done with every hands-on assessment.

Position Statements

University of Illinois Medical Center at Chicago is committed to caring for infants according to the Newborn and Individualized Developmental Care Program (NIDCAP) model of care, which stresses pacing care according to the infant's individual tolerance and behavioral communication. The amount of handling and manipulation done to premature and fragile infants is well known to contribute to their stress and discomfort. As premature infants undergoing a great amount of growth and development are exposed to the environment and stimulation of the NICU, the staff needs to be cognizant and attempt to reduce as much as possible adverse stimuli. Each infant's care should be modified according to individual level of tolerance; if care that taxes the infant must be provided, it should be done in a way that is least costly to the infant. The timing of the assessment is left to the discretion of the nurse, to be presented when the infant is most ready for it; however, the following provides a guideline for the minimum amount of acceptable assessment.

Standards

- All patients whose physiologic condition is labile will be placed on a monitor with trending capability.
- Minimally, all infants in the NICU/ICN will have heart rate and respiratory rate monitored; those receiving oxygen, or who have

recently been on oxygen therapy, should have oxygen saturation levels continuously monitored.

- Monitor reliability for heart rate should be assessed by the caregiver when auscultating the heart at the first hands-on assessment for heart rate. For respirations, a visual inspection of the match between visible breaths and monitor readout should be performed within the first hour of the caregiver's shift. **Note:** Infants on high-frequency ventilation will not have respiratory rate counted. Monitor reliability should be reassessed at any time the caregivers suspect a discrepancy.
- Frequency of "hands-off" assessment will vary depending on the needs and behavior of the infant. Ideally all care is based on the cues of the infant, and all infants should be checked frequently to make sure they are resting comfortably. This may vary from every 15 minutes to every 2 hours. The normal minimum will be hourly checks.
- The RN will plan care based on the infant's clinical condition and behavioral readiness for care.
- Care will be placed to match the tolerance level of the infant.
- Any abnormal finding (vital sign or physical finding) will be reevaluated as necessary and the physician notified immediately if the finding is critical or a mildly abnormal finding is persistent despite intervention.
- For any infant whose baseline vital signs or physical findings are atypical, the physician will specify what values are considered normal for this infant.
- Any intervention will be evaluated for effectiveness and the appropriate personnel notified.

Procedure

A. The following are **minimal** acceptable vital sign measurement and assessment intervals. At the RN or physician's discretion, these can be individualized to meet the patient's needs.
  1. *Basic monitor vital signs* (heart rate, respiratory rate, oxygen saturation): may be read continuously off the monitor; will be documented in the chart at least hourly for NICU patients and every 3 to 4 hours for ICN patients.
  2. Temperature: infants receiving any supplemental heating (incubators, radiant warmers) will have their skin temperature assessed at minimum every 3 to 4 hours.
    a. Infants who have just had supplemental heat removed will have their temperature taken 1 hour after heat has been discontinued and then every 3 to 4 hours until stable.
    b. Infants in cribs without supplemental heat, whose temperatures have been stable more than 24 hours, may have their temperature taken every 6 to 8 hours.

    3. Blood pressure
       a. Invasive arterial and venous pressures can be read off the monitor continuously but will be documented at least hourly on the flow sheet.
       b. Peripheral blood pressure on infants in the ICN is performed daily and every shift on infants in NICU.

B. Physical assessment
    1. Stable patients not on a feeding schedule (NPO or continuous feeding)
       a. Will have complete assessment once each shift
       b. Routine care (diaper change, position change, oxygen probe placement change) should not have interval exceeding 6 hours.
    2. Stable patients on scheduled feedings
       a. Should have a complete assessment once per shift and partial assessment every other feeding
       b. May have "hands-off" assessments every other feeding
       c. "Hands-off" assessment of nasogastric tube placement can be done by any of the following methods: placing tip of tube into sterile water and watching for absence of air bubbles; aspirating gastric contents; checking centimeter marking at taped location.
    3. Stable growing infants on demand feedings
       a. Will have a complete assessment at least once during the caregiver's 8- or 12-hour shift, with a partial assessment at least one other time in the shift
       b. **Note:** Infants for whom feeding volumes are being increased will need to have their abdominal girth measured at least every 6 hours and more frequently if there is any question of feeding intolerance. For infants who are at full feedings, abdominal girth can be measured once every 8 hours.

C. Special situations
    1. Stable chronically, technology-dependent infants or infants beyond 44 weeks' corrected age
       a. As much as possible care will be organized around a normal day/night cycle.
       b. Complete assessment twice per day on day and prn sheet
       c. Medical regimen adjusted as much as possible to promote a long stretch of sleep at night
    2. **Note:** These infants may benefit from being in an environment separate from infants who are receiving intensive care around the clock.

D. Postoperative vital signs
    1. Every 15 minutes × 4, then every 30 minutes × 2, and then hourly until stable
    2. Dressing will be inspected with each vital sign check.

3. A complete physical assessment is performed on return from operating room (OR) and then as condition warrants.

E. Minimal handling: For certain conditions, such as persistent pulmonary hypertension of the newborn (PPHN), infants can be severely compromised by handling. Thus the handling must be carefully controlled for these infants, and an assessment is acceptable every 12 hours. Close collaboration between nursing and medicine is needed to individualize the timing of this care.

F. Micropreemies/sensitive/fragile infants: The timing of sedation should be considered with assessments/procedures scheduled in mind. Individualizing assessment to the infant's tolerance should be collaborative between nursing and medicine.

G. Growth and development monitoring
   1. A growth chart with weekly head circumference, length, and weight will be kept for every infant. The day shift nurse on Mondays will ensure that this is completed.
   2. Weights will be done as ordered by the physician, with the following serving as a guideline:
      a. Infants with acute conditions will be weighed daily.
      b. Stable, growing premature infants will be weighed twice each week.
      c. Long-term hospitalized infants will be weighed twice each week.
   3. **Note:** To encourage parental involvement in care, baths and weights should be coordinated with the parents' presence on the unit; therefore it is most likely to take place on day or evening shift. If the parents have not come on the day the weight is due, then the night shift will be responsible to do the weight.

Tables 3-1 to 3-10 give levels of surveillance of the newborn based on obstetric history, vital functions, and various examinations of the newborn.

Table 3-1	Levels of Surveillance of the Newborn Based on Obstetric History		
	Level of Surveillance		
History	**Normal**	**Alert**	**Alarm**
Pregnancy surveillance	Registered during first trimester	Unregistered during second trimester	Unregistered and in labor
Genetic disease	None known	In family	In sibling of fetus
Uterine volume		Polyhydramnios	Oligohydramnios
Fetal movement		Increased	Decreased
Biochemical		Decreased estriol levels	
Biophysical		Positive oxytocin challenge test	Uterine ultrasound abnormality
Maternal disease		Diabetes and hypertension	Active tuberculosiis
Rupture of membranes	<36 wk		
Labor	36-42 wk	<36 wk, >42 wk	<34 wk
Delivery Vaginal		"Difficult" breech	
Cesarean	Elective (repeat)	Elective (initial)	Emergency
Fetus	Apgar score 8 to 10	Apgar score 4 to 7, visible congenital anomaly	Asphyxia (Apgar score <4), hydrops fetalis

From Nelson NM (2001). Neonatal adaptations. In Hoekelman RA, et al., editors. Primary pediatric care, ed 4, St Louis: Mosby, p. 550. From Seidel HM (1997). Physical examination of the newborn. In Seidel HM, Rosenstein RJ, Pathak A, editors. Primary care of the newborn, ed 2, St Louis: Mosby, p. 41.

Table **3-2**	Levels of Surveillance of the Newborn Based on Vital Functions		
	Level of Surveillance		
Vital Function	**Normal**	**Alert**	**Alarm**
Respiration	Paradoxic	Periodic tachypnea	Apnea, bradycardia, grunting, or gasping
Circulation	Acrocyanosis and heart rate 110-165 beats/min	Tachycardia, hypertension, or cardiac murmur	Central cyanosis, bradycardia, hypotension, enlarged heart, or pallor
Metabolism	Body temperature 95.9°-99.5° F (36.5°-37.5° C)	Hyperthermia	Hypothermia
Digestion	Drooling or "transitional" stools	Spitting	Vomiting or diarrhea
Excretion		No voiding (>24 hr) and no stooling (>24 hr)	Dribbling stream
Behavior	Alert, responsive, reactive startle, or sneeze	Hyperactive, jittery, or yawning	Coma or convulsions

From Nelson NM (2001). Neonatal adaptations. In Hoekelman RA, et al., editors. Primary pediatric care, ed 4, St Louis: Mosby, p. 550.

Table 3-3	Levels of Surveillance of the Newborn Based on Examination of the Skin and its Appendages

	Level of Surveillance		
Characteristic	Normal	Alert	Alarm
Color (age of occurrence)			
Cyanosis	Acrocyanosis (<12 hr)	Central (<1 hr)	Central (>1 hr)
Jaundice	>24 hr	18-24 hr	<18 hr
Pallor			>30 min
Epidermis	Dermatoglyphics	Excoriations	Sloughing
Hair	Lanugo	Lumbosacral tuft and scalp defect	
Texture	Soft and moist	Dry and scaling	Thickened and crusting
Vascular pattern	Harlequin, mottling (cold)	Persistent mottling	
Cysts	Milia and Epstein's pearls		
Papules	Acne and miliaria		
Desquamation	Delicate scaling (>2 days)	Peeling (<2 days)	Denuded sheets (anytime)
Hemangiomas	Telangiectatic (forehead, lids, lips, nape)	Telangiectatic (trigeminal) and angiomatous (few)	Angiomatous (multiple)
Hemorrhage	Petechiae (head or upper body)	Petechiae (elsewhere)	Ecchymoses and purpura
Macules	Mongolian spots	Café au lait spots (<6 spots)	Café au lait spots (>5 spots) and "mountain ash-leaf"
Pustules	Erythema toxicum		Large and dermal
Vesicles			Any
Nodules		Subcutaneous fat necrosis	Sclerema

From Nelson NM (2001). Neonatal adaptations. In Hoekelman RA, et al., editors. Primary pediatric care, ed 4, St Louis: Mosby, p. 555.

Table **3-4**	Levels of Surveillance of Newborn Based on Head and Neck Examination		
	Level of Surveillance		
Location	**Normal**	**Alert**	**Alarm**
Skull	Caput succedaneum, molding, or occipital overhang	Cephalhematoma, craniotabes, large fontanel, or forceps mark	Craniosynostosis, transillumination or bruit
Facies		Hypoplasia or palsy	
Eyes		Mongoloid slant	Aniridia and enlarged cornea
Nose		Nasal obstruction	
Mouth		High-arched palate or macroglossia	Cleft palate and/or lip or micrognathia
Ears		"Simple" structure or low set	
Neck	Rotation ±90 degrees	Dimple or webbing	

From Nelson NM (2001). *Neonatal adaptations*. In Hoekelman RA, et al., editors. *Primary pediatric care, ed 4*, St Louis: Mosby, p. 556.

| Table **3-5** | Levels of Surveillance of the Newborn Based on Chest Examination |

| | **Level of Surveillance** | | |
Characteristic	**Normal**	**Alert**	**Alarm**
Respiration		Paradoxic, periodic, or retractions	Apnea, expiratory grunt, or flaring alae nasi
Auscultation		Decreased air entry	Bowel sounds
Chest roentgeno-gram		Enlarged heart	Oligemia or plethora
Cardiac			
Impulse	Tapping	Heaving, lifting	
Pulses	Full	Decreased	Absent (femoral) and leg (cardiac-radial)
Rate and rhythm	110-165, sinus arrhythmia	Sinus bradycardia	Persistent sinus tachycardia
Sounds	"Tic-toc"	S_2 widely split	S_2 fixed split
Murmurs	Systolic (<24 hr)	Systolic (>24 hr)	
Electrocardio-gram (QRS)			
Vector	+35 to +180 degrees		
Amplitude			0 to −90 degrees: −90 to −180 degrees
V_1	Rs	Rs	rS
V_6	qrS	qRs	qRs

From Nelson NM (2001). Neonatal adaptations. In Hoekelman RA, et al., editors. Primary pediatric care, ed 4, St Louis: Mosby, p. 557.

Table 3-6	Levels of Surveillance of the Newborn Based on Examination of the Abdomen		
	Level of Surveillance		
Characteristics	**Normal**	**Alert**	**Alarm**
Shape	Cylindric	Scaphoid	Distended
Muscular wall	Diastasis recti		Absent
Umbilicus	Amniotic navel or cutaneous navel	Exudation or leakage, granuloma, hernia, inflammation, or <3 cord vessels	Gastroschisis, omphalitis, or omphalocele
Liver	Smooth edge		Enlarged
Spleen	Nonpalpable	Palpable	Enlarged
Kidneys	Lobulated or palpable (lower poles)	Horseshoe	Enlarged

From Nelson NM (2001). Neonatal adaptations. In Hoekelman RA, et al., editors. Primary pediatric care, ed 4, St Louis: Mosby, p. 458.

Table 3-7	Levels of Surveillance of the Newborn Based on Examination of the Perineum		
	Level of Surveillance		
Location	**Normal**	**Alert**	**Alarm**
Anus		Coccygeal dimple	Imperforate, fistula, patulous
Female			
Clitoris		Enlarged, hooded	
Vulva	Bloody secretion, edema, gaping labia or hymenal tags		Hydrometrocolpos
Male			
Gonad	Edema, hydrocele	Bifid scrotum, cryptorchidism, inguinal hernia	
Phallus	Phimosis	Chordee, hypospadia	Microphallus

From Nelson NM (2001). Neonatal adaptations. In Hoekelman RA, et al., editors. Primary pediatric care, ed 4, St Louis: Mosby, p. 559.
From Seidel HM (1997). Physical examination of the newborn. In Seidel HM, Rosenstein RJ, Pathak A, editors. Primary care of the newborn, St Louis: Mosby, p. 47.

Table **3-8**	Levels of Surveillance of the Newborn Based on Examination of the Musculoskeletal System		

| | **Level of Surveillance** | | |
Characteristic	**Normal**	**Alert**	**Alarm**
Fetal posture	Flexor, position of comfort	Frank breech	Extensor
Hand	Webbing	Cortical thumb; overlapping fingers; short, in-curved little finger	Polydactyly, syndactyly
Foot	Dorsiflex 90 degrees, plantar flex 90 degrees, abduct or adduct forefoot 45 degrees, invert or evert ankle 45 degrees	Decreased range of motion	Fixed
Extremities	Tibial bowing		Constriction bands, amputations
Neck	Rotate ±90 degrees		
Joints		Reluctance to use	Subluxation (hips), contracture

From Nelson NM (2001). Neonatal adaptations. In Hoekelman RA, et al., editors. Primary pediatric care, ed 4, St Louis: Mosby, p. 559. From Seidel HM (1997). Physical examination of the newborn. In Seidel HM, Rosenstein RJ, Pathak A, editors. Primary care of the newborn, ed 2, St Louis: Mosby, p. 48.

Table **3-9**	Levels of Surveillance of the Newborn Based on Examination of the Nervous System		
	Level of Surveillance		
Characteristics	**Normal**	**Alert**	**Alarm**
State	Awake: crying, active, quiet alert Asleep: active, indeterminate, quiet		
Motor			
Posture	Flexor, symmetric	Extensor, asymmetric	Obligatory, decerebrate
Tone	Obtuse popliteal angle	Limp in upright suspension	Limp in ventral suspension
Movement	All extremities, nonrepetitive, random, symmetric		
Reflexes	Deep tendon, grasp, Moro, placing and stepping, sucking, tonic neck		Sensory
Sensory	Pinprick response slow (2-3 sec)	Pinprick response equivocal	No response

From Nelson NM (2001). Neonatal adaptations. In Hoekelman RA, et al., editors. Primary pediatric care, ed 4, St Louis: Mosby, p. 561.
From Seidel HM (1997). Physical examination of the newborn. In Seidel HM, Rosenstein RJ, Pathak A, editors. Primary care of the newborn, ed 2, St Louis: Mosby, p. 50.

| Table **3-10** | Levels of Surveillance of the Newborn Based on Examination of the Cranial Nerves |

	Level of Surveillance		
Cranial Nerves	**Normal**	**Alert**	**Alarm**
Forebrain: 2	Fix and follow (visual-evoked potential)	Equivocal (arc <60 degrees)	No response
Midbrain: 3, 4, 5, and 8	Pupillary response, doll's eye response	Unequal, disconjugate, nystagmus	Absent, fixed position
Hindbrain 8	Crib-O-Gram (auditory-evoked potentials)		
5, 7, and 12	Sucking	Weak	Unequal
9 and 10	Swallowing	Uncoordinated	
11	Sternocleido-mastoid muscles	Weak	

From Nelson NM (2001). Neonatal adaptations. In Hoekelman RA, et al., editors. Primary pediatric care, ed 4, St Louis: Mosby, p. 461.
From Seidel HM (1997). Physical examination of the newborn. In Seidel HM, Rosenstein RJ, Pathak A, editors. Primary care of the newborn, ed 2, St Louis: Mosby, p. 46.

BIBLIOGRAPHY

American Academy of Pediatrics (AAP) and American College of Obstetrics & Gynecology (ACOG) (2002). Guidelines for perinatal care, ed 5, Elk Grove Village, Ill: AAP.

Cavaliere T, Sansouci D (2003). Newborn and infant assessment. In Kenner C, Lott JW, editors. Comprehensive neonatal nursing: a physiologic perspective, ed 3, St Louis: WB Saunders.

Kenner C (2003). Resuscitation and stabilization. In Kenner C, Lott JW, editors. Comprehensive neonatal nursing: a physiologic perspective, ed 3, St Louis: WB Saunders.

CHAPTER 4

NEONATAL TRANSPORTS

The transport of a sick infant may be down the hall of the delivering hospital or across the city or state to a regional referral center. The goal is the same: to get the infant to the best possible care in the shortest amount of time. The actual transportation of the infant may be by ground or air, depending on distance, acuity, or economic factors. National guidelines are available that address ground and air transports (James, 2002; NANN, 2000). Guidelines presented here from two institutions outline the roles and responsibilities of transport team members and the nursing care required to stabilize and transport an infant safely.

TRANSPORTS*

Policy

Introduction/general transfer information Level III neonatal intensive care unit (NICU) is a tertiary-level facility staffed and equipped to handle advanced neonatal life support and to provide skilled medical/nursing care to infants, with the commitment to provide the best possible care as determined by medical need without regard to gender, age, religion, political affiliation, ethnic origin, or ability to pay—within limitations of bed space, personnel, and equipment availability.

When situations arise in which the patient's best interests are served by transfer to another department or facility, the infant will be transported by appropriate personnel and means to the facility capable of meeting those needs.

Acceptable reason for transfer No infant may be transported without approval of the attending physician and/or neonatologist; verbal orders are acceptable and documented on transfer order form.

- When medically indicated procedure or service cannot be provided at level III NICU/II special care nursery (SCN) or when patient's best interest is better provided at another facility with appropriate capabilities

*Modified from Altimier L, Brown B, Tedeschi L (2000). Tri-Health's manual of neonatal nursing policies, procedures, competencies, & clinical pathways, Glenview, Ill: National Association of Neonatal Nurses.

- When there is no longer a need for tertiary care, infant is transported to a level I/II facility.
- In rare situations (because of lack of bed space and/or personnel) an infant may be transported to another facility capable of providing the appropriate level of care.
- At request of parent(s) or legal guardian, after explanation is given of the potential risks of transport

Medical Screening Exam

Before transport to NICU/SCN, another institution, or another department, an infant receives an appropriate screening exam. This exam is performed just before transfer from NICU/SCN and/or immediately on arrival to NICU/SCN. The exam includes cardiorespiratory, thermal, and other systems as needed and is documented in patient's chart. Repeat exams, relevant laboratory/radiology evaluations, other diagnostic tests, and any treatment are provided as medically needed.

Selection of receiving hospitals/facilities Selection is made by the transferring physician based on several factors:
- Patient care needs: in most instances provision of medically indicated services or procedures will dictate the appropriate facility to receive patient (i.e., pediatric surgical/subspecialty availability or level II capability for reverse transports).
- Receiving facility: confirmation of bed space, personnel availability, transfer acceptance
- Time and distance factors: if closest appropriate facility is unable to accept transfer, travel time to other facilities capable of providing necessary level of care should be considered.
- Availability of specialized transfer team: infants requiring more advanced life support, air transport capability, or other specialized services en route are also a consideration.

Obtaining acceptance
- Attending physician/neonatologist (resident/certified nurse practitioner [CNP] at direction of attending physician/neonatologist) contacts the receiving physician/CNP.
- Clinical information is exchanged, and verification is made of acceptance.
- Document name, title, date, time person contacted, transfer acceptance on the transfer order form.
- Transport team coordinator contacts receiving unit's transport team member/designated contact to verify bed space, personnel, acceptance.
- Documentation is made on the transfer order form and on the appropriate checklist form.

Selection of transfer mode

- Transferring physician selects appropriate mode of transport, in most instances by ambulance.
- The transport team coordinator contacts the ambulance company to make arrangements.
- For air transports, the regional center is contacted to make arrangements.

Transport Procedures—Nursing

Neonatal transport to surgical center/other appropriate institution/inpatient care When infant is identified as at-risk for medical/surgical complications or needing inpatient diagnostic testing at level III/other appropriate institution requiring transport, the transport system is activated.

1. The transport team coordinator will do the following:
   a. Notify neonatologists on-call of the transport (if not aware).
   b. With neonatologists, assess the infant's condition to determine the transport staffing.
   c. Utilize the registered nurse (RN) staffing plan to determine the transport RN.
   d. Contact admitting unit's transport team coordinator to give patient report in collaboration with attending nurse. Report will include overall plan of care, current patient status, and developmental care needs.
   e. Direct resident/CNP to obtain parental consent for transport as needed.
   f. Verify completion of NICU/SCN transfer orders.
   g. Verify completion of certificate of transfer if infant is unstable or acutely ill.
   h. Have unit clerk/secretary collect recent x-rays, copy pertinent aspects of medical record (last 5 days of progress/nursing notes). If emergency, fax or mail copied chart/x-rays to receiving hospital.
   i. Notify respiratory therapy of the transport with planned departure time.
   j. Notify the ambulance company of the time the crew is needed for the transport.
   k. Direct attending RN to have the infant ready at the scheduled time.
   l. Turn on the Isolette to begin warming.
   m. Obtain placenta (if fresh), available cord blood. Send 10 ml maternal blood in red-top Vacutainer if infant has hydrops fetalis. (Notify L&D [labor and delivery] or postpartum RN to have lab obtain specimen.)
   n. Offer psychosocial support to the family (i.e., notify chaplain, take a picture of infant for family).

o. Give a transfer packet to parents, if appropriate.

p. Notify receiving institution's admitting unit at time of transport team's departure.

2. The attending RN will do the following:

a. Prepare infant for transport.

b. Collaborate with the transport team coordinator in giving report to receiving hospital.

c. Have patient's intravenous (IV) line in place, IV fluids ready if needed.

d. Have patient's airway stabilized.

e. Give report to transport RN.

f. Check ID bands with the transport RN.

g. Offer psychosocial support to family; include information about transport and receiving hospital.

3. The transport RN will do the following:

a. Obtain report from the attending RN.

b. Begin the transport record.

c. Check ID bands with the attending RN.

d. Assist in needed stabilization/preparation of the infant for transport.

e. Perform a pretransport assessment.

f. Open and inspect contents of medication and airway boxes.

g. Transport when stable; take chart, x-rays, placenta, cord blood, maternal blood if appropriate.

h. En route: Provide for and ensure infant's safety and stability; monitor vital signs and IV fluids; keep airway and medication boxes accessible.

i. At receiving institution:

(1) Check ID bands with the admitting RN.

(2) Update on infant's condition, including amount of IV fluids and any medications given en route.

(3) Relinquish care of infant to admitting RN.

(4) Complete the transport record, giving appropriate copy to the admitting RN.

j. On return:

(1) Clean and restock all transport equipment.

(2) Complete transport evaluation, provide input from all team members (evaluation reflects any problems encountered during any part of transport).

(3) Forward to transport coordinator checklists/evaluation, duplicate copy of transport record and ambulance run sheet.

(4) Ensure photocopied chart is complete and mailed to admitting unit (if not taken with infant).

(5) Notify transport coordinator and transport member if transporter is not operating properly so that a transport will not be made until situation is corrected.

(6) Recheck medication/airway boxes, secure with a tamper tag, sign transport checklist.

Neonatal Transport from SCN to NICU/Surgical Center/Inpatient Care

1. Forms and equipment needed: consent to transfer, certificate of transfer (if needed), neonatal transfer order
2. Procedure
   a. Mother's blood draw (10 ml in a red-top tube) labeled and ready for transport
   b. One red-top tube of cord blood, properly labeled
   c. Placenta obtained from L&D or pathology (labeled and double bagged)
   d. All x-rays collected and signed out to accepting hospital
   e. Photocopies of L&D sheet, nursing notes (5 days), physician/CNP notes, transfer summary
   f. Phenylketonuria (PKU) sample drawn before transport and documented in the nursing notes if patient is stable
   g. Record of lab work
   h. One ID bracelet remains on infant; second attached to nursing discharge summary–nursing notes
3. Notify L&D, postpartum floor (wherever the mother is), obstetrician of infant's transfer.
4. The nurse caring for the infant gives parents the telephone number/location where baby will be.

Neonatal Transport to Other Appropriate Institution for Outpatient Testing

Infants requiring outpatient diagnostic tests at another facility are transported by neonatal transport team. Neonatology arranges for diagnostic studies to be done on an outpatient basis. The transport system will then be activated.

1. The transport team coordinator will do the following:
   a. Determine staffing of transport based on infant's condition (collaborating with neonatologists).
   b. Notify transport RN/transport team of scheduled departure time and time of diagnostic test.
   c. Notify the ambulance company of the transport and departure time.
   d. Direct resident to obtain parental consent for transport on the transport consent form.
   e. Direct the attending RN to have infant ready at the scheduled time.
   f. Contact receiving institution's diagnostic department to determine needed preparation of infant.
   g. Turn on the transporter to begin warming.

2. The attending RN will do the following:
   a. Prepare infant for transport.
   b. Give report and check ID bands with the transport RN.
3. The transport RN will do the following:
   a. Obtain report and check ID bands with the attending RN.
   b. Assist in needed preparation of the infant for transport.
   c. Perform a pretransport assessment.
   d. Obtain Addressographed nursing notes/progress notes for needed documentation. Transport notes may be made in nursing notes or on transport record.
   e. Open and inspect the medication and airway boxes before departure.
   f. En route and at receiving institution:
      (1) Provide for and ensure infant's safety and stability; monitor vital signs and IV fluids; at all times be responsible for infant's care.
      (2) Keep airway and medication boxes accessible.
   g. On return:
      (1) Give report to admitting RN on diagnostic tests done and infant's response to procedure.
      (2) Clean and restock all transport equipment.
      (3) Complete transport evaluation, reflect any problems encountered during transport.
      (4) Forward to transport coordinator evaluation forms, copy of documentation (nursing notes and/or pink copy of transport record), and ambulance run sheet.
      (5) Notify transport coordinator if transporter is not operating properly so that a transport will not be made until situation is corrected.
      (6) Recheck/restock medication/airway boxes, secure tamper tag, sign transport checklist.

Neonatal Return Transport

Return transports are routinely completed by the transport team. If transport team or receiving hospital requests the NICU/SCN to return infant on completion of diagnostic studies or stabilization of infant's condition, the transport system will be activated.

1. The transport team coordinator will do the following:
   a. Schedule a time for pick-up.
   b. Notify the transport RN of the scheduled time.
   c. Determine transport staffing (with neonatologists) using information from other institution.
   d. Notify the ambulance company of the time of transport.
   e. Turn on the transporter to begin warming.
2. The transport RN will do the following:
   a. Receive report from the transport team coordinator.

   b. Open and inspect contents of medication and airway boxes.

   c. At other institutions:

     (1) Receive report from the attending personnel.

     (2) Check ID bands with the attending RN.

     (3) Perform pretransport assessment and begin the transport record.

     (4) Prepare/transport infant to NICU/SCN. Monitor vital signs, IV fluids; ensure infant's safety/stability en route.

   d. On return:

     (1) Brief admitting RN of the care, condition, and course of stay at the other institution.

     (2) Check ID bands with the admitting RN.

     (3) Transfer care to the admitting RN.

     (4) Forward to transport coordinator evaluation forms, copy of documentation (nursing notes and/or pink copy of transport record), and ambulance run sheet.

     (5) Recheck, stock, apply tamper tags to medication/airway boxes; sign transport checklist.

     (6) Notify transport coordinator if transporter is not operating properly so that a transport will not be made until the situation is corrected.

Neonatal Incoming/Referral Transport

Infants from an outlying hospital who require level III NICU/SCN care are transported by neonatal transport team. Neonatology receives referral from infant's attending physician and in collaboration with that physician arranges for transfer. The transport system will then be activated.

1. The transport team coordinator will do the following:

   a. Contact referring hospital to obtain detailed report on the infant and schedule a transport time.

   b. Determine staffing in collaboration with neonatologists based on infant's condition and needs.

   c. Notify the transport RN and other team members of the scheduled departure time.

   d. Notify the ambulance company of the transport and departure time.

   e. Turn on the transporter to begin warming.

   f. Contact the receiving hospital at the time of the transport team's departure.

2. The transport RN will do the following:

   a. Obtain report received by the transport team coordinator from the referring hospital.

   b. Check transporter supplies, preparing equipment as necessary.

   c. Open and inspect the medication and airway boxes before departure.

d. On arrival at referring hospital:
   (1) Obtain parental consent with the neonatologist/CNP in attendance for the transport.
   (2) Obtain update on infant's condition from the attending personnel.
   (3) Check ID bands with the attending RN.
   (4) Obtain copy of infant's chart and x-ray.
   (5) Perform a pretransport assessment.
   (6) Initiate the transport record.
   (7) On arrival, contact transport team coordinator/admitting RN to update infant's condition and anticipated needs.
e. En route, ensure infant safety/stability; monitor/document vital signs/IV fluids; keep airway and medication boxes accessible.
f. On return:
   (1) Check ID bands with admitting RN.
   (2) Give copy of completed transport record and chart to admitting RN; assist in admission.
   (3) Complete transport evaluation, reflecting any problems encountered during the transport.
   (4) Forward to transport coordinator evaluation forms, copy of documentation (nursing notes and/or pink copy of transport record), and ambulance run sheet.
   (5) Clean and restock all transport equipment.
   (6) Notify transport coordinator if transporter is not operating properly so that a transport will not be made until the situation is corrected.
   (7) Recheck/restock medication and airway boxes, secure tamper tag, sign transport checklist.

Neonatal Reverse Transport

Infants requiring transport to another NICU/SCN (in transition to discharge) are transported by neonatal transport team. Neonatology arranges for transfer in collaboration with the infant's private pediatrician. The transport system will then be activated.

1. The transport team coordinator will do the following:
   a. Determine staffing of transport based on infant's condition (in collaboration with neonatologist).
   b. Contact receiving hospital admitting unit to give detailed report and schedule transport time.
   c. Notify the transport RN and other team members of the scheduled departure time.
   d. Notify the ambulance company of the transport and departure time.
   e. Direct the unit clerk to have the entire chart photocopied and to obtain recent x-rays.

   f. Direct the attending RN to have infant ready at the scheduled time.

   g. Verify the completion of the NICU/SCN transfer orders.

   h. Turn on the transporter to begin warming.

   i. Contact the receiving hospital at the time of the transport team's departure.

2. The attending RN will do the following:

   a. Prepare infant for transport.

   b. Give report to admitting unit (in collaboration with transport team coordinator). Report includes overall plan of care, current patient status and developmental needs.

   c. Give report to the transport RN.

   d. Check ID bands with the transport RN.

3. The transport RN will do the following:

   a. Obtain report from the attending RN.

   b. Check ID bands with the transport RN.

   c. Assist in preparation of the infant for transport.

   d. Perform a pretransport assessment.

   e. Initiate the transport record.

   f. Open and inspect the medication and airway boxes before departure.

   g. En route and at receiving institution:

     (1) Provide for and ensure infant's safety and stability.

     (2) Monitor vital signs and IV fluids.

     (3) Keep airway and medication boxes accessible.

     (4) Document.

     (5) Give updates to admitting RN on infant's condition and care.

     (6) Give copy of the transport record and chart to admitting RN.

   h. On return:

     (1) Clean and restock all transport equipment.

     (2) Recheck/restock medication and airway boxes, secure tamper tag, sign transport checklist.

     (3) Complete transport evaluation form, reflect any problems encountered during transport.

     (4) Forward to transport coordinator evaluation forms, copy of documentation (nursing notes and/or pink copy of transport record), and ambulance run sheet.

     (5) Notify transport team coordinator if transporter is not operating properly so the situation can be corrected for the next transport.

Neonatal Transports Within the Hospital

Infants requiring testing away from the neonatal area will be transported in heated Isolette with appropriate equipment applied (cardiopulmonary monitor, oximeter, oxygen, infant anesthesia bag and mask, other equipment as needed). The infant must be accompanied by an RN or physician/CNP who will remain with the infant during the entire procedure.

Transport Protocol–Standing Orders

For assistance in any situation, contact the responsible staff neonatologists.

Initial patient assessment and stabilization

1. Ensure airway patency by positioning and suctioning as needed.
2. Assess the stability of infant:
   a. Vital signs on arrival, every 30 minutes or more frequently if condition indicates until stable
   b. Dextrostix on arrival, then every 30 minutes or more frequently if condition indicates until stable
   c. Note color, respiratory pattern, and effort.
3. Attach cardiorespiratory monitor, pulse oximeter, and blood pressure monitor.
4. Assess need to empty infant's stomach—if needed, place orogastric tube to gravity drainage.
5. Stabilize temperature; maintain axillary temperature at 96.8° to 98.6° F.
6. Assess current labs.
7. Obtain IV access for Glucometer <35/Dextrostix <45; administration route for medications if indicated or ordered; NPO infant.
8. For infants needing IV fluids, infuse D10W at 80 ml/kg/day for infants >1 kg; for infants <1 kg use D5W.
9. For hypoglycemia, administer D10W at 2 ml/kg for Dextrostix or blood glucose <25 mg/100 ml, and follow with IV fluids as above.
10. Obtain arterial blood gas (ABG) values for cyanosis, respiratory distress, or oxygen requirement. Notify neonatologists stat of critical results:
    a. pH <7.25 or >7.5; PCO_2 <30 or >55; PO_2 <60 or >100 (if infant <1500 g)
    b. Obtain stat chest x-ray at receiving hospital for cyanosis, respiratory distress, or endotracheal tube placement.
    c. Administer oxygen (Mapleson bag/mask, head hood), adjust FiO_2 to maintain oximeter SaO_2 90% to 94%.
    d. Maintain accurate intake and output (I&O).

Management of Sudden Cardiac Arrest

1. Contact neonatologist on call as soon as condition permits.
2. Assess the infant, perform ABCs (airway, breathing, circulation) or resuscitation.

3. If cardiac arrest or heart rate <80 confirmed by auscultation or palpation:
    a. Begin ventilation with Mapleson using pressures and rate to move chest.
    b. Begin cardiac compression if heart rate (HR) <80 or 60 to 80 and not improving.
    c. Assess performance/infant's response.
    d. Establish IV route for medications:
        (1) Epinephrine, 0.1 to 0.3 ml/kg intravenous push (IVP) or via endotracheal tube (ETT)
        (2) Sodium bicarbonate 4.2%, 1 to 2 mEq/kg IV over at least 2 minutes
        (3) Naloxone (Narcan), 0.1 mg/kg IV or via ETT for known narcotic-induced respiratory depression
        (4) Volume expanders, such as NS or Plasmanate, 10 ml/kg IV over 5 to 10 minutes
    e. Establish endotracheal airway or continue to bag with mask. (Place orogastric tube if needed or if continuing to bag with mask >2 minutes.)
    f. Obtain chest x-ray to rule out pneumothorax.
4. Additional orders from neonatologists will be written on a physician's order sheet by the transport RN, and on return to NICU/SCN, orders must be signed by the neonatologist.

UNIVERSITY OF ILLINOIS MEDICAL CENTER AT CHICAGO CLINICAL CARE GUIDELINE

Subject: Procedure—Transport Activities*

The transport nurse will assess the infant's condition systematically and initiate the appropriate nursing interventions. The transport nurse will obtain and provide, in a professional manner, information about neonate's condition at the referral hospital. The transport nurse along with the staff RN or physician of the referral hospital will identify, band, and take footprints for patient identification. The transport nurse will provide the mother and one other mother-designated significant other with one identification band each. The transport nurse will assist the physician with all special procedures performed at the referring hospital. The transport nurse will remain with and monitor the infant for the duration of the transport. The transport nurse will ensure that all required items for transport have been collected.

Before departure from the referring hospital, the transport nurse will notify the NICU admission nurse or charge nurse regarding condition of the patient.

*From University of Illinois Medical Center at Chicago Women's and Children's Nursing Services. Used with permission by Dharmapuri Vidyasagar, MD; Catherine Theorell, RNC, MSN, NNP; Beena Peters, RN, MS.

The transport nurse will provide psychosocial support to the family.

The transport nurse will check and replace transport equipment as necessary.

The transport nurse will document on the QA for transport form and the neonatal admission/transport flow sheet the following:
1. Vital signs
2. Assessment findings
3. Care provided to neonate during transport

Subject: Transport Standards for NICU/ICN
University of Illinois perinatal center neonatal transport referral call flow
- All calls must be referred to a neonatal fellow/senior resident.
- Obtain information concerning infant and document in the neonatal transport logbook. (Notify the neonatal attending.)
- Make the determination whether the unit will accept or refuse the neonatal transport.

Transport call

REFUSED		ACCEPTED
Network Hospital	Nonnetwork Hospital	Notify Hospital
1. Notify hospital.	1. Notify hospital of refusal.	1. Arrange for transport (inform nursing—call for ambulance).
2. Arrange for placement at another hospital.		2. Notify hospital of estimated time of arrival.

If the refused transport is from within the network and there are no other centers available, University of Illinois Medical Center at Chicago is responsible for accepting and/or placing the infant.

Subject: transport equipment box contents list
Upper tray—right side

Item	Quantity	Size
Bulb syringe	1	
Saline squirts	8	
ECG monitor electrodes	1	
Pulse-ox monitor probe	1	
Stop-cock	3	
Tegaderm	5	
Duo-Derm	2	
IV butterflies	2	23 gauge
Waterproof tape	1	1 inch

Upper tray–left side	Quantity	Size
IV prep kit	3	
Tape	1	½ inch
Tape	1	1 inch
Co-band	1	
Needles	5	16 gauge
Needles	5	19 gauge
Needles	5	25 gauge
0.9% normal saline bag	1	50 ml
5% dextrose bag	1	100 ml
3-cc syringe	5	
0.9% normal saline vials	5	
1-cc syringe	5	
Vaseline gauze dressing	5	
Alcohol wipes	20	

Lower tray–right side		
Item	Quantity	Size
60-cc syringe	1	Catheter tip
60-cc syringe	1	Luer-Lok
30-cc syringe	2	
20-cc syringe	2	
10-cc syringe	2	
5-cc syringe	2	
Instrument tray	1	Disposable

Subject: Transport Drug Bag Contents List

DRUGS   (PATIENT NAME PLATE)

___ (1) Diazepam (5 mg/ml)—2-ml vial

___ (2) Epinephrine 1:10,000 (0.1 mg/ml)—10-ml syringe

___ (3) Phenobarbital (60 mg/ml)—1-ml Tubex (with injector)

___ (4) Sodium bicarbonate 4.2% (0.5 mEq/ml)—infant 10-ml syringe

IV fluids in bags

___ (1) Dextrose 10% in water—250-ml bag

___ (2) Sodium chloride 0.9%—100-ml bag

When drug bag is opened, call pharmacy to restock and relock. For billing purposes, please stamp this sheet with patient name and leave in opened drug bag for pharmacist. Thank you.

Subject: Transport Equipment Check for NICU/ICN

To ensure adequate functioning and availability of transport equipment and supplies. Transport equipment for the NICU includes the following:

• Transport Isolette with built-in ventilator, monitor, and pulse oximeter

• Transport equipment bag/box (stocked and checked before transport)

- Transport drug bag (checked and locked by pharmacy before transport)

Procedure

The charge nurse shall do the following:

- Assign the duty of checking the transport equipment to a registered nurse on each 8-hour shift. The assigned RN is unable to check the equipment within the first 3 hours of the shift. If the assigned RN is unable to check the equipment, she/he shall notify the charge nurse.
- Ensure that the transport Isolette is cleaned and restocked of any used equipment/supplies for the next transport as soon as possible on return from a transport.
- The charge nurse will indicate on the patient assignment sheet the RN assigned to check the transport equipment.
- The charge nurse is responsible for ensuring the transport Isolette and equipment bag/box are checked and will reassign the duty if the assigned RN is not able to complete the check.

The assigned transport RN shall check the transport equipment to ensure the following:

- The transport Isolette is plugged into an electrical source, the battery is charging, and the Isolette is preheated.
- All necessary cables are present (i.e., monitor, pulse oximeter cables).
- The monitors, Isolette, and infusion pumps are charged.
- The contents of the transport bag/box are complete and stocked as necessary.

The clerk shall do the following:

1. The clerk will ensure that the transport paperwork packs are assembled and ready for use.
2. The transport paperwork will include the following:
   a. Authorization for admission
   b. Consent for treatment
   c. Consent for blood transfusion
   d. Consent for operative procedure
   e. University of Illinois Medical Center map
   f. Neonatal transport flow sheet
   g. NICU/ICN admission flow sheet

Documentation

The RN will document that the transport equipment was checked by signing the transport equipment check reporting form.

BIBLIOGRAPHY

Acree CM, et al. (2003). Regionalization in today's health care delivery system. In Kenner C, Lott JW, editors. *Comprehensive neonatal nursing: a physiologic perspective*, St Louis: WB Saunders.

American Academy of Pediatrics (AAP) and American College of Obstetricians and Gynecologists (ACOG) (2002). *Guidelines for perinatal care*, ed 5, Elk Grove, Ill: AAP.

Canadian Institute of Child Health (CICH) (2002). *Childwatch International Research Network: perinatal regionalization.*
http://www.childwatch.uio.no/key_institutions/north_america/ottawa cich.html

Canadian Perinatal Health Surveillance System (CPSS) (2000). *Canadian perinatal health report 2000. http://www.hc-sc.gc.ca/hpb/lcdc/publicat/cphr-rspc00/*

Davis PJ, et al. (2001). Paediatric trainees and the transportation of critically ill neonates: experience, training and confidence. *Acta paediatric*, 90(9), 1068-1072.

Gerber SE, Dobrez DG, Budetti PP (2001). Managed care and perinatal regionalization in Washington state. *Obstetrics & gynecology*, 98(1), 139-143.

Gessner BD, Murth PT (2001). Perinatal care regionalization and low birth weight infant mortality rates in Alaska. *American journal of obstetrics and gynecology*, 185(3), 623-628.

James SE (2002). *Standards for critical care and specialty ground transport.* Denver: Air & Surface Transport Nurses Association.

King BR, Woodward GA (2001). Procedural training for pediatric and neonatal transport nurses. 1. Training methods and airway training. *Pediatric emergency care*, 17(6), 461-464.

L'Herault J, Petroff L, Jeffrey J (2001). The effectiveness of a thermal mattress in stabilizing and maintaining body temperature during the transport of very low-birth weight newborns. *Applied nursing research*, 14(4), 210-219.

National Association of Neonatal Nurses (NANN) (2000). *Neonatal transport standards.* Petaluma, Calif: NANN.

CHAPTER 5

PAIN ASSESSMENT FOR NEWBORNS AND INFANTS

Routine periodic assessment for pain is a mandatory component of health care delivery. Pain assessment is sometimes called the "fifth" vital sign. As late as the 1970s, the prevailing wisdom was that newborns could not feel pain because of an immature central nervous system. Research has revealed that newborns do experience pain. Observant nurses have noted changes in vital signs and decreased oxygen saturation during and following painful procedures. This chapter offers guidelines and the most common pain assessment instruments to aid in the process of pain prevention, assessment, and management.

PAIN PHYSIOLOGY

Noxious mechanical, thermal, or chemical stimuli excite primary afferent fibers that transmit information about the potentially injurious stimuli from the periphery to the dorsal horn of the spinal cord. A-delta (large, myelinated, and fast-conducting) and C (small, unmyelinated, and slow-conducting) fibers are primarily responsible for pain impulse transmission (nociception). However, these signals can be amplified or attenuated by activation of surrounding neurons in the periphery and spinal cord. For example, tissue injury causes the release of inflammatory mediators (e.g., potassium, bradykinin, prostaglandins, cytokines, nerve growth factors, catecholamines, substance P) that sensitize A-delta and C fibers and recruit other neurons (silent nociceptors) resulting in hyperalgesia. Stimulation of A-beta fibers that signal nonpainful touch and pressure can compete with the transmission of nociception in the dorsal horn of the spinal cord, reducing the intensity of the perceived pain (Walden, Franck, 2003).

PAIN ASSESSMENT TOOLS

Pain is a learned experience. We now are gaining evidence that exposure to pain at early ages often leads to changes in the "wiring" of the nervous system. Pain receptors are more dense in those infants who were exposed to repeated pain procedures at an early age. More research is needed in this area before solid conclusions can be drawn. However, pain assessment is essential to prevention of further pain and management of existing pain. No one instrument for measuring pain is right for all situations. Its use must be accompanied by a thorough physical assessment, including lab values such as blood gases and knowledge of the gestational age and diagnosis of the infant. Training on an instrument's use is another essential ingredient of a successful pain management program.

Boxes 5-1 to 5-9 give various scales for rating pediatric pain.

UNIVERSITY OF ILLINOIS MEDICAL CENTER AT CHICAGO CLINICAL CARE GUIDELINE

Subject: Neonatal Pain Assessment And Documentation*

Objective

To assess neonates and infants for pain, provide for the relief of the pain and discomfort, and document the response to pharmacologic and nonpharmacologic interventions.

Definition

For the purpose of this guideline, the following definition applies:

Pain "Pain is an unpleasant sensory and emotional experience, associated with actual or potential tissue damage or described in terms of such damage. Pain is always subjective." (International Society for the Study of Pain)

Position Statements

Neonates may exhibit pain responses differently from older children or adults and often require higher doses of analgesics and anesthetics. The sensory nerve tracts appear in the perioral area during the sev-

---

Box **5-1**

The FLACC Behavioral Scale for Postoperative Pain in Young Children

Overview

The FLACC (Face, Legs, Activity, Cry, Consolability) Behavioral Scale can be used in young children who may not be able to accurately verbalize postoperative pain and discomfort.

Patient Selection

- Children from 2 months to 7 years of age who had undergone a variety of elective surgical procedures
- Children with developmental delay not included

Continued

---

*From University of Illinois Medical Center at Chicago Women's and Children's Nursing Services. Used with permission by Dharmapuri Vidyasagar, MD; Catherine Theorell, RNC, MSN, NNP; Beena Peters, RN, MS.

Box **5-1**

The FLACC Behavioral Scale for Postoperative Pain in Young Children—cont'd

Parameters
1. Face
2. Legs
3. Activity
4. Cry
5. Consolability

Parameter Finding Points
Face
No particular expression or smile: 0
Occasional grimace or frown, withdrawn, disinterested: 1
Frequent to constant quivering chin, clenched jaw: 2
Legs
Normal position or relaxed: 0
Uneasy, restless, tense: 1
Kicking, or legs drawn up: 2
Activity
Lying quietly, normal position, moves easily: 0
Squirming, shifting back and forth, tense: 1
Arched, rigid or jerking: 2
Cry
No cry (awake or asleep): 0
Moans or whimpers, occasional complaints: 1
Crying steadily, screams or sobs, frequent complaints: 2
Consolability
Content, relaxed: 0
Reassured by occasional touching, hugging or being talked to;
distractable: 1
Difficult to console or comfort: 2

Interpretation
FLACC score = sum (points for all 5 parameters)
- Minimum score: 0
- Maximum score: 10
- The higher the score the more the behavior reflecting discomfort and pain.
- Preliminary data showed the scale to be valid and reliable.

*Merkel SI, et al. (1997).The FLACC: a behavioral scale for scoring postoperative pain in young children. Pediatric nursing, 23(3), 293-297.
Source: Medical Algorithms www.medal.org*

Box **5-2**

Modified Behavioral Pain Scale (MBPS) in Infants

Overview
Taddio et al. modified the Behavioral Pain Scale (BPS) of Robieux et al. for use with infants during office procedures such as immunizations. The child is evaluated before the procedure to give a baseline for comparison during and after the procedure.

Parameter Finding Points
Facial Expression
Definite positive expression (smiling): 0
Neutral expression: 1
Slightly negative expression (grimace): 2
Definite negative expression (furrowed brow, eyes closed tightly): 3
Cry
Laughing or giggling: 0
Not crying: 1
Moaning, quiet vocalizing, gentle or whimpering cry: 2
Full-lunged cry or sobbing: 3
Full-lunged cry, more than baseline cry (scored only if child crying at baseline): 4
Movements
Usual movements and activity: 0
Resting and relaxed: 0
Partial movement (squirming, arching, limb tensing, clenching): 2
Attempt to avoid pain by withdrawing the limb where puncture is done: 2
Agitation with complex/generalized movements involving the head, torso, or other limbs: 3
Rigidity: 3

Definitions
- Slightly negative expressions include brow bulging and nasolabial furrow.
- Definitely negative expressions include brow bulging, nasolabial furrow, eyes closed tightly, open lips, with or without a reddened face.

Interpretation
MBPS score = sum (points for all 3 parameters)
- Minimum score: 0
- Maximum score: 10

Reference: Taddio A, et al. (1995). A revised measure of acute pain in infants. Journal of pain and symptom management, 10, 456-463.
Source: Medical Algorithms www.medal.org

Box 5-3

Neonatal Infant Pain Scale (NIPS)

Overview

The Neonatal Infant Pain Scale (NIPS) is a behavioral assessment tool for measurement of pain in preterm and full-term neonates. This can be used to monitor a neonate before, during, and after a painful procedure such as venipuncture. It was developed at the Children's Hospital of Eastern Ontario.

Parameters
1. Facial expression
2. Cry
3. Breathing patterns
4. Arms
5. Legs
6. State of arousal

Parameter Finding Points

Facial Expression
Relaxed: 0
Grimace: 1
Cry
No cry: 0
Whimper: 1
Vigorous crying: 2
Breathing Patterns
Relaxed: 0
Change in breathing: 1
Arms
Restrained: 0
Relaxed: 0
Flexed: 1
Extended: 1
Legs
Restrained: 0
Relaxed: 0
Flexed: 1
Extended: 1
State of Arousal
Sleeping: 0
Awake: 0
Fussy: 1

Box 5-3

Neonatal Infant Pain Scale (NIPS)—cont'd

Definitions
- Relaxed muscles (facial expression): restful face, neutral expression
- Grimace: tight facial muscles, furrowed brow, chin, jaw (negative facial expression—nose, mouth, brow)
- No cry: quiet, not crying
- Whimper: mild moaning, intermittent
- Vigorous cry: loud scream, rising, shrill, continuous (Note: silent cry may be scored if baby is intubated, as evidenced by obvious mouth, facial movements.)
- Relaxed: usual pattern for the baby
- Change in breathing: in-drawing, irregular, faster than usual, gagging, breath holding
- Relaxed/restrained: no muscular rigidity, occasional random movements of limb
- Flexed/extended: tense, straight, rigid, and/or rapid extension, flexion
- Sleeping/awake: quiet, peaceful, sleeping, or alert and settled
- Fussy: alert, restless, and thrashing

Interpretation
NIPS score = sum (points for the 6 parameters)
- Minimum score: 0
- Maximum score: 7

Limitation
- A falsely low score may be seen in an infant who is too ill to respond or who is receiving a paralyzing agent.

Reference: Lawrence J, et al. (1993). The development of a tool to assess neonatal pain. Neonatal network, 12(6, September), 59-66.
Source: Medical Algorithms www.medal.org

enth week of gestation, and connections between sensory neurons and spinal cord dorsal horn cells are completed by the second trimester. Neonates have more cutaneous nerve endings than adults and have an increased sensitivity to pain. The cortical perception of pain is complete before 24 weeks' gestation. Continued stimulation of the pain tract leads to hyperalgesia and leads to the experience of chronic pain. The hormonal and behavioral stress responses to pain may persist during later infancy, resulting in touch aversion, feeding difficulties, impaired parental interaction, and failure to thrive. The sum total effect may lead to permanently affecting neuronal and synaptic brain organization.

Box **5-4**

Children's Hospital of Eastern Ontario Pain Scale (CHEOPS) in Young Children

Overview
The CHEOPS (Children's Hospital of Eastern Ontario Pain Scale) is a behavioral scale for evaluating postoperative pain in young children. It can be used to monitor the effectiveness of interventions for reducing the pain and discomfort.

Patients
- The initial study was done on children 1 to 5 years of age.
- It has been used in studies with adolescents, but this may not be an appropriate instrument for that age-group.
- According to Mitchell (1999) it is intended for ages 0 to 4 years.

Parameter Finding Points
Cry
No cry: 1
Moaning: 2
Crying: 2
Screaming: 3
Facial
Smiling: 0
Composed: 1
Grimace: 2
Child Verbal
Positive: 0
None: 1
Complaints
Other than pain: 1
Pain complaints: 2
Both pain and nonpain complaints: 2
Torso
Neutral: 1
Shifting: 2
Tense: 2
Shivering: 2
Upright: 2
Restrained: 2
Touch
Not touching: 1
Reach: 2
Touch: 2

Box 5-4

Children's Hospital of Eastern Ontario Pain Scale (CHEOPS) in Young Children—cont'd

Touch—cont'd
Grab: 2
Restrained: 2
Legs
Neutral: 1
Squirming, kicking: 2
Drawn up, tensed: 2
Standing: 2
Restrained: 2

Definition

- No cry: child is not crying
- Moaning: child is moaning or quietly vocalizing, silent cry
- Crying: child is crying, but the cry is gentle or whimpering
- Screaming: child is in a full-lunged cry; sobbing may be scored with complaint or without complaint
- Smiling: score only if definite positive facial expression
- Composed: neutral facial expression
- Grimace: score only if definite negative facial expression
- Positive (verbal): child makes any positive statement or talks about other things without complaint
- None (verbal): child not talking
- Complaints other than pain: child complains but not about pain ("I want to see Mommy." or "I am thirsty.")
- Pain complaints: child complains about pain
- Both pain and nonpain complaints: child complains about pain and about other things (e.g., "It hurts; I want Mommy.")
- Neutral (torso): body (not limbs) is at rest; torso is inactive
- Shifting: body is in motion in a shifting or serpentine fashion
- Tense: body is arched or rigid
- Shivering: body is shuddering or shaking involuntarily
- Upright: child is in a vertical or upright position
- Restrained: body is restrained
- Not touching: child is not touching or grabbing at wound
- Reach: child is reaching for but not touching wound
- Touch: child is gently touching wound or wound area
- Grab: child is grabbing vigorously at wound
- Restrained: child's arms are restrained
- Neutral (legs): legs may be in any position but are relaxed; includes gently swinging

Continued

Box **5-4**

Children's Hospital of Eastern Ontario Pain Scale (CHEOPS) in Young Children—cont'd

Definition—cont'd
- Squirming, kicking: definitive uneasy or restless movements in the legs and/or striking out with foot or feet
- Drawn up, tensed: legs tensed and/or pulled up tightly to body and kept there
- Standing: standing, crouching, or kneeling
- Restrained: child's legs are being held down

Interpretation
CHEOPS pain score = sum (points for all 6 parameters)
- Minimum score: 4
- Maximum score: 13

Bibliography
Beyer JE, McGrath PJ, Berde CB (1990). Discordance between self-report and behavioral pain measures in children aged 3-7 years after surgery. *Journal of pain and symptom management,* 5, 350-356.

Jacobson SJ, et al. (1997). Randomized trial of oral morphine for painful episodes of sickle-cell disease in children. *Lancet,* 350, 1358-1361.

McGrath PJ, et al. (1985). CHEOPS: a behavioral scale for rating post-operative pain in children. *Advances in pain research therapy,* 9, 395-402.

McGrath PJ, McAlpine L (1993). Physiologic perspectives on pediatric pain. *Journal of pediatrics,* 122, S2-S8.

Mitchell P (1999). Understanding a young child's pain. *Lancet,* 354, 1708.

Reference: McGrath PJ, Johnson G, et al: CHEOPS: a behavioral scale for rating postoperative pain in children. Adv Pain Research Therapy. 1985; 9:375–402.
Source: Medical Algorithms www.medal.org

Procedure

1. Each infant admitted to the neonatal intensive care or intermediate care nursery will be assessed for evidence of pain or discomfort minimally each time the vital signs are assessed using the Premature Infant Pain Profile (PIPP).

2. The PIPP should be scored for each infant and recorded on a blank column on the nursing care section found on the neonatal intensive care unit (NICU)/intermediate care nursery (ICN) flow sheet. The column should be marked "Pain Assessment" or "PIPP."

3. Using the PIPP, a score of 6 usually indicates no pain and a score >12 reflects moderate to severe pain.

Box **5-5**

Behavioral Pain Scale (BPS) of Robieux et al.

Overview
Robieux et al. developed a behavioral pain scale for use in young children during procedures such as venipuncture. It can be used to monitor the effectiveness of interventions to reduce manifested pain. It was developed as a simplified version of CHEOPS at the Hospital for Sick Children in Toronto, Canada.

Patients
• Infants and toddlers

Parameters
1. Facial expression
2. Cry
3. Movements

Parameter Finding Points
Facial Expression
Positive expression (smiling): 0
Neutral expression: 1
Negative expression (grimace): 2
Cry
Laughing or giggling: 0
Not crying: 1
Moaning: 2
Full-lunged cry or sobbing: 3
Movements
Usual movements (i.e., playing): 0
Neutral, not moving: 1
Attempt to withdraw: 2
Complex agitation involving head, other limbs: 3

Interpretation
BPS score = sum (points for the 3 parameters)
• Minimum score: 0
• Maximum score: 8
• The higher the score, the more severe the pain.

Bibliography
Koren G (1993). Use of the eutectic mixture of local anesthetics in young children for procedure related pain. *Journal of pediatrics,* 122, S30-S35.
Robieux I, et al. (1991). Assessing pain and analgesia with a lidocaine-prilocaine emulsion in infants and toddlers during venipucture. *Journal of pediatrics,* 118, 971-973.

Reference: *Robieux I, Kumar R, et al. Assessing pain and analgesia with a lidocaine-prilocaine emulsion in infants and toddlers during venipuncture. J Pediatr. 1991; 118:971–973.*
Source: *Medical Algorithms www.medal.org*

Box **5-6**

Riley Infant Pain Scale (RIPS)

Overview
The Riley Infant Pain Scale (RIPS) was developed at Riley Hospital for Children in Indiana. It is intended to assess pain in preverbal infants. It was adapted from the Pain Rating Scale
used at Riley Hospital.
Parameters Used to Evaluate Infants
1. Facial
2. Body movement
3. Sleep
4. Verbal/vocal
5. Consolability
6. Response to movement/touch

Parameter Finding Points
Facial
Neutral/smiling: 0
Frowning/grimacing: 1
Clenched teeth: 2
Full cry expression: 3
Body Movement
Calm, relaxed: 0
Restless/fidgeting: 1
Moderate agitation or moderate mobility: 2
Thrashing, flailing, incessant agitation, or strong voluntary immobility: 3
Sleep
Sleeping quietly with easy respirations: 0
Restless while asleep: 1
Sleeps intermittently (sleep/awake): 2
Sleeping for prolonged periods of time interrupted by jerky
    movements or unable to sleep: 3
Verbal/Vocal
No cry: 0
Whimpering, complaining: 1
Pain, crying: 2
Screaming, high-pitched cry: 3
Consolability
Neutral: 0
Easy to console: 1
Not easy to console: 2
Inconsolable: 3

Box 5-6

Riley Infant Pain Scale (RIPS)—cont'd

Response to Movement/Touch
Moves easily: 0
Winces when touched or moved: 1
Cries out when moved or touched: 2
High-pitched cry or scream when touched or moved: 3

Interpretation
RIPS score = sum (points for the 6 parameters)
Average value = RIPS score/6
- Minimum score: 0
- Maximum score: 18
- The higher the score, the more marked the pain.
- An alternative method of scoring is to consider the table as 4 columns graded from 0 to 3 and to assign the infant to the grade with the features matching the child's behavior. This is similar to the use of the Riley Infant Pain Rating Scale.

Bibliography

Joyce BA, et al. (1994). Reliability and validity of preverbal pain assessment tools. *Issues in comprehensive pediatric nursing, 17,* 121-135.
Schade JG, et al. (1996). Comparison of three preverbal scales for postoperative pain assessment in a diverse pediatric sample. *Journal of pain and symptom management, 12,* 348-359.

Source: Medical Algorithms www.medal.org

4. The infant's response to both pharmacologic and nonpharmacologic therapy should be noted within 30 minutes of administration or intervention.
5. Infants receiving continuous analgesic therapy should be assessed for pain with every performance of vital signs and/or with any nursing care.
6. Narrative notes (PIPP) may also be done in the medical record.
7. Physiologic manifestations of pain responses in the neonate are as follows:

Increased		**Decreased**
Heart rate	Skin blood flow	Oxygen saturation
Respiratory rate	Skin color	Arterial oxygen concentration
Blood pressure	Mean airway pressure	Skin temperature
Intracranial pressure	Palmar sweating	Heart rate variability

Box **5-7**

Preverbal, Early Verbal Pediatric Pain Scale (PEPPS)

Overview
The Preverbal, Early Verbal Pediatric Pain Scale (PEPPS) can be used to measure pain in young children based on observed behavior. The score can be used to monitor response to therapeutic interventions. The study was done at the Maine Medical Center in Portland, Maine. Age target is 12-24 months (toddlers).

Parameters
1. Heart rate
2. Facial expression
3. Cry (audible/visible)
4. Consolability/state of restfulness
5. Body posture
6. Sociability
7. Sucking/feeding

Parameter Finding Points
Heart Rate
Baseline range (<10 beats/min above): 0
10-20 beats/min above baseline: 1
21-30 beats/min above baseline: 2
31-40 beats/min above baseline: 3
>40 beats/min above baseline: 4
Facial
Relaxed facial expression: 0
Grimace, brows drawn together, eyes partially closed, squinting: 2
Severe grimace, brows lowered and tightly drawn together, eyes tightly closed: 4
Cry
No cry: 0
Whimpering, groaning, fussiness: 1
Intermittent crying: 2
Sustained crying: 3
Screaming: 4
Consolability, State of Restfulness
Pleasant, well integrated: 0
Distractable, easy to console, intermittent fussiness: 1
Able to console, distract with difficulty, intermittent restlessness, irritability: 2
Unable to console, restlessness, sustained movement: 4
Body Posture
Body at rest, relaxed positioning: 0

Box **5-7**

Preverbal, Early Verbal Pediatric Pain Scale (PEPPS)—cont'd

Body Posture—cont'd
Clenched fists, curled toes, and/or reaching for or touching wound area: 1
Localization with extension or flexion: 2
Stiff and nonmoving: 2
Intermittent or sustained movement with or without periods of rigidity: 3
Sustained arching, flailing, thrashing, and/or kicking: 4
Sociability
Sleeping: 0
Responds to voice and/or touch, makes eye contact and/or smiles,
    easy to obtain and maintain: 0
Responds to voice and/or touch with effort, makes eye contact,
    difficult to obtain and maintain: 2
Absent eye contact, absent response to voice and/or touch: 4
Sucking/Feeding
Not applicable (NA): 0
NPO or oral stimuli not used: 0
Sucking, drinking, and/or eating well: 0
Disorganized sucking: 1
Attempting to eat or drink but discontinues: 1
Lack of sucking, refusing food or fluids: 2

Interpretation
PEPPS score = sum (points for all 7 parameters)
• Minimum score: 0
• Maximum score: 26
• The higher the score, the greater the manifested pain behavior.

*Reference: Schultz AA, et al. (1999). Preverbal, Early Verbal Pediatric Pain
Scale (PEPPS): development and early psychometric testing. Journal of
pediatric nursing, 14, 19-27.*
Source: Medical Algorithms www.medal.org

8. Behavioral manifestations of pain responses in a neonate include
   the following:

Vocalization	**State Changes**	**Facial Expression**
Cry—pitch, length, number	Wakefulness	Grimacing
Whimpering	Fussiness/ irritability	Eye squeeze
Moaning	Difficult to comfort	Brow bulge
Hiccoughs	Feeding difficulties	Quivering chin
Gasps	Listlessness/ lethargy	Taut tongue
Gagging		Open lips
		Pursed lips

Box **5-8**

Premature Infant Pain Profile (PIPP)

Overview
The Premature Infant Pain Profile (PIPP) is a behavioral measure of pain for premature infants. It was developed at the Universities of Toronto and McGill in Canada.

Indicators
1. Gestational age
2. Behavioral state before painful stimulus
3. Change in heart rate during painful stimulus
4. Change in oxygen saturation during painful stimulus
5. Brow bulge during painful stimulus
6. Eye squeeze during painful stimulus
7. Nasolabial furrow during painful stimulus

Scoring Instructions
1. Score gestational age before examining infant.
2. Score the behavioral state before the potentially painful event by observing the infant for 15 seconds.
3. Record the baseline heart rate and oxygen saturation.
4. Observe the infant for 30 seconds immediately following the painful event. Score physiologic and facial changes seen during this time and record immediately.

Indicator Finding Points
Gestational Age
≥36 weeks: 0
32 weeks to 35 weeks, 6 days: 1
28 weeks to 31 weeks, 6 days: 2
<28 weeks: 3
Behavioral State
Active/awake, eyes open, facial movements: 0
Quiet/awake, eyes open, no facial movements: 1
Active/sleep, eyes closed, facial movements: 2
Quiet/sleep, eyes closed, no facial movements: 3
Heart Rate Maximum
0-4 beats/min increase: 0
5-14 beats/min increase: 1
15-24 beats/min increase: 2
≥25 beats/min increase: 3

> ## Box **5-8**
>
> ### Premature Infant Pain Profile (PIPP)—cont'd
>
> *Oxygen Saturation Minimum*
> 0%-2.4% decrease: 0
> 2.5%-4.9% decrease: 1
> 5.0%-7.4% decrease: 2
> ≥7.5% decrease: 3
> *Brow Bulge*
> None (≤9% of time): 0
> Minimum (10%-39% of time): 1
> Moderate (40%-69% of time): 2
> Maximum (≥70% of time): 3
> *Eye Squeeze*
> None (≤9% of time): 0
> Minimum (10%-39% of time): 1
> Moderate (40%-69% of time): 2
> Maximum (≥70% of time): 3
> *Nasolabial Furrow*
> None (≤9% of time): 0
> Minimum (10%-39% of time): 1
> Moderate (40%-69% of time): 2
> Maximum (≥70% of time): 3
>
> ### Interpretation
> PIPP score = sum (points for all 7 indicators)
> - Minimum score: 0
> - Maximum score: 21
> - The higher the score, the greater the pain behavior.

Reference: Stevens B, et al. (1996). *Premature Infant Pain Profile: development and initial validation.* Clinical journal of pain, *12*, 13-22.
Source: Medical Algorithms www.medal.org

Muscle Tone	Body Movements	Skin Color
Fist/toe clenching	Fisting	
	Finger splaying	
Hypertonicity	Diffuse squirming	Pallor
Knee/leg flexion	Restlessness	Flushing
Hypotonicity/flaccidity	Rigidity/extension	
	Trunk arching	
	Thrashing	
	Kicking	

Box **5-9**

The CRIES Scale for Neonatal Postoperative Pain Assessment

Overview
The CRIES (Crying, Requires oxygen, Increased vital signs, Expression, Sleep) Scale is a tool for measuring postoperative pain in the neonate. The scale may be taken over time to monitor the infant's recovery or response to interventions. The authors are from the University of Missouri in Columbia.

Patient Population
- Neonates with study population from 32 to 60 weeks' gestational age.
- The infants were in an intensive care unit following surgery and were evaluated hourly.

Parameters
1. Crying: The characteristic cry of pain is high pitched.
2. Requires oxygen to keep oxygen saturation >95%: neonates experiencing pain show a decrease in oxygenation.
3. Increased vital signs: vital signs are taken last since this may waken the child.
4. Expression: the facial expression most often associated with pain is the grimace. There may be brow lowering, squeezing shut of the eyes, deepening of the nasolabial furrow, and opening of the lips and/or mouth.
5. Sleepless: based on observation during the hour previous to recording score.

Parameter Finding Points
Crying
No: 0
Crying but not high pitched: 0
High pitched but infant consolable: 1
Inconsolable: 2
Requires Oxygen
No: 0
≤30% supplemental oxygen required to keep oxygen saturation >95%: 1
>30% supplemental oxygen required to keep oxygen saturation >95%: 2
Increased Vital Signs
Heart rate and mean blood pressure less than or equal to preoperative values: 0

Box 5-9

The CRIES Scale for Neonatal Postoperative Pain Assessment—cont'd

Heart rate *or* mean blood pressure increased but ≤20% from preoperative levels: 1

Heart rate *or* mean blood pressure increased >20% from preoperative levels: 2

Expression
None: 0
Grimace: 1
Grimace with grunting: 2

Sleepless
No: 0
Wakes at frequent intervals: 1
Constantly awake: 2

Definitions

- Supplemental oxygenation is given as <30% or >30%, with no specification for 30%.
- Vital signs are given as <20% or >20% from preoperative levels, with no specification for 20%.

Interpretation

CRIES score = sum (points for all 5 parameters)
- Minimum score: 0
- Maximum score: 10
- The higher the score, the greater the subjective expression of pain.

Performance

- The results of the CRIES scale correlate well with the OPS score (Box 5-4).
- The authors found the score valid and reliable.

Krechel SW, Bildner J (1995). CRIES: a new neonatal postoperative pain measurement score. Initial testing and reliability. Paediatric anaesthesia, 5, 53-61.

Source: Medical Algorithms www.medal.org

9. Biochemical responses to pain include the following:

Increased	Decreased
Cortisol	Insulin
Epinephrine	
Norepinephrine	
Growth hormone	
Glucagon	
Aldosterone	

10. Pharmacologic intervention for pain is morphine or fentanyl that attenuates the hemodynamic, hormonal, and metabolic responses to pain stress.
    a. Doses are calculated by weight and titrated to clinical response.
    b. Long-term use can result in tolerance—requiring higher doses to achieve similar clinical response.
    c. Physiologic dependency can occur, requiring weaning after long-term use.
    d. Pain associated with surgery should be assessed every 2 to 4 hours with continuous infusions of analgesics for the first 24 hours and additional boluses as needed.
11. Sedation with lorazepam or chloral hydrate does not provide pain relief.
12. Nonpharmacologic interventions attempt to prevent behavioral disorganization by promoting organizing behaviors and include the following:

Environmental Modifications	Behavioral Interventions	Sensory Stimulation
Lower light levels	Nesting	Rocking
Turning down monitor alarm	Swaddling	Talking
Limit telephone ringing	Flexed positioning	Massage
Close incubator doors gently	Boundaries	Soft music
Limit storage on top of incubator	Facilitated tucking	Nonnutritive sucking
Cover incubator	Minimal-handling protocol	Clustering of care
Rounds away from bedside		

13. All procedures should be explained to parents, including a discussion of the plan for the relief of pain.
14. Inform parents of the current medications used for the relief of pain.
15. Guide parents in how they can touch and interact with their infant.
16. Teach parents to understand their infant's manifestations of stress/discomfort or pain.

NICU PAIN AND SEDATION ASSESSMENT AND NURSING MANAGEMENT GUIDELINES*

Purpose

These guidelines outline pain and sedation assessment and nursing management of the infant in pain or being sedated.

*Used with permission from Loyola Medical Center, Maywood, Ill.

Background Information

Assessment and management of a patient's pain are an ethical duty for health care professionals and a primary focus of nursing care. Neonates, both term and preterm, perceive and respond to pain. Untreated pain, whether intermittent or continual, can result in adverse sequelae. Assessment of neonatal pain is difficult because of the neonate's limited verbal and neurologic repertoire. It is difficult to distinguish pain from agitation, distress, or even hunger. Pain should be presumed in neonates in all situations that are usually painful for adults and children. Pain treatment should be instituted in all cases where pain is a possibility. Side effects of this treatment should be monitored for and treated as needed. It is also important to assess infants for sedation. Sedation may be the goal for an infant, or babies may become sedated in response to the administration of analgesics. The desired level of sedation will vary, depending on the clinical goal or situation.

Procedure: Pain Assessment

1. Identify actual or potential sources of pain for the neonate: surgical procedures, invasive/indwelling tubes, heel sticks, suctioning, peritonitis, fractures, renal stones, noxious environment.
2. Pain assessment is the fifth vital sign. Assessment for pain should be included with every vital sign measurement.
3. More frequent pain assessments should be performed in the following situations:
   a. Invasive tubes or lines other than intravenous (IV) lines or feeding tubes: every 2 to 4 hours
   b. Receiving analgesics and/or sedatives: every 2 to 4 hours
   c. One hour after an analgesic is given for pain behaviors—to assess response to medication
   d. Postoperatively: every 2 hours for 24 to 48 hours, then every 4 hours until off medications
4. The N-PASS (Neonatal Pain, Agitation, and Sedation Scale) will be used to assess pain and sedation (Table 5-1).
5. Points are added to the premature infant's pain score based on gestational age to compensate for the neonate's limited ability to behaviorally or physiologically communicate pain.
6. Treatment/interventions should usually be initiated for scores >3. Some older infants may have a higher baseline score; interventions should then be instituted for consistent elevation in scores. Infants being weaned from opioids may also have a higher baseline score.
7. This treatment or intervention can be pharmacologic and/or nonpharmacologic, depending on the clinical situation.
8. The goal of pain treatment/intervention should usually be a score of 3 or less, or a decrease in the pain score.
9. Pain and sedation scores are recorded separately.

Table 5-1   N-PASS: Neonatal Pain, Agitation, and Sedation Scale

Assessment Criteria	Sedation		Normal	Pain/Agitation	
	-2	-1	0	1	2
Crying, Irritability	No cry with painful stimuli	Moans or cries minimally with painful stimuli	Appropriate crying Not irritable	Irritable or crying at intervals Consolable	High-pitched or silent, continuous cry Inconsolable
Behavior State	No arousal to any stimuli No spontaneous movement	Arouses minimally to stimuli Little spontaneous movement	Appropriate for gestational age	Restless, squirming Awakens frequently	Arching, kicking Constantly awake or arouses minimally/no movement (not sedated)
Facial Expression	Mouth is lax No expression	Minimal expression with stimuli	Relaxed Appropriate	Any pain expression intermittent	Any pain expression continual

Extremities, Tone	No grasp reflex Flaccid tone	Weak grasp reflex ↓ Muscle tone	Relaxed hands and feet Normal tone	Intermittent clenched toes, fists or finger splay Body is not tense	Continual clenched toes, fists, or finger spay Body is tense
Vital Signs: HR, RR, BP, SaO$_2$	No variability with stimuli Hypoventilation or apnea	<10% variability from baseline with stimuli	Within baseline or normal for gestational age	↑ 10%-20% from baseline SaO$_2$ 76%-85% with stimulation-quick ↑	↑ >20% from baseline SaO$_2$ ≤75% with stimulation—slow ↑ Out of sync with vent

Premature pain assessment: +3 if <28 weeks' gestation/corrected age; +2 if 28-31 weeks' gestation/corrected age; +1 if 32-35 weeks' gestation/corrected age.

HR, heart rate; RR, respiratory rate; BP, blood pressure; SaO$_2$, oxygen saturation.

Sedation Assessment

1. Sedation is scored to assess the infant's response to stimuli.
2. Sedation does not need to be assessed with every pain score.
3. Sedation assessment should occur with "hands-on" vitals and more frequently as needed. Sedation assessment requires an assessment of response to stimuli; the baby should not be stimulated unnecessarily to accomplish this.
4. The N-PASS is useful when sedation of the infant is the goal, as well as for assessing oversedation related to sedative/opioid administration.
   a. Levels of sedation are noted as negative scores.
   b. Desired levels of sedation vary according to the situation.
   c. For deep sedation, goal is -10 to -5.
   d. For light sedation, goal is -5 to -2.
5. Deep sedation is not recommended unless an infant is receiving ventilator support, related to the high potential for apnea and hypoventilation.
6. A negative score without the administration of opioids/sedatives:
   a. Indicates neurologic depression, sepsis, or other pathology
   b. A premature infant who has experienced prolonged untreated pain and/or stress may also appear sedated, since these infants have been observed to become lethargic and "shut down" in response to their unrelenting pain.
7. Pancuronium (Pavulon)/paralysis
   a. It is impossible to clinically or behaviorally evaluate a paralyzed infant for pain.
   b. Analgesics should be administered continuously by drip or around-the-clock dosing.
      (1) Higher, more frequent dosing may be required if the infant is postoperative, has a chest tube, or has other pathology (e.g., necrotizing enterocolitis [NEC]) that would normally cause pain.
      (2) Increases in heart rate and blood pressure may be the only indicator of a need for more analgesia.
      (3) Opioid doses should be increased by 10% every 3 to 5 days since tolerance will occur without symptoms of inadequate pain relief.

Pain Management

1. If the N-PASS score is above 3 or above the baby's usual baseline score, pain management interventions should occur. Pain management interventions may be instituted with lower scores, as clinically appropriate.
2. Implement nonpharmacologic comfort measures first if the infant has no identifiable cause for pain.

   a. Developmental positioning (knees flexed, arms close to body, hands to mouth), swaddling, nesting, pacifier, reducing environmental stressors (light, noise, handling). Older babies may respond to rocking, holding.

   b. Optimize ventilation: babies become agitated when they are not being adequately ventilated. This should be corrected by optimizing ventilation (suctioning, adjusting ventilator settings).

   c. These measures should always be instituted along with analgesics if the infant has an identifiable pain source (i.e., postoperative, chest tube, etc.).

3. Administer analgesics or sedatives to provide relief of pain in the least painful route possible.

   a. Sedatives do not provide pain relief but do enhance the effects of opioids. Therefore sedatives should rarely be given alone since it is usually not possible to distinguish between pain and agitation in the neonate.

   b. Sedatives are not recommended for use in preterm infants. Seizurelike myoclonic movements have been observed in preterm infants receiving sedatives. Adverse neurologic outcomes have been associated with sedative use in preterm infants.

4. Treat anticipated procedure-related pain prophylactically.

   a. Invasive procedures, such as chest tubes and abdominal drains, should include premedication.

   b. Brief, less invasive procedures, such as IV starts and heel sticks, usually do not require premedication.

   c. Sucrose water attenuates the pain response and should be considered as an adjunctive measure before and during any procedure.

   d. All babies will tolerate procedures better if swaddled or contained by parents or other staff members.

   e. Efforts should be made to calm the baby before and after the procedure.

5. Provide continuous cardiorespiratory monitoring and continual pulse oximetry when using opioids or sedatives for pain relief or to achieve sedation.

6. Correct detrimental side effects of the medications.

7. Evaluate effectiveness of pain medication 30 to 60 minutes after administration.

8. If pain score is not falling as expected, additional medications and nonpharmacologic measures should be instituted and the baby reevaluated for additional causes for pain and agitation.

Parent/Caregiver Education

1. A letter outlining the unit's efforts in pain assessment and management is included in the admission booklet.

2. Parents should be taught infant pain behaviors and be included in the assessment and treatment of the infant's pain.

Documentation

1. N-PASS score will be documented on the appropriate column on the NICU flow sheet.
2. This column is slashed: the top area will be used for pain assessments, and the bottom area will be used to document the sedation score.
3. If management is changed in response to a score (i.e., pain medication, comfort measures, increase or decrease in medication), a response to this intervention is documented in the same column in the next hourly space. This indicates response to the intervention 30 to 60 minutes after the intervention.

Pain Assessment with Painful Procedures

1. Short-lived painful procedures, such as heel sticks, venipuncture, or arterial puncture, do not necessitate pain assessment scores before, during, and after these procedures.
2. Bedside surgical procedures, such as chest tube, abdominal drain insertion, and circumcision, should have pain assessment scores before and during the procedure. For postprocedure scoring, continue to assess pain with each vital sign assessment, since these infants will have more frequent vital signs following these procedures.
3. Assessments will be documented on the NICU flow sheet.

OPIOID WEANING GUIDELINES: NICU

Purpose

These guidelines are for weaning infants from opioids following intrauterine exposure or NICU dependence.

Background Information

At least one half of infants exposed to heroin and/or methadone in utero will exhibit signs of NAS (neonatal abstinence syndrome). In addition, infants in the NICU who received opioids around the clock or as a continual drip for more than 1 week or so will develop tolerance, become dependent, and exhibit signs of NAS when the medication is abruptly discontinued. Gradual weaning of the opioid is outlined in order to minimize withdrawal symptoms.

Procedure
Weaning from fentanyl drip

1. Fentanyl is associated with a higher and more rapid rate of withdrawal as compared with morphine. Use of fentanyl >5 days has been associated with a >50% chance for opiate withdrawal and a

100% chance in infants receiving it for >9 days. For this reason, once the patient is stabilized (i.e., minimal variation in vital signs, oxygen requirements, etc.), fentanyl weaning should begin after 48 to 72 hours in **most** cases.

2. The Finnegan scoring system should be initiated once it is decided that the infant will be weaned off the fentanyl drip in order to assess withdrawal and therefore determine the patient's ability or inability to tolerate weaning. The scoring should be done every 3 or 4 hours, depending on how often the baby is "hands-on."

3. Weaning should be initiated at 0.5 μg/kg/hr (0.1 ml/hr) daily or twice daily (bid) as determined by Finnegan scores:

   a. In general, Finnegan scores of >8 are considered indicative of withdrawal; however, <8 to 11 is generally acceptable for attempting weaning if the patient is otherwise stable.

   b. If average of scores over 24 hours is ≤8, the infant can be weaned by 0.5 μg/kg/hr daily, or every 12 hours if tolerated.

   c. If the patient receiving an infusion has been weaned and subsequent Finnegan scores are >11 for three consecutive scoring periods, increase the infusion back to the rate (i.e., increase by 0.5 μg/kg/hr) before the attempted wean.

4. Once the patient has successfully weaned to 0.5 μg/kg/hr, the patient should be converted back to bolus morphine injections, either 0.1 mg/kg every 2 hours or 0.2 mg/kg every 4 hours (this is equivalent to fentanyl, 0.5 μg/kg/hr).

5. One dose of morphine should be administered **before** the fentanyl drip is discontinued.

6. Once the fentanyl drip is discontinued, the patient should not be weaned from the morphine for 24 hours.

7. If after 24 hours the Finnegan scores are <8 to 11 and the patient is stable, the morphine **dose** should be decreased by 0.05 mg/kg/dose daily as tolerated based on Finnegan scores. The interval should remain every 2, 3, or 4 hours.

8. Once the patient's morphine dose has been weaned to 0.025 mg/kg/dose, the dosing **interval** can be weaned daily, again as determined by Finnegan scores.

9. Once the patient has successfully been weaned down to 0.025 mg/kg every 8 or 12 hours and if Finnegan scores remain stable, the morphine can be discontinued.

10. Finnegan scoring should continue 48 hours after morphine is discontinued to assess any rebound withdrawal symptoms.

11. Weaning may occur more rapidly if the baby has not been on the infusion for a long period or at high doses.

12. Weaning from high-dose prolonged infusion may take weeks. Oral morphine can be added to partially cover the withdrawal before the drip is completely decreased to facilitate discontinuing the drip.

Weaning from IV morphine bolus

1. IV or oral morphine is used to treat NAS or in-unit tolerance.
2. Morphine doses are increased to obtain patient stability and Finnegan scores of 8 to 11.
3. When the baby is stable on morphine, weaning can begin.
4. Weaning of dose, not interval, is recommended overall. However, it may be useful to get the baby to an every 3- or 4-hour schedule to facilitate administration with feedings.
5. The morphine dose is decreased by 10% daily or 20% every 2 to 3 days as tolerated.
6. Finnegan scores should be done with each dose. A score of 8 or less indicates that the baby is probably ready for more weaning.
7. The goal is to avoid a Finnegan score of 0. Babies have to be gently pushed off the opioid. The goal is Finnegan scores of about 8 to 11. The baby should be weaned if the score is less than 8 and the baby is stable.
8. The baby should be changed from IV or oral morphine as soon as feasible, depending on the baby's condition and feeding status.
   a. *Oral morphine doses are three to five times IV doses.*
   b. Oral morphine is obtained from pharmacy diluted to a 1 mg/cc concentration.
9. The oral morphine is weaned to a low dose—usually about 0.05 to 0.1 mg/kg/dose. The baby can then be tried off, or the interval can be further increased before stopping the morphine. IV morphine is weaned to 0.02 to 0.05 mg/kg/dose before stopping it.
10. This process may take a few days or several weeks. In general, the longer the baby has been on the medication, the longer it will take to get off.
11. The infant receiving morphine should be weaned off before discharge if possible.
    a. If this is not possible, the baby can be discharged receiving oral morphine with a weaning plan.
    b. Oral morphine needs to be diluted, however, so this should be obtained only from outpatient pharmacy.
    c. Discharge on paregoric is not desirable, because it contains a large amount of preservatives and alcohol. However, paregoric is already diluted to a usable concentration. The paregoric dose (in cc) is equal to what the baby is receiving of the morphine 1 mg/cc dilution. (Example: if the baby is receiving 0.6 cc of MSO_4 1 mg/cc, the paregoric dose would be 0.6 cc.)
    d. Parents/caretakers should be educated about withdrawal signs and the weaning plan.
    e. The baby should be followed by a home care nurse and be scheduled in the neonatal follow-up clinic about 1 month after discharge.

The following letter regarding pain is sent to parents of our NICU patients*:

> To the parents of our NICU infants:
>
> About pain . . .
>
> We realize that your infant will have some painful experiences while in our unit. We are continually trying to make everything less painful. This is very important to us, and we are sure, important to you. Please let the nurses or doctors know if you think that your baby's pain is not being treated.
>
> It can be difficult to tell if a baby is having pain. Sometimes, especially with premature infants, they are not able to let us know when they are having pain and how bad it is. Signs that your baby may be in pain are: crying, lack of deep sleep, a worried face with a grimace or frown, tightly fisted hands and feet, a rigid or tense body, and higher than normal heart rate and blood pressure. Their oxygen levels may fall rapidly when they are touched or handled. Of course, a hungry baby will cry and be tense and have a high heart rate, but this stops when the baby is fed or given a pacifier.
>
> Some things that cause pain are procedures such as a heel stick, IV, or chest tube placement. Operations, of course, cause pain. Also, being on a ventilator seems to be uncomfortable for some infants, but not all babies need medications for this.
>
> In addition to medications, many other things can be done by you or the nurses to relieve your baby's pain. Keeping the area as dark and quiet as possible will be helpful. Some babies like to be rocked, talked to, massaged, or given a pacifier. Some babies like to be wrapped snugly. Some babies like to be left alone—they can't handle any stimulation at that time. Your baby's nurse will help you decide what works best for your infant.
>
> Some babies that have been receiving pain medications for a long time (>5 to 7 days) will need to be weaned slowly from them. Taking them away too quickly can be bad for your baby. This does not mean that your baby is addicted to the medicine—his or her body has just gotten used to them.
>
> Please be assured that we are doing all we can to keep your infant from being in pain. Your presence at the bedside can be very comforting to your infant. We look forward to working with you.
>
> The NICU staff

PROTOCOL: ORAL SUCROSE SOLUTION USED FOR THE MANAGEMENT OF NEONATAL PROCEDURAL PAIN*

Purpose

This protocol concerns providing nonpharmacologic procedural pain relief.

*Used with permission from Loyola Medical Center, Maywood, Ill.

Background Information

Addressing pain during procedures is an ethical duty for health care professionals. Neonates respond to painful stimuli, and untreated pain can result in adverse sequelae. Nonpharmacologic management of minor procedural pain includes swaddling, facilitated tucking, nonnutritive sucking, and oral sucrose water. The administration of small amounts of concentrated sucrose water via nipple or accompanied by a pacifier reduces the pain-related behaviors seen during minimally invasive procedures. Sucking on a pacifier appears to be synergistic with the sucrose water in providing short-term procedural analgesia.

1. A physician's order is not required for the use of sucrose solution.
2. The infant's ability to suck and swallow should be determined by the nurse.
   a. An inability to suck or swallow is a contraindication to the use of sucrose water.
   b. An infant who is able to suck but has limited ability to swallow (i.e., endotracheal tube [ETT] in place) may have a pacifier dipped in sucrose water but should not be administered any measurable volumes of sucrose water.
3. Sucrose water (SW) should be considered with the following procedures:
   a. Heel sticks
   b. Venipunctures (IV insertions or blood draws)
   c. Arterial punctures
   d. Eye examinations
   e. Nasogastric/orogastric (NG/OG) insertion
   f. IM/SQ (intramuscular/subcutaneous) injections
   g. Adhesive tape removal
   h. Suctioning
   i. Peripheral central venous catheter (PCVC) insertion
4. Sucrose water should be considered adjunctive analgesia with the following procedures:
   a. Circumcision
   b. Lumbar puncture
   c. Chest tube insertion
5. 24% sucrose solution is mixed daily by dietary and stored in the NICU refrigerator.
   a. Approximately 5 cc of the solution should be poured into a medicine cup or 1 to 2 cc drawn into an *oral* syringe.
   b. Do not leave solution at the bedside in an IV syringe to avoid inadvertent IV administration.
6. Single doses have been proven to be safe and efficacious. Repeated administration has not been evaluated.
   a. Infant on full feedings may have repeated doses.

b. Infants who are NPO or on partial feedings may receive sucrose water by dipping the pacifier in the solution. Administration of a larger volume to NPO infants is evaluated with each case.

Procedure

1. Dosing
   a. Full-term infant: 0.5 to 2.0 cc
   b. Preterm infant: 0.1 to 0.4 cc
2. Administration
   a. Nipple or syringe
      (1) 2 minutes before the procedure the solution is sucked through a nipple or squirted onto anterior aspect of the infant's tongue.
      (2) NPO infants may receive sucrose water via nipple or syringe if their GI status is stable—this is determined on a case-by-case basis.
   b. Pacifier
      (1) Dipped into the sucrose solution and given repeatedly during the procedure
      (2) The preferred method if the baby is able to suck but has limited ability to swallow (i.e., ETT) or is NPO
   c. Sucrose solution should not be administered by NG/OG insertion since contact with taste buds is required for analgesia.
3. Monitor the infant during the administration and the procedure to assess the efficacy of the interventions.
4. Documentation: SW for sucrose water as a comfort measure on the NICU flow sheet.

BIBLIOGRAPHY

Anand K (2001). The International Evidence-Based Group for Neonatal Pain. Consensus statement for the prevention and management of pain in the newborn. *Archives of pediatric and adolescent medicine*, 155, 173-180.

Stevens B, Ohlsson A (2001). Sucrose analgesia for newborn infants undergoing painful procedures. *Cochrane database of systematic reviews*, 2.

NEONATAL DRUG WITHDRAWAL

When an infant has been exposed in utero to drugs, withdrawal can occur in the postnatal period. This process of withdrawal is painful and must be carefully supported. The following guideline is offered to help with this process.

Intrauterine exposure to drugs may lead to neonatal intoxication or withdrawal. Please read the statement from the American Academy of Pediatrics, Committee on Drugs, Neonatal Drug

Withdrawal, published in *Pediatrics*, 1998. This is an excellent source of information. More information can be obtained from reading the Self-Study Course: Drug-Exposed Infant at *www.nann.org*.

Important Points

Intrauterine deficits may be compounded by exposure to drugs given after birth to help with the withdrawal. Therefore pharmacologic treatment should be used only if necessary, and a drug from the same class as that causing withdrawal is preferable, if available.

Pharmacologic treatment is often needed for methadone and/or heroin withdrawal. The revised Finnegan score is used to determine treatment and weaning. See Finnegan guidelines for dosage and details. The Finnegan scale is used for opioid withdrawal only. This scale for weaning is also helpful for weaning infants in the unit that have become physiologically dependent on opioids while in the NICU. IV morphine is used when the baby is NPO, and oral morphine is used when the baby is on feedings. The baby should be weaned off morphine before discharge, if possible. If this is not feasible, and the baby is discharged on a weaning dose of morphine, the outpatient supply should be obtained only from outpatient pharmacy in the outpatient pharmacy. A prescription is taken or called to the pharmacy, with a 1 mg/ml dilution, and the dose specified. Enough morphine should be dispensed so that refills are not necessary, if possible.

Pharmacologic treatment of cocaine-exposed infants is rarely necessary. Environmental modification is frequently necessary. Infants that are showing severe withdrawal signs such as seizures, poor feeding, sleeplessness, and failure to gain weight may need treatment. Phenobarbital is usually used in this instance, with a loading dose and bid dosing for 1 to 2 weeks. The phenobarbital should then be discontinued to allow observation of the baby's behaviors and to avoid prolonged exposure to another substance.

Supportive care is always advised. This includes swaddling, frequent feedings, and a dark and quiet environment. High-calorie formula is frequently necessary to facilitate growth in these babies with high caloric expenditure from their activity.

Directions for Using the Modified Finnegan's Scale and Initiation and Weaning of Pharmacologic Therapy

1. These scales are for use in infants with known opiate withdrawal or suspected to be experiencing opiate withdrawal, specifically from heroin, methadone, or opioids administered during the NICU stay. For prenatal exposure, urine and meconium toxicology screens should be collected and sent as quickly as possible to confirm prenatal exposure. These should be sent before postnatal opiates are administered, if at all possible.

2. Pharmacologic treatment should be initiated when the total severity score exceeds 8 for three consecutive scoring periods or when the average of three consecutive scores is >8.

3. Two Finnegan scoring sheets are available: one for use in nonintubated patients and one for use with intubated patients.

4. Pharmacologic therapy will consist of morphine by oral or IV route. These are administered every 3 to 4 hours around the clock. Morphine sulfate is given IV when the infant is NPO, then changed to oral morphine once the baby is stable on feedings.

5. IV morphine is kept in the NICU locked cabinet. This has been diluted in pharmacy to a 1 mg/ml solution. Oral morphine syrup is available from pharmacy. When one or more babies are receiving oral morphine in the NICU, a stock bottle will be ordered from pharmacy daily—this will also be in a 1 mg/ml dilution.

6. Remember, because of first-pass metabolism, oral doses must be three to five times higher than IV doses to achieve the same effect.

7. Dosing
   a. Morphine sulfate IV is given every 4 hours around the clock. Start with 0.05 mg/kg/dose, increasing as needed to keep Finnegan scores less than 8. Doses may be increased as needed—some babies need 0.2 mg/kg/dose or more—if withdrawal symptoms are severe. If the baby has seizures with withdrawal, larger doses will be needed at the beginning.
   b. Oral morphine
      (1) If baby is stable on IV morphine, start with three times the IV dose—five times the IV dose may be needed.
      (2) If the baby is not receiving IV morphine, start with 0.15 mg/kg to 0.25 mg/kg per dose, increasing as needed to keep Finnegan scores less than 8.
      (3) Doses may be increased as needed—some babies need 1 mg/kg/dose or more—if withdrawal symptoms are severe. If the baby has seizures with withdrawal, larger doses will be needed at the beginning.

8. Overdose: if the baby is experiencing side effects from the opiate, do not give Narcan. This will cause severe withdrawal and possibly seizures. Supportive treatment is indicated until the medication is excreted. Apnea should be rare—you will first see that the baby is sleepy and lethargic with very low Finnegan scores; this would indicate that one or more doses should be held and the dosage decreased. It is difficult to overdose a baby that is already so tolerant that he or she is showing abstinence signs, but it can happen. Remember that the goal is not to have Finnegan scores of 0. We have to let the baby have tolerable withdrawal—generally Finnegan scores of less than 8 are acceptable. We have to gently push these infants off the medication.

9. Once the infant is stabilized with scores consistently averaging less than 12 (less than 8 is ideal), the "stabilizing dose" should be maintained for 3 to 5 days. Weaning of the dose can then start.

SYSTEM	SIGNS AND SYMPTOMS	SCORE
CNS	High-pitched cry	2
	Continuous high-pitched cry	3
	Sleeps <1 hr after feeding	3
	Sleeps <2 hr after feeding	2
	Sleeps <3 hr after feeding	1
	Mild tremors disturbed	1
	Moderately severe tremors disturbed	2
	Mild tremors undisturbed	3
	Moderately severe tremors undisturbed	4
	Increased muscle tone	2
	Excoriation (specify area)	1
	Myoclonic jerks	3
	Generalized convulsions	5
Metabolic/ Vasometer/ Respiratory	Fever (37.3° –38.3° C)	1
	Fever (>38.3° C)	2
	Frequent yawning (>3-4 times)	1
	Nasal stuffiness	1
	Sneezing (>3-4 times)	1
	Nasal flaring	2
	Respiratory rate >60/min	1
	Respiratory rate >60/min + retractions	2
Gastrointestinal disturbances	Excessive sucking	1
	Poor feeding	2
	Regurgitation	2
	Projectile vomiting	3
	Loose stools	2
	Watery stools	3

FIGURE **5-1**
Neonatal abstinence syndrome scoring chart. (From Finnegan LP, Kaltenback K (1992). The assessment and management of neonatal abstinence syndrome. In Woekelman, Nelson: *Primary care*, ed 3, Mosby, St Louis.

Avoid a *do not wean interval*—this causes fluctuations in withdrawal symptoms and makes weaning more difficult.

10. After 3 to 5 days of stabilization, the dose can be decreased by 10% daily, as tolerated based on the Finnegan scores. This weaning can take 5 to 40 or more days.

11. The goal is to see the infant growing well, with mild withdrawal signs.

12. Once the baby is weaned to a dose of 0.05 mg/kg/dose of oral morphine or 0.025 mg/kg/dose of IV morphine, pharmacologic therapy can be discontinued. The patient should be observed and Finnegan scoring continued for 2 days following discontinuation of therapy.

13. Every attempt should be made to wean the baby off opioids before discharge. If the baby is being discharged receiving oral morphine to complete weaning at home, the oral morphine 1 mg/ml solution should be obtained only from the outpatient pharmacy. This avoids having community pharmacists dilute the medication, increasing the chance for error. The baby should not need more than one bottle dispensed and should not need refills.

Neonatal Abstinence Score

This neonatal abstinence score (NAS) was developed by Dr. Loretta Finnegan. Many institutions have modified this score. One such modification has been done by the Royal Prince Alfred Hospital (Figure 5-1).

Infants of mothers known or suspected to be drug users who are showing signs of withdrawal should be scored every 4 hours. The scoring should be applied in a consistent manner by personnel who are experienced in dealing with such infants.

Note: Caution must be exercised before symptoms listed here are accepted as part of drug withdrawal. For example, symptoms such as fever, tachypnea, or seizures could be due to sepsis, which should be excluded first with appropriate tests.

BIBLIOGRAPHY

Anand P, Birch R (2002). Restoration of sensory function and lack of long-term chronic pain syndromes after brachial plexus injury in human neonates. *Brain,* 125(pt 1), 113-122.

Anand K, the International Evidence-Based Group for Neonatal Pain (2001). Consensus statement for the prevention and management of pain in the newborn. *Archives of pediatric and adolescent medicine,* 155, 173-180.

Baka NE, et al. (2002). Colostrum morphine concentrations during postcesarean intravenous patient-controlled analgesia. *Anesthesia & analgesia,* 94(1), 184-187, table of contents.

Baos JE, Ruiz G, Guardiola E (2001). An analysis of articles on neonatal pain published from 1965 to 1999. *Pain research management*, 6(1), 45-50.

Bellieni CV, et al. (2002). Effect of multisensory stimulation on analgesia in term neonates: a randomized controlled trial. *Pediatric research*, 51(4), 460-463.

Coutinho SV, et al. (2002). Neonatal maternal separation alters stress-induced responses to viscerosomatic nociceptive stimuli in rat. *American journal of physiology & gastrointestinal liver physiology*, 282(2), G307-G316.

Cuttini M (2001). The European Union Collaborative Project on Ethical Decision Making in Neonatal Intensive Care (EURONIC): findings from 11 countries. *Journal of clinical ethics*, 12(3), 290-296.

Franck L, Lefrak L (2001). For crying out loud: the ethical treatment of infants' pain. *Journal of clinical ethics*, 12(3), 275-281.

Goubet N, Clifton RK, Shah B (2001). Learning about pain in preterm newborns. *Journal of developmental & behavioral pediatrics*, 22(6), 418-424.

Kass FC, Holman JR (2001). Oral glucose solution for analgesia in infant circumcision. *Journal of family practice*, 50(9), 785-788.

Kaufman GE, et al. (2002). An evaluation of the effects of sucrose on neonatal pain with 2 commonly used circumcision methods. *American journal of obstetrics & gynecology*, 186(3), 564-568.

Kawamata T, et al. (2001). Involvement of capsaicin-sensitive fibers in spinal NMDA-induced glutamate release. *Neuroreport*, 12(16), 3447-3450.

Loizzo A, et al. (2002). Naloxone prevents cell-mediated immune alterations in adult mice following repeated mild stress in the neonatal period. *British journal of pharmacology*, 135(5), 1219-1226.

Morison SJ, et al. (2001). Relations between behavioral and cardiac autonomic reactivity to acute pain in preterm neonates. *Clinical journal of pain*, 17(4), 350-358.

Oberlander TF, et al. (2002). Prolonged prenatal psychotropic medication exposure alters neonatal acute pain response. *Pediatric research*, 51(4), 443-453.

Payne MS, et al. (2001). Parathyroid hyperplasia: an unusual cause of neonatal hypercalcemia. *International journal of pediatric otorhinolaryngology*, 61(3), 253-257.

Pollock J, et al. (2002). TNF-alpha receptors simultaneously activate Ca2+ mobilisation and stress kinases in cultured sensory neurons. *Neuropharmacology*, 42(1), 93-106.

Schulman H, et al. (2001). Congenital insensitivity to pain with anhidrosis (CIPA): the spectrum of radiological findings. *Pediatric radiology*, 31(10), 701-705.

Seligmann J, Springen K (1996). Fewer bundles of pain: criticized for causing premature and multiple births, fertility doctors take steps to reform. *Newsweek*, 127(10), 63.

Stevens B, Ohlsson A (2001). Sucrose analgesia for newborn infants undergoing painful procedures. *Cochrane database of systematic reviews*, 2.

Stevens B, Yamada J, Ohlsson A (2001). Sucrose for analgesia in newborn infants undergoing painful procedures (Cochrane review). *Cochrane database systematic reviews*, 4.

Torsney C, Fitzgerald M (2002). Age-dependent effects of peripheral inflammation on the electrophysiological properties of neonatal rat dorsal horn neurons. *Journal of neurophysiology*, 87(3), 1311-1317.

Vendola N, et al. (2001). Low concentration Ropivacaine in labor epidural analgesia: a prospective study on obstetric and neonatal outcome. *Minerva gynecology*, 53(6), 397-403.

Walden M, Franck L (2003). Identification, management, and prevention of newborn/infant pain. In Kenner C, Lott JW, editors. *Comprehensive neonatal nursing care: a physiologic perspective, ed 3*, St Louis: WB Saunders.

CHAPTER 6

GENETIC ASSESSMENT

With the increasing emphasis on genetic linkages to disease and prevention of disease, it is not surprising that genetic information is integrated into nursing care. Taking a genetic history can be easily incorporated into the medical history and assessment of the patient. Ideally a genogram, a pictorial representation of at least three generations of family of the infant, should be done. The genogram may indicate a genetic linkage to the condition that has brought the infant to the neonatal intensive care unit (NICU). If time for this thorough a history is not possible, talk to the family during provision of care. Information about the infant's condition may be similar to conditions of other family members. Presence of certain variables may serve as *red flags* that indicate a need for a genetics consult.

COMMON INDICATIONS FOR REFERRAL*

1. Previous child with multiple congenital anomalies, mental retardation, or an isolated birth defect, such as neural tube defect, cleft lip and palate
2. Family history of a hereditary condition, such as cystic fibrosis, fragile X syndrome, or diabetes
3. Prenatal diagnosis for advanced maternal age or other indication
4. Consanguinity
5. Teratogen exposure, such as to occupational chemicals, medications, alcohol
6. Repeated pregnancy loss or infertility
7. Newly diagnosed abnormality or genetic condition
8. Before undertaking genetic testing and after receiving results, particularly when testing for susceptibility to late-onset disorders, such as cancer or neurologic disease
9. As follow-up for a positive newborn test, such as with phenylketenuria (PKU), or a heterozygote screening test, such as Tay-Sachs

---

*Used with permission from Nussbaum RL, McInnes RR, Willard HF, editors.
*Thompson & Thompson genetics in medicine, ed 6, Philadelphia: WB Saunders,
p. 375.*

GENETIC TESTING

The constitutional chromosomes of an individual can be studied through a process called *chromosome analysis (karyotyping)*, which can be performed only on dividing cells. This process involves obtaining a sample of sterile, living tissue, capable of relatively rapid cell division. Most frequently, blood lymphocytes or skin fibroblasts are used for this purpose. Microscope photographs of metaphase chromosomes are made. From these photographs the chromosomes are karyotyped—grouped in sequences of pairs according to the size of the chromosome pairs and the positions of the centromeres. Each group begins with the largest pair of chromosomes that has the centromeres most centrally located. Subsequent chromosome pairs are ordered according to descending size and more distally located centromeres. Analysis of this type of karyotype can determine numeric chromosome aberrations.

A more accurate chromosome analysis is then obtained when standard cytogenetic techniques are combined with the process of banding. Giemsa banding (G-banding) is the most common of the banding techniques for chromosome analysis. This process involves exposing the fixed slides to a proteolytic enzyme (usually trypsin), which selectively digests areas of the chromosome, and then staining the slide. The areas in which protein is digested do not take up the stain and leave a white space (negative band) on the chromosome. The areas in which protein is not digested do take up the stain and leave a dark area (positive band) on the chromosome. As a result of this process, each chromosome pair has a unique banded or striped appearance, which permits absolute identification of specific chromosomes. It is known that many genetic disorders involve deletions or rearrangements of genes much smaller than 10,000 base pairs.

Molecular testing is also used to determine if there is an aberration. This technique examines the deoxyribonucleic acid (DNA) directly. Another form of testing is to examine the gene directly. This testing depends on the knowledge of which gene alteration results in a specific disease process. Mutation that results in sickle cell anemia can be detected by this method of analysis. This technique can detect fragile X or a breakable area (Scheuerle, 2001). Linkage testing is used when a family member has a known genetic problem and the health professional wants to determine if the condition exists in the infant. The results of linkage testing are not considered diagnostic in the first person affected but only after a second family member is identified who is potentially affected. This testing is useful with cystic fibrosis and Duchenne's muscular dystrophy. Blood tests for DNA analysis are also used. These have been popularized for paternity issues or in criminal cases. The test is considered diagnostic. Protein tests performed on blood examine the structure. This test helps when a suspected protein structural defect is believed involved in the defect or disease process. Examples of conditions where this test would assist in the diagnosis are Ehlers-Danlos syndrome, osteogenesis imperfecta, and Marfan syndrome. Each of these conditions is a connective tissue or protein abnormality (Scheuerle, 2001).

Biochemical testing is used when there is a suspected defect in the metabolic enzymes. The measurement of amino or organic acids results in the identification of an abnormality. This measure is considered a screening test and not a diagnostic test. This test is then followed by direct measurement of the enzymes. These tests are useful if errors of metabolism are suspected (Kenner, 2003).

Patterns of Inheritance

The four types of inheritance patterns associated with single-gene controlled traits include autosomal dominant, autosomal recessive, sex-linked dominant, and sex-linked recessive. Each inheritance pattern for single-gene controlled traits is characterized by specific defining criteria.

Traits with an autosomal dominant pattern of inheritance   Autosomal dominant single-gene traits require that the gene controlling the trait be located on an autosomal chromosome and usually be expressed even when the gene is present on only one chromosome of a chromosome pair. A typical autosomal dominant pattern of inheritance meets all these defining criteria:

1. The trait appears in every generation with no skipping. When the trait is a result of a new mutation (de novo), this criterion is demonstrated only in the branch of the pedigree stemming from the person who first exhibited the new mutation.
2. The risk for affected individuals to have affected children is 50% with each pregnancy.
3. Unaffected individuals do not have affected children; therefore their risk is 0%.
4. The trait is found equally in males and females.

Autosomal dominant patterns of inheritance are associated with many normal variations in body structure, such as brown eye color, widow's peak hairline, and curly hair. In addition, this pattern of inheritance has been demonstrated in a variety of genetically transmitted problems, including achondroplasia, familial hypercholesterolemia, Huntington's disease, dentinogenesis imperfecta, brachydactyly, allergic hypersensitivity, Marfan syndrome, and familial hypercalcemia (Kenner, 2003).

Traits with an autosomal recessive pattern of inheritance   Autosomal recessive single-gene traits require that the gene controlling the trait be located on an autosomal chromosome and that the trait can be expressed only when the gene is present on both chromosomes of a chromosome pair. A typical autosomal recessive pattern of inheritance meets all these defining criteria:

1. The trait appears in alternate generations of any one branch of a kinship.
2. The trait or characteristic usually first appears only in siblings (progeny of unaffected parents) rather than in the parents themselves.
3. Approximately 25% of a kinship is affected and expresses the trait.
4. The children of an affected father and an affected mother are always affected (risk is 100% for each pregnancy). Two affected individuals cannot have an unaffected child.
5. Unaffected individuals who are carriers (have the gene on only one chromosome of a chromosome pair) and do not express the trait themselves, can transmit the trait to their offspring if their mate is also a carrier or is affected. The risk of a carrier having a child who expresses the trait is 25% with each pregnancy when the carrier is married to another carrier, 50% with each pregnancy when the carrier is married to an affected individual, and 0% with each pregnancy when the carrier is married to a noncarrier. The risk of the unaffected carrier having a child who is a carrier for the trait is 50% with each pregnancy.
6. The trait is found equally in males and females.

Autosomal recessive patterns of inheritance are associated with many normal characteristics and variations in body structure and function, such as blue eye color, straight hair, and the Rh-negative blood type. In addition, this pattern of inheritance has been demonstrated in a variety of genetically transmitted conditions, including albinism, sickle cell anemia, cystic fibrosis, phenylketonuria, Tay-Sachs disease, Hurler's syndrome, Bloom's syndrome, Fanconi's anemia, galactosemia, and hyperextensible thumb.

For some of these diseases, the carrier has no symptom of the trait, and in other conditions the carrier does not express the full-blown condition but may express a more mild form when predisposing environmental or personal events are present. For example, carriers of sickle cell anemia may have some sickling of their red blood cells under conditions of extreme hypoxia, although the sickling is never as severe or widespread as it is in the person who is homozygous for sickle cell anemia (Kenner, 2003).

Sex-Linked Patterns of Inheritance

Some genes are present only on the sex chromosomes. The Y chromosome appears to have few genes that are not also present on the X chromosome. However, the X chromosome has many single genes that do not appear to be present elsewhere in the human genome. Thus, for all intents and purposes, the discussion of sex-linked patterns of inheritance is really a discussion of X-linked patterns of inheritance.

Because there is an unequal distribution of X chromosomes between males and females (1:2, respectively), there is an accompanying unequal distribution of the X-linked chromosome genes between the two sexes. Males have only one X chromosome and are said to be hemizygous for any gene on the X chromosome. As a result, X-linked recessive genes have a dominant expressive pattern of inheritance in males and a recessive expressive pattern of inheritance in females. This difference in expression occurs because males do not have a second X chromosome to balance the expression of any recessive gene on the first X chromosome.

Dominant Patterns

Sex-linked (X-linked) dominant single-gene traits require that the gene controlling the trait be located on only one of the X chromosomes for the trait to be expressed. A typical sex-linked dominant pattern of inheritance will meet certain criteria that are obvious in the pedigree. The defining criteria are as follows:

1. There is no carrier status; all individuals with the gene are affected.
2. Female children of affected males are all affected (risk is 100%), whereas male children of affected males are unaffected (risk is 0%). Therefore the overall risk of an affected male having affected children is 50% for each pregnancy, since the probability of having a female is also 50%. It is the inheritance of the trait by female offspring of affected males that defines the problem as X-linked dominant, since the inheritance pattern among the offspring of affected females identically resembles an autosomal dominant pattern.
3. The trait appears in every generation.
4. For homozygous females, the risk of having an affected child is 100% with each pregnancy, and offspring of both sexes are affected equally. For heterozygous females, the risk of having an affected child is 50% with each pregnancy, and children of both sexes are equally at risk.
5. In the general population, X-linked dominant problems affect twice as many females as males, but heterozygous females usually express a more mild form of the problem than do homozygous males.

The most common known X-linked dominant problem is hypophosphatemia (Kenner, 2003).

Recessive Patterns

Sex-linked (X-linked) recessive single-gene traits are among the most well-defined inherited health problems. This pattern of inheritance requires that the gene controlling the trait be present on both X chromosomes for the trait to be fully expressed in females (females must be homozygous for the trait) and on only one of the X chromosomes for the trait to be expressed in males (males must be hemizygous). A typical sex-linked recessive pattern of inheritance meets all these defining criteria:

1. Expression or incidence of the trait is much higher among males in a kinship (and in the general population) than among females.
2. The trait cannot be transmitted from father to son because the father contributes only the Y chromosome to his son's sex chromosome pair.
3. Transmission of the trait is from father to all daughters (who are all carriers but either do not express any of the trait or express it in a very mild form).
4. Female carriers have a 50% risk (with each pregnancy) of transmitting the gene to their offspring. Female offspring inheriting the trait are carriers, and male offspring inheriting the trait are affected.

Sex-linked recessive inheritance patterns may be responsible for normal variation of some secondary female sex characteristics. In addition, this pattern of inheritance has been associated with a variety of disorders including hemophilia (A and B), Duchenne's muscular dystrophy, ichthyosis, Lesch-Nyhan syndrome, color blindness and, probably, fragile X syndrome. For some of these disorders, females who are heterozygous for the gene express no overt symptoms (e.g., color blindness). For other disorders, female heterozygotes do express some mild aberrations (increased bleeding tendency with carriers of hemophilia, mild retardation in fragile X syndrome). Few females expressing homozygosity for these disorders have been found. It is probable that the homozygosity leads to such a severe disorder that it is lethal in embryonic or early fetal life (Kenner, 2003).

Multifactorial Inheritance

Some single-gene traits have a consistently predictable pattern of gene expression that follows strict mendelian law for patterns of inheritance and degree of expression in affected individuals. Other single-gene traits have a relatively high level of variability (especially autosomal dominant traits), with no established reason for this variation of expression. Some proposed theories include the concept of evolution. This concept suggests that developmental interactions over time (generations) may modify the response of the individual to an abnormal gene. Another theory is that although a particular trait may be the result of the expression of one gene, other genes may act in concert to regulate the activity and expression of that one gene. This theory suggests that for the expression of an aberrant gene to cause severe problems, a regulating gene or genes must also have abnormal expression.

In addition to variation in the expression of single genes, it is now known that a single gene may be responsible for the expression of many effects that appear unrelated. This concept is known as *pleiotropy* and probably involves changes or aberrations in regulatory genes rather than in structural genes. One example of pleiotropy is Marfan syndrome. This syndrome is transmitted as an autosomal dominant trait, but the expression involves a variety of aberrations in unrelated tissue types. These aberrations include excessive growth of long bones, the presence (or predisposition to the development of) an aortic aneurysm, and severe nearsightedness.

Some inheritable problems are associated with more than one gene. For example, congenital deafness is an outcome associated with a variety of abnormal genes, although not all the genes have to be abnormal for deafness to result. A possible explanation for this phenomenon is that ear development and hearing involve complex structures and functions that require the input of many genes working in concert for proper development during embryonic and fetal life. An aberration in any one of these genes may result in a failure of one specific aspect of development that leads to overt deafness, although the exact mechanism causing the deafness is different for each gene aberration. Therefore more than one factor can cause the aberrant development. When more than one gene is responsible for a specific characteristic or trait, the trait is controlled through polygenic expression. Other examples of developing tissues that require polygenic expression for normal development and that can develop abnormally if any of the required genes is not normal include cleft palate and neural tube defects (Kenner, 2003).

Numeric Aberrations

The normal diploid number of human chromosomes at metaphase of mitosis is 46—that is, 23 pairs. Some individuals have missing or extra whole chromosomes. This type of aberration usually is the result of abnormal or delayed disjunction in gamete formation during meiosis I or meiosis II. Thus, instead of resulting in the formation of all gametes that each contains 23 chromosomes, some gametes have 24 chromosomes, some have 22 chromosomes, and some have 23 chromosomes. When a 24-chromosome gamete is united with a 23-chromosome gamete of the opposite sex during fertilization, the resulting new individual has 47 chromosomes. One chromosome set contains three copies of a chromosome instead of the normal two copies; this situation is termed a *trisomy*. When a 22-chromosome gamete from one parent is united with a 23-chromosome gamete of the other parent during fertilization, the resulting new individual has 45 chromosomes. One chromosome set contains only one copy of a chromosome instead of the normal two copies; this situation is termed a *monosomy*. Whenever the individual has more or fewer chromosomes than normal, some malformations and abnormal developmental processes are expressed. Nondisjunction is most commonly associated with advanced maternal age at the time of conception, presumably as a result of primary oocytes spending years in prophase of meiosis I. Nondisjunction can occur at any age.

The most common chromosomal aberration found among all conceptuses is a missing X chromosome—Turner's syndrome (45,XO). Evidently most conceptuses with a chromosome constitution of 45,XO do not survive beyond the embryonic period. The most common chromosomal aberration observed among newborns is trisomy 21 (Down syndrome) (47,XX or XY,+ 21). Other syndromes of trisomy that can be observed among newborns include trisomy 13, trisomy 15, trisomy 18, and sex chromosome trisomies (47,XXX; 47,XXY; 47,XYY). Trisomy 16 has been identified in embryonic and early fetal wastage, but this abnormality does not usually lead to a fully developed individual. Autosomal monosomes may be conceived but rarely survive to the stage of birth, although monosomy 21 has been reported among newborns.

All individuals with autosomal trisomies experience some degree of mental retardation. In addition, each trisomy is associated with a specific set of abnormalities, malformations, and unique developmental patterns. This is why although individuals with trisomy share heritable characteristics in common with their normal family members (e.g., hair color and texture, skin tone, eye color), many structural features in these individuals tend to resemble other nonrelated individuals who have the same trisomy.

Individuals with missing or extra whole sex chromosomes tend to be intellectually normal and have fewer recognizable physical malformations when compared with individuals with autosomal numeric aberrations. Somewhat controversial is the concept that these individuals have behavioral patterns that are not completely normal, such as attention deficit problems and other learning disorders.

Structural Aberrations

Structural aberrations can occur in either of two ways. Parts of chromosomes can break off and either become lost or attach themselves to other chromosomes, an actual translocation of chromosome material from one chromosome to another. Also, one whole chromosome can become joined to another whole chromosome, a translocation of chromosomes called *robertsonian translocation*.

When chromosomes are broken and translocated to other chromosomes, the total amount of chromosome material may be balanced (normal) or unbalanced (abnormal). If the total amount of chromosome material present in the individual's cells is normal (balanced), even though it is not located in the usual positions, the individual is phenotypically normal. Problems do not arise until this individual reproduces. Because some of this individual's gametes are not normal (i.e., not balanced) as a result of random assortment and independent segregation of chromatids during gametogenesis, the person is at risk for having chromosomally unbalanced and abnormal offspring. This individual should be referred for genetic counseling. The same situation is true for individuals with robertsonian translocations. As long as the normal amount of chromosome material is present in all the individual's cells, the individual is phenotypically normal, even though chromosome locations might be abnormal (Kenner, 2003).

PRENATAL TESTING AND SCREENING

Many tests can be done during the preconceptual or prenatal period. A few of the more common ones are presented below.

Preimplantation genetic diagnosis (PGD) is used with in vitro fertilization (IVF) often to determine if the zygote has any readily detectable genetic abnormalities.

Fetal ultrasonography involves the use of high-frequency sound waves that are reflected differently in various media and in tissues of different densities.

Tests on fetally derived cells include amniocentesis and chorionic villus sampling. The ideal gestational age for safe amniocentesis is 16 weeks after conception has occurred. At this time, there is considerable amniotic fluid, and the fetus is capable of shedding many viable cells. Once the needle is in place, approximately 20 ml of amniotic fluid is withdrawn. Some viable fetal cells will be present in the fluid. Chorionic villus sampling involves removing a piece of tissue from the growing placenta after its location has been identified through ultrasonography. The needle can be inserted either through the cervical os (more common method) or by transabdominal puncture. This procedure can be performed during the first trimester, as early as 9 to 10 weeks' gestation.

Enzyme analysis of the cells or culture fluid or both can determine whether a specific enzyme is present at all or whether it is present in normal concentrations. Some genetic metabolic problems that can be identified through enzyme analysis of fetal cells include Tay-Sachs disease, Hurler's syndrome, metachromatic leukodystrophy, galactosemia, and homocystinuria.

Maternal serum alpha fetoprotein (MSAFP) is one of the most common prenatal screening tests used. The accuracy of the test requires exact identification of gestational age at the time the fluid or serum is obtained.

AFP levels are considered elevated if they are at least twice the value of the mean for that specific gestational age. The most common problem associated with elevated AFP levels is an open neural tube defect (the open tube provides a means for extra AFP to leak into the amniotic fluid). Lower than normal AFP levels also have been associated with fetal developmental problems, although this phenomenon shows more variability. The most common condition consistently associated with low AFP values is Down syndrome (although this phenomenon is not consistent enough to be used as the only screen for Down syndrome). Other conditions associated with a low AFP level include gestational diabetes and spontaneous abortion.

Multiple-marker screen, or triple screen, is more sensitive for aneuploidy than is AFP by itself. This screen can detect changes in the maternal AFP, human chorionic gonadotropin (hCG), and unconjugated estriol (uE_3). The multiple-marker screen is performed between 15 and 20 weeks' gestation. If an abnormality is found, it should be followed by ultrasonography for confirmation of a problem.

Percutaneous umbilical blood sampling (PUBS) is a very invasive procedure that offers fetal blood for karyotyping, but the fluorescence in situ hybridization (FISH) test is replacing PUBS in many perinatal centers. It can be used after 18 weeks' gestation.

Fluorescence in situ hybridization (FISH) uses DNA probes that resemble chromosomal sequences or regions. These probes are fluorescent so when they bind with areas within or on the chromosome they are visible when viewed 24 hours later. FISH probes are available for chromosomes 13, 18, 21, and X and Y (Harris, Verp, 2001).

GENETIC INFORMATION AND PRIVACY

Access to information and the use of genetic information are a growing concern today. Genetic information can be used to discriminate when it comes to insurance, employment, or other forms of access to services. The ethical, legal, and social implications (ELSI) branch of the Human Genome Research Institute at the National Institutes of Health (NIH) is concerned with these issues. The following points should be considered when working with genetic information.

SOME CRITICAL ETHICAL ISSUES IN MEDICAL GENETICS*

Genetic Testing
Prenatal diagnosis especially for nondisease traits or sex
Testing for genes that predispose to late-onset disease
Testing children for a carrier state

Privacy of Genetic Information
Access to an individual's genetic information

---

*Used with permission from Nussbaum RL, McInnes RR, Willard HF, editors. Thompson & Thompson genetics in medicine, ed 6, Philadelphia: WB Saunders, p. 393.

Misuse of Genetic Information

Discrimination in employment based on an employee's genotype

Discrimination in life insurance underwriting

Discrimination in health insurance underwriting

Genetic Screening

Stigmatization and privacy

BIBLIOGRAPHY

Bennett R (1999). *The practical guide to the genetic family history.* New York: John Wiley & Sons, Inc.

Good WV, Gendron RL (2001). Gene therapy for retinopathy of prematurity: the eye is a window to the future. *British journal of ophthalmology,* 85(8), 891-892.

Harris CM, Verp MS (2001). Prenatal testing and interventions (pp. 59-71). In Mahowald MB, et al., editors. *Genetics in the clinics: clinical, ethical, and social implications for primary care,* St Louis: Mosby.

Kenner C (2003). Human genetics. In Kenner C, Lott JW, editors. *Comprehensive neonatal nursing care: a physiologic perspective,* ed 3, St Louis: WB Saunders.

Scheuerle AE (2001). Diagnosis of genetic disease. (pp. 15-30). In Mahowald MB, et al., editors. *Genetics in the clinics: clinical, ethical, and social implications for primary care,* St Louis: Mosby.

CHAPTER 7

RESPIRATORY CARE

Respiratory stability of the critically ill or preterm newborn is a major concern in the neonatal intensive care unit (NICU). Premature and sick term infants often experience respiratory problems ranging from apnea to tachypnea. Therapies range from supplemental head hood (HH) oxygen to high-frequency ventilation (HFV). This chapter includes common procedures, algorithms, and guidelines for care of the infant in the NICU with respiratory difficulties.

NURSING ASSESSMENT

An infant experiencing respiratory distress does not always have underlying respiratory disease but may have other pathophysiologic conditions that cause respiratory distress. Causes may include congenital heart disease, temperature instability, sepsis, electrolyte imbalance, hyperviscosity syndrome, hypoglycemia, or drug withdrawal. Assessment should be based on the prenatal/intrapartal/postpartal history, Apgar score, gestational age, and physical examination.

CLINICAL MANIFESTATIONS

The clinical manifestations of respiratory distress vary. Peripheral cyanosis in the immediate postnatal period is not specific; this may be due to the transition in the cardiopulmonary system from intrauterine to extrauterine life. Cyanosis of nail beds or mucous membranes with accompanying central duskiness is a better indicator of low arterial oxygen saturation. Decreased peripheral perfusion may be a sign of respiratory distress, but it also may result from the normal transition from intrauterine to extrauterine existence, so it must be considered in light of the gestational and postnatal ages. Signs of increased respiratory effort (grunting, retracting, nasal flaring, stridor, apnea, tachypnea) all indicate respiratory distress. On chest x-ray areas of ground glass, infiltrates, and edema may all be present in this infant.

DIAGNOSTIC TESTS

Tests to help in the evaluation and diagnostic phase of treatment should include the following:
• Complete blood count (CBC) with differential to rule out sepsis
• Serum glucose and electrolytes

- Arterial blood gas
- Chest x-ray
- Other tests as warranted by the infant's symptoms and history

As part of the diagnostic work-up consideration must be given to different causes of respiratory failure (Table 7-1 and Box 7-1). Table 7-2 gives techniques for applying distending pressure.

Apnea

Apnea is the cessation of breathing for more than 20 seconds. Figure 7-1 offers an assessment, differential diagnosis, and evaluative pathway for the infant with apnea.

Table **7-1**	Causes of Respiratory Failure in Neonates

Pulmonary

    Respiratory distress syndrome
    Aspiration syndrome
    Pneumonia
    Transient tachypnea of the newborn
    Persistent pulmonary hypertension
    Pulmonary edema
    Bronchopulmonary dysplasia
    Diaphragmatic hernia
    Tumors
    Pleural effusion
    Congenital lobar emphysema

Airway

    Laryngomalacia
    Tracheomalacia
    Choanal atresia, stenosis
    Pierre Robin syndrome (sequence)
    Micrognathia
    Tumors and cysts
Respiratory muscles
    Phrenic nerve palsy
    Spinal cord injury
    Myasthenia gravis
Central nervous system
    Apnea of prematurity
    Drugs: sedatives, analgesics, magnesium
    Seizures
    Birth asphyxia

Continued

Table 7-1	Causes of Respiratory Failure in Neonates—cont'd

Airway—cont'd

Hypoxic encephalopathy
Central nervous system hemorrhage
Ondine's curse

Miscellaneous

Cyanotic heart disease
Patent ductus arteriosus
Congestive heart failure
Anemia/polycythemia
Postoperative state
Asphyxia neonatorum
Tetanus neonatorum
Extreme immaturity
Shock
Sepsis

From Carlo WA (2001). Assisted ventilation. In Klaus MH, Fanaroff AA, editors. Care of the high-risk neonate, ed 5, Philadelphia: WB Saunders, p. 278.

OXYGEN THERAPY

Martin et al. (2001) offer some practical considerations for use of oxygen in the premature infant. Oxygen must be considered a medication and used with the same precautions as other drugs. The nurse is the key person to protect the infant from harm from improperly administered oxygen.

Practical considerations are as follows*:
1. *Peripheral* cyanosis may be present in a neonate with a normal or high arterial oxygen tension.
2. Environmental (or inspired) oxygen should be continuously monitored in all infants receiving supplemental oxygen or assisted ventilation.
3. Oxygen therapy without concurrent assessments of arterial oxygen tension is dangerous. A noninvasive monitoring device to measure oxygen saturation by pulse oximetry or transcutaneous PO_2 should be used continuously in preterm infants receiving any supplemental oxygen. In the presence of an arterial line during the acute phase of illness, measure PaO_2 at least every 4 hours if the infant is receiving oxygen.

---

*From Martin RJ, Sosenko I, Bacalari E (2001). Respiratory problems. In Klaus MH, Fanaroff AA, editors. Care of the high-risk neonate, ed 5, Philadelphia: WB Saunders, pp. 246-247.

Table **7-2**		Techniques of Applying Continuous Distending Pressure	
Method*	**Advantages**	**Effective for Infants <1500 g**	**Disadvantages**
Endotracheal	Effective	No	Requires intubation; nursing and medical skills as for ventilator
Head box	Noninvasive	No	Neck seal a problem; suction Difficult nerve palsies
Face mask	Simple, inexpensive	Yes	Abdominal distention, pressure on face and eyes, CO_2 retention, cerebellar hemorrhage
Nasal prongs	Simple	No	Trauma to turbinates and septum, excessive crying, variation in Fio_2, increased work of breathing
Nasopha-yngeal	Relatively simple, fixation easy	Yes	May become blocked or kinked
Face chamber	Good seal, minimal trauma to face	Yes	Expensive; baby inaccessible

From Carlo WA (2001). Assisted ventilation. In Klaus MH, Fanaroff AA, editors. Care of the high-risk neonate, ed 5, Philadelphia: WB Saunders, p. 283.
The practice of oxygen hoods varies in different parts of the world; in some areas oxygen hoods are not used at all. Some countries use nasal prongs on all babies with CPAP for all forms of respiratory distress. Oxygen by simple prongs is only for those going home on oxygen or those 36 weeks' gestation who will require oxygen.

Box **7-1**

Differential Diagnosis of Neonatal Respiratory Distress

Pulmonary Disorders
Respiratory distress syndrome
Transient tachypnea of the newborn
Meconium aspiration syndrome
Pneumonia
Air leak syndromes
Pulmonary hypoplasia

Systemic Disorders
Hypothermia
Metabolic acidosis
Anemia/polycythemia
Pulmonary hypertension
Congenital heart disease

Anatomic Problems Compromising Respiratory System

Upper airway obstruction	Rib cage anomalies
Airway malformations	Phrenic nerve injury
Space-occupying lesions	Neuromuscular disease

From Martin RJ, Sosenko I, Bancalari E (2001). Respiratory problems. In Klaus MH, Fanaroff AA, editors. Care of the high-risk neonate, ed 5, Philadelphia: WB Saunders, p. 251.

4. In preterm infants, arterial oxygen tension should be maintained between 50 and 80 mm Hg during the acute phase of respiratory failure.
5. The development of retinopathy of prematurity (ROP) is related to high arterial oxygen tension levels, and these may rise above the normal range even with relatively low inspired oxygen concentrations.
6. When infants receiving supplemental oxygen require mask-and-bag ventilation, both oxygen concentration and inflating pressures must be monitored closely.
7. Use of a nasal cannula for prolonged oxygen therapy allows greater mobility for the infant and enables oral feeding without manipulating oxygen concentration. Both inspired oxygen concentration and flow rate are precisely adjusted and the infant's oxygenation is closely monitored, typically via pulse oximetry. Administration of oxygen by nasal cannula requires close monitoring because in active infants the cannula is easily displaced

Continued

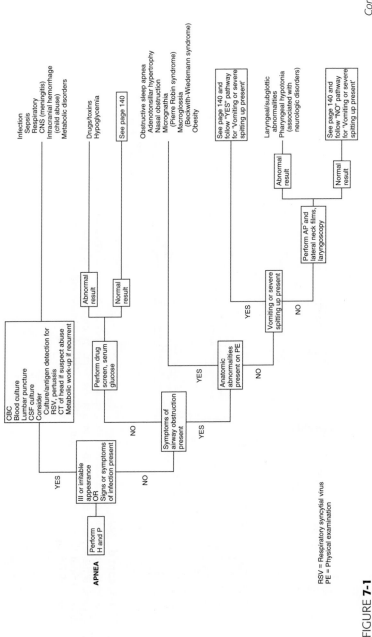

APNEA

Perform H and P

Ill or irritable appearance OR Signs or symptoms of infection present

YES →
CBC
Blood culture
Lumbar puncture
CSF culture
Consider
  Culture/antigen detection for RSV, pertussis
  CT of head if suspect abuse
  Metabolic work-up if recurrent

Infection
Sepsis
Respiratory
CNS (meningitis)
Intracranial hemorrhage (child abuse)
Metabolic disorders

NO ↓

Symptoms of airway obstruction present

NO → Perform drug screen, serum glucose

Abnormal result → Drugs/toxins
Hypoglycemia

Normal result → See page 140

YES ↓

Anatomic abnormalities present on PE

YES →
Obstructive sleep apnea
Adenotonsillar hypertrophy
Nasal obstruction
Micrognathia (Pierre Robin syndrome)
Macroglossia (Beckwith-Wiedemann syndrome)
Obesity

NO ↓

Vomiting or severe spitting up present

YES → See page 140 and follow "YES" pathway for "Vomiting or severe spitting up present"

NO → Perform AP and lateral neck films, laryngoscopy

Abnormal result → Laryngeal/subglottic abnormalities
Pharyngeal hypotonia (associated with neurologic disorders)

Normal result → See page 140 and follow "NO" pathway for "Vomiting or severe spitting up present"

RSV = Respiratory syncytial virus
PE = Physical examination

FIGURE 7-1

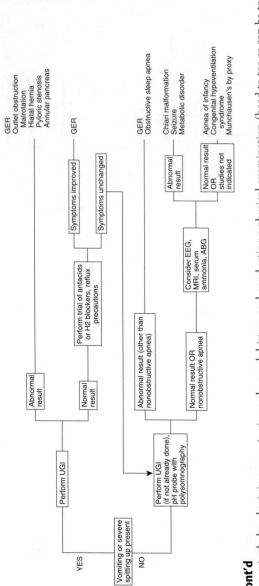

FIGURE 7-1, cont'd

Nursing assessment includes obtaining or reviewing a thorough history and conducting a physical examination (head to toe as can be tolerated). The tests listed above are part of the normal assessment. An important nursing function is to explain the purpose of the tests to the family. (Modified from Pomeranz AJ, et al., editors [2002]. *Pediatric decision-making strategies to accompany Nelson textbook of pediatrics*, ed 16, Philadelphia: WB Saunders, pp. 47, 49.)

from the nose. Also, changes in respiratory pattern may entrain different amounts of room air around the prongs, changing the true inspired oxygen concentration. Finally, high gas flows through the prongs can produce positive airway pressure if the prongs are fitted tightly.

8. When the infant with respiratory distress syndrome (RDS) is improving, environmental oxygen should be lowered in small decrements while continuously monitoring oxygenation.

9. Any inspired oxygen concentration above room air can be damaging to pulmonary tissue if maintained over several days. Oxygen therapy is continued only if necessary.

10. Premature infants receiving additional oxygen for extended periods of time should be examined by an experienced ophthalmologist by 4 to 6 weeks after birth to screen for treatable ROP.

UNIVERSITY OF ILLINOIS MEDICAL CENTER AT CHICAGO CLINICAL CARE GUIDELINE

Subject: Oxygen Therapy for Infants in the NICU/ICU*

Objectives

- To provide clinical guidelines for the safe administration of oxygen to neonates.
- To ensure that the patient has supplemental oxygen available to treat hypoxemia and to decrease the exertion of breathing and the stress on the myocardium.

Monitor infant status with oxygen and decrease oxygen to prevent retinopathy of prematurity, oxygen toxicity, respiratory diseases, and hyperoxygenation.

Definitions

For the purposes of this guideline, the following definitions apply:

Oxygen Therapy—Providing supplemental oxygen to the infant by means of a nasal cannula, head hood, mask, nasopharyngeal continuous positive airway pressure, or endotracheal tube.

Pulse Oximeter—A biomedical device that noninvasively measures arterial oxygen saturation.

Oxygen Saturation—The percent of hemoglobin that is fully saturated by oxygen.

Retinopathy of Prematurity—Vascular pathology of the developing retina thought to be associated with the provision of oxygen.

The nurse shall obtain a physician's written order for the initiation, changes, or discontinuation of oxygen therapy.

---

*From University of Illinois Medical Center at Chicago Women's and Children's Nursing Services. Used with permission by Dharmapuri Vidyasagar, MD; Catherine Theorell, RNC, MSN, NNP; Beena Peters, RN, MS.

The nurse shall institute oxygen therapy without a physician's order in those situations where a delay could be detrimental to the neonate. Following the intervention, the nurse shall document the rationale for his/her action and shall obtain a physician's order.

The nurse shall notify respiratory therapy each time that oxygen is initiated, oxygen is discontinued, or parameter adjustment is indicated.

Procedures

1. All infants receiving oxygen therapy will be continuously monitored with cardiopulmonary and pulse oximeter monitors.
   a. All neonates requiring oxygen therapy will have an infant resuscitation bag with an appropriately sized mask at their bedside.
   b. The nurse will assess the infant for any changes in respiratory status and notify the physician appropriately.
   c. The nurse will reassess the respiratory status of the neonate within 20 minutes of oxygen or ventilatory changes to determine the effectiveness of therapy and need for further intervention.
   d. Blood gases will be obtained as ordered by the physician and prn (as needed) as infant's condition warrants.
   e. The neonate's parent(s) will be provided education regarding the need for oxygen therapy and safety precautions to be followed.
   f. The nurse will facilitate family attachment by allowing parent(s) to hold their neonate as condition allows.
2. Oxygen weaning process
   a. The physician may order the infant to be weaned from FiO_2 or liter flow based on the oxygen saturation values.
   b. The weaning order will provide the following:
      (1) Range of oxygen saturation values that should be maintained
      (2) Parameter (i.e., FiO_2/liter flow) and how fast the oxygen should be decreased
   c. The nurse may decrease the FiO_2 or liter flow only after the neonate has demonstrated a consistent oxygen saturation value above the range within which the physician has ordered.
   d. The nurse will assess the neonate's response to all changes in oxygen therapy.
   e. If the neonate does not tolerate the change, the changed parameter will be returned to its previous setting and the physician will be notified of the failed attempt to wean.
3. The registered nurse (RN) will document the initiation, changes, or discontinuation of oxygen therapy.
   a. The nurse shall document at the beginning of the shift and at each vital sign check:

(1) Concentration of oxygen
(2) Mode of administration
(3) Other ventilator parameter, if appropriate.
(4) Pulse oximeter value
(5) Temperature of humidifier
(6) Blender concentration for resuscitation bag and mask
(7) Presence of bag and mask at bedside (beginning of shift only)

b. The nurse will document the respiratory assessment findings after a change has been made.

c. This documentation should include the oxygen saturation value or blood gas values as ordered by the physician.

d. Documentation of blood gases should include the following:
(1) The time drawn
(2) Oxygen therapy settings
(3) Oxygen saturation value

UNIVERSITY OF ILLINOIS MEDICAL CENTER AT CHICAGO CLINICAL CARE GUIDELINE

Subject: Pulse Oximetry Use in the Neonatal Intensive Care Unit*

Objective

Pulse oximetry should be used to facilitate the safe and efficient monitoring of arterial oxygen saturation in infants at risk for alterations in oxygenation.

Definitions

For the purposes of this guideline, the following definitions apply:

Oxygen Saturation—The percentage level that hemoglobin is saturated with oxygen.

Pulse Oximetry—The biomedical device that noninvasively measures hemoglobin saturation of blood. The probe, which emits and receives refracted light, must be located over an arterial pulse to accurately detect the level of hemoglobin saturation.

Position Statements

All infants should have arterial oxygen saturation monitored with pulse oximetry if supplemental oxygen is administered.

Infants with respiratory distress with or without apnea and/or bradycardia should have arterial oxygen saturation monitored.

Convalescing infants who are undergoing the transition from gavage to nipple feedings should be continuously monitored for oxygen saturation.

*From University of Illinois Medical Center at Chicago Women's and Children's Nursing Services. Used with permission by Dharmapuri Vidyasagar, MD; Catherine Theorell, RNC, MSN, NNP; Beena Peters, RN, MS.

Infants with suspected cardiovascular dysfunction should have arterial oxygen saturation monitored from preductal and postductal sites.

A physician should assess or reevaluate any infant requiring a significant change in oxygen therapy including initiating or restarting oxygen therapy, if more than a 10% increase in oxygen is required or if two or more increases in FiO_2 are necessary.

The order for oxygen therapy must be documented in the medical record.

Procedures

1. Guidelines for oxygenation saturation monitoring
   a. RNs, RNs—license pending, LPN IIs, and nursing students supervised by an RN shall monitor the oxygenation saturation continually, record the oxygen saturation hourly on the flow sheet, and document the infant's status at a minimum of every 8 hours in the medical record.
   b. Respiratory therapists or physical or occupational therapists working with infants shall monitor the oxygen saturation before, during, and in the immediate posttherapy period.
   c. Documentation of the infant's tolerance to the treatment shall be communicated in the note.
   d. Oxygen saturation default alarm limits should be set for the following:
      (1) Low limit for arterial oxygen saturation should be set at 85%.
      (2) High limit for arterial oxygen saturation should be set at 95%.
      (3) Any changes to the above limits require a physician order.
      (4) Examples of conditions of infants in whom the oxygen saturation default alarm limits may need to be altered include the following:
         (a) Cyanotic cardiac disease. The desired saturation limits must be specified in the medical record.
         (b) Persistent pulmonary hypertension. The oxygen saturation default alarm limits may vary depending on the status of the infant and the clinical stage of the disease.
         (c) Normal infants breathing room air. Oxygen saturation levels in these infants are frequently greater than 95% without supplemental oxygen. Thus the upper default alarm limits of saturation may be reset to 100%.
2. Guideline for increasing or decreasing FiO_2
   a. Oxygen weaning orders should be specified in the medical record and reviewed daily on rounds. For example, "wean FiO_2 by 2% to 3% every 15 minutes maintaining arterial oxygen saturation between 85% and 95%."
   b. FiO_2 can be quickly increased by observing the infant at the bedside.

c. To maintain the infant's oxygen saturation within acceptable limits, the level of inspired oxygen may need to be adjusted by the nurse, physician, occupational therapist, physical therapist, or respiratory therapist.

d. Documentation of changes in FiO_2 must be recorded in the medical record and communicated to the nurse and/or respiratory therapist caring for that infant.

e. Assessment of the infant's oxygenation includes an evaluation of heart rate, respiratory rate, respiratory effort, blood pressure, tissue perfusion, and color.

f. Oxygen saturation limits for a critically ill infant may differ from that of stable, recovering, or convalescing infant.

g. Weaning orders should be reassessed for each infant and renewed every 24 hours.

h. Frequency of ordered blood gases should be individualized to the infant's condition utilizing sound clinical assessment and judgment of the nurse and physician caring for the infant.

3. Guidelines for oximeter probes
   a. Some manufacturers' saturation cables are permanent, nondisposable cables.
   b. Oximeter light probes are a single–patient use item.
   c. Anatomic location of the saturation oximeter probes should be changed every 4 to 6 hours depending on the clinical and skin condition of the infant.
   d. Anatomic location of the saturation probe shall be documented in the flow sheet.

Although in these protocols the orders are done by a physician in many institutions these are done by neonatal nurse practitioners. Policies may vary slightly among institutions, but the general guideline parameters remain the same.

Figure 7-2 gives the pathophysiology of neonatal respiratory distress syndrome. Endotracheal tube guidelines are given in Tables 7-3 and 7-4. Table 7-5 lists effects of ventilator settings on blood gases, and Table 7-6 gives supportive care for respiratory distress syndrome.

UNIVERSITY OF ILLINOIS MEDICAL CENTER AT CHICAGO CLINICAL CARE GUIDELINE

Subject: Guidelines for Care of Stable Neonates Requiring Mechanical Ventilation*

Objective

To provide for the safe and efficient care of stable neonates requiring mechanical ventilation.

*From University of Illinois Medical Center at Chicago Women's and Children's Nursing Services. Used with permission by Dharmapuri Vidyasagar, MD; Catherine Theorell, RNC, MSN, NNP; Beena Peters, RN, MS.

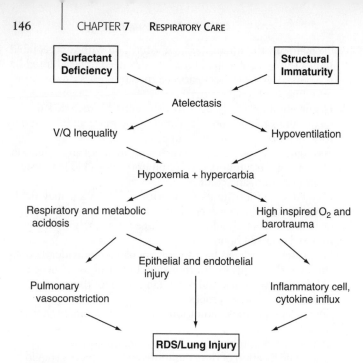

FIGURE **7-2**
Pathophysiology of neonatal respiratory distress syndrome. (From Martin RJ, Sosenko I, Bancalari E [2001]. Respiratory problems. In Klaus MH, Fanaroff AA, editors. *Care of the high-risk neonate*, ed 5, Philadelphia: WB Saunders, p. 254.)

Definitions

For the purpose of this guideline the following definitions apply:

Mechanical Ventilation—Mechanical devices used to support the ventilation and oxygenation requirements of patients. Mechanical ventilation may include continuous positive airway pressure (CPAP) or various types of intermittent mandatory positive pressure ventilation (IMV) modes.

Stable Neonate Requiring Mechanical Ventilation—A neonate in whom spontaneous respiratory efforts are insufficient to sustain ventilation and oxygenation requirements. Infants are considered to be stable when the parameters of the ventilatory support are low to moderate and few changes are required.

Position Statements

The nurse will demonstrate knowledge of the care for stable neonates requiring mechanical ventilation by initiating appropriate nursing interventions based on in-depth nursing assessments of vital signs,

Table **7-3**	Guidelines for Endotracheal Tube Size
Gestational Age (wk)	**Endotracheal Tube Internal Diameter (mm)**
<30	2.5
30-34	3.0
35	3.5

From Jobe AH (2002). The respiratory system. In Fanaroff AA, Martin RJ, editors. Neonatal-perinatal medicine: diseases of the fetus and infant, ed 7, St Louis: Mosby, p.1017.

Table **7-4**	Endotracheal Tube Insertion Length
Infant Weight (g)	**Endotracheal Tube Insertion Length (tip to lip, cm)**
1000	7
2000	8
2001	9
2002	10

From Carlo WA (2001). Assisted ventilation. In Klaus MH, Fanaroff AA, editors. Care of the high-risk neonate, ed 5, Philadelphia: WB Saunders, p. 279.

Table **7-5**	Effects of Ventilator Setting Changes on Blood Gases	
	Effects on Blood Gas Tensions	
Ventilator Setting Changes	**Paco₂**	**Pao₂**
Increase positive inspiratory pressure	Decrease	Increase
Increase positive end expiratory pressure	Increase	Increase
Increase frequency	Decrease	Minimal effect—might increase
Increase inspiratory/expiratory ratio	—	Increase
Increase Fio₂	—	Increase
Increase flow	Minimal effect—decrease	Minimal effect—might increase

From Jobe AH (2002). The respiratory system. In Fanaroff AA, Martin RJ, editors. Neonatal-perinatal medicine: diseases of the fetus and infant, ed 7, St Louis: Mosby, p. 1019.

Table 7-6	Supportive Care for Infants with Respiratory Distress Syndrome

Treatment	Logic
1. (a) Trained staff nurses (ratio of 1:2), respiratory therapists, and monitoring equipment (b) Available trained physicians, nurse practitioners	1. Early management of complications and notification of change in course (e.g., apnea, bleeding from catheter)
2. Precise temperature control to maintain infant in neutral temperature (includes oxygen hood)	2. Maintains minimal oxygen consumption and carbon dioxide production
3. (a) pH, Pao_2, $Paco_2$, and HCO_3^- measurements at least every 4 hr. Maintain Pao_2 at 50-80 mm Hg. *Continuous* Pao_2 or Sao_2 is optimal.	3. (a) To determine requirements for oxygen and additional HCO_3^-. Permits continued assessment of infant's condition and limits toxic effects of oxygen.
(b) Monitor blood pressure.	(b) Recognize hypoperfusion, hypovolemia, patent ductus arteriosus
(c) Attempt to keep pH >7.25. If $Paco_2$ >60 or Pao_2 <50 mm Hg, change treatment.	(c) Same as (a)
(d) Lower environmental oxygen slowly when RDS infant is still ill.	(d) Prevents greater than expected decrease in Pao_2 when environmental oxygen is reduced (right-to-left shunt etiology?)
(e) Limit $NaHCO_3$ to 8 mEq/kg/day.	(e) Prevents hypernatremia with possible brain damage
4. Surfactant therapy (requires endotracheal tube)	4. Therapeutic approach to underlying etiology of RDS
5. IV glucose 50 ml/kg first day, 80-100 ml/kg second day with body weight determination for small infants to calculate if larger amounts of H_2O required. May require 150 ml/kg or more.	5. Need to balance fluid and partial caloric requirements while minimizing the risk of fluid overload problems (e.g., patent ductus arteriosus)

Table **7-6**	Supportive Care for Infants with Respiratory Distress Syndrome—cont'd

Treatment	**Logic**
6. Controlled oxygen administration: warmed and humidified, using a hood	6. Prevents large swings in environmental oxygen concentration and temperature and decreases water requirements
7. Continually monitor respiration, heart rate, and temperature as well as blood pressure, 3(b).	7. Prevents hypoxemia and acidemia with apneic episodes
8. Frequent determinations of blood sugar and hematocrit (Na, K, and Cl every 12-24 hr)	8. Necessary for calculating general metabolic requirements
9. Transfuse if central hematocrit <35 during acute phase of illness	9. For adequate oxygen-carrying capacity
10. Record all observations (laboratory, nurse's notes, etc.)	10. Permits immediate correlation of many variables
11. Urinary output, blood urea nitrogen, creatinine, and when indicated urinary pH, electrolytes, and osmolality	11. Evaluation of renal function and blood flow to the kidney. An increase in output occurs as the infant starts to improve.
12. Obtain blood culture; treat with ampicillin and gentamicin until cultures available.	12. Cannot radiographically separate RDS from group B streptococcal (or other) pneumonia.
13. Minimize routine procedures, such as suctioning, handling, and auscultation.	13. Prevents iatrogenic decreases in Pao_2.

From Martin RJ, Sosenko I, Bancalari E (2001). Respiratory problems. In Klaus MH, Fanaroff AA, editors. Care of the high-risk neonate, ed 5, Philadelphia: WB Saunders, p. 258.

physical and behavioral manifestations, physiologic monitoring parameters, ventilatory requirements, oxygenation, growth, and nutrition. Documentation of nursing care is placed on the bedside flow sheet and medication administration record (MAR) on a continual basis.

Procedures

1. Assessment
   a. Vital signs
      (1) Temperature (axillary), apical pulse, respiration are assessed every 2 hours, if patient is NPO (nothing by mouth) or being fed continuously; otherwise vital signs are assessed with the feeding schedule to minimize disruption of sleep.
      (2) Blood pressure (BP) is obtained every shift. If abnormal, BP is rechecked within 1-2 hours when the infant is quiet and resting.
   b. Physical assessment
      (1) Anterior fontanel status (soft, flat, bulging)
      (2) Muscle tone (limp, rigid, normal)
      (3) Activity level
      (4) Breath sounds (equal, unequal, diminished)
      (5) Color (central vs. peripheral cyanosis, pink, jaundice, pale)
      (6) PMI (point of maximal impulse)
      (7) Quality of apical pulse (presence or absence of murmurs)
      (8) Peripheral pulses assessed (faint, easily palpable, bounding)
      (9) Capillary refill time (number of seconds noted)
      (10) Abdominal appearance (soft, rounded, distended, loops)
      (11) Measure girth before every feeding if on enteral feedings, otherwise every shift
      (12) Check bowel sounds before every feeding, if taking nasogastric (NG) feedings; otherwise every shift
      (13) Skin appearance (rash, ecchymosis, edema, discoloration)
      (14) Weight once per day (usually on night shift or with bath)
      (15) Head circumference every day
      (16) Maintain accurate intake and output record; weigh every diaper
      (17) Elimination status recorded on flow sheet
   c. Routine tests
      (1) Chemstrip every shift if on parenteral fluids.
      (2) If results <40 mg/100 ml, notify physician, obtain serum glucose, and monitor Chemstrip every 1 hour until results are 40 to 80 mg/100 ml × 2 or until further orders.
      (3) Blood gases should be obtained as ordered.
   d. Physiologic monitoring of infants on mechanical ventilation

(1) Cardiorespiratory monitors (electrocardiogram [ECG], respiratory Rate [RR], oxygen saturation)

(2) Set alarm limits as follows:
  (a) ECG: 100 to 200 beats/min (lower ECG limit for term infants may be set to 80 beats/min if needed)
  (b) RR: 20 to 90 breaths per minute (apnea set to 15 seconds)
  (c) Assess alarm limits at the beginning of shift.
  (d) Ensure that alarms are on at all times.

(3) Reposition reusable gel electrodes to achieve contact. Reposition by wetting electrode pad with sterile water and placing on infant.

(4) Oxygen saturation monitor
  (a) Change O_2 saturation monitor site every 2 to 3 hours.
  (b) Monitor the circulation distal to sensor.
  (c) Ensure that infant's heart rate (on ECG) is equal to heart rate displayed on O_2 saturation monitor.

2. Ventilatory support
  a. At the beginning of the shift, verify the ventilator settings with current physician orders.
    (1) Check ventilator settings with each set of vital signs.
    (2) Ensure resuscitation bag with appropriate mask is present at the bedside and connected to oxygen blender.
    (3) Check FiO_2 of blender to make sure oxygen is not >10% off from set FiO_2.
    (4) Obtain order from physician for weaning parameters for O_2.
    (5) Check the stability of the endotracheal tube (ETT). Follow procedure for retaping ETT if tape is deemed to be necessary.
  b. All ventilator settings are changed by the Respiratory Therapist and recorded on Respiratory Therapy flow sheets.
  c. Obtain blood gases as ordered or prn if respiratory distress occurs.

3. Pulmonary suctioning
  a. Perform endotracheal suctioning on individual basis, based on assessment of the neonate.
  b. Assessment of the need for ETT suctioning includes the following:
    (1) Visible secretions in ETT or nares
    (2) Increase in respiratory effort or oxygen requirement
    (3) Coarse breath sounds
  c. Suction ETT at least once per shift, noting characteristics of secretions on flow sheet.
  d. Perform ETT suctioning before feedings.

4. Nutrition (parenteral and enteral)

a. Parenteral nutrition
   (1) At the beginning of shift, double check the name and contents of intravenous (IV) bags against physician orders.
   (2) Syringe pumps should be programmed to allow no more than a 1-hour volume of parenteral fluid to infuse before alarming.
   (3) IV site shall be checked every 1 hour for evidence of infiltration and inflammation.
   (4) Assistance from another RN, fellow, or resident shall be obtained for peripheral central venous catheter (PCVC), dressing changes, or patency problems.
b. Enteral feedings
   (1) Ascertain the current feeding time schedule by reviewing patient's chart and compare with patient care plan.
   (2) If NG tube is composed of PVC, change NG tube every 24 hours. If enteral feeding tube is Silastic, it may be left in place per manufacturer's recommendations. Label tube with date, time, and initials.
   (3) Verify placement of enteral feeding tube tip before each feeding.
       (a) Aspirate for residual using a maximum size of a 5-ml syringe.
       (b) If residual is >10% of total feeding, notify physician and wait for further orders.
       (c) If residual is <10% of the previous feeding, refeed the residual plus the ordered fresh formula/breast milk to complete the desired amount of feeding.
       (d) After feeding, place infant in either prone or right lateral position with head of bed slightly elevated.
c. Continuous enteral feedings
   (1) Place an amount of formula or breast milk in syringe equal to only 4 hours volume for continuous enteral feedings.
   (2) Flush tubing through with fresh formula or sterile H_2O every 4 hours.
   (3) Change tubing at least every 24 hours for formula feedings. Label tubing with date, time, and initials.
   (4) Change tubing every 4 hours for breast milk feedings. Label tubing with date, time, and initials.
   (5) Check residuals every 2 hours for infants receiving continuous enteral feedings. If residual less than or equal to 1 hour's volume of feedings, refeed residual and continue feeding.
   (6) If residual is more than 1 hour's volume of feeding, hold residual, check with physician for further orders.

5. Documentation
   a. Document in nursing flow sheet or medical record:
      (1) Findings of physical assessment at least once per shift, and whenever a change in status is observed
      (2) Follow-up care of abnormal physical findings prn
      (3) Vital signs
      (4) All care activities and patient's response
      (5) Medication administration

HIGH-FREQUENCY VENTILATION*

Sometimes a neonate requires more than conventional ventilation. In those cases one form of high-frequency ventilation (HFV; Table 7-7) may be used.

Purpose

HFV is a rapid rate, low tidal volume ventilation. Reasons for using HFV include the following:
1. To reduce ventilator-associated lung injury:
   a. Prevent pneumothoraces and interstitial emphysema
   b. Reduce the incidence of bronchopulmonary dysplasia
2. To provide a method of assisted ventilation that allows severe pulmonary air leaks to heal

*From Altimier L, Brown B, Tedeschi L (2000). Tri-Health's manual of neonatal nursing policies, procedures, competencies, & clinical pathways, Glenview, Ill: National Association of Neonatal Nurses.

Table 7-7	Techniques for High-Frequency Ventilation			
	HFPPV	**Jet Ventilation**	**Flow Interruption**	**Oscillatory Ventilation**
Tidal volume	> Dead space	> or < Dead space	> or < Dead space	< Dead space
Expiration	Passive	Passive	Passive	Active
Airway pressure waveform	Variable	Triangular	Triangular	Sine wave
Frequency	609-150/min	60-600/min	300-900/min	300-900/min

From Carlo WA (2001). Assisted ventilation. In Klaus MH, Fanaroff AA, editors. Care of the high-risk neonate, ed 5, Philadelphia: WB Saunders, p. 294.

HFPPV, High-frequency positive pressure ventilation; <, smaller; >, larger.

3. In infants when adequate pulmonary gas exchange cannot be achieved by conventional ventilation

Initiating High-Frequency Ventilation

- Obtain chest x-ray and blood gas for baseline comparison while patient is still on conventional ventilation when ordered.
- Establish continuous measurement of infant's oxygenation and ventilation (i.e., pulse oximetry, transcutaneous oxygen monitor).
- Establish continuous monitoring of the arterial BP when possible; otherwise monitor BP
- Initiate inline suctioning system.

Auscultation, Ultrasound, and Chest Radiography

- Chest auscultation for breath or heart sounds is virtually impossible in HFV mode. Infant may need to be disconnected from the ventilator for a short period in order to assess breath/heart sounds.
- Chest x-rays (CXRs) can be performed without concern of HFV.

Blood Gas Interpretation
$PaCO_2$

- Change amplitude (start minimum setting, increase until chest seems to be vibrating). Watch $tcCO_2$ (if available) for trend. If possible get blood gas within 5 minutes to see if $PaCO_2$ warrants increase or decrease in amplitude.
- Reduction of mean pressure will reduce CO_2 if signs of hyperinflation exist.
- Change sigh rate/peak inspiratory pressure.

PaO_2

- FiO_2
- Change mean airway pressure (follow with blood gases; be careful of air trapping, check CXR and observe thorax for signs of hyperinflation).
- Change inspiratory time (IT)/peak inspiratory pressure (PIP).

Troubleshooting Blood Gas Changes on High-Frequency Ventilation
Rapid increase in $PaCO_2$

- Tension pneumothorax
- Obstruction of ETT with change in distal amplitude and reduction in amount of chest vibration
- ETT placement (too far down or leak with change in head positioning)
- Apnea

Gradual increase in PaCo$_2$
- Pulmonary interstitial emphysema (PIE) development
- Atelectasis
- Apnea
- Patent ductus arteriosus (PDA)
- Amplitude drift, change in amplitude 2 degrees to change compliance
- Change in patient sedation, agitation

Rapid decrease in Pao$_2$
- Tension pneumothorax
- Precipitous drop in BP
- Obstruction of endotracheal tube (ETT) (seen with change in distal amplitude and reduction in chest vibration)
- ETT placement (too far down or leak with change in head positioning)

Gradual decrease in Pao$_2$
- Pulmonary interstitial emphysema (PIE) development
- Microatelectasis
- Silent PDA (may not always be silent)
- Change metabolic rate (e.g., hyperthermia)
- Subtle change in BP
- Change in patient sedation, agitation

Comments
Do not use proximal positive end expiratory pressure (PEEP)/continuous positive airway pressure (CPAP) below 3 cm H$_2$O while in the HFV mode (tracheal pressure may be subatmospheric). High-frequency oscillations are negative as well as positive around PEEP. Be aware that there are negative flows and pressures below PEEP when using HFV.

RETINOPATHY OF PREMATURITY*

Retinopathy of prematurity is considered a side effect of oxygen therapy; thus the guideline for follow-up care is presented here.

Eye Screening Exam for Retinopathy of Prematurity (ROP)
Eye exams are required on all infants that meet one or both of these requirements:
- <1500 g birth weight

*From Altimier L, Brown B, Tedeschi L (2000). Tri-Health's manual of neonatal nursing policies, procedures, competencies, & clinical pathways, Glenview, Ill: National Association of Neonatal Nurses.

- Screen infants >1500 g for cyanotic heart disease, for extracorporeal membrane oxygenation (ECMO), or at neonatologist's discretion.

Timing for First Examination
- Perform screening examination during thirty-second week after conception or during the fifth or sixth week after birth—whichever is later.
- After discharge, only if circumstances prevent exam in the hospital. All infants meeting criteria and not examined should have appointments made at the time of discharge.

Follow-Up Examination*

Zone I	Immature	1 week
	Any disease	1 week
Zone II	Up to stage II without plus	2 weeks
	Stage III plus (threshold)	1 week
	Regressing	4 weeks[†]
Zone III	Any disease	4 weeks

How
- Orders for ROP screening exam and eye drop medication orders required for exam will be written by attending physician/pediatric resident/certified nurse practitioner (CNP).
- Drops are given approximately 1 hour before arrival of examining ophthalmologist.
- In each eye, apply one drop of Cyclomydril and repeat × 1 in 15 minutes. After instilling drops into eye, apply pressure over lacrimal sac (pinching upper nasal bridge) for 20 seconds. Each infant should have a unit dose bottle of eye drops at bedside.
- Check pupils for dilation 15 minutes after dosage and repeat drops if needed.
- Infant is to be bundled with arms down, and RN will hold baby's head during eye exam.

PULMONARY INTERSTITIAL EMPHYSEMA

Pulmonary interstitial emphysema (PIE) is a complication of respiratory distress that often leads to chronic lung disease (Figure 7-3). High-frequency ventilation is used in infants that have severe respiratory distress because of surfactant deficiency. Their lungs are stiff, and they respond better to a low peak pressure, PEEP, and quick,

---

*Follow-up times can vary.
†If reconfirming examination documents stable regressing disease and further improvement, follow-up is 6 months.

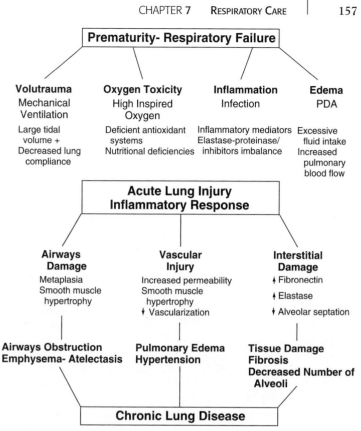

FIGURE **7-3**
Pathogenesis of chronic lung disease. (From Martin RJ, Sosenko I, Bancalari E [2001]. Respiratory problems. In Klaus MH, Fanaroff AA, editors. *Care of the high-risk neonate*, ed 5, Philadelphia: WB Saunders, p. 265.)

rapid breaths to help blow off the carbon dioxide. Infants may require high-frequency ventilation upward to 150 breaths/min.

PERSISTENT PULMONARY HYPERTENSION OF THE NEWBORN (PPHN)

Persistent pulmonary hypertension of the newborn (PPHN) is commonly associated with meconium aspiration syndrome (Figure 7-4). This infant has normal lungs, but there is hypertension at the level of the pulmonary tree that prevents adequate pulmonary circulation and subsequent oxygenation. The infant with PPHN is hard to ventilate with normal ventilation pressures, and high pressures via conventional ventilation place the infant at high risk for pulmonary air leaks. High-frequency ventilation is an alternative therapy for

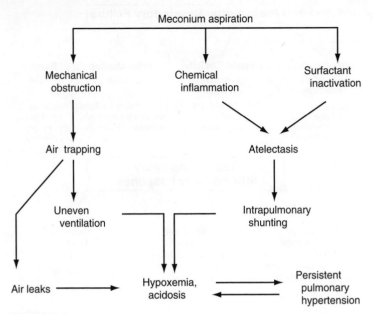

FIGURE **7-4**
Pathophysiology of cardiorespiratory problems accompanying meconium aspiration. (From Martin RJ, Sosenko I, Bancalari E [2001]. Respiratory problems. In Klaus MH, Fanaroff AA, editors. *Care of the high-risk neonate*, ed 5, Philadelphia: WB Saunders, p. 260.)

PPHN. Inhaled nitric oxide, a powerful vasodilator, may offer a better alternative. Extracorporeal membrane oxygenation (ECMO) is reserved for those cases that do not respond to these other therapies. This infant is quite ill and requires good nursing assessment and care. The principles of oxygenation and ventilation described in preceding sections are important in the care of the infants with PPHN. Close monitoring of arterial blood gases is essential. Maintenance of alkalosis promotes pulmonary vasodilation and is generally part of the overall management. Typically the pH should be kept between 7.45 to 7.55 with a $PaCO_2$ of 25 to 30 mm Hg. Suggested ventilator settings are as follows: PIP 30 to 40, PEEP 4 to 5 cm H_2O, and ventilatory rates of 100 breaths/min (Cifuentes et al. 2003).

BIBLIOGRAPHY

Anninos P, et al. (2002). A survey of albuterol administration practices in intubated patients in the neonatal intensive care unit. *Respiratory care*, 47(1), 31-38.

Brion LP, Primhak RA, Ambrosio-Perez I (2002). Diuretics acting on the distal renal tubule for preterm infants with (or developing) chronic lung disease (Cochrane Review). *Cochrane database systematic reviews*, 1.

Carbonell-Estrany X, Quero J (2001). Hospitalization rates for respiratory syncytial virus infection in premature infants born during two consecutive seasons. *Pediatric infectious diseases journal*, 20(9), 874-879.

Chien LY, et al. (2002). Variations in antenatal corticosteroid therapy: a persistent problem despite 30 years of evidence. *Obstetrics & gynecology*, 99(3), 401-408.

Cifuentes J, Segars AH, Carlo WA (2003). Respiratory system management and complications. In Kenner C, Lott JW, editors. *Comprehensive neonatal nursing care: a physiologic perspective*, ed 3, St. Louis, WB Saunders.

Clark RH, Auten RL, Peabody J (2001). A comparison of the outcomes of neonates treated with two different natural surfactants. *Journal of pediatrics*, 139(6), 828-831.

Cordero L, et al. (2002). Surveillance of ventilator-associated pneumonia in very-low-birth-weight infants. *American journal of infection control*, 30(1), 32-39.

Davies MW, Davis PG (2002). Nebulized racemic epinephrine for extubation of newborn infants (Cochrane Review). *Cochrane database systematic reviews*, 1.

Dimitriou G, et al. (2002). Rescue high frequency oscillation and predictors of adverse neurodevelopmental outcome in preterm infants. *Early human development*, 66(2), 133-141.

Durand M, et al. (2002). A randomized trial of moderately early low-dose dexamethasone therapy in very low birth weight infants: dynamic pulmonary mechanics, oxygenation, and ventilation. *Pediatrics*, 109(2), 262-268.

Elbourne D, Field D, Mugford M (2002). Extracorporeal membrane oxygenation for severe respiratory failure in newborn infants (Cochrane Review). *Cochrane database systematic reviews*, 1.

Elgellab A, et al. (2001). Effects of nasal continuous positive airway pressure (NCPAP) on breathing pattern in spontaneously breathing premature newborn infants. *Intensive care medicine*, 27(11), 1782-1787.

Fuloria M, Kreiter S (2002). The newborn examination. I. Emergencies and common abnormalities involving the skin, head, neck, chest, and respiratory and cardiovascular systems. *American family physician*, 65(1), 61-68.

Giannakopoulou C, et al. (2002). Comparative randomized study: administration of natural and synthetic surfactant to premature newborns with respiratory distress syndrome. *Pediatrics international*, 44(2), 117-121.

Hofmeyr GJ, Kulier R (2002). Piracetam for fetal distress in labour (Cochrane Review). *Cochrane database systematic reviews*, 1.

Lassus P, et al. (2001). Pulmonary vascular endothelial growth factor and Flt-1 in fetuses, in acute and chronic lung disease, and in persistent pulmonary hypertension of the newborn. *American journal of respiratory critical care medicine*, 164(10 Pt 1), 1981-1987.

Lewis V, Whitelaw A (2002). Furosemide for transient tachypnea of the newborn (Cochrane Review). *Cochrane database systematic reviews*, 1.

Rehan VK, et al. (2001). Effects of continuous positive airway pressure on diaphragm dimensions in preterm infants. *Journal of perinatology*, 21(8), 521-524.

Sreenan C, et al. (2001). Isolated mental developmental delay in very low birth weight infants: association with prolonged doxapram therapy for apnea. *Journal of pediatrics*, 139(6), 832-837.

Swingler GH (2001). Observer variation in chest radiography of acute lower respiratory infections in children: a systematic review. *British medical center medical imaging*, 1(1), 1.

Trittenwein G, et al. (2001). Neonatal and pediatric extracorporeal membrane oxygenation using nonocclusive blood pumps: the Vienna experience. *Artificial organs*, 25(12), 994-999.

Verklan MT (2002). Physiologic variability during transition to extrauterine life. *Critical care nursing quarterly*, 24(4), 41-56; quiz 2 pp. following p. 83.

Wijnberger LD, et al. (2002). Comparison of single and repeated antenatal corticosteroid therapy to prevent neonatal death and morbidity in the preterm infant. *Early human development*, 67(1-2), 29-36.

Wilson BJ, et al. (2002). A 16-year neonatal/pediatric extracorporeal membrane oxygenation transport experience. *Pediatrics*, 109(2), 189-193.

CHAPTER 8

CARDIAC CARE

Cardiovascular problems are common in the neonate. The infant with cardiovascular problems must be distinguished from one that has respiratory problems. Some cardiac problems do not manifest until several days of life; unfortunately since many infants are born close to term they may already be discharged before a problem is identified.

NURSING ASSESSMENT

Below is an overview of the cardiac cycle.

Cardiac Valves
1. Semilunar valves
   a. Pulmonary valve
   b. Aortic valve
2. Atrioventricular valves
   a. Tricuspid valves
   b. Mitral valves

Cardiac Cycle
1. Systole
   a. Contraction of the heart increases ventricular pressure.
   b. Aortic and pulmonary valves open.
   c. Blood is ejected from ventricles.
   d. Pressure decreases.
   e. Valves close.
2. Diastole
   a. Mitral and tricuspid valves open.
   b. Seventy percent of blood flows from atria to ventricles.
   c. Coronary perfusion of the heart occurs.
   d. Mitral and tricuspid valves close.

Cardiac Output

Cardiac output (CO) = Stroke volume × Heart rate

CO is influenced by the following:
1. Changes in heart rate
   a. Pulmonary vascular resistance
   b. Systemic resistance to flow

2. Frank-Starling law: within physiologic limits, the heart will pump all the blood that enters it, without allowing excessive accumulation of blood in the veins

Pressure and resistance
1. Pressure and resistance are inversely related.
2. Size of the vessel influences resistance.
3. The greater the radius of the vessel, the lower the resistance.
4. If there is increased pressure in the arterial bed, there are the following:
   a. Decreased resistance
   b. Improved flow

Local factors that influence venous return
1. Hypoxia
2. Acidosis
3. Hypercarbia
4. Hyperthermia
5. Increased metabolic demand
6. Increased metabolites
   a. Potassium
   b. Adenosine triphosphate (ATP)
   c. Lactic acid

Autonomic cardiac control Baroreceptors and chemoreceptors in the aorta and carotid sinus provide feedback to the autonomic nervous system (ANS). This feedback stimulates the parasympathetic or sympathetic nervous system (SNS).

Stimulation of the SNS
1. Through ganglionic chain
2. Releases norepinephrine and epinephrine
3. Acts on sinoatrial (SA) node, atrioventricular (AV) node, and ventricles
4. Alpha effects
   a. Rate: 250 to 300 beats/min (chronotropic)
   b. Contractility: 100% (ionotropic)
5. Beta effects
   a. Vasodilation
   b. Bronchodilation
   c. Smooth muscle relaxation

Cardiac Assessment
1. History
2. Physical assessment
3. Diagnostic tests

Physical Assessment
1. Inspection
2. Palpation
3. Auscultation
4. Percussion

Look for the following:
1. Activity
2. Respiratory effort
3. Color
4. Presence of sweating
5. Precordial activity

Palpate for the following:
1. Precordium
   a. Hyperactivity
   b. Thrill
   c. Point of maximal impulse
2. Peripheral pulses
   a. Carotid, brachial, femoral, pedal
   b. Equality or irregularity of volume, rate, intensity

Palpate abdomen for the following:
1. Size, consistency, and location
   a. Liver
   b. Spleen

Auscultate for the following:
1. Heart rate
2. Regularity
3. Heart sounds
   a. Systolic sounds
   b. Diastolic sounds
4. Heart murmurs

Individual heart sounds are as follows:
1. **S1:** closure of mitral and tricuspid valves
2. **S2:** closure of aortic and pulmonary valves
3. **S3:** blood flowing into nearly filled ventricles
4. **S4:** late diastole or presystole; always abnormal in infants and children

Auscultatory findings are as follows:
1. Intensity
2. Timing
3. Quality
4. Location
5. Radiation
6. Accessory features

Cardiac assessment includes history taking, physical assessment, and interpretation of diagnostic tests. Review of the maternal, fetal, and neonatal history is helpful in cardiac evaluation of the newborn.

Associated with congenital heart diseases (CHDs) are (1) maternal infections, especially viral and protozoal infections early in pregnancy; (2) maternal use of tobacco, alcohol, or drugs; and (3) maternal diseases. Birth weight may also aid in the identification of a CHD. Macrosomia is associated with maternal diabetes and transposition of the great arteries (TGA), whereas infants of mothers with viral diseases are frequently small for gestational age (Lott, 2003).

A neonatal history of cyanosis, tachypnea without pulmonary disease, sweating, poor feeding, edema, or, in older infants, failure to gain weight is suggestive of congenital heart disease. Careful evaluation of the maternal, fetal, and neonatal history, in conjunction with a thorough physical assessment, identifies infants for whom further diagnostic testing is indicated (Lott, 2003).

The following states of the newborn should be observed: sleeping or awake, alert or lethargic, anxious or relaxed. Respiratory effort, including signs of respiratory distress such as nasal flaring, expiratory grunting, stridor, retractions, or paradoxic respirations, should be observed. Tachypnea and tachycardia are early signs of left ventricular failure. Severe left ventricular failure also causes dyspnea and retractions.

Cyanosis is the bluish color of the skin, mucous membranes, and nail beds that occurs when there is at least 5 g/100 ml of deoxygenated hemoglobin in the circulation. If cyanosis is present, note whether it is peripheral or central cyanosis and whether it improves with crying, does not change, or becomes worse with crying. Cyanosis can result from pulmonary, hematologic, central nervous system, or metabolic diseases, as well as from cardiac defects. Pulmonary and cardiac defects are the two most common causes of central cyanosis in the newborn.

Pallor may indicate vasoconstriction resulting from congestive heart failure (CHF) or circulatory shock caused by severe anemia. Prolonged physiologic jaundice may occur in infants with CHF or congenital hypothyroidism, which is associated with patent ductus arteriosus (PDA) and pulmonary stenosis (PS). A ruddy or plethoric appearance is often seen in polycythemia. These infants may appear cyanotic without significant arterial desaturation.

The presence of sweating is very suggestive of a CHD in the newborn. The cause of sweating is sympathetic overactivity as a compensatory mechanism for decreased cardiac output. Precordial activity is a reliable parameter of cardiac dysfunction. Precordial bulging is suggestive of chronic cardiac enlargement. Precordial activity without bulging may be associated with acute onset of cardiac dysfunction. Pectus excavatum may cause a pulmonary systolic ejection murmur or a large cardiac silhouette on an anteroposterior chest radiograph because of the decreased anteroposterior chest diameter. Pectus excavatum does not cause cardiac dysfunction (Park, 1996).

Palpation includes the palpation of the precordium and peripheral pulses. Palpation of the precordium detects hyperactivity, thrill, and the point of maximal impulse (PMI). Irregularities or inequalities of rate or volume can be detected by counting the peripheral pulse rate. Evaluation of the carotid, brachial, femoral, and pedal pulses detects differences between sides and upper and lower extremities. If pulses are unequal, four extremity blood pressures should be measured. Weak leg pulses with strong arm pulses suggest coarctation of the aorta (COA). If the right brachial pulse is stronger than the left, supravalvular aortic stenosis or coarctation proximal to or near the origin of the left subclavian artery may be present (Park, 1996).

Heart defects that lead to "aortic runoff" include PDA, aortic insufficiency, large arteriovenous fistula, or persistent truncus arteriosus; these defects cause bounding pulses. However, preterm newborns frequently have a bounding pulse secondary to relatively decreased subcutaneous tissue. Also, preterm infants frequently have PDA secondary to their prematurity. Cardiac failure or circulatory shock causes weak or thready pulses (Park, 1996).

The hyperactive precordium indicates a heart defect with increased volume, such as CHDs with large left-to-right shunts (e.g., PDA, ventricular septal defect [VSD]) or heart disease with valvular regurgitation (e.g., aortic regurgitation, mitral regurgitation). The location of the PMI depends on whether the right or left ventricle is dominant. With right ventricular dominance, the PMI is at the lower left sternal border. Left ventricular dominance places the PMI at the apex. A diffuse, slow-rising PMI is called a *heave*. Heaves are associated with volume overload. A sharp, fast-rising PMI is called a *tap* and is associated with pressure overload. The normal newborn has a right ventricular dominance (Park, 1996).

The apical impulse of the newborn is normally felt in the fourth intercostal space to the left of the midclavicular line. Displacement of the apical impulse downward or laterally may indicate cardiac enlargement (Park, 1996).

The presence and location of a thrill provide important diagnostic information. The palms of the hands, rather than the fingertips, should be used to feel for a thrill, except in the suprasternal notch and carotid arteries. The examiner should palpate for the presence of thrills in the upper left, upper right, and lower left sternal border; in the suprasternal notch; and over the carotid arteries. A thrill in the upper left sternal border is derived from the pulmonary valve or pulmonary artery. Thrills in the lower left sternal border suggest pulmonary stenosis, pulmonary artery atresia, or occasionally PDA. A thrill felt in the upper right sternal border signifies aortic origin, usually aortic stenosis or, less frequently, PS, PDA, or COA. A thrill over the carotid arteries along with a thrill in the suprasternal notch suggests COA, aortic stenosis, or other defects of the aorta or aortic valve (Park, 1996).

Palpation of the abdomen is performed to determine the size, consistency, and location of the liver and spleen. Increased liver size is a frequent finding with CHF (Park, 1996).

Careful auscultation by a skilled evaluator is an essential component of any cardiovascular assessment. Auscultation includes heart rate and regularity, heart sounds, systolic and diastolic sounds, and heart murmurs. The skillful evaluation of cardiac sounds requires systematic auscultation and much practice.

Part of the nursing assessment is determining the rate, rhythm, pulse pressure, and equality of pulses throughout the body. Another part of the assessment is the determination of murmurs.

Cardiac murmurs should be evaluated for intensity (grades 1 to 6), timing (systolic or diastolic), location, transmission, and quality (musical, vibratory, or blowing).

The grade scale for murmurs is as follows:
Grade 1: barely audible
Grade 2: soft but easily audible
Grade 3: moderately loud; no thrill
Grade 4: loud; thrill present
Grade 5: loud; audible with stethoscope barely on chest
Grade 6: loud; audible with stethoscope near chest

The murmur grade is recorded as 1/6, 2/6, and so on. Again, practice in auscultation improves the listener's evaluation skills. The intensity of the murmur is affected by cardiac output; anything that increases cardiac output (e.g., anemia, fever, exercise) increases the intensity of the murmur.

Figure 8-1 gives a pediatric nursing assessment including possible tests.

CLINICAL MANIFESTATIONS

Clinical manifestations will depend on whether blood flow is diminished or increased. The signs will also depend on how long the problem has existed before diagnosis and other co-morbidities the infant may have.

DIAGNOSIS

Diagnosis is usually made on physical examination, arterial blood gas results, chest x-ray, ultrasound, and echocardiogram.

The more common congenital heart defects will be discussed below.

PATENT DUCTUS ARTERIOSUS IN THE TERM NEONATE

In extrauterine life, the flow of blood through the ductus arteriosus is reversed. The PDA allows blood to flow from left to right, thereby reentering the pulmonary circuit and increasing pulmonary blood flow. The amount of blood flow through the PDA and the effects of the

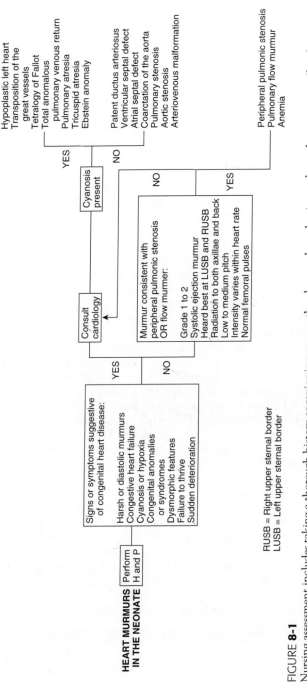

FIGURE **8-1**

Nursing assessment includes taking a thorough history or reviewing one on the chart and conducting a physical examination (head to toe as can be tolerated). If you are a nurse practitioner you may order the tests listed here; otherwise you may wish to make sure these tests are ordered. Follow the results to help the family understand what is being done. (Modified from Pomerzanz AJ, et al., editors (2002). *Pediatric decision-making strategies to accompany Nelson textbook of pediatrics*, ed 16, Philadelphia: WB Saunders, p. 69.)

ductal flow depend on the difference between systemic and pulmonary vascular resistance and the diameter and length of the ductus. High pulmonary blood flow causes increased pulmonary vascular resistance, pulmonary hypertension, and right ventricular hypertrophy.

Clinical Manifestations

A small PDA may be asymptomatic. A large PDA with significant shunting may cause signs of CHF with tachypnea, dyspnea, and hoarse cry. Frequent lower respiratory tract infections, coughing, and poor weight gain are common in older infants with PDA.

Diagnosis

The diagnosis of PDA is based on history and physical examination findings, radiograph, and echocardiogram. Characteristic findings on physical examination include bounding peripheral pulses, widened pulse pressure (>25), and a hyperactive precordium. A systolic thrill may be felt at the upper left sternal border. A grade 1/6 to 4/6 continuous "machinery" murmur is audible at the upper left sternal border or left intraclavicular area. The murmur is heard throughout the entire cardiac cycle because of the pressure gradient between the aorta and the pulmonary artery in both systole and diastole. In severe PDA with large shunt, the S_2 may be accentuated because of pulmonary hypertension (Park, 1996).

A small PDA may not be distinguishable on radiograph. With more severe shunting, there may be cardiomegaly and increased pulmonary vascularity. Electrocardiogram (ECG) may show left atrial and ventricular enlargement and an abnormal QRS axis for age. The definitive diagnosis is made by echocardiogram. With two-dimensional echocardiogram, PDA can be directly visualized. A ductus is considered to be hemodynamically significant if the left atrium (LA)/aortic root (AO) ratio is greater than 1:3 in term newborns or greater than 1:0 in preterm newborns (Park, 1996).

Nursing Management

Nursing management includes prophylactic antibiotics against bacterial endocarditis. There are no exercise restrictions in the absence of pulmonary hypertension. Definitive treatment is surgical ligation through a posterolateral thoracotomy. Corrective surgery is performed in patients between 1 and 2 years of age, unless there is CHF, recurrent pneumonia, or pulmonary hypertension. The mortality rate is less than 1% (excluding preterm newborns). The prognosis is excellent, and complications are rare (Park, 1996).

PATENT DUCTUS ARTERIOSUS IN THE PREMATURE NEONATE

The ductus ateriosus in the preterm newborn is not as responsive (compared with term newborns) to increased oxygen content and does not close. Decreased pulmonary vascular resistance causes blood to shunt from left to right and reenter the pulmonary circuit, leading to increased pulmonary venous congestion, which decreases lung compliance and stiff lungs. Consequences of large shunts include symptoms of CHF, inability to wean from ventilatory support, or increased oxygen requirement.

Clinical Manifestations
Clinical findings include bounding peripheral pulses, hyperactive precordium, widened pulse pressures (>25), and a continuous murmur, best heard at the upper left and middle sternal border. Radiographic findings include increased pulmonary vascularity and cardiomegaly. PDA can be directly visualized by two-dimensional echocardiogram and Doppler flow studies (Park, 1996).

Nursing Management
Management of PDA depends on the severity of the symptoms. Conservative management consists of fluid restriction and diuretic therapy. Use of cardiac glycosides is controversial in the preterm newborn. The preterm newborn's myocardium has a higher amount of connective tissue and water, which may decrease the left ventricular distensibility; thus digitalis would have no effect. Digitalis toxicity may occur because of poor elimination of the drug. If digitalis is used, the dose should be decreased and monitored carefully (Park, 1996).

Indomethacin, a prostaglandin synthetase inhibitor, may be used to close the ductus arteriosus. Indomethacin works best if used in newborns younger than 13 days of life; it is not effective past 4 to 6 weeks after birth. Indomethacin dosage is 0.2 mg/kg intravenously every 12 hours for three doses. Indomethacin is highly nephrotoxic, so the blood urea nitrogen (BUN) and creatinine levels must be monitored. Contraindications to using indomethacin include renal failure, low platelet count, bleeding disorders, necrotizing enterocolitis, and hyperbilirubinemia (Park, 1996).

Surgical ligation is reserved for cases in which indomethacin fails or is contraindicated.

VENTRICULAR SEPTAL DEFECT

A VSD is a defect or opening in the ventricular septum that results from imperfect ventricular division during early fetal development. The defect can occur anywhere in the muscular or membranous ventricular septum. The size of the defect and the degree of pulmonary vascular resistance are more important in determining the severity than the location. With a small defect, there is a large resistance to the left-to-right shunt at the defect and the shunt is not dependent on the pulmonary vascular resistance. With a large VSD, there is little resistance at the defect and the amount of left-to-right shunt depends on the level of pulmonary vascular resistance (Park, 1996; Turner et al., 1999).

Small VSDs produce minimal shunting and may not be symptomatic. Chest radiograph and ECG are generally normal. A loud, harsh pansystolic heart murmur may be best heard in the third and fourth left intercostal spaces at the sternal border (Park, 1996; Turner et al., 1999).

With moderate-sized VSDs, the blood is shunted from the left to right ventricle because of higher pressure in the left ventricle and higher systemic vascular resistance. The shunt of blood occurs during systole, when the right ventricle contracts, so that the blood enters the pulmonary artery rather than remaining in the right ventricle. This prevents the development of right ventricular hypertrophy.

With large VSDs, blood is shunted from the left to right ventricle. The larger the VSD will result in a greater volume of blood shunted in the right side of the heart. The pressures found in the right ventricle and pulmonary artery will be higher than normal. If pulmonary artery pressure is significantly increased, thickening of the walls of the pulmonary arterioles may develop and the increased resistance may decrease the left-to-right shunt. Pulmonary vascular disease can lead to right-to-left shunting and cyanosis.

Clinical Manifestations
Manifestations of VSD depend on the degree of shunting. Small VSDs may produce no hemodynamic compromise and be asymptomatic. Larger defects are associated with decreased exertional tolerance, recurrent pulmonary infections, poor growth, and symptoms of CHF. With severe VSD, there may be pulmonary hypertension and cyanosis.

Diagnosis
In VSD, a systolic thrill may be palpated at the lower left sternal border. There may be a precordial bulge with very large VSDs. A grade 2/6 to 5/6 regurgitant systolic murmur is heard at the lower left sternal border. There may also be an apical diastolic rumble, and the pulmonary heart sound may be loud.

Radiographs show cardiomegaly involving the left atrium, the left ventricle, and possibly the right ventricle, as well as increased pulmonary vascularity. Electrocardiogram may reveal left ventricular hypertrophy. Right ventricular hypertrophy may also be present in severe cases. Echocardiogram (M-mode) shows a large left atrium. Two-dimensional echocardiogram shows other defects and the size and location of the VSD (Park, 1996).

Physical examination of infants with a large VSD not detected in the neonatal period may reveal inadequate weight gain, cyanosis, and clubbing of the digits.

Nursing Management

Treatment of the VSD depends on the severity of the defect and the symptoms produced. Spontaneous closure of the VSD can occur, so that defects that cause no compromise may be observed to allow time for spontaneous closure to occur. Small VSDs generally spontaneously close by approximately 6 years of age. Muscular VSDs have a higher spontaneous closure rate than do perimembranous VSDs (29% vs. 69%) (Turner et al., 1999).

Initial management of the hemodynamically significant VSD includes monitoring for signs of CHF and prompt initiation of therapy. CHF in the older infant is treated with diuretics and digitalis. Unless there is pulmonary hypertension, there is no need to restrict activities. Prophylaxis against bacterial endocarditis is indicated.

Surgical management involves direct closure of the VSD. Cardiopulmonary bypass is required for the surgical correction. The timing of the surgery depends on the severity of the circulatory and pulmonary compromise. Infants with significant left-to-right shunting with evidence of severe compromise require surgery. Signs of CHF that do not respond to conservative medical management or increasing pulmonary vascular resistance is an indication for surgical correction. Asymptomatic children with a moderate VSD usually have surgical correction between 2 and 4 years of age.

The mortality rate for VSD correction is approximately 5%. The mortality rate is higher among smaller infants, those with other defects, and those with multiple VSDs.

ATRIAL SEPTAL DEFECT

An atrial septal defect (ASD) is a defect or opening in the atrial septum that develops as a result of improper septal formation early in fetal cardiac development.

An ASD usually does not produce symptoms until pulmonary vascular resistance begins to decrease and right ventricular end-diastolic and right atrial pressures decline.

With an ASD, blood shunts from left to right across the defect because the right ventricle offers less resistance to filling because it is more compliant than the left. Any factors that decrease right ventricular distensibility or obstruct flow into the right ventricle (e.g., pulmonary stenosis, tricuspid stenosis) can reduce or reverse the shunt direction. The left-to-right shunt increases right ventricular volume, but pulmonary vascular resistance decreases, so pulmonary artery pressure is almost normal. The large pulmonary blood flow gradually leads to increased pulmonary artery pressures.

Clinical Manifestations

Newborns with ASDs are usually asymptomatic, although there may be a grade 2/6 to 3/6 systolic ejection murmur, which can best be heard at the upper left sternal border. S_2 may be widely split and fixed. With a large ASD, there may be a mid-diastolic rumble caused by the relative tricuspid stenosis audible at the lower left sternal border (Park, 1996). On chest radiograph, the heart is enlarged, with a prominent main pulmonary artery segment and increased pulmonary vascularity. Electrocardiogram enhances detection of ASD, showing right axis deviation and mild right ventricular hypertrophy. There may be incomplete right bundle branch block (Danford et al., 1999; Park, 1996).

Echocardiogram by M-mode shows increased right ventricular dimension and paradoxic movement of the ventricular septum. Diagnosis can be made by two-dimensional echocardiogram, which shows the location and size of the defect. Children with ASDs are usually thin and may be easily fatigued. By late infancy, there may be a precordial bulge caused by enlargement of the right side of the heart.

Nursing Management

Untreated ASD can lead to CHF, pulmonary hypertension, and atrial arrhythmias in adults. Spontaneous closure of ASDs occurs in the first 5 years of age in up to 40% of children (Park, 1996). Medical management of ASD consists of prevention or treatment of CHF. There is no need to limit activity. Surgical correction is accomplished by a simple patch or with direct closure during open-heart surgery using cardiopulmonary bypass. Timing of surgery depends on the severity of the defect. The presence of a significant left-to-right shunt is an indication for surgical correction. Surgery is performed when the patient is between 2 and 5 years of age. The surgery is not performed in infants unless there is CHF that is unresponsive to medical management. The mortality rate of the surgery is less than 1%. The highest risk is for small infants with CHF or increased pulmonary vascular resistance (Park, 1996).

ENDOCARDIAL CUSHION DEFECTS

Endocardial cushion defects result from inappropriate fusion of the endocardial cushions during fetal development. Endocardial cushion defects produce abnormalities of the atrial septum (ostium primum), ventricular septum, and AV valves. Endocardial cushion defects take many forms and are characterized by downward displacement of the AV valves as a result of deficiency in ventricular septal tissue and an elongation of the left ventricular outflow tract. The term *complete AV canal* describes the large opening in the center of the heart between the atria and the ventricles. The following defects can occur in the AV canal: (1) an ostium primum ASD, (2) a VSD in the inlet portion of the ventricular septum, (3) a cleft in the anterior mitral valve leaflet, and (4) a cleft in the septal leaflet of the tricuspid valve, which results in common anterior and posterior cusps of the AV valve (Park, 1996).

The hemodynamic consequences of endocardial cushion defects depend on the type and severity. There may be interatrial and interventricular shunts, left ventricle–to–right atrium shunts, or AV valve regurgitation.

Clinical Manifestations

The manifestations of endocardial cushion defects result from the increased pulmonary blood flow caused by the abnormal connection between both ventricles and the atria and by absent or malformed AV valves. The newborn may have respiratory distress, signs of CHF, tachycardia, and a cardiac murmur. The mitral regurgitation may be heard as a grade 3/6 to 4/6 holosystolic regurgitant murmur audible at the lower left sternal border, which transmits to the left back and may be audible at the apex. There is also a mid-diastolic rumble at the lower left sternal border or at the apex caused by the relative stenosis of tricuspid and mitral valves. S_1 is accentuated, and S_2 is narrowly split and the sound intensified.

Chest radiograph reveals generalized cardiomegaly with increased pulmonary vascularity and a prominent main pulmonary artery segment. ECG shows left axis deviation with a prolonged P-R interval, right and left atrial enlargement, right ventricular hypertrophy, and incomplete right bundle branch block. An infant with an endocardial cushion defect may demonstrate signs of CHF, recurrent respiratory infections, and failure to thrive.

Nursing Management

Initial medical management is aimed at preventing or treating CHF with diuretics and digitalis. Prophylaxis against bacterial endocarditis is required before and after surgical correction. Definitive management consists of surgical closure of the ASD and VSD, with reconstruction of AV valves with the patient under cardiopulmonary bypass, deep hypothermia, or both. In some cases, pulmonary artery banding may be performed as a palliative procedure if there is not significant mitral regurgitation. This procedure carries a slightly higher mortality risk than when primary surgical repair is performed.

Surgery is indicated when there is CHF that is unresponsive to medical therapy, recurrent pneumonia, failure to thrive, or a large shunt with development of pulmonary hypertension and increasing pulmonary vascular resistance. The repair is performed in patients aged approximately 6 months to 2 years. The mortality rate has declined in recent years to approximately 5% to 10%. The mortality rate for patients who undergo pulmonary banding is approximately 15%. Factors that increase the risks of this procedure include (1) very young age, (2) severe AV valve incompetence, (3) hypoplastic left ventricle, and (4) severe symptoms before surgery (Park, 1996).

PERSISTENT TRUNCUS ARTERIOSUS (PTA)

The truncus arteriosus is a large vessel located in front of the developing fetal heart. The truncus arteriosus gives rise to the coronary and pulmonary arteries and the aorta. The persistence of the truncus arteriosus results from inadequate division of the common great vessel into a separate aorta and pulmonary artery during fetal cardiac development. A single, large great vessel arises from the ventricles and gives rise to the systemic, pulmonary, and coronary circulations. Inadequate closure of the conal ventricular septum results in a VSD.

Desaturated blood from the right ventricle and oxygenated blood from the left ventricle are received in the truncus arteriosus. The pressures of both ventricles are equal. The truncus arteriosus supplies blood to the systemic and pulmonary circuits. The amount of flow depends on the resistance of the two circulations. Pulmonary vascular resistance is high at birth, so pulmonary flow and systemic flow are relatively equal initially. Pulmonary resistance gradually decreases over time, causing increased pulmonary blood flow. CHF may develop as a result of increased pulmonary blood flow. If the CHF is not corrected, pulmonary vascular disease develops in response to high pressure and increased pulmonary blood flow, subsequently decreasing pulmonary blood flow. These changes, although compensatory initially, complicate the hemodynamics after surgical correction. The volume overload is compounded by incompetent truncal valves, which allow regurgitation of blood into the ventricles.

Clinical Manifestations

The presence of cyanosis depends on the amount of pulmonary blood flow. Signs of CHF may be the first indication of PTA. On auscultation, there may be a systolic click at the apex and upper left sternal border. The VSD may produce a harsh, grade 2/6 to 4/6 systolic murmur heard along the lower sternal border. Increased pulmonary blood flow may produce an atrial rumble. Truncal valve insufficiency produces a high-pitched, early diastolic decrescendo murmur. There may be bounding arterial pulses and a widened pulse pressure. S_2 is single. If truncus arteriosus is not detected in the newborn period, symptoms of poor feeding, failure to thrive, frequent respiratory infections, and signs of CHF appear.

Diagnosis

On x-ray the heart size is increased and pulmonary blood flow may be increased. Fifty percent of cases have a right aortic arch (Park, 1996). Electrocardiography reveals a normal QRS axis and ventricular hypertrophy. Echocardiography demonstrates the presence of the truncus arteriosus overriding a VSD and the absence of the pulmonary valve (Park, 1996).

Nursing Management

Medical management consists primarily of treatment of CHF and prophylaxis with antimicrobials. Pulmonary artery banding, instituted as a palliative measure, may be performed in small infants with increased pulmonary blood flow and CHF unresponsive to medical management. The mortality rate for this group of infants is close to 30% (Park, 1996).

The definitive surgical correction is Rastelli's procedure. Surgery is performed in infants because there is a high mortality rate for uncorrected truncus arteriosus. The mortality rate associated with surgery is also high, ranging from 20% to 60%. Repeated surgery may be required to enlarge the conduit as growth occurs (Park, 1996).

AORTIC STENOSIS

Aortic stenosis is one of a group of defects that produce obstruction to ventricular outflow. Aortic stenosis may be valvular, subvalvular, or supravalvular. Valvular stenosis is the most common, and supravalvular is the least common (Park, 1996).

In valvular stenosis, there is usually a bicuspid valve. Subvalvular stenosis can involve either a simple diaphragm or a long tunnel-like ventricular outflow tract. Idiopathic hypertrophic subaortic stenosis is a form of subvalvular stenosis that presents as a cardiomyopathy. Supravalvular stenosis is associated with Williams syndrome, or elfin facies, characterized by mental retardation, short palpebral fissures, and thick lips (Park, 1996).

Aortic stenosis causes increased pressure load on the left ventricle, leading to left ventricular hypertrophy. The resistance to blood flow through the stenosis gradually causes a pressure gradient between the ventricle and the aorta. Eventually, coronary blood flow decreases.

Clinical Manifestations

Symptoms depend on the severity of the defect. Mild aortic stenosis may not cause symptoms. With more severe defects, there is activity intolerance, chest pain, or syncope. With severe defects, CHF develops.

Diagnosis

Physical examination reveals normal development without cyanosis. There may be a narrow pulse pressure and a higher systolic pressure in the right arm with severe supravalvular aortic stenosis. There is a systolic murmur of approximately grade 2/6 to 4/6, best heard at the second right or left intercostal space with transmission to the neck. With valvular aortic stenosis, there may be an ejection click. With severe aortic stenosis, there may be paradoxic splitting of S_2. Aortic insufficiency may cause a high-pitched, early diastolic decrescendo murmur if there is bicuspid aortic valve or subvalvular stenosis (Park, 1996).

Chest radiographs may be normal, may show a dilated ascending aorta, or, in the case of valvular stenosis, may show a prominent aortic "knob" caused by poststenotic dilation (Park, 1996).

Cardiomegaly is present if there is CHF or severe aortic regurgitation. ECG may be normal or may show mild left ventricular hypertrophy and inverted T waves. Echocardiogram shows prominent thickening of the septum and abnormal mitral valve motions. Two-dimensional echocardiogram shows the anatomy of the aortic valve (bicuspid, tricuspid, or unicuspid) and that of subvalvular and supravalvular aortic stenosis.

Cardiac catheterization may be performed. Its purpose is to identify the exact anatomy and to analyze pressure gradients.

Nursing Management

Management is aimed at preventing or treating the CHF with fluid restriction, diuretics, and digitalis. In children with moderate to severe aortic stenosis, activity is restricted to prevent increased demand on the heart. Balloon valvuloplasty is sometimes performed at the time of cardiac catheterization to improve circulation. In critical aortic stenosis, maintenance of the patency of the ductus arteriosus with prostaglandin E_1 (PGE$_1$) is necessary to prevent hypoxia.

The type of surgical correction depends on the exact location and severity of the defect. The procedure may consist of aortic valve commissurotomy or valve replacement with a prosthetic valve or a graft. The placement of prosthetic valves is usually deferred until adult-sized prosthetic valves can be inserted. The timing of the surgery depends on the severity of the defect. Infants with critical aortic stenosis with CHF must have corrective surgery. Surgery is performed on children when there is a peak systolic pressure gradient greater than 80 mm Hg or when there are symptoms of chest pain.

The mortality risk for infants and small children is 15% to 20%.

TETRALOGY OF FALLOT

Tetralogy of Fallot (TOF) was first described in 1888. Tetralogy of Fallot develops as a result of lack of development of the subpulmonary conus during fetal life. TOF consists of a large VSD, pulmonary stenosis or other right ventricular outflow tract obstruction, overriding aorta, and hypertrophied right ventricle. The right ventricle may not be hypertrophied initially. In the most severe form, there is pulmonary valve atresia.

In TOF, the VSD causes equalization of pressure in the ventricles. Unsaturated blood flows through the VSD into the aorta because of the obstruction to blood flow from the right ventricle into the pulmonary artery.

Clinical Manifestations

Cyanosis, hypoxia, and dyspnea are the cardinal signs of TOF. Newborns can present with just a loud murmur, or they may be cyanotic. Severe decompensation or "tet" spells are common in infants or children but can also occur in neonates. Children instinctively assume a squatting position, which traps venous blood in the legs and decreases systemic venous return to the heart. Chronic arterial desaturation stimulates erythropoiesis, causing polycythemia. Increased viscosity of the blood caused by the increased red blood cells and microcytic anemia may lead to cerebrovascular accident (stroke). Brain abscesses may also occur as a result of bacteremia and compromised cerebral flow in the microcirculation. The chronic hypoxemia and polycythemia cause (1) an increased risk of hemorrhagic diathesis because decreased platelet survival time and reduced platelet aggregation cause thrombocytopenia and (2) impaired synthesis of vitamin K–dependent clotting factors.

Diagnosis

Neonates with TOF exhibit varying degrees of cyanosis, depending on the severity of the obstruction of blood flow through the right ventricular outflow tract. A long, loud, grade 3/6 to 5/6 systolic ejection murmur is heard at the middle and upper left sternal border. There may also be a ventricular tap along the lower left sternal border and a systolic thrill at the lower and middle left sternal border. A PDA murmur may also be heard in severe TOF (Park, 1996).

Chest radiograph demonstrates decreased or normal heart size with decreased pulmonary vascularity. The contour of the heart may be a typical boot shape caused by the concave main pulmonary artery segment with upturned apex. There may also be right atrial enlargement and a right aortic arch.

Echocardiography shows a large VSD and overriding aorta. The anatomy of the right ventricular outflow tract and pulmonary valve can be identified by two-dimensional echocardiogram.

In addition to the manifestations present in the neonate, clubbing of the fingers may be present in the infant or child with TOF.

Nursing Management

The definitive therapy for TOF is surgical repair with the patient under cardiopulmonary bypass. The surgical correction can sometimes be delayed with careful medical management. Neonates with only mild cyanosis improve when the pulmonary vascular resistance decreases. Medical management is aimed at prevention or treatment of hypoxemia, polycythemia, infection, and microcytic hypochromic anemia. Careful follow-up is essential to detect signs of clinical deterioration.

Dehydration must be avoided to prevent increased risk of cerebral infarcts caused by hemoconcentration. Polycythemia develops as a compensatory mechanism to increase the oxygen-carrying capacity of the blood. In the presence of decreased volume, however, the increased viscosity of the blood may further impede cerebral circulation.

Parents must be taught how to recognize the early signs and symptoms of decompensation. They must also be taught to recognize and treat hypercyanotic or "tet" spells. Tet spells are precipitated by events that lower the systemic vascular resistance, producing a large right-to-left ventricular shunt. Increased activity, crying, nursing, or defecation may trigger a hypoxemic episode. The right-to-left shunt causes a decreased partial pressure of oxygen (PO_2), increased partial pressure of carbon dioxide (CO_2), and decreased pH, which stimulates the respiratory center, causing increased rate and depth of respirations (hyperpnea). The hyperpnea causes increased systemic venous return by increasing the efficiency of the thoracic pump. The right ventricular outflow tract obstruction prevents the increased blood flow from entering the pulmonary artery, so the increased flow is shunted through the aorta, which further decreases the arterial PO_2. Severe, uninterrupted hypercyanotic spells lead to loss of consciousness, hypoxemia, seizures, and death.

Surgical treatment is indicated in the presence of hypercyanotic spells (tet spells) that result in increased hypoxemia, metabolic acidosis, inadequate systemic perfusion, increased cyanosis, or polycythemia. Systemic perfusion can be evaluated by observing peripheral pulse intensity, urine output, capillary filling time, blood pressure, or peripheral vasoconstriction.

Surgical management can be either palliative or corrective. Palliative procedures are undertaken to improve pulmonary blood flow by creating a pathway between the systemic and pulmonary circulation. In addition, these procedures allow time for the right and left pulmonary arteries to grow. Palliative procedures are indicated for newborns with TOF and pulmonary atresia, severely cyanotic infants younger than 6 months old, infants with medically unmanageable tet spells, or children with a hypoplastic pulmonary artery, in whom corrective surgery is difficult (Park, 1996).

Surgical correction is performed with the patient under cardiopulmonary bypass after the infant is 6 months old. Surgery may be delayed until age 2 to 4 years in asymptomatic children or in children who undergo palliative procedures. The defect is repaired by patch closure of the VSD and resection and widening of the right ventricular outflow tract. The mortality rate for TOF varies with the severity of the circulatory compromise caused by the defect. The postoperative mortality rate is 5% to 10% in the first 2 years for uncomplicated

TOF. More severe cases have a higher mortality rate, exhibit residual pulmonary outflow tract obstruction, and may require further surgery. Because myocardial damage may occur from the restriction of the right ventricular blood flow during the surgery, cardiac support is needed to ensure adequate myocardial perfusion. Extracorporeal membrane oxygenation (ECMO) is being used by some centers to support the cardiovascular perfusion. ECMO is also being attempted after surgical procedures for transposition of the great arteries (TGA) and total anomalous pulmonary venous return (TAPVR), but infants with TOF make up the largest group of patients who benefit from its use. Many of these infants experience pulmonary hypertension secondary to the cardiac problem or the surgical correction. With ECMO, management of cases can focus on decreasing pulmonary vascular resistance and diminishing right-to-left shunting during the immediate postoperative period.

PULMONARY ATRESIA

Pulmonary atresia results in the absence of communication between the right ventricle and the pulmonary artery. The atresia can be at the level of the main pulmonary artery or the pulmonary valve. Atresia of the pulmonary valve, with a diaphragm-like membrane, is the most common type. The right ventricle is usually hypoplastic, with thick ventricular walls. Less frequently, the right ventricle is of normal size with tricuspid regurgitation. The presence of a PDA, ASD, or patent foramen ovale to allow mixing of blood is crucial for survival.

Pulmonary atresia with ASD results in a small, hypoplastic right side of the heart. The absence of a right ventricular outflow tract results in high right ventricular end-diastolic pressures. Tricuspid insufficiency occurs, and right atrial pressures increase, causing systemic venous blood to shunt from the right to the left atrium through the patent foramen ovale or ASD. Mixed venous blood flows into the left ventricle and aorta. The PDA produces the only pulmonary blood flow. Closure of the PDA causes severe cyanosis, hypoxemia, and acidosis.

In the presence of a VSD, right ventricular size is usually adequate. Systemic venous blood shunts from the right ventricle through the VSD to the left ventricle and enters the aorta. The PDA still provides the only pulmonary blood flow.

Clinical Manifestations

Pulmonary atresia usually is seen with cyanosis at birth. Tachypnea is present, but there is no obvious respiratory distress. S_2 is single, and a soft systolic PDA murmur can be heard in the upper left sternal border. Tricuspid insufficiency may produce a harsh systolic murmur along the lower right and left sternal border (Park, 1996).

Heart size may be normal or enlarged on radiograph. The main pulmonary artery segment is concave and similar to the radiographic appearance of tricuspid atresia. Pulmonary vascular markings are decreased and continue to decrease as the PDA closes.

ECG may reveal a normal QRS axis, left ventricular hypertrophy (type I), or, less frequently, right ventricular hypertrophy (type II). Right atrial hypertrophy is seen in approximately 70% of cases (Park, 1996). Two-dimensional echocardiogram reveals the atretic pulmonary valve and the hypoplastic right ventricular cavity and tricuspid valve. The location and size of the atrial communication are estimated by echocardiogram.

Nursing Management

Immediate management of pulmonary atresia is administration of prostaglandin to maintain ductal patency. PGE_1 (Prostin) is given as a continuous intravenous infusion. The initial dose is started at 0.1 µg/kg/min. When the desired effect is achieved, the dose is incrementally decreased to a maintenance dose of 0.01 µg/kg/min. Careful attention to the site of the infusion is important.

A balloon atrial septostomy is performed at cardiac catheterization to promote better mixing of systemic and pulmonary venous blood in the atria. As soon as the newborn is stabilized, surgical correction is performed. Initially, a systemic-pulmonary artery shunt using Gore-Tex between the left subclavian artery and the left pulmonary artery (Blalock-Taussig procedure) is performed. If pulmonary valve atresia is present, a closed heart pulmonary valvotomy (Brock's procedure) may be performed. The mortality rate for these procedures is 10% to 25%.

If the initial systemic-pulmonary shunt is not effective, a second shunt is attempted in another location. Right ventricular outflow tract reconstruction can be attempted if the right ventricle size is adequate. This procedure has a mortality rate of 25%. The Fontan procedure is attempted in the presence of a hypoplastic right ventricle in late childhood. The mortality rate for this procedure can be as high as 40%.

The prognosis for pulmonary atresia depends on the size of the pulmonary outflow tract established through surgery and the degree of fibrosis of the right ventricle. If there is severe fibrosis and significant outflow tract obstruction, there is an increased risk of development of arrhythmias and right ventricular dysfunction (Park, 1996).

PULMONARY STENOSIS

Pulmonary stenosis is caused by abnormal formation of the pulmonary valve leaflets during fetal cardiac development. Pulmonary stenosis can be valvular, subvalvular (infundibular), or supravalvular. Valvular pulmonary stenosis is the most common, accounting for

90% of cases. Pulmonary stenosis is frequently seen in Noonan's syndrome. It is one of the four defects found in TOF. Isolated infundibular pulmonary stenosis is uncommon.

Pulmonary stenosis results in obstruction to blood flow from the right ventricle to the pulmonary artery. The right ventricle hypertrophies in response to the increased pressure caused by the obstruction to outflow. Pulmonary blood flow volume is normal in the absence of intracardiac shunting.

Clinical Manifestations
Pulmonary stenosis may be asymptomatic if it is mild. Moderate pulmonary stenosis may cause easy tiring. Severe or critical pulmonary stenosis causes CHF.

Diagnosis
The findings of pulmonary stenosis depend on the severity of the defect. A pulmonary systolic ejection click can be heard at the upper left sternal border. S_2 may be widely split, and the pulmonary component may be soft and delayed. A systolic ejection murmur (grade 2/6 to 5/6) is audible at the upper left sternal border and transmits across the back. The severity of the pulmonary stenosis is directly related to the loudness and duration of the murmur. A systolic thrill can sometimes be felt at the upper left sternal border. Hepatosplenomegaly may be present along with CHF.

The ECG is normal in mild pulmonary stenosis. There may be right axis deviation and right ventricular hypertrophy with moderate stenosis. Right atrial hypertrophy and right ventricular strain occur with severe pulmonary stenosis.

On radiographic examination the heart size is normal, with a prominent main pulmonary artery segment. In mild to moderate pulmonary stenosis, pulmonary markings are normal. The critical type of pulmonary stenosis causes decreased pulmonary markings. CHF results in increased heart size. Echocardiogram demonstrates decreased motion of the pulmonary valve leaflets and poststenotic dilation of the main pulmonary artery segment (Danford et al., 1999; Park, 1996).

Nursing Management
Management of pulmonary stenosis is determined by the severity of the obstruction to flow. The mild type generally requires no therapy except antimicrobial prophylaxis against subacute infective endocarditis (SAIE). Moderate pulmonary stenosis is treated through balloon valvuloplasty during cardiac catheterization. Surgical correction is performed in children when the right ventricular pressure measures 80 to 100 mm Hg and balloon valvuloplasty is not successful or when the pulmonary stenosis is infundibular in origin. Infants

with critical pulmonary stenosis and CHF require PGE$_1$ infusion to maintain ductal patency until surgery is performed (Park, 1996). Careful fluid and electrolyte management requires balancing the need for fluids against the prevention of further expansion of the extracellular fluid volume and consequent strain on the heart's ability to pump (Burlet et al., 1999).

The overall prognosis for pulmonary stenosis is excellent. The mortality rate is less than 1% in older infants. The mortality rate is higher in newborns with critical pulmonary stenosis and CHF (Park, 1996).

HYPOPLASTIC LEFT HEART SYNDROME

Hypoplastic left heart syndrome (HLHS) consists of a group of cardiac defects, including a small aorta, aortic and mitral valve stenosis or atresia, and a small left atrium and ventricle. The great vessels are usually normally related.

Left ventricular output is greatly reduced or eliminated secondary to the valvular obstruction and small size of the left ventricle. Left atrial and pulmonary venous pressures are elevated, and there is pulmonary edema and pulmonary hypertension. With a PDA, blood shunts from the pulmonary artery into the aorta. The PDA provides the only cardiac output because there is little or no flow across the aortic valve. Retrograde flow through the aortic arch supplies the head, upper extremities, and coronary arteries.

Although circulation is abnormal in utero, the high pulmonary vascular resistance and the low systemic vascular resistance make survival possible. The right ventricle maintains normal perfusion pressure in the descending aorta by a right-to-left ductal shunt. At birth, the onset of pulmonary ventilation causes the pulmonary vascular resistance to decrease. The systemic vascular resistance increases because the placenta is eliminated. Closure of the ductus arteriosus further decreases systemic cardiac output and aortic pressure, leading to metabolic acidosis and circulatory shock. Increased pulmonary blood flow causes increased left atrial pressure and pulmonary edema (Park, 1996).

Clinical Manifestations
Progressive cyanosis, pallor, and mottling are presenting symptoms of HLHS. Tachycardia, tachypnea, dyspnea, and pulmonary rales are present. The S$_2$ is loud and single. Poor peripheral pulses and vasoconstriction of the extremities are noted on examination. A cardiac murmur may be absent, or there may be a grade 1/6 to 3/6 nonspecific systolic murmur (Park, 1996).

Diagnosis
On radiographic study of HLHS, there is mild to moderate heart enlargement and pulmonary venous congestion or pulmonary edema.

Metabolic acidosis found on arterial blood gas study is a result of decreased cardiac output. Right ventricular hypertrophy is the characteristic finding on ECG. Echocardiography is usually diagnostic. Findings demonstrate the components of the small left-sided heart structures and the dilated or hypertrophied right-sided heart structures. Findings include a small left ventricle, small ascending aorta and aortic root, absent or abnormal mitral valve, and enlarged right ventricle. An abnormal left ventricle/right ventricle end-diastolic ratio is present (Park, 1996).

Nursing Management

Medical management of HLHS is aimed at prevention of hypoxemia and correction of metabolic acidosis. PGE_1 is administered through continuous infusion to maintain ductal patency. Balloon atrial septostomy may be performed to decompress the left atrium.

Surgical correction of the HLHS is experimental and has a high mortality rate. However, this defect was once considered 100% fatal. Surgical correction is performed in stages. The first stage, the modified procedure, is performed in the neonatal period to maintain pulmonary blood flow and create interatrial mixing of blood. The second stage, a modified Fontan procedure, is performed in patients at 6 to 24 months of age. This procedure closes the Gore-Tex shunt, closes the atrial communication, and forms a direct anastomosis of the right atrium and pulmonary artery.

The mortality rate for HLHS remains high. The first-stage surgical repair has a mortality rate of nearly 75%. For the survivors, there is a 50% mortality rate with the second-stage operation (Park, 1996). Nursing care is critical after the first-stage repair. Nursing care must focus on assessment of homeostasis and pulmonary blood flow during the immediate postoperative period. Attention to nutritional status is important for the long-term recovery. These changes require close monitoring of the following:

1. Vital signs for symptoms of blood loss
2. Chest tube output more than 10% of the total blood volume per hour, lasting over a period of several hours
3. Platelet counts that may require treatment with fresh-frozen plasma, platelets, or cryoprecipitate at 10 ml/kg until the patient is stable
4. Daily liver function studies that may indicate vitamin K treatment
5. Guaiac testing of body fluids, such as stool and gastric drainage
6. Ventilatory status, with maintenance of mean airway pressure of less than 10 cm H_2O or peak inspiratory pressure of less than 25 cm H_2O
7. Blood gases for persistent acidosis or systemic hypotension as evidenced by arterial oxygen pressures more than 45 mm Hg or saturations more than 85%

Use of dopamine at 5 to 10 µg/kg/min may be necessary to decrease pulmonary vasoconstriction. Dobutamine and isoproterenol are avoided because they dilate the pulmonary arterioles making the situation worse. Fentanyl may be used to balance pulmonary vascular resistance. Diuretics or peritoneal dialysis may be necessary to maintain a fluid balance. High-frequency ventilation is sometimes used to support pulmonary function when there is acidosis and stiffening lungs. ECMO has also been used in these infants.

Initially, nutritional support is provided through total parenteral nutrition (TPN). Monitoring of daily weights; of urine for ketones, glucose, and protein; and of serum levels of electrolytes and trace minerals is necessary to adjust the parenteral fluids. Enteral feedings may be started in the first 2 weeks postoperatively if the infant is stable and when the greatest danger of necrotizing enterocolitis is past.

Pericardial effusion may occur several days or weeks after the Fontan procedure; alterations in tissue perfusion and changes in systemic blood flow return may be present if pericardial effusion occurs. Cardiac transplantation, although experimental, may provide improved prognosis for infants with HLHS. It is essential that parents be informed of all available treatments, including risks and prognosis if surgical intervention is an option.

COARCTATION OF THE AORTA

Coarctation is a narrowing or constriction of the aorta in the aortic arch segment. The most common location is below the origin of the left subclavian artery. Coarctation may occur as a single lesion caused by improper development of the aorta, or it may occur secondary to constriction of the ductus arteriosus. The severity of the circulatory compromise depends on the location of the constriction and the degree of constriction. Coarctation proximal to the ductus arteriosus (preductal COA) has associated defects in 40% of cases. Associated defects include VSD, TGA, and PDA. Collateral circulation is poorly developed with preductal COA. Postductal COA is usually not associated with other defects, and collateral circulation is more effective. Infants with postductal COA may not be symptomatic. More than one half of infants with COA have a bicuspid aortic valve (Park, 1996).

Coarctation causes obstruction to flow, which leads to varying pressure across the aortic segment. The portion of aorta proximal to the constriction has an elevated pressure, which leads to increased left ventricular pressure. The increased left ventricular pressure results in left ventricular hypertrophy and dilation. Collateral circulation develops from the proximal to distal arteries, bypassing the constricted segment of the aorta. This is a compensatory mechanism to increase flow to the lower extremities and abdomen, producing lower pulses in the lower extremities.

Clinical Manifestations

The severity and time of appearance of symptoms of coarctation depend on the location and degree of constriction, as well as the presence of associated cardiac defects. Symptoms of coarctation include signs of CHF and absent, weak, or delayed pulses in the lower extremities with bounding pulses in the upper extremities. In the presence of CHF, however, all pulses may be weak. With severe COA, S_2 is loud and single. A systolic thrill may be felt in the suprasternal notch. An ejection click may be audible at the apex if there is a bicuspid aortic valve or if systemic hypertension is present. A systolic ejection murmur of grade 2/6 to 3/6 can be heard at the upper right and middle or lower left sternal border, and at the left interscapular area in the infant's back; however, no murmur is heard in more than one half of infants with COA. Correction of CHF may produce the murmur (Park, 1996).

Diagnosis

Diagnosis of COA is based on history, physical findings, radiograph, ECG, and echocardiographic data. In asymptomatic infants and children, radiographs may show a normal or slightly enlarged heart. Dilation of the ascending aorta may be evident. The E sign on barium swallow is characteristic but is usually not evident until at least 4 months of age. The E appearance is due to the large proximal aortic segment or prominent subclavian artery above and the poststenotic dilation of the descending aorta below the constricted segment (Park, 1996). In symptomatic infants and children, radiographs show cardiomegaly and increased pulmonary venous congestion.

The ECG of asymptomatic children may show left axis deviation of the QRS and left ventricular hypertrophy. In symptomatic children, the ECG reveals normal or right axis deviation of the QRS. Right ventricular hypertrophy or right bundle branch block is present in infants, whereas left ventricular hypertrophy is present in older children (Park, 1996). Two-dimensional echocardiogram demonstrates the location and degree of the constriction and the presence of associated defects.

Nursing Management

Surgical correction of COA is the definitive treatment. Surgery is performed in patients aged 3 to 5 years if signs and symptoms can be medically controlled. Earlier surgery is indicated if medical management is not successful.

Medical management is aimed at providing adequate oxygenation, preventing or treating CHF, and preventing SAIE. PGE_1 may be needed to maintain ductal patency if the constricted segment is at the level of the ductus arteriosus (Park, 1996).

Surgical intervention of COA involves the excision of the constricted segment of the aorta with end-to-end anastomosis, patch graft, bypass tube graft, or Dacron graft (Park, 1996). Alternatively, a subclavian flap aortoplasty may be performed. Surgery is indicated in the presence of CHF with or without circulatory shock. In the presence of a large VSD, pulmonary artery banding may be performed at surgery to reduce pulmonary blood flow in an attempt to prevent pulmonary hypertension. The pulmonary artery banding is removed and the VSD is repaired at 6 to 24 months of age. The mortality rate for surgical corrections is less than 5%. Postoperative complications include renal failure and recoarctation.

COMPLETE TRANSPOSITION OF THE GREAT ARTERIES OR VESSELS

Complete transposition of the great arteries or vessels (TGA or TGV) is the result of inappropriate septation and migration of the truncus arteriosus during fetal cardiac development. TGA may be dextrotransposition of the great arteries (D-TGA) or levotransposition of the great arteries (L-TGA). In D-TGA, the aorta arises from the right ventricle and the pulmonary artery arises from the left ventricle. The aorta receives unoxygenated systemic venous blood and returns it to the systemic arterial circuit. The pulmonary artery receives oxygenated pulmonary venous blood and returns it to the pulmonary circulation.

In L-TGA, the great vessels are transposed, with the aorta arising from the right ventricle and the pulmonary artery arising from the left ventricle. The aorta is to the left and anterior to the pulmonary artery. This type of transposition is called *corrected*, because functionally the hemodynamics are normal. The oxygenated blood comes into the left atrium, enters the right ventricle, and goes through the aorta to the systemic circulation. Frequently there are other associated cardiac defects (Park, 1996).

Hemodynamically, two separate parallel circulations result from complete D-TGA. Oxygenated blood from the lungs is returned to the left atrium, enters the left ventricle, and goes through the pulmonary artery to the lungs again. Desaturated blood from the systemic circulation enters the right atrium, goes to the right ventricle, enters the aorta, and is directed back into the systemic circulation. The end result is that the heart and brain and other vital tissues are perfused with desaturated blood. This defect is incompatible with life. A communication between the two circulations must exist to allow mixing of the oxygenated and desaturated blood. This communication can be at the ductal, atrial, or ventricular level. The best mixing occurs with a large VSD.

Clinical Manifestations

Marked cyanosis is the prominent sign of TGA. The degree of cyanosis varies with the amount of communication between the two circulations. Signs of CHF are present. S_2 is loud and single. If a VSD is present, there is a loud, harsh systolic murmur of variable intensity. Hypoglycemia, hypocalcemia, and metabolic acidosis are frequently present.

Diagnosis

On radiographic study of TGA, the heart is enlarged and has a narrow base because the aorta is over the pulmonary artery. The heart is described as egg shaped (Park, 1996). Pulmonary blood flow is increased. On ECG, there is right axis deviation of the QRS and right ventricular hypertrophy. Echocardiography reveals the abnormal origin of the great arteries from the ventricles. Associated defects can also be visualized by echocardiography.

Nursing Management

TGA is a cardiac emergency. Immediate medical management includes correction of acidosis, hypoglycemia, hypocalcemia, administration of oxygen and infusion of PGE_1, and treatment of CHF. A cardiac catheterization is performed and a balloon atrial septostomy is carried out to promote mixing of oxygenated and desaturated blood in the atria. If the septostomy and PGE_1 infusion do not sufficiently improve oxygenation, surgical excision of the posterior aspect of the atrial septum (Blalock-Hanlon procedure) is performed without cardiopulmonary bypass as a palliative measure. This procedure has a 10% to 25% mortality rate (Park, 1996).

Definitive surgical correction involves switching the right- and left-sided structures at the ventricular level (Rastelli's procedure), the artery level (Jatene's procedure), or the atrial level (Senning's or Mustard's procedure).

The prognosis for TGA without surgical intervention is poor; 90% of patients die within the first year of life. The surgical procedures have high mortality rates and a high rate of postoperative complications (e.g., arrhythmias, obstruction to systemic or pulmonary venous return, right ventricular dysfunction). Jatene's procedure is newer but seems to minimize many complications associated with the intraatrial repair operations. Long-term results of this procedure must be evaluated. The type and timing of surgical correction depend on the condition of the patient and the anatomic defect, so each case must be decided individually.

TOTAL ANOMALOUS PULMONARY VENOUS RETURN

With TAPVR, the pulmonary veins drain into the right atrium (rather than the left atrium) directly or through connection with the systemic veins. There no direct connection between the pulmonary veins and the left atrium.

If there is an ASD or patent foramen ovale in TAPVR, a portion of the mixed blood from the right atrium can cross into the left atrium, into the left ventricle, and on into the systemic circulation. The direction of the blood flow and the amount that crosses the atrial communication into the left atrium or that enters the left ventricle are determined by the compliance of the ventricles.

Two clinical hemodynamic states exist with TAPVR. If there is no obstruction to pulmonary blood flow, this flow is greatly increased. The result is highly saturated blood in the right atrium and mild cyanosis. If there is obstruction to pulmonary blood flow, the volume of flow is decreased and cyanosis is severe. Pulmonary edema often occurs secondary to elevated pulmonary venous pressure. Obstruction to pulmonary blood flow is a common occurrence when the TAPVR is below the diaphragm (Park, 1996).

Clinical Manifestations

The manifestations of TAPVR depend on the presence of pulmonary venous obstruction (PVO). TAPVR without PVO includes a history of mild cyanosis, frequent pulmonary infections, poor growth, and CHF. TAPVR with PVO involves severe cyanosis and respiratory distress in the neonatal period, with progressive growth failure. Feeding is associated with increased cyanosis secondary to the compression of the common pulmonary vein by the filled esophagus (Park, 1996). Signs and symptoms of CHF are also present.

Diagnosis

TAPVR without PVO produces a precordial bulge with hyperactive right ventricular impulse. The PMI is at the xiphoid process or lower left sternal border. S_2 is widely split and fixed; the pulmonic sound may be pronounced. A grade 2/6 to 3/6 systolic ejection murmur can be heard at the upper left sternal border, and there is always a mid-diastolic rumble at the lower left sternal border. The rhythm is a quadruple or quintuple gallop (Park, 1996).

TAPVR with PVO may produce minimal cardiac findings. S_2 is loud and single, and there is a gallop rhythm. There may be a faint systolic ejection murmur at the upper left sternal border. Pulmonary rales may be audible.

Radiographic findings of TAPVR without PVO include mild to moderate cardiomegaly and increased pulmonary markings. The characteristic "snowman" sign occurs because of the anatomic appearance of the left superior vena cava, the left innominate vein, and the right superior vena cava. This sign is seldom visible before the patient is 4 months of age. With TAPVR with PVO, the heart size is normal on radiograph and there are signs of pulmonary edema (Park, 1996).

On ECG, TAPVR without PVO has right axis deviation of the QRS and sometimes, right atrial hypertrophy. TAPVR with PVO has right axis deviation for age and right ventricular hypertrophy in the form of tall R waves in the right precordial leads.

Echocardiography of TAPVR without PVO reveals the pulmonary veins draining into a common chamber posterior to the left atrium. The ASD and small left atrium and left ventricle are visualized. A dilated coronary sinus protruding into the left atrium or a dilated innominate vein and superior vena cava can be visualized, if present. Two-dimensional echocardiography of TAPVR with PVO shows the small left atrium and left ventricle. Anomalous pulmonary venous return below the diaphragm can be directly visualized. Doppler echocardiography can be used to detect the venous flow pattern (Park, 1996).

Nursing Management

Management of TAPVR is surgical, and surgery is emergent when PVO is below the diaphragm. Medical management is aimed at preventing or treating CHF and preventing hypoxemia. Diuretics may be required to manage pulmonary edema. Balloon atrial septostomy at cardiac catheterization is performed to enlarge the interatrial communication and promote better mixing of blood. Surgery may be delayed when response to medical management is good, but it is usually performed when the patients are infants (Park, 1996).

The surgical procedure depends on the site of the anomalous drainage. Cardiopulmonary bypass is required. Surgery involves the anastomosis of the pulmonary veins to the left atrium, closure of the ASD, and division of the anomalous connection. The surgical mortality rate is high (10% to 25%), but it is lower than with medical management alone. The highest mortality rate is with the infracardiac type.

EXPERIMENTAL TREATMENTS IN THE POSTOPERATIVE PERIOD

As discussed, morbidity and mortality rates remain high after surgery in many of the cardiac defects. Treatments that are aimed at decreasing pulmonary vascular resistance, decreasing persistent pulmonary hypertension, and improving cardiac output are being tried at many centers. These include ECMO, especially in infants with TOF, and high-frequency jet ventilation in infants who have undergone stage-one repair of the Norwood procedure for stage 1 HLHS. Other newer treatments include nitric oxide (NO) and ultrafiltration.

Inhaled NO acts as a pulmonary dilator. It directly impacts pulmonary and systemic vascular resistance. Its use is being researched in infants who have undergone procedures that require cardiac bypass, such as bidirection Glenn or Fontan procedures.

Ultrafiltration is an experimental procedure undertaken after open-heart surgery. This process is similar to peritoneal dialysis in that it removes water and solutes to increase the hematocrit and blood pressure and to decrease cardiac workload and pulmonary vascular resistance. The action is probably due to a change in the pressure gradient between the blood and the dialysing solution. The result is restoration or maintenance of blood volume, which reduces the need for transfusions. The better perfusion lessens the edema. As contractility of the heart improves, cardiac workload decreases, possibly because cardiodepressant proteins that are present after cardiac surgery are removed. The exact action of this procedure is being researched. It does appear to be a potential treatment for capillary leak syndrome that is prevalent after cardiac surgery.

CONGENITAL COMPLETE HEART BLOCK

The AV node and the bundle of His arise as separate structures that join together. Congenital heart block is a result of a discontinuity between the atrial musculature and the AV node or the bundle of His and the AV node. For the majority of cases, the exact cause of the discontinuity is unknown and the remainder of the heart anatomy is normal. Certain antibodies passed from mothers with systemic lupus erythematosus (SLE) are associated with congenital heart block. Congenital heart block can be a manifestation of congenital heart defects, including congenitally corrected transposition of the great arteries.

Congenital complete heart block can be diagnosed by detection of consistent fetal bradycardia (heart rate of 40 to 80 beats/min) by auscultation, fetal echocardiography, or electronic monitoring. A newborn with a ventricular rate less than 50 beats/min and an atrial rate greater than 150 beats/min is at significant risk. If the newborn has an associated heart defect, the risk for mortality is higher.

Nursing Management

Asymptomatic infants do not require treatment. If the infant is in congestive heart failure, digitalization is generally the first line of treatment. Insertion of a pacemaker is necessary for infants in congestive heart failure that does not respond to digitalization. Close follow-up because of complications or adverse effects of the pacemakers is required.

SUPRAVENTRICULAR TACHYCARDIA

Supraventricular tachycardia (SVT) can arise in utero or in the neonatal period. The most common arrhythmias that produce signs are paroxysmal SVT with or without ventricular preexcitation, atrial flutter, and junctional tachycardia. If the SVT occurs in utero, it can lead to heart failure and hydrops fetalis. SVT in the fetus is treated through maternal administration of digitalis. If digitalization is not successful, propranolol, quinidine, felcainide, or amiodarone is used. The fetus is delivered if there is evidence of fetal lung maturity.

In most cases of SVT, no cause is found. Long-acting thyroid stimulators and immune gamma-2-globulin from hyperthyroid mothers, hypoglycemia, and Ebstein's anomaly of the tricuspid valve can be the cause in other cases. Ten to fifty percent of infants with SVT have Wolfe-Parkinson-White (WPW) syndrome in which the atrial impulse activates the whole or some part of the ventricle or the ventricular impulse activates the whole or some part of the atrium earlier than would be expected if the impulse traveled via the normal pathway. WPW is characterized by a normal QRS, regular rhythm, ventricular rates of 150 to 200 beats/min, sudden onset, and sudden termination.

Symptoms produced by the SVT after birth are subtle and often are undetected until signs of CHF have been present for 24 to 36 hours. Treatment with digitalis or adenosine, cardioversion, transesophageal atrial pacing, or an elicitation of a diving reflex by covering the face with a cold washcloth for 4 to 5 seconds generally is successful in establishing normal sinus rhythm. After conversion, digitalis is continued for 9 to 12 months. Therapy is discontinued abruptly, without weaning dosages.

Recurrence in patients with WPW is more likely and is treated with the above drugs, alone or in combination. Recurrence decreases between ages 2 and 10 years of age. Prognosis for SVT is good.

CONGESTIVE HEART FAILURE

CHF is a condition in which the blood supply to the body is insufficient to meet the metabolic requirements of the organs. CHF is a manifestation of an underlying disease or defect, rather than a disease itself. Before development of CHF, compensatory mechanisms are activated to maintain adequate cardiac output (Park, 1996).

Increased volume may be caused by fluid overload or fluid retention. In the normally functioning myocardium, fluid retention does not cause CHF; however, fluid retention complicates CHF from other causes. In neonates, the most common cause of increased volume is CHD or altered hemodynamics, as in PDA.

CHF caused by obstruction to outflow occurs when the normal myocardium pumps against increased resistance. This increased resistance may be caused by structural defects, such as valvular stenosis or COA, or by pulmonary disease or pulmonary hypertension. CHF caused by pulmonary disease is called *cor pulmonale*. Severe systemic hypertension can also cause increased resistance.

CHF in the neonate usually results from abnormal stresses placed on the heart rather than from an ineffective myocardium. However, electrolyte imbalances, acidosis, and myocardial ischemia affect the ability of the heart to function effectively. Conditions such as rheumatic fever, infectious myocarditis, Kawasaki disease, and anomalous origin of the left coronary artery reduce the effectiveness of the heart.

Arrhythmias that may produce CHF include complete AV block or sustained primary tachycardia. AV block results in a severe bradycardia that prohibits adequate circulation of blood. Tachycardia causes insufficient time for ventricular filling, decreasing cardiac output.

Severe anemia can cause CHF because of excessive demand for cardiac output. Because the oxygen-carrying capacity of the blood is diminished, the heart must pump more blood per minute to meet the tissue oxygenation requirements. If the heart cannot meet the excessive demand, CHF develops (Park, 1996).

Compensatory mechanisms function to meet the body's increased demand for cardiac output. These mechanisms are regulated by the sympathetic nervous system and mechanical factors. The compensatory mechanisms can sustain adequate cardiac output for only a short period of time. If the underlying condition is not corrected, CHF develops.

Sympathetic Nervous System Compensatory Mechanisms

Decreased blood pressure stimulates vascular stretch receptors and baroreceptors in the aorta and carotid arteries, which trigger the sympathetic nervous system. Decreased systemic blood pressure inactivates baroreceptors, causing (1) increased sympathetic stimulation, (2) increased heart rate, (3) increased cardiac contractility, and (4) increased arterial blood pressure. Catecholamine release and beta-receptor stimulation increase the rate and force of myocardial contraction. Catecholamines also increase venous tone, so that blood is returned to the heart more effectively. Circulation to the skin, kidneys, extremities, and splanchnic bed is decreased, allowing better circulation to the brain, heart, and lungs. Decreased renal blood flow stimulates the release of renin, angiotensin, and aldosterone. This release causes retention of sodium and fluid, resulting in increased circulating volume. The increased volume puts additional work on the heart.

Mechanical Compensatory Mechanisms

The heart muscle thickens to increase myocardial pressure. The hypertrophy is effective in the early stages, but as soon as the muscle mass increases, compliance decreases. This change in compliance requires greater filling pressure for adequate cardiac output. The hypertrophied heart eventually becomes ischemic because it does not receive adequate circulation to meet its metabolic needs. Ventricular dilation occurs as myocardial fibers stretch to accommodate heart volume. Initially, this increases the force of the contraction, but it, too, fails after a point.

Effects of Congestive Heart Failure

When the right ventricle is unable to pump blood into the pulmonary artery, the lungs oxygenate less blood, there is increased pressure in the right atrium and systemic venous circulation, and edema occurs in the extremities and viscera. When the left ventricle is unable to pump blood into the systemic circulation, there is increased pressure in the left atrium and pulmonary veins. The lungs become congested with blood, causing elevated pulmonary pressures and pulmonary edema.

The end effects of CHF are the following:

1. Decreased cardiac output. This stimulates the sympathetic nervous system, causing tachycardia, increased contractility, increased vasomotor tone, peripheral vasoconstriction, and diaphoresis.
2. Decreased renal perfusion. This stimulates the renin–angiotensin–aldosterone mechanism, causing sodium and water retention.
3. Systemic venous engorgement. This results in hepatomegaly, jugular venous distention, periorbital and facial edema, and, occasionally, ascites and dependent edema.
4. Pulmonary venous engorgement. This results in tachypnea; decreased tidal volume; decreased lung compliance; increased airway resistance; early closure of the small airways with air trapping; increased work of breathing; and increased respiratory effort, grunting, and rales. Stimulation of the j-receptors in the lung causes the infant to become apprehensive.

Diagnosis

The diagnosis of CHF is based on clinical signs and symptoms, laboratory data, and chest radiography. In contrast to infants with cyanotic heart disease, infants with CHF usually have significant respiratory distress with tachypnea, grunting, and retractions. They exhibit peripheral pallor, appearing to be ashen or gray in color. The precordium is active, and there are usually loud murmurs heard throughout systole and diastole. Pulses are usually full, but there may be a difference between the upper and the lower extremities. Hepatomegaly is common. The infants are irritable.

In addition to demonstrating hypoxemia, arterial blood gas may reveal a metabolic acidosis resulting from the decreased systemic blood flow. If acidosis is severe, there may be concurrent respiratory acidosis because of the pulmonary edema caused by left-sided heart failure. Pulmonary ventilation–perfusion mismatch may cause hypoxemia. Hypocalcemia is often present in infants with CHF because they have an inappropriate response to stress. In addition, infants with DiGeorge syndrome may have hypocalcemia because of absent parathyroids. Aortic arch abnormalities (e.g., interrupted aortic arch, hypoplastic left heart, COA) are commonly associated with DiGeorge syndrome (Park, 1996).

Hypoglycemia may be present in infants with severe CHF. The myocardium is dependent on glucose; decreased glucose levels diminish the ability of the heart to compensate for CHF. On chest radiograph, the heart is enlarged and there is increased pulmonary congestion. ECG is not generally diagnostic, unless the CHF is caused by an arrhythmia. There may be nonspecific changes in the T waves, changes in the ST segment, and an increase in the height of the P wave.

Electrolyte imbalances usually include relative hyponatremia, which is due to the increase in free water. Hypochloremia and increased bicarbonate may result from respiratory acidemia and the use of loop diuretics. Hyperkalemia results from the release of intracellular cations, which is related to poor tissue perfusion. Elevated lactic acid levels are also indicative of tissue hypoxia. Atrial natriuretic factor (ANF), a peptide hormone, may be important in the regulation of volume and blood pressure. ANF is released from the atria when they are distended. ANF release causes natriuresis, diuresis, and vasodilation. ANF acts with other volume regulators, such as renin, aldosterone, and vasopressin. An increased ANF level may be found when there is increased pulmonary blood flow, increased left atrial pressure, or pulmonary hypertension.

Children with corrected or noncorrected congenital heart defects frequently have abnormal homeostasis, suggesting a chronic compensated disseminated intravascular coagulopathy, with reduced synthesis of clotting factors and/or deranged platelet aggregation (Goel et al., 2000), so bleeding problems may be present.

Nursing Management

The goal of management of CHF is to improve cardiac function while identifying and correcting the underlying cause. General measures that decrease the demand on the heart are helpful; however, pharmacologic intervention is the most efficacious therapy.

General measures General measures to manage CHF include the administration of oxygen to improve ventilation and perfusion at the alveolar level. Ventilation with positive end-expiratory pressure at 6 to 10 cm H_2O may relieve the effects of CHF by reducing pulmonary edema.

Fluid restriction may decrease the circulating volume. Careful monitoring of serum electrolytes, intake and output, and weight is essential. It is imperative that *all* fluid be counted in the total daily fluid volume. Infants with CHF do not usually feed well and may require caloric supplementation with hyperalimentation or gavage feedings (Park, 1996).

Infants with CHF are irritable and agitated, which further complicates their status. Sedation with continuous infusions of morphine sulfate or fentanyl may improve the infant's comfort and oxygenation. Other measures that reduce cardiac demand include maintenance of a normal hematocrit, maintenance of a thermoneutral environment, and minimal stimulation. Cautious use of sedation may reduce anxiety and agitation, increasing comfort and decreasing the demand for oxygen.

The mainstay of management of CHF beyond the neonatal period is digitalis (digoxin). Digoxin slows conduction through the AV node, prolongs the refractory period, and slows the heart rate through vagal effects on the SA node.

The use of digoxin in preterm or term neonates is controversial. The preterm newborn is at risk for digitalis toxicity because of the narrow range between therapeutic and toxic drug levels. The preterm infant requires a lower maintenance dose because of limited renal excretion of the drug. If digoxin is used, the neonate must be carefully monitored for signs and symptoms of digitalis toxicity. Lead II ECGs should be obtained before each dose for the first 3 days; the dose should be withheld if the P-R interval is greater than 0.16 second or if there is an arrhythmia present. Digoxin levels should be monitored and should be less than 2.0 ng/ml (Park, 1996). Blood samples for digoxin levels should be drawn after the drug has achieved equilibrium in the body, approximately 6 to 8 hours after administration.

Other inotropic agents can be used to improve cardiac output. Dopamine, a norepinephrine precursor, has direct and indirect beta-adrenergic effects that are dose dependent. At low doses (2 to 5 µg/kg/min), there is increased renal blood flow with minimal effect on heart rate, blood pressure, or contractility. Medium doses (5 to 10 µg/kg/min) increase renal blood flow, heart rate, blood pressure, and contractility. Pulmonary artery pressure may be increased; peripheral resistance is not affected. High doses (10 to 20 µg/kg/min) cause alpha effects, resulting in peripheral vasoconstriction, increased cardiac rate, and increased contractility (Park, 1996).

Dobutamine is a synthetic catecholamine that acts on beta- and alpha-adrenergic receptors. Dobutamine (2 to 10 µg/min) has decreased effects on the heart rate and rhythm and causes less peripheral vasoconstriction.

Isoproterenol (Isuprel), a synthetic epinephrine-like substance, has $beta_1$- and $beta_2$-adrenergic effects. The usefulness of Isuprel in the neonate is limited because it produces increased heart rate, arrhythmias, and decreased systemic vascular resistance, which may worsen the hypotension (Park, 1996).

Diuretics   Diuretics are useful in the treatment of CHF to decrease sodium and water retention. The primary goal is to increase renal perfusion (with inotropic agents or vasodilators) and to increase sodium delivery to distal diluting sites of the renal tubules. Diuretic agents increase the renal excretion of sodium and other anions by inhibition of tubular reabsorption of sodium (Park, 1996).

Furosemide (Lasix) is a loop diuretic that blocks sodium and chloride reabsorption in the ascending limb of the loop of Henle. Loop diuretics interfere with the formation of free water and free water reabsorption by preventing the transport of sodium, potassium, and chloride into the medullary interstitium. Loop diuretics cause increased excretion of potassium by delivering increased quantities of sodium to sites in the distal nephron where potassium can be excreted. Furosemide also increases excretion of calcium but does not affect the ability of the kidney to regulate acid-base balance.

An aldosterone antagonist such as spironolactone (Aldactone) may be useful because it is a potassium-sparing diuretic. Spironolactone works by binding to the cytoplasmic receptor sites and blocking aldosterone action, thus impairing the reabsorption of sodium and the secretion of potassium and hydrogen ion. Spironolactone has no effect on free water production and absorption. Thiazide diuretics (chlorothiazide, hydrochlorothiazide) inhibit sodium and chloride reabsorption along the distal tubules. They are not as effective as the loop diuretics and are infrequently used (Park, 1996).

Complications of diuretic therapy. The complications of diuretic therapy include (1) volume contraction, (2) hyponatremia, (3) metabolic alkalemia or acidemia, and (4) hypokalemia or hyperkalemia. When using diuretics, fluid and electrolyte balance must be maintained by administration of water and electrolytes. The adequacy of the volume can be determined by monitoring serum electrolytes, BUN, creatinine, urinary output, weight, specific gravity, and skin turgor.

The increased renal losses of sodium can lead to hyponatremia unless adequate amounts of sodium are provided. There may also be increased antidiuretic hormone release secondary to changes in the osmoreceptors or inhibition of antidiuretic hormone action. Decreasing the amount of total water and improving the cardiac output, thus increasing renal perfusion, can best manage this condition.

Metabolic alkalosis can result from administration of loop diuretics that interfere with sodium- and potassium-dependent chloride reabsorption. Hypochloremia results in a greater aldosterone production and an increase in bicarbonate concentration. Hypokalemia is a frequent complication of loop diuretic therapy. An increased ratio of intracellular to extracellular potassium results in the clinical signs and symptoms of hypokalemia. Hypokalemia increases the risk for digoxin toxicity. In contrast, hyperkalemia may result when the cardiac output is low and tissue perfusion is severely compromised. Other complications of diuretic therapy include increased calcium excretion, hyperuricemia, and glucose intolerance.

Vasodilators may be used in severe CHF to reduce the right and left ventricular preload and afterload to improve cardiac function.

Vasodilators cause arterial and venous dilation, resulting in decreased systemic and pulmonary vascular resistance. Sodium nitroprusside (Nipride) is a smooth muscle relaxant that decreases ventricular afterload by decreasing pulmonary and systemic vascular resistance and decreases venous return and ventricular preload. This leads to decreased ventricular end-diastolic volume, increased ejection fraction, increased heart rate and cardiac index, and decreased pulmonary and systemic resistance. Sodium nitroprusside is sensitive to light and must be stored in dark containers. Side effects are cyanide toxicity and decreased platelet function (Park, 1996). The prognosis for CHF depends on the severity of the underlying condition and on the degree of CHF.

SUBACUTE INFECTIVE ENDOCARDITIS

SAIE can be a complication of CHD. Two factors are important in the development of SAIE: (1) structural abnormalities that create turbulent flow or pressure gradients and (2) bacteremia. All cardiac defects that produce turbulent flow or have a significant pressure gradient predispose the patient to bacterial invasion of the cardiac endothelium. The turbulent flow damages the endothelial lining and platelet–fibrin thrombus formation. Prevention of bacterial SAIE requires scrupulous daily oral care as well as prophylactic antimicrobials for dental procedures (Park, 1996). All CHDs, except secundum-type ASDs, predispose the patient to SAIE. VSDs, TOF, and aortic stenosis are the CHDs most commonly associated with SAIE (Park, 1996).

Vegetation of SAIE is usually on the low-pressure side of the defect, where endothelial damage is established by the jet effect of the defect. More than 90% of SAIE cases are caused by *Streptococcus viridans*, *Streptococcus faecalis* (enterococcus), and S*taphylococcus aureus*. Other organisms include *Haemophilus influenzae, Pseudomonas, Escherichia coli, Proteus, Aerobacter,* and *Listeria. Candida* may infect infants who have been receiving long-term antimicrobial or steroid therapy.

Prevention

Procedures for which SAIE prophylaxis is indicated include (1) all dental procedures, (2) tonsillectomy or adenoidectomy, (3) surgical procedures involving the respiratory mucosa, (4) bronchoscopy, (5) incision and drainage of infected tissue, and (6) gastrointestinal or genitourinary procedures.

HYPERTENSION

For many different reasons an infant may experience hypertension. Table 8-1 gives the most common antihypertensive medications that can be used.

Table 8-1	Antihypertensive Medications	
Drug	**Dose**	**Route**
Sodium nitro- prusside	0.5-80 μg/kg/min	IV
Labetalol	0.25-3 mg/kg/hr	IV
	0.20-1.0 mg/kg	IV
Diazoxide	2-5 mg/kg (bolus)	IV
Hydralazine	0.1-0.4 mg/kg/dose	IV
Enalaprilat	5-30 μg/kg/day	IV
Captopril	0.03-2.0 mg/kg/day	PO
Nifedipine	0.2-0.3 mg/kg	PO/SL
Propranolol	0.5-4.0 mg/kg/day	PO
Furosemide	1-10 mg/kg/day	PO/IV/ continuous drip
Chlorothiazide	20-40 mg/kg/day	PO/IV

From Vogt BA, Davis ID, Avner ED (2001). The kidney. In Klaus MH, Fanaroff AA, editors. Care of the high-risk neonate, ed 5, Philadelphia: WB Saunders, p. 439.
IV, Intravenously; PO, orally; SL, sublingually.

BIBLIOGRAPHY

Bevilacqua L, Hordof A (1998). Cardiac pacing in children. *Current opinion in cardiology*, 13(1), 48-55.

Botto LD, Correa A, Erickson JD (2001). Racial and temporal variations in the prevalence of heart defects. *Pediatrics*, 107(3), 1-8.

Bradley SM, Simsic JM, Atz AM (2001). Hemodynamic effects of inspired carbon dioxide after the Norwood procedure. *Annals of thoracic surgery*, 72(6), 2088-2093; discussion 2093-2094.

Burlet A, Drukker A, Guignard JP (1999). Renal function in cyanotic congenital heart disease. *Nephron*, 81(3), 296-300.

Centers for Disease Control and Prevention (CDC) (1998). Trends in infant mortality attributable to birth defects—United States, 1980-1995. *Morbidity and mortality weekly reports (MMWR)*, 47(37), 773-778.

Colucci WS, Braunwald E (2001). Pathophysiology of heart failure. (pp. 503-533). In Braunwald E, editor. *Heart disease: a textbook of cardiovascular medicine*, Philadelphia: WB Saunders.

Dosing Interval	Action	Comment
Continuous	Vasodilator	Drug of choice
Continuous Bolus every 6 hr	Alpha-, beta-blockade	Drug of choice
Every 12 hr	Vasodilator	Second-line drug
Bolus every 4 hr	Vasodilator	Second-line drug
Every 6-24 hr	ACE (angiotensin-converting enzyme) inhibitor	Second-line drug
Every 6-12 hr	ACE inhibitor	
Every 30 min–4 hr	Calcium channel antagonist	PO/SL administration
Every 6-12 hr	Beta-blockade	Contraindicated in heart block and heart failure
Every 8-24 hr	Loop diuretic	
Every 12 hr	Distal tubule diuretic	Give 30 min before furosemide

Cooley DA (1997). Early development of congenital heart surgery: open heart procedures. *Annals of thoracic surgery*, 64(5), 1544-1548.

Danford DA, et al. (1999). Pulmonary stenosis: defect-specific diagnostic accuracy of heart murmurs in children. *Journal of pediatrics*, 134(1), 76-81.

Devine PC, Malone FD (2000). Noncardiac thoracic anomalies. *Clinics in perinatology*, 27(4), 865-899.

Dodge-Khatami A, et al. (2001). Neonatal complete correction of tetralogy of Fallot versus shunting and deferred repair: is the future of the right ventriculo-arterial junction at stake, and what of it? *Cardiology of the young*, 11(5), 484-490.

Goel M, et al (2000). Haemostatic changes in children with cyanotic and acyanotic congenital heart disease. *Int House of Japan* 559-563.

Holper K (2001). Results of biventricular repair of congenital cardiac malformations: definitive corrective surgery? *European journal of cardiothoracic surgery*, 20(6), 1207-1213.

Lott JW (2003). Assessment and management of the cardiac system. In Kenner C, Lott JW, editors. *Comprehensive neonatal nursing care: a physiologic perspective*, ed 3, St Louis: WB Saunders.

Park MK (1996). *Pediatric Cardiology for Practitioners*, ed 3, St Louis, Mosby, p. 408.

Tchervenkov CI, et al. (2001). Neonatal aortic arch reconstruction avoiding circulatory arrest and direct arch vessel cannulation. *Annals of thoracic surgery*, 72(5), 1615-1620.

Turner SW, Hunter S, Wyllie JP (1999). The natural history of ventricular septal defects. *Archives of disease in childhood*, 81(5), 413-416.

Welch KK, Brown SA (2000). The role of genetic counseling in the management of prenatally detected congenital heart defects. *Seminars in perinatology*, 24(5), 373-379.

CHAPTER 9

NEONATAL INFECTIONS

Fetal and neonatal infections are the most common cause of morbidity and mortality in the neonatal intensive care unit (NICU) population. Prevention, early recognition, and effective treatment are imperative if neonatal health outcomes are to improve. Nurses are often the health professionals who have the most consistent contact with an infant. Thus it is the nurse who often identifies a problem long before there are changes in vital signs or in lab values. A subtle sign of infection can be as simple as an infant not "looking quite right" or not feeding as well as in the past. Nursing assessment, along with a knowledge of the risk factors present from the maternal and neonatal histories, is imperative.

CLINICAL MANIFESTATIONS

1. Temperature instability or hypothermia or hyperthermia
2. Lethargy
3. Poor feeding
4. Decreased reflexes
5. Abdominal distention
6. Diarrhea
7. Failure to thrive, poor weight gain
8. Hypoglycemia or hyperglycemia, glycosuria
9. Decreased vascular perfusion, poor capillary refill
10. Color—pale, cyanotic, or mottled
11. Petechiae
12. Thrombocytopenia
13. Prolonged prothrombin time (PT), partial thromboplastin time (PTT)
14. Increased split fibrin products
15. Hemolytic anemia
16. Apnea
17. Bradycardia
18. Cardiovascular shock
19. Sclerema
20. Sudden purpura, rash, or petechiae indicating systemic infection

DIAGNOSTIC LABS

1. Complete blood count (CBC) with differential
2. PT, PTT times
3. Split fibrin products

INDICATIONS OF BACTERIAL INFECTION*

- Increased total neutrophils—neutrophilia
- Decreased total neutrophils—neutropenia
- Increased immature forms (bands, metamyelocytes, sometimes promyelocytes and myeloblasts)
- Increased band/segmented neutrophil ratio equal to or greater than 0:3 or immature neutrophil/total neutrophil ratio greater than or equal to 0:2
- Presence of Döhle bodies (aggregates of reticuloendothelial system)
- Presence of vacuoles in nucleus
- Toxic granules in cell
- CD11b found on neutrophils
- Increased interleukin 8 (IL-8) levels

RECENT CHANGES IN EPIDEMIOLOGY AND MANAGEMENT OF INFECTIOUS DISEASES OF THE FETUS AND NEWBORN INFANT†

Epidemiology

- Increased viability of very low–birth weight infants at risk for invasive infectious disease
- Increased number of multiple births (often of very low birth weight) because of successful techniques for management of infertility
- Global perspective of vertically transmitted infectious diseases
- Early discharge from the nursery mandated by insurance programs leading to concern for decreased time of observation for infants at risk for sepsis

Diagnosis

- Polymerase chain reaction (PCR) for diagnosis of infection in mother, fetus, and neonate
- Decreased use of fetal blood sampling and chorionic villus sampling for diagnosis of infectious diseases

Prevention

- Peripartum antibiotics to prevent early-onset group B streptococcal infection

*From Lott JW, Kenner C (2003). Assessment and management of the immune system. In Kenner C, Lott JW, editors. Comprehensive neonatal nursing: a physiologic perspective, St Louis: WB Saunders.
†From Klein JO, Remington JS (2001). Current concepts of infections of the fetus and newborn infant. In Remington JS, Klein JO, editors. Infectious disease of the fetus and newborn infant. Philadelphia: WB Saunders, p. 2.

- Antiretroviral therapy in pregnancy to prevent transmission of human immunodeficiency virus (HIV) to fetus (Figure 9-1 and Table 9-1)

Treatment
- Antiretroviral therapy in the mother to treat the HIV-infected fetus
- Antitoxoplasmosis therapy in the mother to treat the infected fetus
- Spread within nurseries of antibiotic-resistant bacterial pathogens
- Increased use of vancomycin for multidrug-resistant gram-positive infections
- Increased use of acyclovir for infants with suspected herpes simplex meningoencephalitis

Location
Tuberculosis is on the rise in the United States so it has to be considered a potential infectious agent for neonates. With the recent

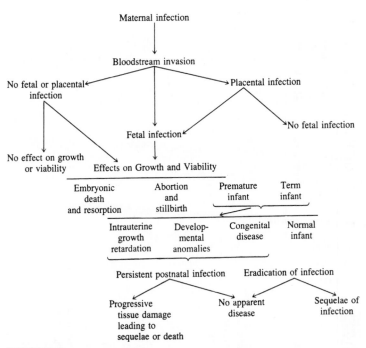

FIGURE **9-1**
Pathogenesis of hematogenous transplacental infections. (From Klein JO, Remington JS [2001]. Current concepts of infections of the fetus and newborn infant. In Remington JS, Klein JO, editors. *Infectious diseases of the fetus and newborn infant*, Philadelphia: WB Saunders, p. 4.)

Table 9-1 Effects of Tranplacental Fetal Infection on the Fetus and Newborn Infant

Organism or Disease	Prematurity	Intrauterine Growth Retardation and Low Birth Weight	Developmental Anomalies	Congenital Disease	Persistent Positive Infection
Viruses					
Rubella	–	+	+	+	+
Cytomegalovirus	+	+	+	+	+
Herpes simplex	+	–	–	+	+
Varicella–zoster	–	(+)	+	(+)	–
Mumps	–	–	–	(+)	–
Rubeola	+	–	–	+	–
Vaccinia	–	–	–	+	–
Smallpox	+	–	–	+	–
Coxsackieviruses B	–	–	(+)	–	–
Echoviruses	–	–	–	+	–
Polioviruses	–	–	–	–	–
Influenza	+	–	–	+	–
Hepatitis B	(+)	(+)	–	–	+
Human immunodeficiency virus	–	–	(+)	+	+
Lymphocytic choriomeningitis virus	–	–	–	+	–
Parvovirus	–	–	–	+	–

Bacteria				
Treponema pallidum	+	–	+	+
Mycobacterium tuberculosis	+	–	+	+
Listeria monocytogenes	+	–	+	–
Campylobacter fetus	+	–	+	–
Salmonella typhosa	+	–	+	–
Borrelia burgdorferi	–	–	+	–
Protozoa				
Toxoplasma gondii	+	+	+	+
Plasmodium	(+)	+	+	+
Trypanosoma cruzi	+	+	+	–

From Klein JO, Remington JS (2001). Current concepts of infections of the fetus and newborn infant. In Remington JS, Klein JO, editors. Infectious disease of the fetus and newborn infant. Philadelphia: WB Saunders, p. 6.
+, Evidence for effect; –, no evidence for effect; (+), association of effect with infection has been suggested and is under consideration.

emphasis on bioterrorism smallpox, a disease that was once thought to be eradicated has come to the forefront in health care again. Thus we have included it in this listing of possible infectious agents (Table 9-2).

The neonate is conferred some passive immunity (Table 9-3) from the mother to the fetus through the placenta. This immunity depends on maternal exposures and whether the mother has certain antibodies. Another factor to consider that influences maternal immunity is the mother's own health and nutritional status. A woman who is in a compromised state will not be able to pass on much protection to her fetus and neonate. Table 9-3 indicates the usual protection from mother to fetus and illustrates that some agents do not readily pass through the placenta.

Immunologic factors are produced in thymus, bone marrow, blood, and tissues (Figure 9-2).

Neonatal infections are a global issue. The causative agents depend on those organisms that are endemic in that part of the world. However, the factors that increase an infant's susceptibility to infection are slightly different in developing vs. developed countries. For example, in parts of Africa neonatal tetanus is an increasing problem. Table 9-4 has information for nurses working in a developing country.

The following are suggested interventions for decreasing the incidence of neonatal infections in developing countries.

INTERVENTIONS TO REDUCE NEONATAL INFECTIONS OR TO REDUCE INFECTION AND ASSOCIATED MORTALITY IN DEVELOPING COUNTRIES

Antenatal Care
- Tetanus immunization
- Maternal immunization with new vaccines in the future (e.g., group B streptococci, *Haemophilus influenzae* type B, pneumococcus)
- Primary prevention of sexually transmitted disease, urinary tract infection, malaria, tuberculosis, other infections
- Plan for clean and safe delivery

Intrapartum/Delivery Care
- Prevent prolonged labor
- Optimal management of complications, including fever, premature rupture of membranes, puerperal sepsis
- Clean delivery
- Clean cutting of cord/optimal cord care

Breast-Feeding
- Promote early and exclusive breast-feeding (HIV dilemma noted)

Table 9-2	Clinical Manifestations of Neonatal Infection Acquired in Utero or at Delivery						
	Microorganism						
Clinical Sign	Rubella Virus	Cytomegalo-virus	Toxoplasma Gondii	Herpes Simplex Virus	Treponema Pallidum	Entero-viruses	Group B Streptococcus or Escherichia Coli
Hepatosplenomegaly	+	+	+	+	+	+	+
Jaundice	+	+	+	+	+	+	+
Adenopathy	+	–	+	–	+	+	–
Pneumonitis	+	+	+	+	+	+	+
Lesions of Skin or Mucous Membranes							
Petechiae or purpura	+	+	+	+	+	+	+
Vesicles	–	+	–	++	+	–	–
Maculopapular exanthems	–	–	+	+	++	+	–
Lesions of Nervous System							
Meningoencephalitis	+	+	+	+	+	+	+
Microcephaly	–	++	+	+	–	–	–
Hydrocephalus	+	+	++	+	–	–	–
Intracranial calcifications	–	++	++	–	–	++	–
Paralysis	–	–	–	–	+	–	–
Hearing deficits	+	+	–	–	+	–	–

Continued

Table 9-2 Clinical Manifestations of Neonatal Infection Acquired in Utero or at Delivery—cont'd

	Microorganism						
Clinical Sign	Rubella Virus	Cytomegalo-virus	Toxoplasma Gondii	Herpes Simplex Virus	Treponema Pallidum	Entero-viruses	Group B Streptococcus or Escherichia Coli
Lesions of Heart							
Myocarditis	+	-	+	+	-	++	-
Congenital defects	++	-	-	-	-	-	-
Bone lesions	++	-	+	-	++	-	-
Eye Lesions							
Glaucoma	++	-	-	-	+	-	-
Chorioretinitis or retinopathy	++	+	++	+	+	-	-
Cataracts	++	-	+	+	-	-	-
Optic atrophy	-	+	+	-	-	-	-
Microophthalmia	+	-	+	-	-	-	-
Uveitis	-	-	+	-	+	+	-
Conjunctivitis or keratoconjunctivitis	-	-	-	++	-	-	-

From Klein JO, Remington JS (2001). Current concepts of infections of the fetus and newborn infant. In Remington JS, Klein JO, editors. Infectious diseases of the fetus and newborn infant, Philadelphia: WB Saunders, p. 8.
−, Either not present or rare in infected infants; +, occurs in infants with infection; ++, has special diagnostic significance for this infection.

Table 9-3	Neonatal Passive Immunity: Placental Passage of Maternal Antibodies		
Good Passive Transfer (Immunoglobulin G [IgG])	**Poor Passive Transfer**	**No Passive Transfer***
Tetanus antitoxin	*Bordetella pertussis* Ab	*Salmonella* somatic (O) Ab
Diphtheria antitoxin	*Shigella flexneri* Ab	*Escherichia coli* H and O Ab
Bordetella pertussis agglutinin	*Streptococcus* Mg Ab	Heterophil Ab
Antistreptolysin Ab		Wassermann AB
Antistaphylolysin Ab		Natural (anti-A, anti-B) iso-agglutinins
Poliomyelitis Ab		Rh saline (complete) agglutinins
Measles, mumps, rubella Ab		Reaginic Ab (IgE)
Herpes simplex Ab		
Haemophilus influenzae Ab		
Group B streptococcal Ab		
Salmonella flagellar (H) Ab		
Rh incomplete (Coombs') Ab		
Immune (anti-A, anti-B) isoagglutinins		
VDRL Ab		
Long-acting thyroid stimulator		
Antinuclear Ab (ANA)		

Modified from Miller ME, Stiehm ER (1983). Immunology and resistance to infection. In Lewis DB, Wilson CB (2001). Developmental immunology and role of host defenses in fetal and neonatal susceptibility to infection. In Remington JS, Klein JO, editors. Infectious disease of the fetus and newborn infant, Philadelphia: WB Saunders, p. 68.
Ab, Antibodies; VDRL, Venereal Disease Research Laboratories.
Mostly immunoglobulin M (IgM).

Gender Issues
- Promote gender equality.
- Encourage education of girls.

INTERVENTIONS TO DECREASE LOW BIRTH WEIGHT AND/OR PREMATURITY
- Delay child-bearing in young adolescents
- Promote maternal education

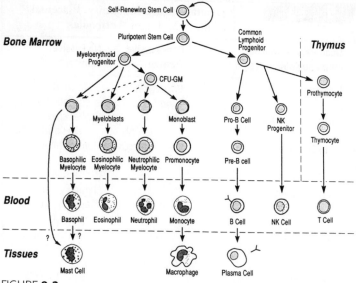

FIGURE **9-2**
The myeloid and lymphoid differentiation and tissue compartments in which they occur. CFU-GM, Colony-forming unit–granulocyte-monocyte. (From Lewis DB, Wilson CB [2001]. Developmental immunology and role of host defenses in fetal and neonatal susceptibility to infection. In Remington JS, Klein JO, editors. *Infectious diseases of the fetus and newborn infant*, Philadelphia: WB Saunders, p. 75.)

- Improve maternal nutrition: caloric supplementation before and during pregnancy
- Reduce tobacco use
- Diagnose and treat sexually transmitted diseases
- Malaria prophylaxis and treatment
- Limit maternal workload during pregnancy
- Maternal support to decrease stress/anxiety

Community-Based Interventions
- Train birth attendants to identify problems in the newborn, treat similar problems, refer newborns with serious illness
- Promote and support breast-feeding (HIV dilemma noted)
- Maternal education regarding personal and domestic hygiene, newborn care, childhood immunization
- Home-based diagnosis and treatment of newborn infections

EARLY IDENTIFICATION AND IMPROVED TREATMENT OF NEONATES WITH INFECTION

- Integrated approach to the sick young infant (WHO/UNICEF)
- Improved newborn care at all levels: home, village, health center, district hospital, referral hospital

Table **9-4**	Direct and Indirect Causes of Infection-Related Neonatal Death in Less Developed Countries
Direct Causes of Death	**Indirect Causes of Death**
Medical	Sociocultural
Sepsis	Poverty
Meningitis	Illiteracy
Omphalitis with sepsis	Low social status of women
Tetanus	Lack of political power
Pneumonia	Gender discrimination (for mother and newborn)
Tuberculosis	Harmful traditional practices
Diarrhea	Poor hygiene
Malaria	Lack of clean water and sanitation
HIV/AIDS	Cultural belief that a sick newborn is doomed to die
	Inability to recognize danger signs in sick newborn
	Poor care-seeking behavior
	Inadequate access to high-quality medical care
	Lack of transport for emergency care
	Lack of appropriate drugs
	Maternal death
	Medical
	Poor maternal health
	Untreated maternal infections, including sexually transmitted diseases, urinary tract infection, chorioamnionitis
	Failure to fully immunize mother against tetanus
	Inappropriate management of labor and delivery
	Unsanitary cutting and care of the umbilical cord
	Failure to promote early and exclusive breast-feeding (HIV dilemma noted)
	Prematurity/low birth weight

Modified from Stoll BJ (1997). The global impact of neonatal infection. Journal of clinical perinatology, 24, 1-21. In Stoll B (2001). Neonatal infections: a global perspective. In Remington JS, Klein JO, editors. Infectious diseases of the fetus and newborn infant. Philadelphia: WB Saunders, p. 155.

NEONATAL IMMUNIZATION

Box 9-1 gives interventions to reduce neonatal infections and associated mortality.

Box **9-1**

Interventions to Reduce Neonatal Infections or to Reduce Infection-Associated Mortality in Developing Countires

Antenatal Care
Tetanus immunization
Maternal immunization with new vaccines in the future (e.g, group B streptocci, *Haemophilus influenzae* type B, pneumoccocus)
Primary prevention of sexually transmitted diseases, including HIV, through maternal education and safer sex using condoms
Diagnosis and treatment of sexually transmitted diseases, urinary tract infection, malaria, tuberculosis, other infections
Plan clean and safe delivery

Intrapartum/Delivery Care
Prevent prolonged labor
Optimal management of complications, including fever, premature rupture of membranes, puerperal sepsis
Clean delivery
Clean cutting of cord/optimal cord care

Breast-Feeding
Promote early and exclusive breast-feeding (HIV dilemma noted)
Gender Issues
Promote gender equality
Encourage education of girls

Interventions to Decrease Low Birth Weight and/or Prematurity
Delay child-bearing in young adolescents
Promote maternal education
Improve maternal nutrition: caloric supplementation before and during pregnancy
Reduce tobacco use
Diagnose and treat sexually transmitted diseases
Malaria prophylaxis and treatment
Limit maternal workload during pregnancy
Maternal support to decrease stress/anxiety

Box 9-1

Interventions to Reduce Neonatal Infections or to Reduce Infection-Associated Mortality in Developing Countires—cont'd

Community-Based Interventions
Train birth attendants to identify problems in the newborn, treat similar
   problems, refer newborns with serious illness
Promote and support breast-feeding (HIV dilemma noted)
Maternal education regarding personal and domestic hygiene,
   newborn care, childhood immunization
Home-based diagnosis and treatment of newborn infections

***Early Identification and Improved Treatment of Neonates with
Infection***
Integrated approach to the sick young infant (WHO/UNICEF)
Improve newborn care at all levels: home, village, health center, district
   hospital, referral hospital

Neonatal Immunization
Bacillus Calmette-Guérin, hepatitis B, other new vaccines (e.g.,
   rotavirus)

*Adapted from Stoll BJ (1997). The global impact of neonatal infection.
Clinics in Perinatology, 24, 1-21; Stoll BJ: Neonatal infections: a global
perspective. In Remington JS, Klein JO, editors. Infectious disease of the fetus
and newborn infant. Philadelphia: WB Saunders, p. 156.*

DIFFERENTIAL DIAGNOSIS

Since there are many reasons why an infant may present with clinical
symptoms described above it is important to consider the most likely
causes.

Differential Diagnosis of Clinical Signs Associated with Neonatal Sepsis and Some Noninfectious Conditions*

1. **Respiratory distress** (apnea, cyanosis, costal and sternal retrac-
   tion, rales, grunting, diminished breath sounds, tachypnea)
   a. Transient tachypnea of the newborn
   b. Respiratory distress syndrome

*From Klein JO (2001). Bacterial sepsis and meningitis. In Remington JS, Klein JO,
editors. Infectious diseases of the fetus and newborn infant, ed 5, Philadelphia: WB
Saunders, p. 966.

  c. Atelectasis
  d. Aspiration pneumonia, including meconium aspiration
  e. Pneumothorax
  f. Pneumomediastinum
  g. Central nervous system disease: hypoxia, hemorrhage
  h. Congenital abnormalities, including tracheoesophageal fistula, choanal atresia, diaphragmatic hernia, hypoplastic lungs
  i. Congenital heart disease
  j. Cardiac arrhythmia
  k. Hypothermia (neonatal cold injury)
  l. Hypoglycemia
  m. Neonatal drug withdrawal syndrome
  n. Medication error with inhaled epinephrine

2. **Temperature abnormality** (hyperthermia or hypothermia)
  a. Altered environmental temperature
  b. Disturbance of central nervous system thermoregulatory mechanism, including anoxia, hemorrhage, kernicterus
  c. Hyperthyroidism or hypothyroidism
  d. Neonatal drug withdrawal syndrome
  e. Dehydration
  f. Congenital adrenal hyperplasia
  g. Vaccine reaction

3. **Jaundice**
  a. Breast milk jaundice
  b. Blood group incompatibility
  c. Red cell hemolysis, including blood group incompatibility, G6PD deficiency
  d. Reabsorption of blood from closed-space hemorrhage
  e. Gastrointestinal obstruction, including pyloric stenosis
  f. Extrahepatic or intrahepatic biliary tract obstruction
  g. Errors of metabolism, including galactosemia, glycogen storage disease type IV, tyrosinemia, disorders of lipid metabolism, paroxysmal disorders, defective bile acid synthesis (trihydroxycoprostanic acidemia)

4. **Hepatomegaly**
  a. Red cell hemolysis, including blood group incompatibility, G6PD deficiency
  b. Infant of a diabetic mother
  c. Errors of metabolism, including galactosemia, glycogen storage disease, organic acidemias, urea cycle disorders, hereditary fructose intolerance, paroxysmal disorders
  d. Biliary atresia
  e. Congestive heart failure
  f. Benign liver tumors, including hemangioma, hamartoma
  g. Malignant liver tumors, including hepatoblastoma, metastatic neuroblastoma, congenital leukemia

5. **Gastrointestinal abnormalities** (anorexia, regurgitation, vomiting, diarrhea, abdominal distention)
   a. Gastrointestinal allergy
   b. Overfeeding, aerophagia
   c. Intestinal obstruction (intraluminal or extrinsic)
   d. Necrotizing enterocolitis
   e. Hypokalemia
   f. Hypercalcemia or hypocalcemia
   g. Hypoglycemia
   h. Errors of metabolism, including galactosemia, urea cycle disorders, organic acidemias
   i. Ileus secondary to pneumonia
   j. Congenital adrenal hyperplasia
   k. Gastric perforation
   l. Neonatal drug withdrawal syndrome
6. **Lethargy**
   a. Central nervous system disease, including hemorrhage, hypoxia, or subdural effusion
   b. Congenital heart disease
   c. Neonatal drug withdrawal syndrome
   d. Hypoglycemia
   e. Hypercalcemia
   f. Familial dysautonomia
7. **Seizure activity** (tremors, hyperactivity, muscular twitching)
   a. Hypoxia
   b. Intracranial hemorrhage or kernicterus
   c. Congenital central nervous system malformations
   d. Neonatal drug withdrawal syndrome
   e. Hypoglycemia
   f. Hypocalcemia
   g. Hyponatremia, hypernatremia
   h. Hypomagnesemia
   i. Errors of metabolism, including urea cycle disorders, organic acidemias, galactosemia, glycogen storage disease, paroxysmal disorders
   j. Pyridoxine deficiency
8. **Petechiae and purpura**
   a. Birth trauma
   b. Blood group incompatibility
   c. Neonatal isoimmune thrombocytopenia
   d. Maternal idiopathic thrombocytopenic purpura
   e. Maternal lupus erythematosus
   f. Drugs administered to mother
   g. Giant hemangioma (Kasabach-Merritt syndrome)
   h. Thrombocytopenia with absent radii (RAR) syndrome
   i. Disseminated intravascular coagulopathy

   j. Coagulation factor deficiencies
   k. Congenital leukemia
   l. Child abuse

Table 9-5 gives characteristics of cerebrospinal fluid in normal very low–birth weight infants.

MENINGITIS

One of the most serious conditions in the neonatal is an inflammation of the meninges, meningitis. This condition can be caused by infectious and noninfectious factors (Table 9-6). In fact the meningitis may be considered aseptic in some instances, meaning that there is no known bacterial agent causing the inflammation.

NEONATAL INFECTIONS

Neonatal infections can arise from a variety of organisms as indicated in previous sections. The following sections will highlight the most common causes, clinical symptoms, and treatments of neonatal infections.

TORCH Infections

The cluster of sexually transmitted infections (STIs) is still a major concern during the fetal/neonatal period. The TORCH infections are toxoplasmosis, others, rubella, cytomegalovirus (CMV), and herpes.

TOXOPLASMOSIS

Toxoplasmosis is caused by the parasite *Toxoplasma gondii*. It is generally spread by perinatal transmission that takes place when the mother contracts the protozoa and the subsequent protozoemia transmits the organism transplacentally to the fetus. The microorganisms then invade and multiply within the placenta and eventually enter the fetal circulation. The life cycle of *Toxoplasma* is complicated. The predominant host of this organism is the ordinary house cat; however, other animals can serve as hosts (Lott, Kenner, 2003).

Clinical Manifestations

The most common clinical manifestations are as follows:
- Prematurity
- Dysmaturity or intrauterine growth restriction
- Chorioretinitis
- Hydrocephalus
- Hypotonia
- Anemia
- Intracranial calcifications
- Jaundice
- Hepatomegaly

Table 9-5	Hematologic and Chemical Characteristics of Cerebrospinal Fluid in Normal Very Low–Birth Weight Infants					
Birth Weight (g)	Age (Days)	Red Blood Cells (mm³) Mean (Range)	White Blood Cells (mm³) Mean (Range)	Polymorphonuclear Leukocytes (%) Mean (Range)	Glucose (mg/dl) Mean (Range)	Protein (mg/dl) Mean (Range)
<1000	0-7	335 (0-1780)	3 (1-8)	11 (0-50)	70 (41-89)	162 (115-222)
	8-28	1465 (0-19,050)	4 (0-14)	8 (0-66)	68 (33-217)	159 (95-370)
	29-84	808 (0-6850)	4 (0-11)	2 (0-36)	49 (29-90)	137 (76-260)
1000-1500	0-7	407 (0-2450)	4 (1-10)	4 (0-28)	74 (50-96)	136 (85-176)
	8-28	1101 (0-9750)	7 (0-44)	10 (0-60)	59 (39-109)	137 (54-227)
	29-84	661 (0-3800)	8 (0-23)	11 (0-48)	47 (31-76)	122 (45-187)

From Klein JO (2001). Bacterial sepsis and meningitis. In Remington JS, Klein JO, editors. Infections diseases of the fetus and newborn infant, ed 5, Philadelphia: WB Saunders, p. 973. Modified from Rodriguez AF, Kaplan SL, Mason EO (1990). Cerebralspinal fluid values in the very low birth weight infant. J Pediatric 116:971.

Table 9-6	Infectious and Noninfectious Causes of Aseptic Meningitis* in the Neonate
Agent	**Disease**
Infectious	
Bacteria	Partially treated meningitis
	Parameningeal focus (brain or epidural abscess) tuberculosis
Viruses	Herpes simplex meningoencephalitis
	Cytomegalovirus
	Enteroviruses
	Rubella
	Acquired immunodeficiency syndrome
	Lymphocytic choriomeningitis
	Varicella
Spirochetes	Syphilis
	Lyme disease
Parasites	Toxoplasmosis
	Chagas' disease
Mycoplasma	*Mycoplasma hominis* infection
	Ureaplasma urealyticum infection
Fungi	Candidiasis
	Coccidioidomycosis
	Cryptococcosis
Noninfectious	
Trauma	Subarachnoid hemorrhage
	Traumatic lumbar puncture
Malignancy	Teratoma
	Medulloblastoma
	Choroid plexus papilloma and carcinoma

From Klein JO (2001). Bacterial sepsis and meningitis. In Remington JS, Klein JO, editors. Infectious diseases of the fetus and newborn infant, ed 5, Philadelphia: WB Saunders, p. 978.
*Aseptic meningitis is defined as meningitis in the absence of evidence of bacterial pathogen detectable in cerebrospinal fluid by usual laboratory techniques.

- Splenomegaly
- Fever
- Vomiting
- Diarrhea
- Erythroblastosis

- Hydrops fetalis
- Microcephaly
- Seizures
- Abnormal computed tomography scan and/or head ultrasound
- Abnormal cerebrospinal fluid—xanthochromia and mononuclear pleocytosis, high protein count
- PCR positive for *T. gondii*
- Enzyme-linked immunosorbent assay (ELISA) and immunofluorescent assay (IFA) tests positive for *T. gondii*

Long-Term Consequences
- Hearing impairment
- Visual problems
- Hydrocephalus
- Mental retardation
- Seizures
- Spasticity

Guidelines for Evaluation of Newborn of Mother Who Acquired Her Infection During Gestation to Determine Whether Infant Has Congenital Toxoplasma Infection and to Assess Degree of Involvement*
- History and physical examination
- Pediatric neurologic evaluation
- Pediatric ophthalmologist's examination of retinae
- Complete blood cell count with differential, platelet count
- Liver function test (bilirubin, gamma-glutamyltranspeptidase [GGTP])
- Urinalysis, serum creatinine
- Serum quantitative immunoglobulins
- Serum Sabin-Feldman dye test (immunoglobulin G [IgG]), IgM, ISAGA, IgA, ELISA, IgE, ISAGA/ELISA† (with maternal serum, perform same tests as for infant except substitute IgM, ELISA for the IgM ISAGA, and also obtain AC/HS†)
- Cerebrospinal fluid cell count, protein, glucose, and *T. gondii*–specific IgG and IgM antibodies as well as quantitative IgG to calculate antibody load: Subinoculate into mice or tissue culture 1 ml peripheral blood buffy coat or clot and digest of 100 g placenta.

*From Remington JS, et al. (2001). Toxoplasmosis. In Remington JS, Klein JO, editors. Infectious disease of the fetus and newborn infant, Philadelphia: WB Saunders, p. 276.
†When performed in combination in our laboratories, these tests have demonstrated a high degree of specificity and sensitivity in establishing the diagnosis of acute infection in the pregnant woman and congenital infection in the fetus and newborn.

Consider PCR of buffy coat from approximately 1 ml of blood, cell pellet from approximately 1 ml of cerebrospinal fluid, and cell pellet from 10 to 20 ml of amniotic fluid.
- Brain computed tomography scan with and without contrast medium enhancement
- Auditory brain-stem response to 20 dB

Nursing Management

Nursing management is supportive care aimed at prevention of complications and assisting the newborn to overcome the infection (Table 9-7). Education of the family focuses on the occurrence of toxoplasmosis and the prevention of future infections.

RUBELLA

Rubella is a result of transmission of the rubella virus, the one responsible for German measles. It is effectively transmitted across the placenta to the fetus. The clinical manifestations vary according to the timing of the in utero exposure.

Clinical Manifestations

The most common clinical manifestations include the following:
- Anemia
- Cataracts
- Chorioretinitis
- Microophthalmia
- Glaucoma
- Hearing deficits—sensorineural deafness is the most common
- Cardiac—patent ductus arteriosus, peripheral pulmonary artery stenosis, atrial or ventricular septal defects
- Neurologic—microcephaly, meningoencephalitis, mental retardation, intrauterine growth restriction
- Radiolucent bone defects
- Thrombocytopenia with or without purpura

The typical presentation includes mild disease with malaise, low-grade fever, headache, and conjunctivitis. In 1 to 5 days, a macular rash appears on the face and usually disappears after 3 or 4 days. Natural viremia is necessary for placental and fetal rubella infection. Most cases occur following primary disease. Frequently, skin rashes that resemble rubella may occur as a result of adenovirus, enterovirus, or other respiratory virus infections. Laboratory titers are recommended to confirm the diagnosis of rubella infection (Lott, Kenner, 2003).

Diagnosis

Confirmation of the diagnosis is by demonstration of the rubella antibody.

Table 9-7   Guidelines for Treatment of *Toxoplasma gondii* Infection in the Pregnant Woman and Congenital *Toxoplasma* Infection in the Fetus, Infant, and Older Child

Manifestation of Infection	Medication	Dosage	Duration of Therapy
In pregnant women with acute toxoplasmosis			
First 21 wk of gestation or until term if fetus not infected	Spiramycin*	1 g every 8 hr without food	A = until fetal infection documented or excluded at 21 wk; if documented, in alternate months with pyrimethamine, leucovorin, and sulfadiazine†
If fetal infection confirmed after wk 18 of gestation	Pyrimethamine	Loading dose: 100 mg per day in two divided doses for 2 days, then 50 mg per day	As in A†
	plus		
	Sulfadiazine	Loading dose: 75 mg/kg per day in two divided doses (maximum 4 g per day) for 2 days, then 100 mg/kg per day in two divided doses (maximum 4 g per day)	As in A†
	plus		
	Leucovorin (folinic acid)	10–20 mg daily‡	During and for 1 wk after pyrimethamine therapy

Continued

Table 9-7 Guidelines for Treatment of *Toxoplasma gondii* Infection in the Pregnant Woman and Congenital *Toxoplasma* Infection in the Fetus, Infant, and Older Child—cont'd

Manifestation of Infection	Medication	Dosage	Duration of Therapy
Congenital *Toxoplasma* infection in the infant	Pyrimethamine[§]	Loading dose: 2 mg/kg per day for 2 days, then 1 mg/kg per day for 2 or 6 mo,[‖] then this dose every Monday, Wednesday, Friday[§]	1 yr[¶]
	plus		
	Sulfadiazine[§]	100 mg/kg per day in two divided doses	1 yr[¶]
	plus		
	Leucovorin[§]	10 mg three times weekly[‡]	During and for 1 wk after pyrimethamine therapy
	Corticosteroids[#] (prednisone) have been used when cerebrospinal fluid protein ≥1 g/dl and when active chorioretinitis threatens vision	B = 1 mg/kg per day in two divided doses	C = Until resolution of elevated (≥1 g/dl) cerebrospinal fluid protein level or active chorioretinitis that threatens vision
Active chorioretinitis in older children	Pyrimethamine	Loading dose: 2 mg/kg per day (maximum 50 mg) for 2 days, then maintenance, 1 mg/kg per day (maximum 25 mg)	D = Usually 1-2 wk beyond the time that signs and symptoms have resolved
	plus		

Sulfadiazine	Loading dose: 75 mg/kg, then maintenance, 50 mg/kg every 12 hr	As in D
plus		
Leucovorin	10-20 mg three times weekly[c]	During and for 1 wk after pyrimethamine therapy
Corticosteroids	As in B	As in C

Modified from information appearing in Daffos F, et al. (1988). Prenatal management of 746 pregnancies at risk for congenital toxoplasmosis. New England Journal of medicine, 31, 271-275. Cited in Remington JS, et al. (2001). Toxoplasmosis. In Remington JS, Klein JO, editors. Infectious disease of the fetus and newborn infant, Philadelphia: WB Saunders, p. 293.

*Available only on request from the U.S. Food and Drug Administration, telephone number 301-443-5680.

†The only studies are those of Daffos et al. However, because Daffos and colleagues found pyrimethamine-sulfadiazine therapy to be superior to spiramycin for treatment of the fetus, continuous therapy with pyrimethamine, sulfadiazine, and leucovorin should be considered in the third trimester. This regimen has been used extensively in France and appears to be safe and feasible. Alternatively, in the United States, daily administration of pyrimethamine (50 mg/day) and sulfadiazine (1 g each 6 hr) plus leucovorin (10 mg) administered every other day to the mother has been used in the treatment of a limited number of fetuses in utero. This treatment was begun after the eighteenth week of gestation and continued until birth of the infant. Subsequent treatment of the infant is the same as that described under treatment of congenital infection. This appears to have been feasible and safe treatment for a small number of patients. When the diagnosis of infection in the fetus is established earlier, we suggest that sulfadiazine be used alone until approximately 20 wk of gestation, at which time pyrimethamine should be added to the regimen.

‡Adjusted for megaloblastic anemia, granulocytopenia, or thrombocytopenia; blood cell counts, including platelets, should be monitored as described in text.

§Optimal dosage, feasibility, and toxicity currently being evaluated or planned in ongoing Chicago-based National Collaborative Treatment Trial, telephone number 773-834-4152.

‖These two regimens are currently being compared in a randomized manner in the National Collaborative Treatment Trial. Data are not yet available to determine which, if either, is superior. Both regimens appear to be feasible and relatively safe.

¶The duration of therapy is unknown for infants and children, especially those with AIDS. See discussion in the Congenital Toxoplasma Infection and AIDS section.

#Corticosteroids should be used only in conjunction with pyrimethamine, sulfadiazine, and leucovorin treatment and should be continued until signs of inflammation (high cerebrospinal fluid protein >1 g/dl) or active chorioretinitis that threatens vision have subsided—dosage can then be tapered and discontinued; use only with pyrimethamine, sulfadiazine, and leucovorin.

Nursing Management

Prevention is the ideal goal to eradicate congenital rubella. That means immunization of all child-bearing women.

When a congenital infection is present or a neonatal infection is detected treatment is symptomatic. Currently, treatment in the nursery of the rubella-infected infant is rare. Therapy for identified problems, such as respiratory, cardiac, or neurologic deficits, is supportive, and there is no specific recommended therapy. Caretakers should have known immune titers and not be pregnant. Rubella-specific IgM can usually accurately identify these infants. Persistent shedding of the virus may last until 1 year of life; thus pregnant women should avoid contact with these patients. Follow-up care for surgical corrections of heart defects and cataracts as well as special schooling may be needed for these infants (Lott, Kenner, 2003).

Nursery Exposure to Rubella

Sometimes nurseries are exposed to rubella or measles. The guidelines in Table 9-8 should be followed if this occurs.

GONOCOCCAL INFECTION

Neisseria gonorrhoeae is the gram-negative diplococcus bacterium responsible for gonococcal infections.

Clinical Manifestations

The main symptom in the newborn is conjunctivitis. Gonococcal ophthalmia neonatorum is the condition that results. It can spread to a full-blown septicemia if not properly and promptly treated.

If the infection has disseminated then the signs and symptoms may include conjunctivitis, pyuria, pharyngitis, scalp abscess, or sepsis with an onset of 3 to 21 days.

Diagnosis

The diagnosis is made on the basis of a positive Gram stain.

Nursing Management

Gonococcal infections of infants and children Child abuse should be carefully considered and evaluated for any child with documented gonorrhea.

Treatment of infants born to mothers with gonococccal infection* Infants born to mothers with untreated gonorrhea are at high risk of infection (e.g., ophthalmia and disseminated gonococcal infection [DGI])

---

*Modified from Centers for Disease Control and Prevention (1998). Sexually transmitted diseases treatment guidelines. MMWR morbidity & mortality weekly report, 47 (RR-1). Cited in Gutman LT (2001). Gonococcal infections. In Remington JS, Klein JO, editors. Infectious diseases of the fetus and newborn infant, ed 5, Philadelphia: WB Saunders, p. 1206.

Table 9-8	Guidelines for Preventive Measures After Exposure to Measles in the Nursery or Maternity Ward		
	Measles Present (Prodrome or Rash)*		
Type of Exposure or Disease	**Mother**	**Neonate**	**Disposition**
A. Siblings at home with measles* when neonate and mother are ready for discharge from hospital	No	No	1. *Neonate:* Protective isolation and IG indicated unless mother had unequivocal history of previous measles or measles vaccination.† 2. *Mother:* With history of previous measles or measles vaccination, she may either remain with neonate or return to older children. Without previous history she may remain with neonate until older siblings are no longer infectious, or she may receive IG prophylactically and return to older children.
B. Mother without history of measles or measles vaccination exposed during period 6-15 days antepartum‡	No	No	1. *Exposed mother and infant:* Administer IG to each and send home at earliest date unless there are siblings at home with communicable measles. Test mothers for susceptibility if possible. If susceptible, administer live measles vaccine 5 months after IG (see text).

Continued

Table 9-8 Guidelines for Preventive Measures After Exposure to Measles in the Nursery or Maternity Ward—cont'd

Type of Exposure or Disease	Measles Present (Prodrome or Rash)*		Disposition
	Mother	Neonate	
			2. *Other mothers and infants:* Same unless clear history of previous measles or measles vaccination in the mother.
			3. *Hospital personnel:* Unless clear history of previous measles or measles vaccination administer IG within 72 hr of exposure. Vaccinate 5 mo or more later.
C. Onset of maternal measles antepartum or postpartum§	Yes	Yes	1. *Infected mother and infant:* Isolate together until clinically stable, then send home.
			2. *Other mothers and infants:* Same as B-3 except infants should be vaccinated at 15 mo of age.
			3. *Hospital personnel:* Same as B-3.

| D. Onset of maternal measles antepartum or postpartum§ | Yes | No | 1. *Infected mother:* Isolate until no longer infectious.§
2. *Infected mother's infant:* Isolate separately from mother. Administer IG immediately. Send home when mother is no longer infectious. Alternatively, observe in isolation for 18 days for modified measles,‡ especially if IG administration was delayed more than 4 days.
3. *Other mothers and infants:* Same as C-2.
4. *Hospital personnel:* Same as B-3. |

*Catarrhal stage or less than 72 hours after onset of exanthem.

†Vaccination with live attenuated measles virus (see text).

‡With exposure less than 6 days antepartum, mother would not be potentially infectious until at least 72 hours postpartum.

§Considered infectious from onset of prodrome until 72 hours after onset of exanthem.

‖Incubation period for modified measles may be prolonged beyond the usual 10 to 14 days.

From Gershon AA (2001). Chickenpox, measles, and mumps. In Remington JS, Klein JO, editors. Infectious diseases of the fetus and newborn infant, ed 5, Philadelphia: WB Saunders, p. 717.

and should be treated with a single injection of ceftriaxone (50 mg/kg intravenously [IV] or intramuscularly [IM], not to exceed 125 mg). Ceftriaxone should be given cautiously to hyperbilirubinemic infants, especially premature infants. Topical prophylaxis for neonatal ophthalmia is not adequate treatment for documented infections of the eye or other sites.

Treatment of infants with gonococcal infection Infants with documented gonococcal infections at any site (e.g., eye) should be evaluated for DGI. This evaluation should include a careful physical examination, especially of the joints, as well as blood and cerebrospinal fluid cultures. Infants with gonococcal ophthalmia or DGI should be treated for 7 days (10 to 14 days if meningitis is present) with one of the following regimens.

Recommended regimen
- Ceftriaxone, 24 to 50 mg/kg/day IV or IM in a single daily dose
- Cefotaxime, 24 mg/kg IV or IM every 12 hours

Alternative regimen Limited data suggest that uncomplicated gonococcal ophthalmia among infants may be cured with a single injection of ceftriaxone (50 mg/kg up to 125 mg). A few experts use this regimen for children who have no clinical or laboratory evidence of disseminated disease.

Infants with gonococcal ophthalmia should receive eye irrigations with buffered saline solutions until discharge has cleared. Topical antibiotic therapy alone is inadequate. Simultaneous infection with *Chlamydia trachomatis* has been reported and should be considered for patients who do not respond satisfactorily. Therefore the mother and infant should be tested for chlamydial infection.

Gonococcal infections of children Children who weigh more than 45 kg should be treated with adult regimens. Children who weigh less than 45 kg who have uncomplicated vulvovaginitis, cervicitis, urethritis, pharyngitis, or proctitis should be treated as follows.

Recommended regimen Ceftriaxone, 125 mg IV once, is recommended. Patients who cannot tolerate ceftriaxone may be treated with spectinomycin, 40 mg/kg IM once.

Patients weighing less than 45 kg with bacteremia or arthritis should be treated with ceftriaxone, 50 mg/kg (maximum 1 g) once daily for 7 days. For meningitis, treatment is for 10 to 14 days and the maximum dose is 2 g.

Children older than 8 years of age should also be given doxycycline, 100 mg bid for 7 days. All patients should be evaluated for coinfection with syphilis and *C. trachomatis*. Follow-up cultures are unnecessary if ceftriaxone has been used.

Prevention of Ophthalmia Neonatorum

Instillation of a prophylactic agent into the eyes of all newborns is recommended to prevent gonococcal ophthalmia neonatorum and is required by law in most states to prevent gonococcal eye disease; the efficacy of prophylactic agents in preventing chlamydial eye disease is not clear.

Further, they do not eliminate nasopharyngeal colonization with *C. trachomatis*. Treatment of gonococcal and chlamydial infections in pregnant women is the best method for preventing neonatal gonococcal and chlamydial disease.

Recommended regimen Erythromycin (0.5%) ophthalmic ointment once *or* tetracycline (1%) ophthalmic ointment once *or* silver nitrate (1%) aqueous solution once is recommended.

One of these agents should be instilled into the eyes of every neonate as soon as possible after delivery and definitely within 1 hour after birth. Single-use tubes or ampules are preferable to multiple-use tubes. The efficacy of tetracycline and erythromycin in the prevention of TRNG and penicillin-producing *N. gonorrhoeae* (PPNG) ophthalmia is unknown, although both are probably effective because of the high concentrations of drug in these preparations. Bacitracin is *not* recommended.

CYTOMEGALOVIRUS

Cytomegalovirus (CMV), a member of the herpes family, is common. CMV is a deoxyribonucleic acid (DNA) virus covered with a glycoprotein coat that closely resembles the herpes and varicella-zoster viruses.

Clinical Manifestations

The common clinical manifestations of CMV are as follows:
- Intrauterine growth restriction
- Microcephaly
- Periventricular calcifications
- Deafness
- Blindness
- Cataracts
- Profound mental retardation
- Hepatosplenomegaly
- Jaundice
- Blueberry muffin syndrome—petechiae

Diagnosis

Urine culture for CMV is the most sensitive indicator. IgG and IgM antibody titer levels with IgM elevations indicate exposure, but IgG indicates perinatally acquired infection. Negative maternal IgG titer and a positive neonatal titer indicate postnatal transmission.

Nursing Management

General supportive therapy is based on the presence of these clinical manifestations. Specific therapy for CMV is still in the experimental stage but includes immunoglobulin therapy, vaccines, and chemotherapy. IV immunoglobulin therapy provides passive immunity to at-risk infants but not to those already infected. Two live attenuated vaccines for CMV have been developed and tested on renal transplant patients. Theoretically, these vaccines would be useful preconceptually or perinatally to prevent vertical transmission; however, only limited research has been done with this population. Chemotherapy offers the most promise for treatment of neonatal CMV infection; however, clinically, it has not been shown to be effective in improving outcome. These agents include doxuridine, cytosine arabinoside, adenine arabinoside, acyclovir, leukocyte interferon, interferon stimulators, and ganciclovir (Lott, Kenner, 2003).

SYPHILIS

Syphilis is caused by the organism *Treponema pallidum*.

Clinical Manifestations

Common manifestations can range from very mild to severe symptoms. They include pale mottling, temperature instability, irritability, "blueberry muffin spots" caused by small hemorrhages, hepatosplenomegaly, intrauterine growth restriction, and, on ultrasound of some infants, cerebral ventriculomegaly. Some infants exposed in utero will have no symptoms at birth.

Diagnosis

The diagnosis is made on the basis of the Venereal Disease Research Laboratory (VDRL) test or the rapid plasma reagin (RPR) (nontreponemal antibody) tests used to detect the anticardiolipin antibody. FTA-ABS (fluorescent treponemal antibody, absorbed with non-*pallidum* treponemes) will also detect the *T. pallidum* antibody. The ELISA test will detect both nontreponemal and treponemal antibodies. PCR will detect *T. pallidum* DNA in tissues or body fluids. When there is a positive VDRL or RPR in the presence of snuffles or a vesiculobullous eruption accompanied by hepatosplenomegaly, lymphadenopathy, bony changes, and lesions, then syphilis is probably the correct diagnosis (Ingall, Sanchez, 2001).

Nursing Management

The cornerstone of treatment is antibiotic therapy (Tables 9-9 and 9-10).

HUMAN PARVOVIRUS B19

Human parvovirus (HPV) B19 is a DNA viral agent that has been associated with fifth disease in children. That disease is characterized by a bright red rash—erythema infectiosum. In adults it can cause a self-limiting infection. Some people harbor the virus and carry a chronic infection, especially if they are immunosuppressed. This infection can be transmitted transplacentally.

Clinical Manifestations
The most common symptoms are anemia, nonimmune fetal hydrops, myocarditis, and possible structural anomalies, especially of the eye and central nervous system.

Diagnosis
The diagnosis is made when anti-B19 antibodies are detected, usually through PCR tests.

Nursing Management
The nursing management is symptomatic. Depending on when the fetus was exposed, this can be a self-limiting disease. If there is organ compromise or structural abnormalities the treatment is aimed at those specific problems.

FUNGAL INFECTIONS

The most common forms of fungal infections found in the neonate are candidiasis. *Candida albicans* is the general form. *Candida* organisms are oval, yeastlike cells that can bud to reproduce. *C. albicans* produces endotoxins, hemolysis, pyrogens, and proteolytic enzymes that are damaging to tissues. Early recognition and treatment of fungal sepsis are imperative to prevent severe central nervous system complications and death. Prolonged broad-spectrum antibiotic treatment for small premature infants may predispose infants to *Candida* overgrowth in the gastrointestinal tract. This overgrowth may predispose the infant to disseminated fungemia. Administration of hyperalimentation, frequent use of indwelling venous lines, and invasive procedures may also predispose the infant to *C. albicans* infection (Lott, Kenner, 2003).

Clinical Manifestations
The symptoms at first may be vague. Later the infant may experience feeding intolerance, abdominal distention, guaiac-positive stools, temperature instability, hypotension, and respiratory distress.

Diagnosis
The diagnosis is made on the basis of the fungus in a culture.

Nursing Management
Fungal infections are life threatening and require aggressive therapies. Unfortunately the medications are not without the potential for

Table **9-9**		Recommended Treatment of the Newborn*†
Maternal Rx‡	**Clinical Findings in Newborn**	**Drug (Penicillin G)**
None or inadequate§	Present	Aqueous *or* Procaine
None or inadequate§	Absent	Aqueous *or* Procaine *or* Benzathine
Adequate (during pregnancy)	Absent	Benzathine (CDC) *or* Follow-up only (AAP)
Adequate (before pregnancy)	Absent	Follow-up only *or* Benzathine (only if follow-up cannot be ensured)

From Ingall D, Sanchez PJ (2001). Syphilis. In Remington JS, Klein JO, editors. Infectious diseases of the fetus and newborn infant, ed 5, Philadelphia: WB Saunders, p. 669.

IM, Intramuscular; IV, intravenous; CDC, Centers for Disease Control; AAP, American Academy of Pediatrics.

*See text.

†Close and frequent follow-up, including serologic test for syphilis, is essential.

‡Test mother for HIV antibody.

§Inadequate maternal treatment: Rx not documented; Rx within 4 wk of delivery; Rx with erythromycin or nonpenicillin drug; or serologic antibody titers do not fall appropriately (see text).

serious side effects. The most effective drug for treatment of C. albicans infection is amphotericin B. This toxic, potent antifungal agent must be used cautiously. The initial dose is 0.1 to 0.3 mg/kg IV over a period of 2 to 6 hours. The maintenance dosage is 0.5 to 1.0 mg/kg/day over 2 to 6 hours. Lower doses are started until higher doses can be tolerated. Increments of 0.1 mg/kg/day are used to increase the daily dose slowly. Many infants tolerate a total dose of 25 to 30 mg/kg if titrated over approximately 1 month (Khoory et al., 1999; Miller, 2001). Often, if organ involvement is minimal, infants can be successfully given lower doses. If meningitis is suspected, 5-fluorouracil (5-FU) may be used. This antifungal agent acts to inhibit DNA syn-

Route	Dose (50,000 units/kg)
IM or IV	Daily × 10-14 days in two (<7 days), three (8-30 days), or four (>1 mo) doses
IM	Daily dose × 10-14 days
IM or IV	Daily × 10-14 days in two (<7 days), three (8-30 days), or four (>1 mo) doses
IM	Daily dose × 10-14 days
IM	Single dose
IM	Single dose
IM	Single dose

thesis so that *Candida* replication cannot occur. Dosage recommendations for this drug are based on extrapolated data from adults; there is no clearly established recommendation. Average daily dosage is 100 mg/kg/day in four divided doses, in conjunction with amphotericin B.

Miconazole has also been used to treat systemic candidiasis in newborns. Dosage guidelines for this drug have not been established; however, 10 mg/kg/day in two divided doses, IV, followed by oral therapy, is generally given.

Safety and efficacy of these drugs in the treatment of newborns have not been established.

Renal toxicity is a major side effect of amphotericin B therapy because it causes renal vasoconstriction and decreases both renal blood flow and glomerular filtration rate. This damage can result in hyponatremia, hypokalemia, increased blood urea nitrogen, and increased creatinine, as well as acidosis. If the medication makes the patient oliguric, most physicians recommend stopping the drug until the next day. Thrombocytopenia, granulocytopenia, fever, nausea, and vomiting are the common side effects associated with amphotericin B. One major side effect of 5-FU is bone marrow depression, resulting in a decreased platelet count.

Table 9-10	Follow-Up After Treatment or Prophylaxis for Congenital Syphilis
Patient Category	**Follow-Up Procedures**
Patients diagnosed as having congenital syphilis	RPR testing every 2-3 mo until negative or decreased fourfold; if RPR is stable or increasing after 6-12 mo of treatment, reevaluate and re-treat Treponemal antibody test after 15 mo of age If initial CSF was abnormal or infant showed sings of central nervous system disease, repeat every 6 mo until normal Careful developmental evaluation, vision testing, and hearing testing
Patients treated in utero or at birth because of maternal syphilis	RPR testing at birth and then every 3 mo until test is negative Treponemal antibody test after 15 mo of age
Women treated for syphilis during pregnancy	RPR testing as often as monthly until delivery, then every 6 mo until negative or decreased fourfold Retreatment any time there is a fourfold rise in RPR titer

From Ingall D, Sanchez PJ (2001). Syphilis. In Remington JS, Klein JO, editors. Infectious diseases of the fetus and newborn infant, ed 5, Philadelphia: WB Saunders, p. 671. Modified from Rathburn KC (1983). Congenital syphilis: a proposal for improved surveillance, diagnosis and treatment. Sexually transmitted diseases, 10, 103; (1998). MMWR morbidity & mortality weekly report, 47, 45.
RPR, Rapid plasmid reagin; CSF, cerebrospinal fluid.

Because of the insidious onset of candidiasis, the infant with sepsis who is not responding to traditional antibiotic treatment may have Candida. Catheter tips at IV sites and percutaneous lines should be changed and cultured. Urine can easily be cultured for the presence of Candida. Thrush and monilial rashes are indicative of candidiasis. These can easily be treated with oral and local antifungal agents.

Monitoring of infants receiving amphotericin B is challenging, because infants may have reactions to this medication. Blood pressure should be monitored every half hour, and urine output should be observed closely. Vital signs and laboratory work, including liver enzyme tests, should be done daily to detect early signs of neonatal toxicity (Khoory et al., 1999; Miller, 2001).

GROUP B STREPTOCOCCAL INFECTION

Group B streptococcus is a bacterial agent, a gram-positive diplococcus responsible for a large proportion of neonatal sepsis. Risk factors for congenital infection (early onset) are maternal positive infection, prolonged rupture of membranes, chorioamnionitis, intrapartal fever, use of intrapartal internal fetal monitor, twin pregnancy, maternal age under 20 years; premature delivery; and previous history of a child with group B strep. Late-onset infection (after the first 7 days of life) risk factors are respiratory infection as well as the other risk factors listed for early onset.

Clinical Manifestations
For early-onset group B strep the symptoms usually occur in the first 24 hours of life. The presenting signs may include respiratory distress, grunting and retracting, pneumonia, cyanosis or mottling, poor peripheral perfusion, hypotension, and cardiovascular collapse. Meningitis may or may not be present.

In late-onset strep, the signs include all of the signs of early onset but in this instance meningitis is a usual finding. Bacteremia and osteoarthritis may also be present.

In either case, long-term consequences include mental retardation, deafness, blindness, seizures, spastic quadriplegia, and diabetes insipidus.

Diagnosis
The diagnosis is based on clinical symptoms and cultures of blood, cerebrospinal fluid, and other fluid or tissue, such as umbilical cord. A lumbar puncture should be done if meningitis is suspected. Counterelectrophoresis and latex particle agglutination can be used to get results quickly because they will detect the presence of antigens.

Nursing Management
The main treatment is antimicrobial therapy (Table 9-11). Support for the infant's cardiovascular status is critical, but the infection must be treated or the child will not survive. Some infants will require extracorporeal membrane oxygenation (ECMO) for support. Nonsteroidal antiinflammatory agents can assist those infants experiencing pulmonary hypertension. Indomethacin or dazmegrel may be used. Intravenous immune globulin (IGIV) is used in some centers to boost the immune system. This medication needs future research to determine its efficacy.

Table 9-11 Antimicrobial Regimens Recommended for Treatment of Group B Streptococcal Infections in Infants*

Site of Infection	Drug	Dose per Day (Intravenous)	Duration
Bacteremia without meningitis	Ampicillin plus gentamicin	150-200 mg/kg plus 7.5 mg/kg	Initial treatment before culture results (48-72 hr)
	Penicillin G	200,000 units/kg	Complete a total treatment course of 10 days
Meningitis	Ampicillin plus gentamicin	300-400 mg/kg plus 7.5 mg/kg	Initial treatment (until cerebrospinal fluid is sterile)
	Penicillin G	500,000 units/kg	Complete a minimum total treatment course of 14 days[†]
Septic arthritis	Penicillin G	200,000 units/kg	2-3 wk
Osteomyelitis	Penicillin G	200,000 units/kg	3-4 wk
Endocarditis	Penicillin G	400,000 units/kg	4 wk[‡]

From Edwards MS, Baker CJ (2001). Group B streptococcal infections. In Remington JS, Klein JO, editors. Infectious diseases of the fetus and newborn infant, ed 5, Philadelphia: WB Saunders, p.1125.

No modification of dose by postnatal age is recommended. Oral therapy is never indicated.

[†]*Longer treatment (up to 4 wk) may be required for ventriculitis.*

[‡]*In combination with gentamicin for the first 14 days.*

Group B strep guidelines* for patient care are as follows:

- All pregnant women should be screened at 35-37 weeks' gestation for vaginal and rectal GBS colonization. At the time of labor or rupture of membranes, intrapartum chemoprophylaxis should be given to all pregnant women identified as GBS carriers. Colonization during a previous pregnancy is not an indication for intrapartum prophylaxis in subsequent deliveries. Screening to detect GBS colonization in each pregnancy will determine the need for prophylaxis in that pregnancy.

- Women with GBS isolated from the urine in any concentration (e.g., 10^3) during their current pregnancy should receive intrapartum chemoprophylaxis because such women usually are heavily colonized with GBS and are at increased risk of delivering an infant with early-onset GBS disease. Labels on urine specimens from prenatal patients should clearly state the patient's pregnancy status to assist laboratory processing and reporting of results. Prenatal culture-based screening at 35-37 weeks' gestation is not necessary for women with GBS bacteriuria. Women with symptomatic or asymptomatic GBS urinary tract infection detected during pregnancy should be treated according to current standards of care for urinary tract infection during pregnancy.

- Women who have previously given birth to an infant with invasive GBS disease should receive intrapartum chemoprophylaxis; prenatal culture-based screening is not necessary for these women.

- If the result of GBS culture is not known at the onset of labor, intrapartum chemoprophylaxis should be administered to women with any of the following risk factors: gestation <37 weeks, duration of membrane rupture ≥18 hours, or a temperature of ≥100.4° F (≥38.0° C). Women with known negative results from vaginal and rectal GBS screening cultures within 5 weeks of delivery do not require prophylaxis to prevent GBS disease even if any of the intrapartum risk factors develop.

- Women with threatened preterm (<37 weeks' gestation) delivery should be assessed for need for intrapartum prophylaxis to prevent perinatal GBS disease. An algorithm for management of women with threatened preterm delivery is provided. Other management approaches, developed by individual physicians or institutions, may be appropriate.

- Culture techniques that maximize the likelihood of GBS recovery are required for prenatal screening. Collection of specimens for culture may be conducted in the outpatient clinic setting by either the patient, with appropriate instruction, or health care provider. This involves swabbing the lower vagina and rectum (i.e., through the

*From U.S. Centers for Disease Control and Prevention www.cdc.gov

anal sphincter). Because lower vaginal as opposed to cervical cultures are recommended, cultures should not be collected by speculum examination. Specimens should be placed in a nonnutritive transport medium (e.g., Amies or Stuart's without charcoal). Specimen labels should clearly identify that specimens are for group B streptococcal culture. If susceptibility testing is ordered for penicillin-allergic women, specimen labels should also identify the patient as penicillin allergic and should specify that if GBS is isolated, it should be tested for susceptibility to clindamycin and erythromycin. Specimens should be inoculated into a selective broth medium (examples of appropriate commercially available media include Trans-Vag Broth supplemented with 5% defibrinated sheep blood or LIM broth), incubated overnight, and subcultured onto solid blood agar medium. Methods of testing prenatal isolates from penicillin-allergic women for susceptibility to clindamycin and erythromycin are outlined. Laboratories should report culture results (positive and negative) and susceptibility testing results to the anticipated site of delivery (when known) and to the health care provider who ordered the test.

- Health care providers should inform women of their GBS screening test result and the recommended interventions. In the absence of GBS urinary tract infection, antimicrobial agents should not be used before the intrapartum period to treat GBS colonization. Such treatment is not effective in eliminating carriage or preventing neonatal disease and may cause adverse consequences.

- GBS-colonized women who have a planned cesarean delivery performed before rupture of membranes and onset of labor are at low risk for having an infant with early-onset GBS disease. These women should not routinely receive intrapartum chemoprophylaxis for perinatal GBS disease prevention.

- For intrapartum chemoprophylaxis, the following regimen is recommended for women without penicillin allergy: penicillin G, 5 million units intravenously initial dose, then 2.5 million units intravenously every 4 hours until delivery. Because of its narrow spectrum of activity, penicillin is the preferred agent. An alternative regimen is ampicillin, 2 g intravenously initial dose, then 1 g intravenously every 4 hours until delivery.

- Intrapartum chemoprophylaxis for penicillin-allergic women takes into account increasing resistance to clindamycin and erythromycin among GBS isolates. During prenatal care, history of penicillin allergy should be assessed to determine whether a patient is at high risk for anaphylaxis, i.e., has a history of immediate hyper-sensitivity reactions to penicillin (e.g., anaphylaxis, angioedema, or urticaria) or history of asthma or other conditions that would make anaphylaxis more dangerous. Women who are not at high risk for anaphylaxis should be given cefazolin, 2 g intravenously initial dose, then 1 g intravenously every 8 hours until delivery. For women at high risk for anaphylaxis, clindamycin and erythromycin susceptibility testing, if available, should be performed on isolates obtained during GBS prenatal carriage screening. Women with clindamycin- and erythromycin-susceptible isolates should be given either clindamycin, 900 mg intravenously every 8 hours until delivery; or erythromycin, 500 mg intravenously every 6 hours until delivery. If susceptibility testing is not possible, susceptibility results are not known, or isolates are resistant to erythromycin or clindamycin, the following regimen can be used for women with immediate penicillin hypersensitivity: vancomycin, 1 g intravenously every 12 hours until delivery.

- Routine use of antimicrobial prophylaxis for newborns whose mothers received intrapartum chemoprophylaxis for GBS infection is not recommended. However, therapeutic use of these agents is appropriate for infants with clinically suspected sepsis. An updated algorithm for management of infants born to mothers who received intrapartum chemoprophylaxis for GBS infection is provided. This revised algorithm is not an exclusive approach to management; variation that incorporates individual circumstances or institutional preferences may be appropriate.

- Local and state public health agencies, in conjunction with appropriate groups of hospitals, are encouraged to establish surveillance for early-onset GBS disease and to take other steps to promote perinatal GBS disease prevention and education to reduce the incidence of early-onset GBS disease in their states. Efforts to monitor the emergence of perinatal infections caused by other organisms are also encouraged.

Before full implementation of this strategy can be expected in all health care settings, all members of the health care team will need to improve protocols for isolation and reporting of GBS culture results, to improve information management to ensure communication of screening results, and to educate medical and nursing staff responsible for prenatal and intrapartum care. Within institutions, such efforts may take several months.

Even with ideal implementation, cases of early-onset GBS disease will continue to occur. Tools to help promote prevention and educate parents of infants with early-onset GBS disease are available at http://www.cdc.gov/groupbstrep. Additional tools available to assist with prevention implementation are available at http://www.acog.org, http://sales.acog.com, http://www.aap.org and http://www.health. state.mn.us/divs/dpc/ades/invbact/strepb.htm Multiple copies of educational materials published by CDC are available at the Public Health Foundation, 1220 L St., NW Suite 350, Washington, DC 20005, telephone 877-252-1200, or online at http://www.phf.org.

HEPATITIS

There are several forms of hepatitis (A, B, C, D, E) that have the potential for fetal and neonatal infections. Hepatitis B is the most common one. The hepatitis B virus (HBV) is a fairly large (approximately 42 mm in diameter), double-stranded, DNA-containing virus.

Infection early in pregnancy with HBV causes a 50% risk of neonatal HBV infection. Ninety percent of infants born to women who are positive for both hepatitis B surface antigen (HBsAg) and hepatitis E antigen (HBeAg) are at risk for development of HBV infection by their first birthday if they are not given treatment. Infants born to women who are positive for HBsAg but negative for HBeAg have lower rates of perinatal infection (20%). Infants who do not receive treatment are likely to become carriers, which may eventually lead to primary hepatocellular carcinoma (Crumpacker, 2001).

Clinical Manifestations

The most common clinical manifestations are prematurity, low birth weight, and hyperbilirubinemia. Hepatosplenomegaly may or may not be present.

Diagnosis

HBsAg is an important test in assessing a woman's risk of transmitting HBV to her unborn child. The presence of HBsAg and HBeAg is the best indication of infectiousness. It is currently recommended that all pregnant women be screened at their first prenatal visit for HBsAg and HBeAg to prevent prenatal transmission (Crumpacker, 2001). HBV has a long incubation period—50 to 190 days, average 90 days. Current recommendations are for all pregnant women to be screened initially and again before delivery. Screening is essential to identify potential risk for perinatal transmission and for protection of those who are exposed to antigen-positive blood. Family clustering of HBV has been identified through spread via household contact (Crumpacker, 2001). The surface antigen can be detected in the newborn as well.

Nursing Management

Treatment for infants whose mothers are known to be positive should be HBV vaccine along with hepatitis B immunoglobulin (HBIG). For neonates whose mothers are HBsAg positive or exposed, HBV vaccine, 0.5 ml, should be given IM in the anterolateral part of the thigh at or within 24 hours of birth. Vaccination should be repeated at 1 and 6 months: 0.5 ml; booster injections are suggested at 12 months and may need repeating at 5-year intervals. The vaccine can be used in infants who have been exposed to HIV. There is usually an immune response in these infants despite an altered CD4 count. The response does appear to be somewhat diminished. If HBIG is not available, standard immune serum globulin (ISG) should be given at birth (2.0 ml) and at age 1 month (Crumpacker, 2001).

HUMAN PAPILLOMA VIRUS

Human papilloma virus (HPV) is a sexually transmitted disease that is responsible for genital warts. It is a DNA virus that is easily transmitted across the placenta.

Clinical Manifestations

The virus often attacks the upper airway, resulting in inflammation of the larynx—laryngeal papillomatosis. The result is a weak, squeaky, or hoarse cry. Respiratory stridor is possible.

Diagnosis

The diagnosis is made based on viral cultures producing HPV.

Nursing Management

The management is symptomatic. Respiratory support may be necessary if upper airway obstruction is present.

HUMAN IMMUNODEFICIENCY VIRUS

We have made great strides in decreasing the perinatal transmission of human immunodeficiency virus (HIV), a dreaded and often lethal disease. In some parts of the world, nearly 100% of the population is infected with this virus. HIV is a viral agent that replicates and mutates once it is in the cell. The mutations have created a problem in trying to develop an effective vaccine. This section will review the guidelines set forth by the U.S. Centers for Disease Control and Prevention for the classification, diagnosis, and treatment of infants with HIV.

1994 Revised Human Immunodeficiency Virus Pediatric Classification System: Clinical Categories*

Category N: not symptomatic Category N includes children who have no signs or symptoms considered to be the result of HIV infection or who have only one of the conditions listed in category A.

---

*From Centers for Disease Control and Prevention (CDC) (1998). Guidelines for the use of antiretroviral agents in pediatric HIV infection, Atlanta: CDC. Modified from CDC (1994). 1994 Revised classification system for human immunodeficiency virus infection.

Category A: mildly symptomatic Category A includes children with two or more of the following conditions but none of the conditions listed in categories B and C:

- Lymphadenopathy ($\geq$0.5 cm at more than two sites; bilateral = one site)
- Hepatomegaly
- Splenomegaly
- Dermatitis
- Parotitis
- Recurrent or persistent upper respiratory infection, sinusitis, or otitis media

Category B: moderately symptomatic Category B encompasses children who have symptomatic conditions other than those listed for category A or category C that are attributed to HIV infection. Examples of conditions in clinical category B include but are not limited to the following:

- Anemia (<8 g/100 ml), neutropenia (<1000/mm^3), or thrombocytopenia (<100,000/mm^3) persisting at least 30 days
- Bacterial meningitis, pneumonia, or sepsis (single episode)
- Candidiasis, oropharyngeal (i.e., thrush) persisting longer than 2 months in children aged 6 months
- Cardiomyopathy
- Cytomegalovirus infection with onset before age 1 month
- Diarrhea, recurrent or chronic
- Hepatitis
- Herpes simplex virus (HSV) stomatitis, recurrent (i.e., more than two episodes within 1 year)
- HSV bronchitis, pneumonitis, or esophagitis with onset before age 1 month
- Herpes zoster (i.e., shingles) involving at least two distinct episodes or more than one dermatome
- Leiomyosarcoma
- Lymphoid interstitial pneumonia (LIP) or pulmonary lymphoid hyperplasia complex
- Nephropathy
- Nocardiosis
- Fever lasting 1 month
- Toxoplasmosis with onset before age 1 month
- Varicella, disseminated (i.e., complicated chickenpox)

Category C: severely symptomatic Category C includes children who have any condition listed in the 1987 surveillance case definition for acquired immunodeficiency syndrome, with the exception of LIP (which is a category B condition).

Table **9-12**	1994 Revised Human Immunodeficiency Virus Pediatric Classification System: Immune Categories Based on Age-Specific CD4+ T-Lymphocyte Count And Percentage		
Immune Category	**<12 mo**	**1-5 yr**	**6-12 yr**
	No./μl (%)	**No./μl (%)**	**No./μl (%)**
Category 1—no suppression	≥1500 (≥25%)	≥1000 (≥25%)	≥500 (≥25%)
Category 2— moderate suppression	750-1499 (15%-24%)	500-999 (15%-24%)	200-499 (15%-24%)
Category 3— severe sup-pression	<750 (<15%)	<500 (<15%)	<200 (<15%)

Modified from CDC (1994). Revised classification system for human immunodeficiency virus infection in children less than 13 years of age. MMWR morbidity and mortality weekly report, 43 (no. RR-12), 1-10. In Centers for Disease Control and Prevention (CDC) (1998). Guidelines for the use of antiretroviral agents in pediatric HIV infection, Atlanta: CDC.

Table 9-12 gives the 1994 revised HIV pediatric classification categories.

Indications for Initiation of Antiretroviral Therapy in Children with Human Immunodeficiency Virus (HIV) Infection[*][†]

Clinical symptoms associated with HIV infection (i.e., clinical categories A, B, or C) are as follows:

1. Evidence of immune suppression, indicated by CD4+ T-lymphocyte absolute number or percentage (i.e., immune category 2 or 3)
2. Age younger than 12 months regardless of clinical, immunologic, or virologic status
3. For asymptomatic children aged at least 1 year with normal immune status, two options can be considered:
   a. Preferred approach: Initiate therapy regardless of age or symptom status.

---

[*]*From Centers for Disease Control and Prevention (CDC) (1998). Guidelines for the use of antiretroviral agents in pediatric HIV infection. Atlanta: CDC.*
[†]*Indications for initiation of antiretroviral therapy in postpubertal HIV-infected adolescents should follow the adult guidelines (Office of Public Health and Science, Department of Health and Human Services [1997]. Availability of report of NIH panel to define principles of therapy of HIV infection and guidelines for the use of antiretroviral agents in HIV-infected adults. Federal register, 62, 33417-33418)*

b. Alternative approach: Defer treatment in situations in which the risk for clinical disease progression is low and other factors (e.g., concern for the durability of response, safety, adherence) favor postponing treatment. In such cases, the health care provider should regularly monitor virologic, immunologic, and clinical status. Factors to be considered in deciding to initiate therapy include the following:

(1) High or increasing HIV ribonucleic acid (RNA) copy number

(2) Rapidly declining CD4+ T-lymphocyte number or percentage to values approaching those indicative of moderate immune suppression (i.e., immune category 2)

(3) Development of clinical symptoms

Recommended Antiretroviral Regimens for Initial Therapy for Human Immunodeficiency Virus (HIV) Infection in Children*

Preferred regimen There is evidence of clinical benefit and sustained suppression of HIV RNA in clinical trials with this regimen in HIV-infected adults; clinical trials in HIV-infected children are ongoing.

- One highly active protease inhibitor plus two nucleoside analogue reverse transcriptase inhibitors (NRTIs)
- Preferred protease inhibitor for infants and children who cannot swallow pills or capsules: nelfinavir or ritonavir; alternative for children who can swallow pills or capsules: indinavir
- Recommended dual NRTI combinations: The most data on use in children are available for the combinations of zidovudine (ZDV) and dideoxyinosine (ddI) and for ZDV and lamivudine (3TC). More limited data are available for the combinations of stavudine (d4T) and ddI, d4T and 3TC, and ZDV and zalcitabine (ddC).[†]

Alternative regimen This regimen is less likely to produce sustained HIV RNA suppression in infected adults; the combination of nevirapine, ZDV, and ddI produced substantial and sustained suppression of viral replication in two of six infants first treated at age younger than 4 months[‡]

---

*From Luzuiraga K et al. (1997). Combination treatment with zidovudine, didanosine, and nevirapine in infants with human immunodeficiency virus type 1 infection. New England journal of medicine, 336, 1343-1349. From Centers for Disease Control and Prevention (CDC) (1998). Guidelines for the use of antiretroviral agents in pediatric HIV infection, Atlanta: CDC.

[†]ddC is not available in a liquid preparation commercially, although a liquid formulation is available through a compassionate use program of the manufacturer (Hoffman-LaRoche Inc., Nutley, N.J.). ZDV and ddC are a less preferred choice for use in combination with a protease inhibitor.

[‡]A liquid preparation of nevirapine is not available commercially but is available through a compassionate use program of the manufacturer (Boehringer Ingelheim Pharmaceuticals, Inc., Ridgefield, Conn.).

- Nevirapine and two NRTIs

  Secondary alternative regimen Clinical benefit was demonstrated with this regimen in clinical trials involving infected adults and/or children, but initial viral suppression may not be sustained.
- Two NRTIs

  Not recommended Evidence is against use of these agents because of overlapping toxicity and/or because use may be virologically undesirable.
- Any monotherapy[*]
- d4T and ZDV
- ddC and ddI
- ddC and d4T
- ddC and 3TC

Considerations for Changing Antiretroviral Therapy for Human Immunodeficiency Virus (HIV)–Infected Children[†]
Virologic considerations[‡]

- Less than a minimally acceptable virologic response after 8 to 12 weeks of therapy. For children receiving antiretroviral therapy with two nucleoside analogue reverse transcriptase inhibitors

  (NRTIs) and a protease inhibitor, such a response is defined as a less than tenfold (1.0 log10) decrease from baseline HIV RNA levels. For children who are receiving less potent antiretroviral therapy (i.e., dual NRTI combinations), an insufficient response is defined as a less than fivefold (0.7 log10) decrease in HIV RNA levels from baseline.
- HIV RNA not suppressed to undetectable levels after 4 to 6 months of antiretroviral therapy[§]
- Repeated detection of HIV RNA in children who initially responded to antiretroviral therapy with undetectable levels[||]

---

[*]*Except for ZDV chemoprophylaxis administered to HIV-exposed infants during the first 6 weeks of life to prevent perinatal HIV transmission; if an infant is identified as HIV infected while receiving ZDV prophylaxis, therapy should be changed to a combination antiretroviral drug regimen.*

[†]*From Centers for Disease Control and Prevention (CDC) (1998). Guidelines for the use of antiretroviral agents in pediatric HIV infection, Atlanta: CDC.*

[‡]*At least two measurements (taken 1 week apart) should be performed before considering a change in therapy.*

[§]*The initial HIV RNA level of the child at the start of therapy and the level achieved with therapy should be considered when contemplating potential drug changes. For example, an immediate change in therapy may not be warranted if there is a sustained 1.5 to 2.0 log10 decrease in HIV RNA copy number, even if RNA remains detectable at low levels.*

[||] *More frequent evaluation of HIV RNA levels should be considered if the HIV RNA increase is limited (e.g., if when using an HIV RNA assay with a lower limit of detection of 1000 copies/ml, there is a L0.7 log10 increase from undetectable to approximately 5000 copies/ml in an infant aged <2 years).*

- A reproducible increase in HIV RNA copy number among children who have had a substantial HIV RNA response but still have low levels of detectable HIV RNA. Such an increase would warrant change in therapy if, after initiation of the therapeutic regimen, a greater than threefold (0.5 log10) increase in copy number for children aged at least 2 years and a greater than fivefold (0.7 log10) increase are observed for children aged younger than 2 years.

Immunologic considerations[*]

- Change in immunologic classification (Table 9-12)
- For children with CD4+ T-lymphocyte percentages below 15% (i.e., those in immune category 3), a persistent decline of five percentiles or more in CD4+ cell percentage (e.g., from 15% to 10%)
- A rapid and substantial decrease in absolute CD4+ T-lymphocyte count (Table 9-13) (e.g., a 30% decline in <6 months)

Clinical considerations

- Progressive neurodevelopmental deterioration
- Growth failure defined as persistent decline in weight-growth velocity despite adequate nutritional support and without other explanation
- Disease progression defined as advancement from one pediatric clinical category to another (e.g., from clinical category A to clinical category B)[†]

ENTEROVIRUSES

Enteroviruses are a group of RNA viral agents that encompass coxsackieviruses, echoviruses, enteroviruses, and polioviruses. All are capable of infecting a neonate, usually perinatally through the placenta (fetal infection) or human contact (neonatal infection). The respiratory route is the most likely culprit. The enteroviruses reproduce rapidly, but all are killed by heat.

---

[*]Minimal changes in CD4+ T-lymphocyte percentile that may result in change in immunologic category (e.g., from 26% to 24%, or 16% to 14%) may not be as concerning as a rapid substantial change in CD4+ percentile within the same immunologic category (e.g., a drop from 35% to 25%).

[†]In patients with stable immunologic and virologic parameters, progression from one clinical category to another may not represent an indication to change therapy. Thus, in patients whose disease progression is not associated with neurologic deterioration or growth failure, virologic and immunologic considerations are important in deciding whether to change therapy.

Table 9-13   Recommendations for *Pneumocystis carinii* Pneumonia (PCP) Prophylaxis and CD4 Monitoring in HIV-Exposed Infants and HIV-Infected Children

Age/HIV Infection Status	PCP Prophylaxis	CD4+ Monitoring
Birth to 4-6 wk/HIV exposed or infected	No prophylaxis (because PCP is rare and due to concerns regarding kernicterus with TMP/SMX)	1 mo
4-6 wk to 4 mo/HIV exposed	Prophylaxis	3 mo
4-12 mo	Prophylaxis	6, 9, 12 mo
HIV infected or indeterminate		None
HIV infection reasonably excluded*	No prophylaxis	None
	No prophylaxis	
1-5 yr/HIV infected	Prophylaxis if CD4+ count <500 cells/mm³ or CD4+ percentage <15%	Every 3-4 mo (more frequently if indicated)
Older than 6 yr/HIV infected	Prophylaxis if CD4+ count <2000 cells/mm³ or CD4+ percentage <15%	Every 3-4 yr

From Centers for Disease Control and Prevention (1995). 1995 Revised guidelines for prophylaxis against Pneumocystis carinii pneumonia for children infected with or perinatally exposed to human immunodeficiency virus. MMWR morbidity & mortality weekly report, 44, 1-12. Cited in Mueller BU, Pizzo PA (2001). Acquired immunodeficiency syndrome in the infant. In Remington JS, Klein JO, editors. Infectious diseases of the fetus and newborn infant, ed 5, Philadelphia: WB Saunders, p. 456.

HIV, Human immunodeficiency virus; TMP/SMX, trimethoprim/sufamethoxazole; IgG, immunoglobulin G.

*Two or more negative HIV diagnostic tests (i.e., HIV culture or polymerase chain reaction), both performed at ≥1 mo of age and one of which was performed at ≥4 mo of age; or at least two negative HIV IgG antibody tests performed at ≥6 mo of age among children without clinical evidence of HIV disease.

Clinical Manifestations

These viruses often attack the central nervous system. Infiltrates of the anterior horn cells and glial matter are noted with poliomyelitis. Coxsackieviruses (mainly form B) result in myocarditis or meningoencephalitis. There can be systemic organ involvement as well. Echoviruses result in hemorrhages of the adrenals, spleen, liver, renal system, and cerebellum secondary to disseminated intravascular coagulation (DIC) in its most severe form. Each of these types of viruses can also produce mild symptoms of fever and malaise. Respiratory symptoms are the more common with coryza, pneumonia, and pharyngitis present. Gastrointestinal symptoms include vomiting or diarrhea. Other signs of mild sepsis are possible. In some infants necrotizing enterocolitis may be present.

Diagnosis

The diagnosis is based on positive tissue cultures; ELISA and other similar tests are not helpful in the diagnosis if the disease is in the early stages. PCR can detect the virus in cerebrospinal fluid, blood, and urine. Because the symptoms are similar to bacterial infections, this type of infection must be ruled out.

Nursing Management

The treatment for enteroviruses is symptomatic and supportive.

LYME DISEASE (LYME BORRELIOSIS)

Lyme disease, although thought of as a pediatric or adult disease, is capable of perinatal transmission to the fetus and neonate. It is a tick-borne pathogen.

Clinical Manifestations

The spirochete organism attacks major organ systems resulting in systemic infection. It is responsible for meningoencephalitis, cardiac anomalies (e.g., ventricular septal defect, patent ductus arteriosus, coarctation of the aorta, atrial septal defect), intrauterine growth restriction, syndactyly, clubfoot, contractures, radial dysplasia, cryptorchidism, hypospadias, renal dysplasia, omphalocele, tracheoesophageal fistula, and developmental delays.

Diagnosis

The diagnosis is made by cultures and use of PCR to detect *Borrelia burgdorferi* growth. The ELISA test along with the Western blot can be used as well. The differential diagnosis includes other general infectious agents (e.g., rubella, echoviruses, hepatitis, herpes simplex, cytomegalovirus, toxoplasmosis, syphilis) and other conditions (e.g., idiopathic congenital heart disease, congenital hypotonia, failure to thrive).

Nursing Management

Antibiotics are the mainstay of treatment for Lyme disease (Table 9-14).

LISTERIOSIS

Listeria monocytogenes is a gram-positive, motile bacterium. It is responsible for perinatal infections that easily cross the placenta to the fetus.

Clinical Manifestations

If contracted during the first or early second trimester of pregnancy, listeriosis can result in early fetal demise, premature birth, and severe infection. If contracted later in pregnancy it can result in pneumonia. If born prematurely the infant will usually be meconium stained because of perinatal asphyxial episodes. Infants also may appear flaccid and apneic and have low Apgar scores; if feedings are attempted, poor feeding is noted. A papular erythematous skin rash and hepatosplenomegaly may be present. Early onset of the infection is denoted in the first few hours to weeks of life. Late-onset listeriosis that can occur at 1 month of age can result in meningitis, with resultant mental retardation and developmental delays.

Nursing Management

Ampicillin in combination with an aminoglycoside is the most common treatment for listeriosis.

TUBERCULOSIS

Mycobacterium tuberculosis is a gram-positive rod, bacterial infection that is on the rise in the United States. It is easily passed to the fetus through the placenta.

Clinical Manifestations

The infant with *M. tuberculosis* may present with fever, lethargy, papular skin lesions, respiratory distress, hepatosplenomegaly, and abdominal distention.

Diagnosis

The diagnosis is made on the basis of a chest x-ray that exhibits a miliary pattern and often parenchymal infiltrates. Tissue cultures of the placenta are helpful. Acid-fast staining of tissue and fluid cultures will demonstrate the presence of *M. tuberculosis*.

Nursing Management

Nursing management centers on the treatment of the infection with antituberculosis drugs. Unfortunately little research has been done on the safety and efficacy of these medications in premature and term

Table 9-14 Treatment of Congenital Lyme Borreliosis (CLB)*

Clinical Classification	Age at Time of Antibiotic Therapy		
	Neonate, <1 Wk	Neonate, 1-4 Wks	Infant >4 Wk
Gestational LB exposure: asymptomatic infant, born to adequately treated mother†	No antibiotic *or* Amoxicillin, 40 mg/kg/day PO tid × 10-30 days	No antibiotic *or* Amoxicillin, 50 mg/kg/day PO tid × 10-30 days	No antibiotic *or* Amoxicillin, 50 mg/kg/day PO tid × 10-30 days
Gestational LB exposure: asymptomatic infant, born to inadequately treated mother‡ *or* Early CLB: infant symptomatic in first 2 wk of life‡¶	Ceftriaxone, 50 mg/kg/day IV/IM every 24 hr × 14-30 days *or* Cefotaxime, 100 mg/kg/day IV/IM every 12 hr × 14-30 days	Ceftriaxone§ 75 mg/kg/day IV/IM q24h × 14-30 days *or* Cefotaxime‖, 150 mg/kg/day IV/IM every 8 hr × 14-30 days	Ceftriaxone 100 mg/kg/day IV/IM q12h × 14-30 days *or* Cefotaxime‖, 150 mg/kg/day IV/IM every 8 hr × 14-30 days

Late CLB: infant symptomatic after first 2 wks of life‡ ¶	Ceftriaxone§, 75 mg/kg/day, IV/IM every 24 hr × 14-42 days¶ or Cefotaxime‖, 150 mg/kg/day IV/IM every 8 hr 14-42 days¶	Ceftriaxone§, 100 mg/kg/day IV/IM every 12 hr × 14-42 days¶ or Cefotaxime‖, 150 mg/kg/day IV/IM every 8 hr × 14-42 days¶

From Gardner R (2001). Lyme disease. In Remington JS, Klein JO, editors. Infectious diseases of the fetus and newborn infant, ed 5, Philadelphia: WB Saunders, p. 603.

Recommendations are based on limited data, and lengths of therapy are not well established. Different age-appropriate doses are shown, but treatment is recommended as soon as possible after birth.

†*Because there is a wide range in what is considered adequate therapy, the alternative of oral amoxicillin therapy to be given pending further evaluation of the neonate for CLB is offered.*

‡*Because ceftriaxone should not be used if hyperbilirubinemia is present, cefotaxime is offered as an alternative, although clinical experience in therapy of Lyme borreliosis is not as extensive as with ceftriaxone.*

§*Ceftriaxone dose 50 mg/kg/day IV/IM every 24 hr if weight <2000 g.*

‖*Cefotaxime dose 100 mg/kg/day IV/IM every 12 hr if weight <1200 g.*

¶*Prolonged oral amoxicillin (40 mg/kg/day) after the course of IV antibiotic therapy may be considered, depending on the clinical course of the infant.*

infants. INH (isoniazid) remains the drug of choice at a dosage of 10 to 20 mg/kg/day to a maximum dose of 300 mg/day. Serum aspartate aminotransferase and serum alanine aminotransferase need to be monitored as long as INH is being given because it can lead to hepatotoxicity. Other medications that may be used are rifampin, pyrazinamide, streptomycin, and ethambutol.

RESPIRATORY SYNCYTIAL VIRUS

Respiratory syncytial virus (RSV) is a virus that occurs from time to time in the NICU. The following guideline can be used for care of the infant with RSV.

UNIVERSITY OF ILLINOIS MEDICAL CENTER AT CHICAGO CLINICAL CARE GUIDELINE

Subject: Synagis–Indications for Use Prior to the Time of Discharge from NICU/ICN*

Objective

To ensure that infants at risk for the development of respiratory syncytial viral infections have been administered Synagis to reduce the morbidity and mortality associated with this infection.

Definitions

For the purpose of this guideline, the following definitions apply:

Premature Infants—Infants in whom birth occurs before the completion of 32 weeks of gestation.

Chronic Lung Disease—Defined as infants with an oxygen requirement at 36 weeks of corrected gestational age.

Respiratory Syncytial Virus (RSV)—A viral infection that primarily affects immunocompromised individuals, results in severe pulmonary symptoms, and exacerbates chronic lung disease.

RSV Season—The time period during the year when RSV infections peak, such as from October until April each year.

Synagis—The brand name for monoclonal antibody to RSV. The generic name for the drug is palivizumab.

Position Statements

Premature infants and infants with chronic lung disease are at risk for the development of RSV infections. RSV infection results in increased morbidity and mortality among these infants.

*From University of Illinois Medical Center at Chicago Women's and Children's Nursing Services. Used with permission by Dharmapuri Vidyasagar, MD; Catherine Theorell, RNC, MSN, NNP; Beena Peters, RN, MS.

Infants who are hospitalized in the NICU/ICN and who are at risk for RSV infection will have Synagis administered throughout the RSV season.

Every effort will be made to coordinate services to ensure the continuation of this therapy during RSV season after discharge.

Procedures

1. Infants at risk for the development of RSV infection should be identified. Such at-risk infants may include the following:

   a. Infants born at or less than 28 weeks of gestational age with or without chronic lung disease. These infants should receive monthly doses of Synagis for at least one RSV season. The second RSV season should be individualized according to each patient.

   b. Infants born between 29 and 35 weeks of gestational age who have been diagnosed with chronic lung disease. These infants should receive monthly doses of Synagis for at least one RSV season. The second RSV season should be individualized according to each patient.

   c. Infants born between 29 and 35 weeks of gestational age in whom chronic lung disease is not present. The infants need to have the Synagis protocol individualized according to each patient.

   d. All other infants diagnosed with chronic lung disease who are less than 2 years of age. These infants may be considered for Synagis during the next RSV season even if they do not meet the above indications.

2. The infants identified as meeting the eligibility criteria for Synagis shall have monthly dose of the drug ordered by the pediatric house staff.

3. The nursing staff shall document the administration of Synagis in the medication administration record. In addition, the nurse may make a note of this in the nurse to nurses notes on the infant's care plan.

4. The nurse shall work with the family and health care providers in order to arrange for the continuation of all required doses for the entire RSV season after hospitalization. Family education about monoclonal antibody reduces hospitalization from respiratory syncytial virus infection in high-risk infants. Understanding the importance of this drug is a paramount part of the process of discharge education.

5. All efforts should be made for the follow-up doses for the whole season by arranging with the primary care pediatrician, pulmonologist, or developmental clinics. The drug company will also help to get the patient for follow-up doses with their Reach Program.

REFERENCE

The Impact-RSV Study Group (1998). Palivizumab, a humanized respiratory syncytial virus monoclonal antibody, reduces hospitalization from respiratory syncytial virus infection in high-risk infants. *Pediatrics*, 102, 531-537.

URINARY TRACT INFECTIONS

Urinary tract infections (UTIs) are commonly caused by bacteria. The usual agents are *Escherichia coli*, *Klebsiella*, *Enterobacter*, coagulase-negative staphylococci, and *Candida*.

Clinical Manifestations

The usual signs and symptoms of UTIs include irritability, fever, failure to thrive, diarrhea, jaundice, and lethargy.

Diagnosis

Diagnosis is by urine culture detecting the presence of the bacteria ($>10^4$ colonies/ml). Blood and cerebrospinal fluid cultures may also be indicated to make sure there is no systemic infection present. A urine Gram stain will help determine the causative agent. If this infection is considered to be due to an obstructive or other anomaly a voiding cystourethrogram or ultrasound is in order. Another test that can be used is the renal cortical scintigraphy that uses technetium-99m radioisotope. This test is used if pyeleonephritis is suspected.

Nursing Management

Penicillin and gentamicin are the drugs of choice if septicemia is suspected. If there is a suspected renal abscess methicillin or oxacillin may be used because *Staphylococcus aureus* is the most likely cause. If this is a nosocomial infection then vancomycin and an aminoglycoside may be used. The antimicrobial therapy is given for 10 to 14 days.

BIBLIOGRAPHY

Crumpacker CS (2001). Hepatitis. In Remington JS, Klein JO, editors. *Infectious diseases of the fetus and newborn infant*, ed 5, Philadelphia: WB Saunders, pp. 913-942.

Ingall E, Sanches PI (2001). Syphilis. In Remington JS, Klein JO, editors. *Infectious disease of the fetus and newborn infant*, ed 5, Philadelphia: WB Saunders, p. 58.

Khoory BJ, et al. (1999). *Candida* infections in newborns: a review, *Journal of chemotherapy*, 11(5), 367-378.

Lott JW, Kenner C (2003). Assessment and management of the immune system. In Kenner C, Lott JW, editors. *Comprehensive neonatal nursing care: a physiologic perspective*, ed 3, St Louis: WB Saunders.

Miller MJ (2001). Fungal infections. In Remington JS, Klein JO, editors. *Infectious diseases of the fetus and newborn infant*, ed 5, Philadelphia: WB Saunders, pp. 813-854.

Remington JS, Klein JO, editors. (2001). *Infectious diseases of the fetus and newborn infant*, ed 5, Philadelphia: WB Saunders.

CHAPTER 10

GASTROINTESTINAL CARE

The gastrointestinal (GI) system is made up of upper and lower GI organs. The problems that occur concern ingestion, digestion, and elimination. Many neonatal GI problems require surgical intervention because they are due to functional or mechanical obstructions. These can be in the form of atresia, stenosis, other malformations of the GI tract, or functional plugs, such as meconium plugs. These problems and their care will be discussed in Chapter 16.

NURSING ASSESSMENT

The assessment of the GI system should include a thorough history—prenatal, intrapartal, and postpartal. The key features that are *"red flags"* for GI disturbance are the following:
• Polyhydramnios
• Oligohydramnios
• Increased production of mucus
• Feeding intolerances—vomiting, diarrhea, difficulty sucking or swallowing, cyanosis, large residuals, abdominal distention (this distention can occur even in NPO [nothing by mouth] infants)
• Delayed passage of meconium
• Failure to thrive

CLINICAL MANIFESTATIONS

The clinical manifestations are consistent with the area of the GI tract that is nonfunctional. If it is upper GI then there is a problem with secretions such as excessive saliva, difficulty swallowing or sucking, feeding ingestion problems, visible defects such as a cleft lip or palate, or difficulty breathing if there is a tracheoesophageal fistula in which case respiratory distress and pneumonia may be present. Digestion problems elicit problems with feeding—vomiting, residual amounts of gastric aspirate, abdominal distention, or increased irritability; some infants experience cyanosis with feedings. The color of the vomitus will indicate the level of the obstruction. Problems with elimination also result in abdominal distention, constipation, diarrhea, or failure to pass meconium. The color of the stool will indicate the level of obstruction.

DIAGNOSIS

The diagnosis is made based on a thorough physical examination, and usually abdominal x-rays, ultrasounds, computed tomography (CT) scans, and magnetic resonance imaging (MRI) are used for the definitive diagnosis.

The more common problems will be presented in Box 10-1 along with feeding implications. Although cleft lip and/or palate does require surgical intervention, the feeding aspects of this problem (ingestion) become one of the most challenging problems from a nursing perspective so it is presented here.

UNIVERSITY OF ILLINOIS MEDICAL CENTER AT CHICAGO CLINICAL CARE GUIDELINE*

Subject: Palatal Device Care in the Neonatal Intensive Care Unit (NICU)

Objective
To establish written guidelines for the application, safe use, and care of the palatal device.

Definition
For the purposes of this guideline, the following definition applies:

Palatal Device—A customized, molded plastic device that protects the developing hard palate from pressure and friction caused by the position of the oral endotracheal tube.

Position Statements
The pediatric dentist/dental resident will identify candidates for palatal device regularly and will obtain the palatal impression for eligible infants.

During the period that the palatal impression is being performed or whenever manipulation of the palatal device is necessary, a pediatric resident will be available in the event of accidental extubation.

Registered nurses (RNs), RNs license pending, supervised by an RN preceptor, or nursing students supervised by nursing faculty or staff RN shall do the following:
1. Assist pediatric dentist/dental resident in obtaining the palatal impression
2. Ensure that all impression material is removed before retaping endotracheal tube (ETT) after the palatal impression

---

*From University of Illinois Medical Center at Chicago Women's and Children's Nursing Services.
Used with permission by Dharmapuri Vidyasagar, MD; Catherine Theorell, RNC, MSN, NNP; Beena Peters, RN, MS.

Box 10-1

Cleft Lip and/or Palate: Feeding, Care, and Management/Intervention for Term Infant

General Guidelines
- Feed in upright sitting position. Squeeze formula into mouth, directing flow to sides of mouth and coordinating with swallow.
- Place infant on sides, in infant seat and later on back (1 hour after feeds) but not on abdomen. This eliminates adjustment of cleft lip infants at the time of early surgical correction, which eliminates suture repair trauma.
- Frequent burping (because of excessive air ingestion) will eliminate spitting/possible aspiration.
- Burp in sitting position on lap, which prevents soft tissue trauma on caregiver's shoulder.

Therapeutic
- Mead-Johnson or Haberman feeder—for cleft lip and/or hard palate with or without alveolar ridge, partial or complete defects:
  - Initial oral feedings with nipple: allow for maximal palatal shelf formations, minimize palate and soft tissue trauma, allow for feeding with minimal energy expenditure and prepare for early postoperative lip feeding regimen with minimal adjustment
- Regular nipple feedings—may be attempted in infants with submucosal clefts and/or bifid uvula:
  - Assess for adequate suction achievement.
  - Assess ability to ingest adequate volume in a given time without tiring.
- Breast-feeding—may be attempted in infants with submucosal clefts or bifid uvula and partially in infants with incomplete cleft lip:
  - Assess for adequate suction achievement.
  - Assess intake by monitoring output, weight gain.
  - Half of feedings should be by Ross feeder in preparation for surgical adjustment.
- Pacifiers—discouraged until approved by surgeon postoperatively
- Haberman feeder diaphragm—for severe feeding problems such as Down syndrome, cleft lip/palate, Pierre Robin syndrome or sequence
  - Four holes for disk to bottom, white disk circle up toward nipple. Squeeze nipple with upright and hold to release air, then invert while squeezing (small amount of formula will enter the nipple to fill until full—holds 30 cc. Squeeze for flow with slits as noted above. Usually no. 3 vertical slit is used (centered in mouth).

Box **10-1**

Cleft Lip and/or Palate: Feeding, Care, and Management/ Intervention for Term Infant—cont'd

Social
- Encourage maximal parent interaction for acceptance of the infant as an individual, to decrease anxiety, and to gain confidence with the feeding technique.
- Offer support group information/patient and family counseling.
- Encourage mother to make a written list of her concerns and to take to her first surgical appointment within 1 to 2 days of infant's discharge.
- Arrange for photo conference to reinforce the achievements of surgical intervention and decrease apprehension.

Diagnostic Criteria
- Cleft lip—with or without palatal involvement is a grossly obvious defect, not necessitating a work-up
- Cleft palate—more subtle and identified on physical assessment

Associated Complications (Usually Isolated Occurrence or Genetic Predisposition)
- Pierre Robin syndrome or sequence: severity of micrognathia may cause airway obstruction/aspiration; feed as you would cleft lip/palate
- Trisomy 15 and other chromosomal defects
- Dental and speech pathologic conditions in cleft palate infants
- Otitis media in cleft palate children
- Multisystem or multiple midline anomalies

Prognosis
- Dependent on associated complications
- Excellent cosmetic surgical results: may be single or staged repairs
- Dental, speech and audiology follow-up with or without the craniofacial anomalies team: offers maximal results, depending on infant's potential and associated defects

Discharge Planning
- Plan for discharge with mother or on third or fourth day of life if mother feels confident with feeding technique.
- Surgical intervention for lip is at several weeks of age with demonstrated steady weight gain. Palate repair is deferred until 12 to 18 months and adequate growth.

From Altimier L, Brown B, Tedeschi L (2000). Tri-Health's manual of neonatal nursing policies, procedures, competencies, & clinical pathways, Glenview, Ill: National Association of Neonatal Nurses.

3. Maintain the orotracheal tube in proper placement during palatal device insertion
4. Clean palatal device and assess oral cavity for breakdown
5. Assess breath sounds to ascertain proper tube placement after manipulation of ETT

Infants meeting the following criteria will be considered for use of a palatal device:

1. Birth weight between 500 to 2000 g in whom prolonged intubation is anticipated
2. Infants weighing more than 2000 g with the potential for endotracheal intubation longer than 1week will also be considered for device placement.
3. Infants who are able to maintain SaO_2 greater than 85% with no greater than a 10% increase in FiO_2 during handling
4. Infants who are intubated less than 48 hours are not eligible for palatal devices.
5. Infants who have palatal deformities or micrognathia are not eligible for palatal devices.

Clean technique (incorporating Standard Precautions) shall be maintained when obtaining palatal impression and cleaning the device.

Palatal devices shall be cleaned daily.

Position of the palatal device and ETT stability within the device shall be assessed every shift and as needed.

Procedures

1. Obtaining the palatal impression
   a. Equipment for retaping the endotracheal tube (ETT) (Duoderm and custom cut adhesive tape) should be assembled before the initiation of the impression.
   b. Obtain an order to increase FiO_2 as necessary to prevent desaturation.
   c. Untape ETT.
   d. Note and mark the location of ETT at the upper lip.
   e. Hold infant's forehead with one hand and the ETT at the marked spot with the other hand while securing the chin.
   f. Reposition the ETT down in the mouth to rest on the tongue while keeping the ETT in proper placement.
   g. After impression is made, remove any remaining expression material and retape the ETT according to standard procedure.
2. Placement of the palatal device
   a. Equipment for placement of palatal device (sterile water, sterile 4 × 4s, and denture adhesive powder) should be obtained before procedure.
   b. Dip the device in bottle of sterile water while holding attached string.

    c. Take the palatal device out of the water and place it on a sterile 4×4 with palatal side up.

    d. Sprinkle small amount of adhesive powder over the palatal device, and shake off excess.

    e. While the helper nurse is stabilizing the ETT, place the device sideways into one corner of the mouth holding the device at the point of the string attachment

    f. Slide the device toward the center of the oral cavity between the ETT and the palate.

    g. Apply light pressure upward against the hard palate with the palatal device to promote adhesion.

    h. Assess the oral cavity for the location of the tongue and fit of the device.

    i. After ensuring that the positioning of the palatal device is correct, ease the ETT into the groove.

    j. Placement of the ETT is accomplished by exerting pressure on the tube with the index finger starting at the anterior margin of the device and moving inward along the tube.

    k. Tape the string to the ETT to prevent laceration of the infant's cheek.

3. Daily palatal device cleaning

    a. Equipment required for cleaning (sterile 2×2, sterile water, half-strength hydrogen peroxide, denture adhesive powder, Surgilube jelly [optional], Duoderm, Elastoplast of waterproof tape)

    b. If ETT is not required, only one nurse is needed for this procedure. Secure the ETT in position at the corner of the infant's mouth opposite the side where the string is attached.

       (1) Begin by loosening the orotracheal tube from the palatal groove by pinching the tube and pulling downward gently.

       (2) Exert downward pressure on the front ridge of the device with a finger, and pull gently on the string to allow the device to be removed from the corner of the mouth opposite the orotracheal tube.

       (3) When the device is out, examine the oral cavity for the presence of thrush or irritation of mucous membranes.

    c. If ETT taping is required during cleaning of the palatal device, secure the assistance of another nurse.

       (1) Nurse one removes the tape from ETT and skin.

       (2) Nurse two secures the ETT in position at the corner of the infant's mouth opposite the side where the string is attached.

       (3) Exert downward pressure on the front ridge of the device with a finger, and pull gently on the string to allow the device to be removed from the corner of the mouth opposite the orotracheal tube.

(4) When the device is out, examine condition of the oral cavity for presence of thrush or irritation of mucous membranes.

d. Perform oral hygiene with a 2 × 2 gauze dipped in sterile water.

e. Clean the device with half-strength hydrogen peroxide, and rinse with sterile water.

f. Sprinkle a small amount of denture adhesive on the device. Shake off excess powder.

g. If oral cavity is small, Surgilube jelly can be used to lubricate the corners of the infant's mouth before insertion of the palatal device. While stabilizing the ETT place the device sideways into the corner of the mouth holding the device up and toward the center of the mouth above the orotracheal tube.

h. When the device is in place on the palate, apply gentle pressure upward against the device to promote adhesion.

i. After ensuring that the positioning of the palatal device is correct, ease the orotracheal tube into the groove of the device with a finger.

j. Retape ETT as necessary according to procedure.

4. Parent teaching and documentation

a. Explain the necessity of the device to the parents as simply as possible.

(1) The device prevents the ETT from rubbing against the roof of the mouth, thereby preventing palatal grooving and abnormal tooth development.

(2) The device does not cause the infant discomfort.

(3) Explain the process of oral hygiene and cleaning the device.

(4) Explain the subsequent need for new device as infant grows.

b. Document on nursing flow sheet:

(1) The date and time of initial insertion of the palatal device

(2) The pulse oximeter reading, bradycardic episodes that occur, any need for increased FiO_2, accidental extubations, and overall tolerance to procedure:

(a) During the impression

(b) During the placement of the device

(c) During the cleaning procedure

(3) The condition of the oral mucosa each time the device is removed for cleaning

(4) The date a new impression is made because of growth and/or a change in orotracheal tube size

(5) The date the device is discontinued along with the reason for discontinuation

(6) Parent teaching

Table 10-1	Modified Bell's Staging Criteria for Neonatal Necrotizing Enterocolitis			
Stage	**Systemic Signs**	**Intestinal Signs**	**Radiologic Signs**	**Treatment**
IA—suspected NEC	Temperature instability, apnea, bradycardia, lethargy	Elevated pregavage residuals, mild abdominal distention, emesis, guaiac-positive stool	Normal or intestinal dilation, mild ileus	Nothing by mouth, antibiotics for 3 days pending cultures
IB—suspected NEC	Same as above	Bright red blood from rectum	Same as above	Same as above
IIA—definite NEC: mildly ill	Same as above	Same as above, *plus* diminished or absent bowel sounds with or without abdominal tenderness	Intestinal dilation, ileus, pneumatosis intestinalis	Nothing by mouth, antibiotics for 7-10 days if examination is normal in 24-48 hr
IIB—definite NEC: moderately ill	Above *plus* mild metabolic acidosis and mild thrombocytopenia	Above *plus* definite abdominal tenderness, with or without abdominal cellulitis or right lower quadrant mass, absent bowel sounds	Same as stage IIA with or without portal vein gas, with or without ascites	Nothing by mouth, antibiotics for 14 days, NaHCO$_3$ for acidosis

Continued

Table 10-1	Modified Bell's Staging Criteria for Neonatal Necrotizing Enterocolitis—cont'd			
Stage	Systemic Signs	Intestinal Signs	Radiologic Signs	Treatment
IIIA–advanced NEC: severely ill, bowel intact	Same as IIB, *plus* hypotension, bradycardia, severe apneas, combined respiratory and metabolic acidosis, disseminated intravascular coagulation, neutropenia, anuria	Above *plus* signs of generalized peritonitis, marked tenderness, distention of abdomen, and abdominal wall erythema	Same as stage IIB above, definite ascites	Same as above *plus* fluids, 200 ml/kg/day, fresh frozen plasma, inotropic agents; intubation, ventilation therapy; paracentesis; surgical intervention if patient fails to improve with medical management within 24-48 hr
IIIB–advanced NEC: severely ill, bowel perforation	Same as stage III	Same as stage III	Same as stage IIB above *plus* pneumoperitoneum	Same as above *plus* surgical interventions

From Kalhan SC, Price PT (2001). Nutrition and selected disorders of the gastrointestinal tract. In Klaus MH, Fanaroff AA, editors. Care of the high-risk neonate, ed 5, Philadelphia: WB Saunders, p. 187.

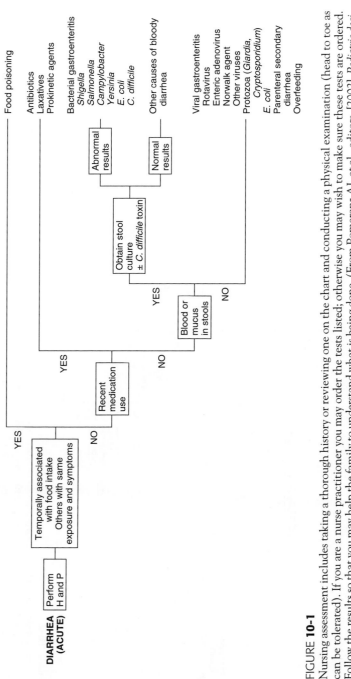

FIGURE 10-1

Nursing assessment includes taking a thorough history or reviewing one on the chart and conducting a physical examination (head to toe as can be tolerated). If you are a nurse practitioner you may order the tests listed; otherwise you may wish to make sure these tests are ordered. Follow the results so that you may help the family to understand what is being done. (From Pomeranz AJ, et al., editors. [2002]. *Pediatric decision-making strategies to accompany Nelson textbook of pediatrics*, ed 16, Philadelphia: WB Saunders, p. 87.)

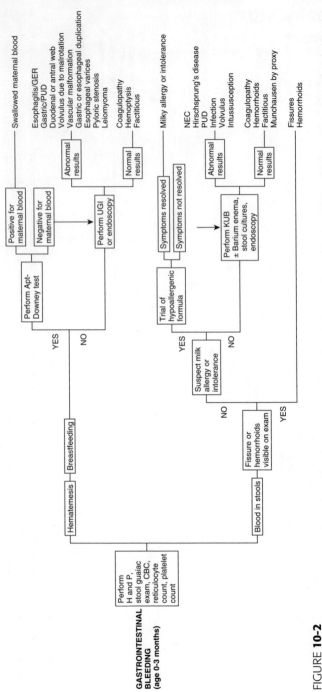

FIGURE 10-2

Nursing assessment includes taking a thorough history or reviewing one on the chart and conducting a physical examination (head to toe as can be tolerated). If you are a nurse practitioner you may order the tests listed; otherwise, you may wish to make sure these tests are ordered. Follow the results so that you may help the family to understand what is being done. (From Pomeranz AJ, et al., editors. [2002]. *Pediatric decision-making strategies to accompany Nelson textbook of pediatrics*, ed 16, Philadelphia: WB Saunders, p. 103.)

NECROTIZING ENTEROCOLITIS

Necrotizing enterocolitis (NEC) can be life threatening. It may or may not require surgical intervention. It is believed to be due to a hypoxic episode that shunts blood away from the GI tract. However, there is a strong indication that infection plays a major role in this condition. *Escherichia coli, Klebsiella, Salmonella, Clostridium, Enterobacter, Staphylococcus,* and *Candida* are the most common agents.

Bell's staging (Table 10-1) indicates the criteria for NEC. It includes the clinical manifestations, diagnostic tests, and treatment. Nursing management focuses on stabilizing the infant and anticipating problems.

DIARRHEA

Another common neonatal problem is diarrhea. Figure 10-1 will assist in your care of the infant with diarrhea.

GASTROINTESTINAL BLEEDING

GI bleeding can be a mild or severe condition. It generally is a symptom of a much larger problem. Figure 10-2 will assist you in your nursing care of the infant with GI bleeding.

BIBLIOGRAPHY

Amin HJ, et al. (2002). Arginine supplementation prevents necrotizing enterocolitis in the premature infant. *Journal of pediatrics,* 140(4), 425-431.

Banieghbal B, et al. (2002). Surgical indications and strategies for necrotizing enterocolitis in low income countries. *World journal of surgery,* 26(4), 444-447.

Bisquera JA, Cooper TR, Berseth CL (2002). Impact of necrotizing enterocolitis on length of stay and hospital charges in very low birth weight infants. *Pediatrics,* 109(3), 423-428.

Butter A, Flageole H, Laberge JM (2002). The changing face of surgical indications for necrotizing enterocolitis. *Journal of pediatric surgery,* 37(3), 496-499.

Foster J, Cole M (2001). Oral immunoglobulin for preventing necrotizing enterocolitis in preterm and low birth-weight neonates. *Cochrane database systematic reviews,* 3.

Jadcherla SR, Kliegman RM (2002). Studies of feeding intolerance in very low birth weight infants: definition and significance. *Pediatrics,* 109(3), 516-517.

Lazzaroni M, et al. (2002). Upper GI bleeding in healthy full-term infants: a case-control study. *American journal of gastroenterology,* 97(1), 89-94.

Martindale J, et al. (2000). Genetic analysis of *Escherichia coli* K1 gastrointestinal colonization. *Molecular microbiology,* 37(6), 1293-1305.

Noel L, et al. (2001). Multiple gastrointestinal tract duplication: a neonatal case report. *Journal of radiology,* 82(6, Pt 1), 676-678.

Powley TL, et al. (2001). Gastrointestinal projection maps of the vagus nerve are specified permanently in the perinatal period. *Brain research of the developing brain,* 129(1), 57-72.

Prasad TR, Bajpai M (2000). Intestinal atresia. *Indian journal of pediatrics*, 67(9), 671-678.

Saiman L, et al. (2000). Risk factors for candidemia in Neonatal Intensive Care Unit patients. The National Epidemiology of Mycosis Survey study group. *Pediatric infectious disease journal*, 19(4), 319-324.

Sandberg DJ, Magee WP, Jr, Denk MJ (2002). Neonatal cleft lip and cleft palate repair. *Association of operating room nurses (AORN) journal*, 75(3), 490-498; quiz 501-504, 506-508.

Thigpen J, Kenner C (2003). Assessment and management of the gastrointestinal system. In Kenner C, Lott JW, editors. *Comprehensive neonatal nursing: a physiologic perspective*, St Louis: WB Saunders.

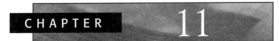

CHAPTER 11

TOTAL PARENTERAL NUTRITION

Total parenteral nutrition (TPN) is a mainstay of neonatal intensive care unit (NICU) care. The nurse is responsible for monitoring the infant who requires TPN as well as ordering the fluids if functioning in an advanced practice role. Before TPN can be ordered and monitored some basic principles of fluids and electrolytes need to be reviewed.

BASIC DEFINITIONS AND PRINCIPLES OF FLUIDS AND ELECTROLYTES

1. Total body water (TBW): all fluid within the body
2. Intracellular fluid (ICF): all fluids contained within cells
3. Extracellular fluid (ECF): all fluid outside cells
4. Proportional changes in ECF, ICF, and TBW with increasing age (Tables 11-1 and 11-2)
   a. TBW: decreases with increasing age
   b. Extracellular water: decreases with increasing age
   c. Intracellular water: increases with increasing age
5. Body fluid compartments
   a. Intracellular fluid: all fluid within cells of the body
   b. Extracellular fluid
      (1) Intravascular fluid
      (2) Interstitial fluid
      (3) Plasma
      (4) Cerebrospinal fluid (CSF)
      (5) Intraocular fluid
      (6) Potential fluid spaces
      (7) Gastrointestinal tract
6. Extracellular fluids
   a. Intravascular fluid
   b. Blood plasma
   c. Interstitial fluid
   d. All fluid in the spaces between cells and outside the blood vessels
7. Lymph and transcellular fluid
   a. CSF
   b. Synovial fluid
   c. Intraocular fluids
   d. Intestinal fluid

Table 11-1	Distribution of Body Water (BW)	
	Body Water	**Volume (L)**
Intracellular fluid	40%	28
Extracellular fluid	20%	14
Interstitial	(15%)	(11)
Intravascular	(5%)	(3)
Total body water	60%	42

Table 11-2	Water Balance
Intake	
Drinking	1400-1800 ml
Food	700-1000 ml
Oxidation	300-400 ml
Total	2400-3200 ml
Output	
Urine	1400-1800 ml
Stool	~100 ml
Insensible water loss	900-1300 (500 + 800)
Skin	300-500
Lungs	600-800
Total	2400-3200

VARIABILITY OF TOTAL BODY WATER

1. Age
   a. Increased in newborns
   b. Decreased in older adults
2. Gender
   a. Males: more muscle mass, less body fat, more TBW
3. Body composition: fat less than or equals TBW%

WATER BALANCE

Body water balance depends on the following:
- Intake
- Output
- Movement of water

IMPORTANT CONCEPTS

- Semipermeable cellular membranes
- Solutes

- Valence
- Osmotic pressure
- Oncotic pressure
- Hydrostatic pressure
- Osmolarity
- Osmolality

Semipermeable Membranes
- Cell membranes are dynamic and composed of individual proteins that are continually being modified.
- Cell membranes allow passage of some water and solutes through the cell wall through active and passive transport mechanisms.

Solutes
1. Electrolytes
   a. Ions
   b. Cations
   c. Anions
2. Nonelectrolytes
   a. Glucose
   b. Urea
   c. Creatinine

Ions
1. Cations
   a. Have positive charge
   b. Migrate toward negative pole (cathode)
2. Anions
   a. Have negative charge
   b. Migrate toward positive pole (anode)

Valence
- Electrical charge
- Number of plus (+) or minus (−) signs
- 1 mEq/L of any cation can combine with 1 mEq of any anion

Pressure

Hydrostatic pressure
- Mechanical pressure of fluids pushing against cellular membranes
- Blood pressure generated in vessels by contraction of heart

Osmosis
- Movement of water from area of higher concentration to area of lower concentration

- Osmolarity is a measure of the number of milliosmoles per liter of solution, or the concentration of molecules per volume of solution

Osmolality
- Osmolality is a measure of the number of milliosmoles per kilogram of water, or concentration of molecules per weight of water
- Total number of solute particles in solution, such as electrolytes and protein molecules

Osmotic pressure
- Osmotic pressure is the amount of hydrostatic pressure required to oppose the osmotic movement of water.
- Osmolality of ICF and ECF tends to equalize and so provides a measure of body fluid concentration and hydration.

Factors that determine osmotic pressure
- Type and thickness of plasma membrane
- Size of molecules
- Concentration of molecules or concentration gradient
- Solubility of molecules within the membrane

Oncotic pressure (colloid osmotic pressure)
- Plasma proteins influence osmolality.
- They do not generally cross cell membranes.
- They carry a negative charge and influence movement of smaller particles to maintain electroneutrality.

REGULATION OF WATER

Water Balance
Filtration is movement of water out of the capillary and into the interstitial space. Starling's hypothesis concerns forces favoring filtration and forces opposing filtration (net filtration).

Filtration
Capillary net filtration forces are as follows:
1. + Filtration
   a. Capillary hydrostatic pressure
   b. Interstitial oncotic pressure
2. − Filtration
   a. Plasma oncotic pressure
   b. Interstitial hydrostatic pressure

Fluid Requirements
The three major components are as follows:
1. Maintenance
2. Replacement of losses (deficits)
3. Replacement of ongoing losses

Factors that increase water requirements
- Increased insensible water loss (IWL)
- Fecal losses
- Surgical and chest tube drainage
- Dehydration
- Increased urinary losses
- Third-spacing of fluids
- Fever

Third-spacing of fluids (capillary leak syndrome)
- Third-spacing is accumulation of fluid and electrolytes in a static body compartment.
- Third-spaced fluids do not contribute to circulatory dynamics.

Weight Loss After Birth
1. Physiologic: isotonic contraction of ECF
2. Pathophysiologic: inadequate nutrition, volume deficits

Physiologic losses
- Insensible water loss
- Renal water loss
- Stool water loss

Renal water loss
1. Quantity depends on the following:
    a. Status of renal function
    b. Renal solute load
2. Renal solute load comes from two sources:
    a. Exogenous
    b. Endogenous

Normal water losses

Evaporative	
Skin and lungs	21 to 30 ml/kg/day
For the infant <1250 g	60 to 120 ml/kg/day
Urinary output	25 to 62 ml/kg/day
Stool	2 ml/kg/day
Average range	48 to 84 ml/kg/day

ASSESSMENT OF FLUID STATUS
- Weight
- Urinary output
- Specific gravity
- Electrolytes, blood urea nitrogen (BUN), creatinine
- Skin turgor
- pH
- Hematocrit
- Fractional excretion of sodium (FENa)

Fluid Changes After Birth

1. Relative oliguria
   a. Low urine volume production (0.5 to 2 ml/kg/hr)
   b. Lasts about 24 hours in healthy term newborns
   c. Lasts longer in preterm or asphyxiated newborns
   d. Caused by elevated levels of arginine vasopressin (AVP) or inadequate response to AVP
   e. Decreased glomerular filtration rate (GFR) because of redistribution of blood flow postnatally
2. Diuresis
   a. Obligatory in all newborns
   b. Amount determined by gestational age
   c. Term: 7% to 10% of birth weight
   d. Preterm: 10% to 15% of birth weight
   e. Very low birth weight (VLBW): up to 20% of birth weight
3. Loss of sodium causes contraction of the extracellular water (ECW).
4. Loss of ECW causes weight loss of newborn.
5. Failure to undergo this diuresis may lead to patent ductus arteriosus (PDA), congestive heart failure (CHF), or pulmonary edema.

Diuresis is a natural process following birth. If the extra fluid that has accumulated during fetal life does not dissipate then complications such as PDA, CHF, and pulmonary edema can occur. The full-term infant is better able to achieve diuresis than the premature infant whose renal system is immature. TBW and ECW decrease with increasing gestational age whereas ICW increases with increasing gestational age.

Causes of Diuresis

- Renal tubules have transient inability to reabsorb normal amount of sodium filtered by glomerulus.
- Sodium diuresis is necessary to allow cardiac atria to contract.
- Diuresis is induced by atrial natriuretic protein (ANP).

IMPORTANCE OF FLUID MANAGEMENT IN PRETERM INFANTS

- Frequent use of parenteral fluid therapy
- Variability in requirements for fluids
- Limitation of renal adjustments in cases of fluid overload or deficit
- Interrelationship of fluid/electrolyte balance and pathophysiologic conditions of preterm infants (respiratory distress syndrome [RDS], bronchopulmonary dysplasia [BPD], patent ductus arteriosus [PDA], necrotizing enterocolitis [NEC])

The goal of fluid and electrolyte therapy is to provide adequate fluid and electrolytes to replace physiologic losses.

Preterm Infants Have Higher Insensible Water Loss
- Greater water permeability through relatively immature epithelial layer
- Higher surface area/body weight ratio
- Relatively higher skin vascularity

Factors that increase insensible water loss
- Low-humidity environment
- Increased respiratory rates
- Radiant energy
- Convection
- Phototherapy
- High environmental temperature
- High body temperature
- Skin breakdown or defect

Ways to reduce insensible water loss
- Provide adequate humidity.
- Use incubators, heat shields, Saran wrap.
- Prevent evaporative, conductive, convective, and radiant heat losses.

Renal Water Loss
1. Quantity depends on the following:
   a. Status of renal function
   b. Renal solute load
2. Renal solute comes from two sources:
   a. Exogenous (enteral and parenteral)
   b. Endogenous (from catabolism)

Basal Energy Requirements
- Low–birth weight (LBW) babies require about 50 kcal/kg/day in the first few days of life. They generally use some endogenous sources for some of this energy.
- The catabolic state produces about 5 mOsm/kg/day of a solute load for the kidney to excrete.
- Five mOsm/kg/day requires about 20 ml/kg/day of free water for excretion.
- By 3 weeks, the normal infant is taking about 120 kcal/kg/day, which requires about 80 ml/kg/day of free water for excretion.

Stool Water Loss
- Stool water loss is minimal during first few days of life.
- After enteral feeding is established, the stool water loss is about 5 to 10 ml/kg/day.

   Table 11-3 gives fluid requirements for infants, and Box 11-1 gives examples of fluid calculations.

Box 11-1

Fluid Calculations for Maintenance

Maintenance*	A
Day 1	Weight × 60-80
Day 2	Weight × 80-100
Day 3	Weight × 100-120
>Day 3	Weight × 100-150

*Total fluid per kilogram per day.

Table 11-3	Fluid Requirement		
Birth Weight (g)	**Days 1 and 2 (ml/kg)**	**Day 3 (ml/kg)**	**Days >15 (ml/kg)**
750-1000	105	140	150
1001-1250	100	130	140
1251-1500	90	120	130
1501-1750	80	110	130
1751-2000	80	110	130

FLUID CALCULATIONS

Maintenance (A)

Day 1	wt × 60-80
Day 2	wt × 80-100
Day 3	wt × 100-120
> Day 3	wt × 100-150

Total fluid/kg/day (maintenance)
- B: Deficit × Estimated dehydration (%)
- C: Ongoing losses
- Radiant warmer: add 20% to 50%
- Phototherapy: 20% to 30%
- Add A + B + C

Subtract: Estimate of flushes or colloids are subtracted from total fluid/kg/day = Total IV fluid/day (D)

IV hourly rate = D/24

INDICATORS OF FLUID STATUS

- Weight
- Urinary output

- Specific gravity
- Electrolytes, blood urea nitrogen (BUN), creatinine
- Skin turgor
- Fontanel
- pH
- Hematocrit
- Fractional excretion of sodium

Fractional Excretion of Sodium
This formula is useful to evaluate oliguria:

$$\frac{\text{Urine sodium x Plasma creatinine}}{\text{Urine creatinine x Plasma sodium}} \times 100$$

A value above 2.5% occurs with acute renal failure, and a value below 1% occurs with prerenal conditions.

Best Indicators for Fluid Status

Weight loss	1% to 2%/day
Maximum of 10% in preterm	
Maximum of 20% in term	
Output	1 to 3 cc/kg/hr
Specific gravity	1.008 to 1.012

Table 11-4 gives the amount of total body water as a percent of body weight, and Table 11-5 gives gestational weight loss as a percent of body weight. Table 11-6 lists the regulatory factors for water in the newborn.

Table **11-4**	Distribution of Total Body Water as Percent of Body Weight		
Weeks' Gestation	**Total Body Water (%)**	**ECW (%)**	**ICW (%)**
24	86	60	26
28	84	57	26
30	83	55	28
32	82	53	29
34	81	51	30
36	80	49	31

From Goetzman BW, Wennberg RP (1999). Neonatal intensive care handbook, ed 3, St Louis: Mosby, p. 35.
ECW, Extracellular water; ICW, intracellular water.

Table 11-5	Gestation Weight Loss as a Percent of Body Weight (BW)
Gestation (wk)	**Weight Loss (% of BW)**
26	15-20
30	10-15
34	8-10
Term	5-10

From Goetzman BW, Wennberg RP (1999). Neonatal intensive care handbook, ed 3, St Louis: Mosby, p. 36.

Table 11-6	Regulatory Factors for Water Levels of the Newborn	
Factor	**Intracellular Water**	**Extracellular Water**
Major ion	Potassium (K+)	Sodium (Na+)
Volume regulated by:	Na-K cellular pump	Kidneys
Volume maintained by:	Potassium salts (KCl, KPO$_4$)	Sodium salts (NaCl, NaHCO$_3$)

ELECTROLYTES

1. Extracellular
   a. Sodium (Na+)
   b. Chloride (Cl–)
   c. Calcium (Ca++)
2. Intracellular: potassium (K+)

Normal Ranges

Sodium	135 to 140 mEq/L
Potassium	4.5 to 6.5 mEq/L
Chloride	100 to 110 mEq/L
CO$_2$	18 to 24 mmol/L
Calcium	7 to 10.5 mg/dl
BUN	3 to 20 mg/dl
Creatinine	0.6 to 2.0 mg/dl

Recommendations

Sodium	2 to 4 mEq/kg/day
Potassium	2 to 3 mEq/kg/day
Chloride	2 to 4 mEq/kg/day
Phosphate	1 to 2 mm/kg/day
Calcium	1 to 2.5 mg/kg/day (500 mg/kg/day)
Magnesium	0.25 to 0.5 mg/kg/day
Base	Variable

Sodium

1. Main extracellular ion
2. Deficiency: hyponatremia (<127 to 130 mEq/L)
3. Excess: hypernatremia (<160 mEq/L)
4. >90% of solutes absorbed in small and large intestines
   a. Passive absorption, after glucose
   b. Active absorption
      (1) Stimulated by glucose and amino acids
      (2) Uncoupled with glucose, part of Na-K pump
5. Excreted by kidneys
6. Filtered by glomeruli and reabsorbed by tubules and collecting ducts
7. 96% to 99% reabsorbed: reabsorption primarily regulated by oncotic and hydrostatic pressure in peritubular capillaries and action of aldosterone

Sodium Imbalance: Hyponatremia

1. Serum Na+ below 127 to 130 mEq/L
2. Symptoms related to central nervous system (CNS) irritability
   a. Lethargy, coma
   b. Seizures
3. Respiratory distress
4. Poor skin turgor
5. Jaundice
6. Shock
7. Types of hyponatremia
   a. Dilutional
   b. Absolute
   c. Onset
      (1) Early
      (2) Late

Early hyponatremia

- First 2 days of life
- Extrinsic perinatal factors
- Perinatal asphyxia most common cause
- Decreased excretion of free water (increased secretion of antidiuretic hormone [ADH])
- Impaired renal function because of hypoxia
- Respiratory distress syndrome (RDS)

Iatrogenic early hyponatremia

- Large volume of hypotonic fluid to mother before delivery
- Nebulized continuous positive airway pressure (CPAP)
- Administration of diuretics with excessive free water replacement
- Excessive total fluid volume

Late hyponatremia
- Can occur in growing preterm infants after first week postbirth on standard infant formulas or human milk
- Inadequate sodium intake
- Small surface area for reabsorption in tubules
- Transient unresponsiveness to aldosterone

Signs of hyponatremia
- Lethargy
- Coma
- Seizures
- Respiratory distress
- Poor skin turgor
- Jaundice
- Shock

Types of hyponatremia
1. Dilutional: result of excess extracellular fluid volume
2. Absolute
   a. Decreased intake of sodium
   b. Increased loss of sodium

Causes of hyponatremia
1. Dilutional
   a. Too much water
   b. Iatrogenic fluid overload
   c. Congestive heart failure
   d. Renal failure
   e. Syndrome of inappropriate ADH secretion (SIADH)
2. Absolute
   a. Inadequate sodium intake
   b. Excessive sodium loss
   Ask the following questions:
- Does the baby have too little sodium or too much water?
- If the baby has too little sodium, is the baby just not getting enough or is the baby losing too much?

Causes of dilutional hyponatremia
1. Iatrogenic fluid overload
   a. Maternal
   b. Neonatal
2. Congestive heart failure
3. Renal failure
4. Inappropriate antidiuretic hormone secretion
   a. Management
   b. Fluid restriction
   c. Diuretics

Absolute hyponatremia

1. Insufficient sodium supplementation
2. Management: adjust sodium supplementation
3. Three presentations
   a. Normal ECF volume
   b. Increased ECF volume
   c. Decreased ECF volume

Increased ICF volume

1. Predisposing factors
   a. Excess intravenous (IV) fluids
   b. SIADH
2. Causes of SIADH
   a. Pain
   b. Opiate administration
   c. Intraventricular hemorrhage (IVH)
   d. Asphyxia
   e. Pneumothorax
   f. Positive pressure ventilation
3. Diagnosis
   a. Increased weight without edema (without SIADH)
   b. History of increased IV fluids
   c. Normal or high urinary output
   d. Normal specific gravity

Syndrome of inappropriate antidiuretic hormone (SIADH)

- Increased urine sodium
- Decreased urine output
- Increased urine osmolality

  SIADH can be diagnosed only if there is normal cardiac output and normal renal, adrenal, and thyroid hormone.

Therapy for normal extracellular fluid volume

- Fluid restriction if more than 120 mEq/L
- If the sodium is less than 120 mEq/L or if neurologic signs are present, faster replacement by replacement of urinary sodium mEq/mEq with 3% sodium followed by Lasix (1 mg/kg IV every 6 hours)
- Results in decreased free water with no change in total body sodium

Hyponatremia with decreased extracellular fluid volume

1. Predisposing factors
   a. Loss of sodium and water from ECF in proportionate amounts
   b. Diuretics
   c. Osmotic fluid administration

    d. VVLBW infants with severe renal water and electrolyte loss
    e. Adrenal or renal tubular disorders
    f. Gastrointestinal (GI) losses
    g. Third-spacing of ECF
2. Diagnosis
    a. Weight loss
    b. Poor skin turgor
    c. Tachycardia
    d. High BUN
    e. Metabolic acidosis
    f. Decreased urinary output
    g. High specific gravity
    h. Low fractional excretion of sodium
3. Therapy
    a. Elimination of ongoing losses
    b. Liberalized sodium and water intake to replace deficits and meet maintenance needs

Hyponatremia with increased ECF volume

1. Predisposing factors
    a. Decreased cardiac output (sepsis, necrotizing enterocolitis [NEC], congenital heart disease [CHD])
    b. Neuromuscular blockade
2. Diagnosis
    a. Weight gain with edema
    b. Decreased urinary output
    c. High specific gravity
    d. Increased BUN
    e. Low fractional excretion of sodium
3. Therapy
    a. Treatment of underlying condition
    b. Fluid restriction
    c. Monitoring cardiac output

Sodium Replacement

- Provide maintenance sodium in amounts to meet daily requirements, using guidelines for maintenance electrolytes.
- If the serum sodium is too low, provide sodium and chloride in excess of maintenance amounts. Add 0.6 mEq of sodium per kilogram for each 1 mEq/L increase in serum sodium desired. About two thirds of this should be sodium chloride.

Rapid sodium replacement

1. Shock
    a. Normal saline (NS) at 10 to 20 ml/kg IV over 20 to 30 minutes; repeat until blood pressure (BP) is normalized

2. Symptomatic hyponatremia
   a. 3% saline solution
      (1) Normal saline = 154 mEq/L
      (2) 3% = ~513 mEq/L
      (3) Correct to 120 to 125 mEq/L over 12 to 24 hours
   b. Monitor electrolytes, vital signs, urine output

Sodium Replacement

- If the serum sodium is below 120 mEq/L replace the deficit using a high concentration of sodium to prevent neurologic effects of hyponatremia.
- Calculate the total body sodium deficit, and replace with 3% sodium chloride solution.
- Subtract the actual sodium from the desired sodium (135 mEq/L), and multiply the remainder by weight in kilograms and by the ECF volume (0.6).
- Give one half the requirement slowly over a 12- to 18-hour period.
- Sodium (3%) has 0.5-mEq sodium per milliliter.
- Observe sodium levels closely.
- Do not correct the deficit too quickly to prevent CNS effects.

$$Na+ \text{ deficit (mEq/L)} = [Normal\ Na+\ (mEq/L) - Actual\ Na+\ (mEq/L)] \times Weight\ (kg) \times 0.3$$

Example: serum sodium 125; weight 2.5 kg

$$[135 - 125] \times 2.5 \times 0.3 = 7.5\text{-mEq deficit}$$

Hypernatremia

1. Serum sodium of 160 mEq/L
   a. Dehydration
   b. Excessive sodium intake
2. GI disturbances
3. Tremors
4. Seizures
5. High fever
6. Dehydration
7. Apnea
8. Lethargy
9. Coma
10. Paralysis
11. Increased free water

Caveat: Hypernatremia alone does not indicate change in total body sodium. Sodium should not be decreased or increased without appropriate evidence.

Hypernatremia with normal or decreased extracellular fluid Predisposing factors include a VLBW infant with increased renal and insensible water losses, skin sloughing, or ADH deficiency caused by intraventricular hemorrhage (IVH).

Diagnosis
- Weight loss
- Metabolic acidosis
- Tachycardia
- Hypotension
- Decreased urine
- Decreased FENa
- Increased BUN and specific gravity

Hypernatremia with increased ECF volume
1. Predisposing factors
    a. Excessive isotonic or hypertonic solutions
    b. Decreased CO
2. Diagnosis
    a. Weight increase with edema
    b. Normal heart rate, BP, urine output, specific gravity, and FENa
3. Therapy
    a. Reduction of sodium concentration in IV fluids
    b. Possible restriction of IV fluid volume

Potassium

Potassium is the principal intracellular ion. *Hypokalemia* is an abnormally low concentration of potassium in the blood:
1. Serum level below 4 mEq/L
2. Signs occur with level below 3 mEq/L
3. Dilutional hypokalemia
    a. Increased intravascular volume
    b. Acute
4. Absolute hypokalemia
    a. Inadequate potassium intake
    b. Excessive potassium losses
    c. Chronic diuretic therapy

Hypokalemia Therapy for hypokalemia is potassium supplementation as follows:
- Provide maintenance potassium *after* establishment of urinary output.
- Supplement when on chronic diuretic therapy.
- Use of Aldactone with Diuril may decrease the amount of potassium excreted in the urine.

Signs of hypokalemia
- Skeletal and smooth muscle weakness

- Depressed deep tendon reflexes
- Paralytic ileus
- Cardiac arrhythmias
- Electrocardiogram (ECG) changes: broad, flat T waves, depressed ST segment, prolonged PR interval, prominent P waves

Hyperkalemia

Hyperkalemia is a serum K+ level above 6mEq/L from a non-hemolyzed blood sample.

If red blood cells (RBCs) are hemolyzed, the intracellular potassium is released from within the cells, falsely elevating the serum potassium. Causes of hyperkalemia are as follows:

- Lysis of RBCs
- Decreased renal excretion of potassium
- Transcellular shifts of potassium
- High potassium intake

Signs of hyperkalemia

- Arrhythmias
- Ventricular fibrillation
- Asystole
- Tachycardia
- ECG changes: prolonged PR interval, widened QRS, sine wave, fusion of T and QRS

Therapy for hyperkalemia

- Sodium polystyrene sulfonate enema (Kayexalate) at 0.5 to 2 g/kg in mineral oil
- Peritoneal hemodialysis or hemodialysis
- Glucose with insulin
- Titrate with ECG
- Discontinue potassium
- Acute: if on ventilator, increase ventilatory rate to induce respiratory alkalosis
- Calcium gluconate (100 to 200 mg/kg/dose IV) *or*
- Sodium bicarbonate (2 to 4 mEq/kg)

Chloride

1. Metabolism closely follows sodium
2. Absorbed in small intestine with sodium and potassium, through active diffusion
3. Transported in blood and lymphatics under force of heart and skeletal muscles
4. Secreted in sweat, bile, pancreatic and intestinal fluids (with sodium), and gastric juice (with hydrogen ions)
5. Excretion
   a. Depends on body's need for sodium bicarbonate
   b. Absorbed primarily with sodium in the ascending loop of Henle

6. Increased serum sodium, increased chloride
7. Inversely related to bicarbonate levels

Hypochloremia
1. Increased secretion and loss of gastric juice
2. Increased renal excretion
3. Disorders of regulation
   a. Hemodilution
   b. Hyponatremia
   c. Acidosis

Hyperchloremia
- Hypernatremia
- Decreased production of bicarbonate secondary to respiratory alkalosis or renal tubular acidosis
- Dehydration
- Excessive reabsorption from the GI tract

Calcium
- Most abundant mineral in body
- Component of skeleton
- Role in muscle contraction
- Neural transmission
- Blood coagulation
- Transported in intestine by active and passive processes
- Absorption depends on an acid pH for ionization of Ca compounds, such as Ca caseinate and phosphate in the stomach
- Active transport requires carriers called *calcium-binding proteins*
- Vitamin D (1,25-dihydroxyvitamin D) is essential
- Parathyroid hormone stimulates production of 1,25-dihydroxyvitamin D, which increases calcium concentration
- Calcitonin decreases serum calcium
- Excreted by kidneys
- Filtered calcium reabsorbed in most segments of renal tubules
- Parathyroid hormone increases reabsorption of calcium
- Calcitonin decreases calcium reabsorption

Calcium supplementation
- Need more calcium enterally than parenterally
- Calcium directly related to phosphorus
- Cannot achieve fetal accretion rates in parenteral nutrition because high calcium concentrations will precipitate in IV lines

Hypocalcemia
- Ionized serum calcium below 4.4 or total serum calcium below 7
- Early hypocalcemia: first 48 hours
- Late hypocalcemia: after 48 hours; ~ 1 week

Early hypocalcemia

1. Caused by perinatal factors
   a. Abrupt termination of maternal calcium supply
   b. Temporary functional hypoparathyroidism (infants of diabetic mothers [IDMs])
   c. Increased calcitonin (asphyxiated and preterm infants)
   d. 1,25-dihydroxyvitamin D resistance (preterm infants)
2. Prevalence
   a. 30% of preterm infants
   b. 35% of asphyxiated infants
   c. 17% to 32% IDMs
   d. 90% VLBW infants

Late hypocalcemia

- End of first week
- Increased dietary phosphate load
- Much less common because of better commercial infant formulas with more natural phosphate content
- Phototherapy may increase risk for hypocalcemia
- Hypomagnesemia

Treatment of hypocalcemia

1. May complicate other perinatal complications, such as hypoglycemia or asphyxia (have similar signs)
2. May be associated with seizures (without being the cause)
3. Generally asymptomatic and self-limited
4. Asymptomatic
   a. 10% calcium gluconate (elemental calcium, 9.4 mg/ml) at 75 mg/kg/day in six doses
5. Symptomatic
   a. 10% calcium gluconate IV at 2 ml/kg over 10 minutes
   b. Monitor heart rate
6. Maintenance
   a. Appropriate calcium in TPN or enteral feeds

Hypercalcemia

1. Serum calcium above 11 mg/dl
2. Generally iatrogenic: excessive administration of calcium or vitamin D
3. Primary disorders—rare
   a. Subcutaneous fat necrosis
   b. Congenital hyperparathyroidism
   c. Hyperprostaglandin E syndrome
   d. Familial hypocalciuric hypercalcemia
4. Nonspecific signs
   a. Constipation
   b. Polyuria
   c. Bradycardia

Treatment
- Stop the calcium!
- Stop vitamin D
- Increased fluid volume
- If vitamin D intoxication is the cause, glucocorticoids to decrease intestinal absorption and bone resorption of calcium

Phosphorus
- Absorbed mainly in jejunum by active and passive diffusion
- Depends on relative concentration of calcium and phosphorus
- Absolute amount of phosphorus intake
- Presence of substances that bind to phosphorus and make it unavailable for absorption
- Excreted by kidneys: 10% to 15% of filtered phosphorus is excreted
- Parathyroid hormone directly influences phosphorus excretion
- Phosphorus concentration in TPN is recommended at ~390 to 470 mg/L to prevent precipitation

Hypophosphatemia
1. Serum level below 4 mg/dl
2. Osteopenia of prematurity
3. Inadequate TPN phosphorus
4. Familial hypophosphatemias
   a. Vitamin D–resistant rickets
   b. Fanconi's syndrome
   c. X-linked hypophosphatemia

Hyperphosphatemia
- Serum level above 7.0 mg/dl
- Infant formulas with too high phosphate load
- Excessive phosphate in TPN
- Impaired excretion (renal failure)
- Hypoparathyroidism

Treatment
- Decrease phosphorus supplementation
- Treat underlying cause

Magnesium
1. Skeleton and intracellular space
   a. Energy production
   b. Cell membrane function
   c. Mitochondrial function
   d. Protein synthesis
2. 50% to 70% of dietary magnesium absorbed by passive diffusion in small intestine
3. Serum concentration regulated by kidney

4. 3% to 5% of filtered magnesium excreted
5. Parathyroid hormone: increases serum concentration
6. Acute decrease in magnesium: increases parathyroid hormone secretion
7. Chronic magnesium deficiency: decreases secretion and may cause hypocalcemia
8. Recommended TPN levels to prevent precipitation: 36 to 48 mg/L

Hypomagnesemia
- Serum level below 1.6 mg/dl
- Infants of diabetic mothers: decreased maternal magnesium
- Small for gestational age: placental insufficiency
- Malabsorption syndromes
- Isolated intestinal magnesium malabsorption

Hypermagnesemia
1. Serum level above 2.8 mg/dl
2. Maternal treatment with magnesium sulfate for pregnancy-induced hypertension (PIH)
3. Excessive magnesium administration with TPN
4. Signs
   a. Hyporeflexia
   b. Apnea
   c. Lethargy

Glucose
1. Substrate of glycolysis that is sole pathway that produces adenosine triphosphate (ATP) in anaerobic life; red blood cells depend on glycolysis for ATP (they have no mitochondria)
2. Major substrate for brain metabolism
3. Used by all tissues of body
4. Penetration into muscle and adipose tissue dependent on insulin
5. Liver: primary regulator of glucose
   a. Takes up glucose and converts it to glycogen
   b. Uses fatty acids for energy
6. Breakdown of glycogen and gluconeogenesis: provides glucose to the blood to be used by brain, red blood cells, and other tissues during periods of fasting
7. Serum glucose: stimulus that elicits glucose uptake or output by liver

Hypoglycemia
1. Blood sugar: below 40 mg/dl term and preterm infant if >72 hours of age
2. Maintenance: 6 to 8 mg/kg/min

Signs of hypoglycemia

1. Jitteriness
2. Brisk Moro's reflex
3. Lethargy
4. Poor feeding
5. Irritability
6. Hypothermia
7. Respiratory distress
8. Apnea
9. Bradycardia
10. Seizure
11. Coma
12. Sudden death
13. Disorders of underproduction
    a. Inadequate stores
    b. Prematurity
    c. Small for gestational age
    d. Starvation
    e. Ketotic hypoglycemia
    f. Disorders of hepatic glucose production
       (1) Glucose-6-phosphatase deficiency
       (2) Galactosemia
    g. Hormonal abnormalities (e.g., growth hormone deficiency)
14. Disorders of excessive glucose utilization
    a. Hyperinsulinism
    b. Defects in glucose utilization
    c. Sepsis or other hypermetabolic state

Treatment of hypoglycemia

Acute treatment of hypoglycemia consists of IV dextrose 10%, 2.5 mg/kg, followed by IV infusion to match normal hepatic glucose production. In an infant this is approximately 6 to 8 mg/kg/min.

WEB RESOURCES

http://www.neonatology.org/syllabus/calcium2.html
http://www.neonatology.org/syllabus/feeding.premature.html
http://www.cs.nsw.gov.au/rpa/neonatal/html/newprot/hyperk.htm
http://www.cs.nsw.gov.au/rpa/neonatal/html/newprot/hypogly.htm
http://www.vh.org/Providers/Simulations/VirtualPedsPatients/Case08/Case08.html

• • •

The next sections will present guidelines for fluid and TPN administration.

MONITORING INTRAVENOUS FLUID THERAPY*

Table 11-7 gives guidelines for initial fluid administration, and Table 11-8 gives electrolyte requirements.

The following assessments of hydration should be obtained as frequently as needed (often every 8 to 12 hours in tiny infants with high insensible water loss):
1. Body weight
2. Blood chemistries
   a. Electrolytes: Sodium tends to be lower in premature infants; 132 mEq is acceptable. In very small infants, diuresis may exceed the ability of renal tubules to concentrate sodium, resulting in hypernatremia. Free water should be increased to maintain serum sodium less than 145 mEq/L.
   b. Plasma osmolality: 240 to 280 mOsm/kg H_2O. In the first week of life it must be measured directly. After 1 week of age, it can be estimated by the following: mOsm/kg water = 5 + 1.86 Na + 2.8 BUN + G/18 (Na in milliequivalents per liter, BUN and glucose [G] in milligrams per deciliter).

---

*From Goetzman BW, Wennberg RP (1999). Neonatal intensive care handbook, ed 3, St Louis: Mosby, p. 37.

Table **11-7**	Guidelines for Initial Fluid Administration (ml/kg/24 hr)		
	Birth Weight		
Age	**<1000 g**	**1000-1500 g**	**1500-2500 g**
First 24 hr	100-150	80-100	60-80
Second 24 hr	120-150	110-130	90-110
>48 hr	140-180	140-180	120-140

From Goetzman BW, Wennberg RP (1999). Neonatal intensive care handbook, ed 3, St Louis: Mosby, p. 36.

Table **11-8**	Electrolyte Requirements (mEq/kg/24 hr)	
Electrolyte	**Parenteral**	**Oral**
Sodium	3-5	8
Potassium	2-5	7
Calcium	2	2-3

From Goetzman BW, Wennberg RP (1999). Neonatal intensive care handbook, ed 3, St Louis: Mosby, p. 36.

   c. Serum creatinine and BUN levels reflect both renal function and metabolism and may be elevated over the first 24 hours because of a normally low glomerular filtration rate (GFR) and increased production.

3. Urine
   a. Urine volume is typically 2 to 5 ml/kg/hr (40 to 100 ml/kg/24 hr).
   b. Urine electrolytes do not assess hydration but are useful in assessing requirements (e.g., by comparing sodium intake, output, and changes in serum sodium concentration).
   c. Osmolality is typically 75 to 300 mOsm/kg/24 hr if the renal solute load is between 7.5 and 15 mOsm/kg/24 hr (assumes normal renal, adrenal, and posterior pituitary function).
   d. Specific gravity is proportional to osmolality if no protein or glucose is present in urine. Osmolality can be estimated by multiplying the decimal number of the specific gravity (sp gr) by 20:
     (1) If sp gr = 1.003, mOsm = $20 \times 3 = 60$
     (2) If sp gr = 1.015, mOsm = $20 \times 15 = 300$
     (3) Normal range of sp gr: 1.003 to 1015

*Interpretation of Data**

1. *Appropriate monitoring period* should be decided depending on the patient's gestational age and condition (e.g., 6, 12, 24 hours).
2. *Laboratory data* should be obtained close to the time when fluids are to be assessed.
3. *Predicted change in weight*: Predict (guess!) the expected change in weight over the monitoring period.
   a. For a 1000-g infant at birth, expected to lose about 15% of its birth weight, one might predict a 2% to 4% weight loss over the first 12 hours.
   b. Given a 1200-g infant receiving 150 ml/kg/24 hr, but only given 40 kcal/kg/24 hr, one might expect a calorie deficit of about 20 kcal/kg/24 hr. Since the infant has little fat, 4 to 5 g of protein would need to be burned to make up the calorie deficit, and thus 4 to 5 g in weight would be lost over 24 hours even though fluid intake was adequate.
4. *Conditions that may alter fluid requirements*
   a. Acute tubular necrosis (ATN) following asphyxia may produce oliguria.
   b. Reduced glomerular filtration rate (GFR) with hyaline membrane disease (HMD) or respiratory distress syndrome (RDS) decreases urine output.

---

*From Goetzman BW, Wennberg RP (1999). Neonatal intensive care handbook, ed 3, St Louis: Mosby, p. 38.

   c. Shock and pituitary and renal dysfunction can all affect urine output.

   d. Third-spacing after bowel surgery

   e. Inappropriate antidiuretic hormone secretion

   f. Decreased extracellular saline at birth

   g. Adrenal insufficiency

   h. Phototherapy

   i. Extended losses, for example, nasogastric suction, diarrhea, external ventriculostomy

Correction of Abnormalities*

1. Hyponatremia may be due to excess sodium loss (usually renal or gut) or excess water gain (usually renal failure, third-spacing, or intracellular shifts).

   a. Estimate extracellular volume (ECV), which includes postnatal or recent weight change.

   b. Calculate sodium deficit: $(140 - [Na+]) \times ECV$ (in liters); and estimate ongoing loss (or water gain if third-spacing).

   c. Replace deficit + anticipated loss over net 12- to 24-hour period.

   d. If serum sodium is less than 120 mEq/L, replace sodium with 3% NaCl solution (0.513 mEq/ml) to achieve an estimated serum sodium of 124 mEq/L.

   e. Rarely, hyponatremia is due to excess free water administration, in which case fluid restriction is indicated.

2. Hypernatremia may be due to excess insensible water loss, inability of kidney to concentrate sodium during postnatal diuresis (common in micropremature infants), or, infrequently, inadvertent excess sodium administration.

   a. Estimate ECV (in liters).

   b. Water deficit = $(ECV \times [Na+]/140 - ECV)$.

   c. If serum sodium greater than 165 mEq/L, correct slowly over 24 hours.

3. Hypokalemia may be due to renal or intestinal loss, or, rarely, intracellular shifts.

   a. If potassium is less than 2 mEq/L, administer 0.5 mEq/kg IV over 2 hours.

   b. If patient is symptomatic, potassium may be given at a maximum infusion rate of 1 mEq/kg/hr.

4. Hyperkalemia may be due to renal failure, adrenal disease, injury, excess administration, or exchange transfusion.

---

*From Goetzman BW, Wennberg RP (1999). *Neonatal intensive care handbook*, ed 3, St Louis: Mosby, pp. 38-39.

a. Infants frequently tolerate potassium levels of 7.5 to 8.5 mEq/L without cardiac effects (peaked T waves, widened QRS complex).

b. Exchange resin (sodium polystyrene sulfonate [Kayexalate]) may be given as an enema, 1 g/kg. One gram will exchange 2 to 3 mEq sodium for 1 mEq potassium, lowering the serum level by about 1 mEq/L. Hypernatremia is a complication of excessive use. Exchange resins work slowly and are best used for potassium levels less than 7.0 in the absence of ECG changes.

c. Sodium bicarbonate, 2 mEq/kg IV, should be given if T waves are peaked.

d. Glucose, 2 to 5 ml/kg of 10% dextrose, together with 0.2 U insulin, will shift potassium intracellularly. Maintain GFR 3 to 5 mg/kg/min higher than normally tolerated and add insulin, 0.2 U/kg/hr, monitoring glucose levels to prevent excessive hyperglycemia or hypoglycemia.

e. Major ECG changes should be treated initially with 10% calcium gluconate (0.5 ml/kg), given slowly, followed by sodium bicarbonate.

f. Dialysis is indicated if hyperkalemia with cardiotoxicity is not rapidly corrected by these means.

A QUICK ALGORITHM FOR TREATMENT OF SYMPTOMATIC HYPONATREMIA

Use 3% saline solution (normal saline = 154 mEq/L; 3% = ~513 mEq/L). Correct to 120 to 125 over 12 to 24 hours. Monitor electrolytes, vital signs, and urine output.

Steps

1. If the serum sodium is below 120 mEq/L replace the deficit using a high concentration of sodium to prevent neurologic effects of hyponatremia.

2. Calculate the total body sodium deficit, and replace with 3% sodium chloride solution.

3. Subtract the actual sodium from the desired sodium (135 mEq/L) and multiply the remainder by weight in kilograms and by the ECF volume (0.6).

4. Give one half the requirement slowly over a 12- to 18-hour period.

5. Three percent sodium has 0.5 mEq sodium per milliliter.

6. Observe sodium levels closely.

7. Do not correct the deficit too quickly to prevent CNS effects.

8. Formula:

$$\text{Na+ deficit (mEq/L)} = [\text{Normal Na+ (mEq/L)} \\ \text{Actual Na+ (mEq/L)}] \times \text{Weight (kg)} \times 0.3$$

9. Example: serum sodium, 125; weight, 2.5 kg

$$[135 - 125] \times 2.5 \times 0.3 = 7.5\text{-mEq deficit}$$

TOTAL PARENTERAL NUTRITION GUIDELINES*

1. Glucose
   a. Infusion generally begins at 6 to 8 mg/kg/min and is increased daily by 0.6 to 1.2 mg/kg/min (approximately 1.0 to 2.0 g/kg/day) as tolerated. Most infants do not tolerate more than 12 to 15 mg/kg/min.
   b. Dextrostix readings may be obtained every 12 hours and more often if changes in glucose infusion are made or if the infant's glucose level is elevated. If the serum glucose level is greater than 130 mg/dl, or urine glucose level is greater than 2+, then glucose concentration should be decreased.
   c. Insulin (0.25 to 0.5 U/kg) may be used if lowering the glucose concentration does not produce the desired effect.
2. Amino acids
   a. Begin at 0.5 g/kg and increase by 0.25 to 0.5 g/kg/day to a maximum of 3.0 g/kg/day (3.5 g/kg/day for body weight less than 1000 g).
   b. Ratio of nonprotein to protein calories should be approximately 10:1.
   c. Total protein, ammonia (NH_3), BUN, serum pH, ALT (alanine aminotransferase), AST (aspartate aminotransferase), and bilirubin values and urine output should be monitored.
   d. The contents of amino acid solutions vary by manufacturer. Both FreAmine III 10% and Travasol 10% contain the percentages of essential amino acids required by neonates. TrophAmine 6% is specifically formulated for neonates and is preferred.
      (1) Arginine is present in sufficient quantities to reduce the incidence of hyperammonemia.
      (2) Chloride contents are low, an important consideration with respect to metabolic acetate per gram of amino acid, and FreAmine III 10% contains insignificant amounts of chloride and 0.7 mEq of acetate per gram of amino acid. Supplement with L-cysteine acetate per gram of amino acid. Supplementation with L-cysteine HCl, 2 mmol/kg/day, is recommended.

*From Goetzman BW, Wennberg RP (1999). Neonatal intensive care handbook, ed 3, St Louis: Mosby, p. 55.

(3) Branched-chain amino acids are present and are anticatabolic. They provide the substrate to meet the necessary energy requirements that occur during stress.

(4) TrophAmine plus L-cysteine has pH 5.5. Increases Ca and P solubility (Ca/P ratio of 1.7:1).

(5) Pharma Thera, Inc., of Memphis, Tenn., will formulate amino solutions to fulfill special needs of infants with inherited metabolic disorders. Nepramine should be used for all urea cycle defects. Aminosyn should be used for disorders of leucine metabolism (isovaleric acidemia, maple syrup urine disease, hydroxyl methyl glutamyl-CoA lyase deficiency). TrophAmine can be used for all other metabolic disorders as a protein source.

3. Lipid
   a. Intralipid infusion is begun at 0.5 g/kg/day and increased to 3 g/kg/day for preterm infants and begun at 4 g/kg/day for term infants with increments of 0.5 g/kg/day. The infusion rate should not exceed 0.8 ml/kg/hr (20% emulsion = 20 g/100 ml, 2 kcal/ml) in preterm infants less than 33 weeks' gestation and no more than 1.5 ml/kg/hr in other infants. The preferred 20% solution is cleared by premature infants better than the 10% solution.
   b. Lipids should be given to avoid essential fatty acid deficiency. This may be accomplished by a dose of 2% to 4% of total calories by fat or 0.5 g/kg/day three or four times per week, at a minimum.
   c. Obtain a baseline serum triglyceride level before starting parenteral nutrition and weekly thereafter. Maintain at less than 150 mg/dl.
   d. Heparin, 1 U/ml, in TPN improves lipid clearance but may increase free fatty acid levels.
   e. Calories from fat should not exceed 45% of total daily caloric intake.
   f. Risk for bacterial and fungal growth may increase when a lipid bottle is open longer than 12 hours. When it is not possible to infuse a daily requirement in 12 hours or less, then two 30-ml bottles should be ordered and changed after 12 hours. When possible, infuse total dose over 20 to 24 hours.
   g. Addition of lipids to parenteral nutrition solution in pharmacy is not practical. TPN solution compounding is not a standard practice because of concerns with solubility and the small catheter size used in neonates.

4. Vitamins
   a. MVI-Pediatric concentrate solution provides the following per 5 ml: vitamin A (0.7 mg), vitamin B_1 (1.2 mg), vitamin B_2 (1.4 mg), vitamin B_6 (91 mg), niacin (17 mg), vitamin C (80 mg),

vitamin D (10 μg), vitamin E (7 mg), biotin (20 μg), folic acid (140 μg), vitamin B_{12} (1 μg), vitamin K_1 (200 μg), and pantothenic acid (5 mg).

b. MVI-Pediatric daily dosage is based on infant size: 1.5 ml for less than 1 kg; 3.25 ml for 1 to 3 kg; 5 ml for greater than 3 kg.

   (1) Begin on day 1 of parenteral nutrition.

   (2) If other vitamin preparations are used, different volumes will need to be administered. Be aware of preservatives (i.e., propylene glycol) used in adult IV vitamin preparations. Neonates cannot tolerate high doses of these preservatives.

   (3) Remember MVI-Pediatric contains vitamin K. If the patient is receiving Coumadin, dosing may be difficult, especially if parenteral nutrition is cycled.

5. Trace minerals

   a. For premature infants, zinc and copper, 0.3 mg/kg/day, are added as the sulfates when caloric goals are being met or at about 2 weeks of age.

   b. For term infants, the Zn and Cu requirements are less 0.1 mg/kg/day.

   c. Selenium should be added at a dose of 2 to 3 μg/kg/day. It should be withheld if renal output is impaired or if renal failure is present.

   d. Copper and manganese should be withheld in the presence of cholestasis (i.e., conjugated [direct] hyperbilirubinemia). They accumulate in the liver with impaired bile secretion and are hepatotoxic.

   e. The addition of iron to parenteral nutrition is discouraged.

Table 11-9 gives laboratory tests for monitoring infants receiving parenteral nutrition.

DETERMINING THE INFUSION RATE OF INTRAVENOUS SOLUTIONS IN DROPS PER MINUTE*

Overview

Several methods have been developed to determine the drops per minute required to deliver a given quantity of infusion solution. The first method was presented as a nomogram that allowed for the increase in drop size as the dropping rate increases.

*From Medical Algorithms www.medal.org.

Table 11-9	Laboratory Tests for Monitoring Infants Receiving Parenteral Nutrition
Test	**Suggested Frequency**
Urine specific gravity, glucose, protein, pH	Each shift until stable, then once per day
Glucose oxidase strip	As needed to check blood glucose stat
Hematocrit	Once every 1-2 wk, then monthly when stable
CBC, platelets with differential	Once every 1-2 wk, then monthly when stable
CBG or ABG	As indicated
Serum Na, K, Cl, Ca, BUN	Daily first week, then twice per week when stable
Total/direct bilirubin	Once per week; more often if jaundiced; serum and urine osmolality as indicated
Magnesium	Once per week
24-hr factor automated chemical analysis, particularly for liver enzymes, albumin, phosphate, creatinine, total protein	Once per week until stable, then every 2-4 wk
Blood glucose	Daily first week and if glycosuria 2+ and/or Chemstrip >130 mg/dl
Serum triglycerides	Daily first week or with increased dosage of lipids, then once or twice per week

From Goetzman BW, Wennberg RP (1999). *Neonatal intensive care handbook*, ed 3, St Louis: Mosby, p. 57.
CBC, Complete blood count; CBG, capillary blood gases; ABG, arterial blood gases; Na, sodium; K, potassium; Cl, chloride; Ca, calcium; BUN, blood urea nitrogen.

Method 1

Drops per Milliliter	Milliliters per Minute											
	1	2	3	4	5	6	7	8	9	10	11	12
20	20.5	41	60	78	96	114	131	147	164	180	196	214
19	20	39	57	75	92	108	125	141	156	171	186	202
18	19.5	37	54	71	87	103	119	134	148	163	177	192
17	18	35	52	67	83	98	113	127	141	154	166	180
16	17.5	33	49	64	78	92	106	120	133	145	158	170
15	17	32	47	60	74	87	100	113	124	137	148	160
14	15	30	43	56	69	82	94	106	117	128	139	149
13	14.5	29	41	53	65	76	87	99	110	120	129	139

Approximated from Illustration 2, p. 11, of Jeanneret VP, et al. (1957). Tropfengrosse und Dauertropfinusion. Pharmaceutica acta helvetica, 32, 118-124.
Where 1 cubic centimeter = 1 ml.

Second-degree polynomial equations matching the data are as follows:

Drops per Milliliter	Milliliters per Minute 2	Milliliters per Minute	Intercept
13	-0.169456	13.463412	1.875
14	-0.18981	14.628372	0.8636364
15	-0.169081	15.124625	2.4318182
16	-0.18469	16.24538	1.5340909
17	-0.222278	17.546953	0.8181818
18	-0.17545	17.883991	1.9659091
19	-0.193806	18.925075	1.8181818
20	-0.168207	19.541583	2.2159091

A line matching the data offers simpler calculations but is less accurate at high drip rates.

Drops per Milliliter	Milliliters per Minute	Intercept
13	11.26049	7.0161616
14	12.160839	6.6212121
15	12.926573	7.5606061
16	13.844406	7.1363636
17	14.657343	7.5606061
18	15.603147	7.2878788
19	16.404494	7.6969697
20	17.354895	7.3181818

Method 2

Based on the formula at the bottom of p. 7 of Droste and von Planta (1997) and formula 1, p. 118 of Jeanneret et al. (1957):

$$K = 60/(drops/ml)$$

Drops per minute = (infusion volume in ml)/(infusion duration in hours) * K

This is related to the drip rate formula in the previous section.

REFERENCES

Diem K, Lentner C, editors (1970). *Documenta Geigy scientific tables*, ed 7, Basel, Switzerland, Geigy Pharmaceuticals, p. 529, Figure 3.

Droste C, von Planta M (1997). *Memorix clinical medicine*. Philadelphia, Williams & Wilkins, p. 7.

Jeanneret VP, Essellier AF, Schneider E (1957). Tropfengrosse und Dauertropfinusion. *Pharmaceutica acta helvetiae*, 32, 118-124.

BIBLIOGRAPHY

Ainsworth SB, Furness J, Fenton AC (2001). Randomized comparative trial between percutaneous long lines and peripheral cannulae in the delivery of neonatal parenteral nutrition. *Acta paediatrics*, 90(9), 1016-1020.

Cairns PA, Stalker DJ (2002). Carnitine supplementation of parenterally fed neonates. *Cochrane review, the Cochrane library*, 1, http://www.cochrane.org/cochrane/revabstr/ab000950.htm

des Robert C, et al. (2002). Acute effects of intravenous glutamine supplementation on protein metabolism in very low birth weight infants: a stable isotope study. *Pediatric research*, 51(1), 87-93.

Mason-Wyckoff M, et al. (2003). Nutrition: physiologic basis of metabolism and management of enteral and parenteral nutrition. In Kenner C, Lott JW, editors. *Comprehensive neonatal nursing: a physiologic perspective*, ed 3, St Louis: WB Saunders.

Tyson JE, Kennedy KA (2002). Minimal enteral nutrition for promoting feeding tolerance and preventing morbidity in parenterallly fed infants. Cochrane review, *the Cochrane library*, 1, http://www.cochrane.org/cochrane/revabstr/ab000504.htm

CHAPTER 12

ENTERAL NUTRITION

Enteral nutrition is important to support growth and development of the neonate, yet it is one of the most challenging aspects of neonatal care. For the very immature infant consumption of calories is at a high rate. Couple this with the attempts to feed and the small gastric capacity of the infant and you have an oxymoron situation—you are trying to increase calories by giving enteral feeding at a time that the act of feeding itself may be burning more calories than are actually being given.

Infants who are left NPO (nothing by mouth) for long periods seem to do better at later feeding attempts if nonnutritive sucking activities are started early in life. This sucking also has been reported to increase growth and weight gains. Another aspect of feeding the very immature infant is use of minimal enteral feedings. These feedings stimulate the gut and help prime it for absorption of nutrients.

This chapter will review the recommendations for weight gains (Table 12-1 and Figures 12-1 to 12-4), dietary allowances (Table 12-2), and minimal enteral feeding rates (Table 12-3), as well as compare formulas and breast milk. Guidelines for care are included.

Table **12-1**	Approximate Daily Weight Gain for Infants
Gestational Age	**g/kg/day**
24-28 wk	15-20
29-32 wk	17-21
33-36 wk	14-15
37-40 wk	7-9
Corrected Age	**g/day**
40 wk to 3 mo	30
3-6 mo	20
6-9 mo	15
9-12 mo	10
12-24 mo	6

From Kalhan SC, Price PT (2001). Nutrition and selected disorders of the gastrointestinal tract. In Klaus MH, Fanaroff AA, editors. Care of the high-risk neonate, ed 5, Philadelphia: WB Saunders, p. 172.

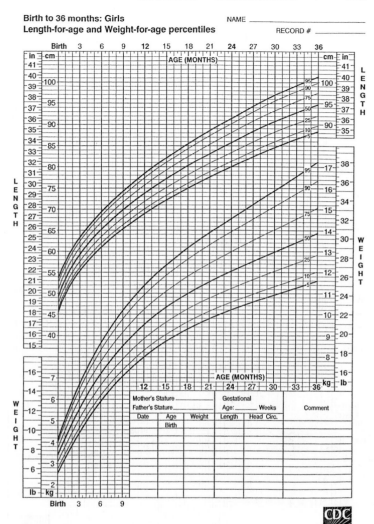

FIGURE 12-1

Girls from birth to 36 months: length-for-age and weight-for-age percentiles. (Developed by the National Center for Health Statistics in collaboration with the National Center for Chronic Disease Prevention and Health Promotion [2000]. http://www.cdc.gov/growthcharts)

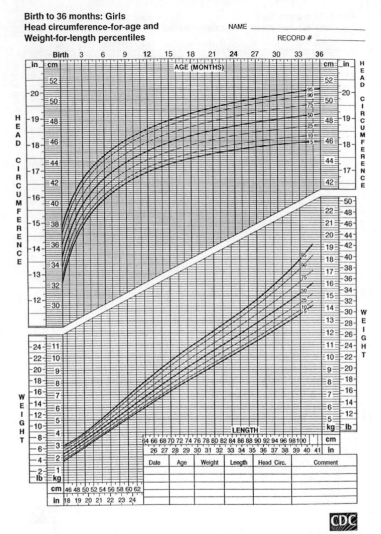

FIGURE **12-2**

Girls from birth to 36 months: head circumference-for-age and weight-for-length percentiles. (Developed by the National Center for Health Statistics in collaboration with the National Center for Chronic Disease Prevention and Health Promotion [2000]. http://www.cdc.gov/growthcharts)

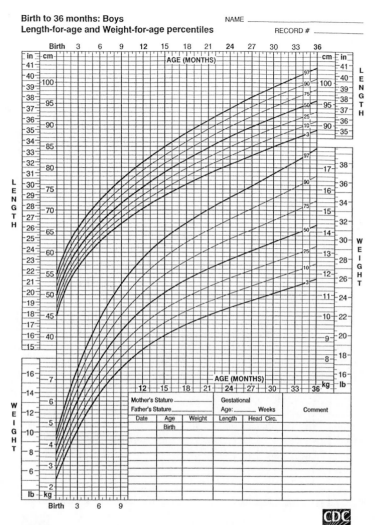

FIGURE 12-3

Boys from birth to 36 months: length-for-age and weight-for-age percentiles. (Developed by the National Center for Health Statistics in collaboration with the National Center for Chronic Disease Prevention and Health Promotion [2000]. http://www.cdc.gov/growthcharts)

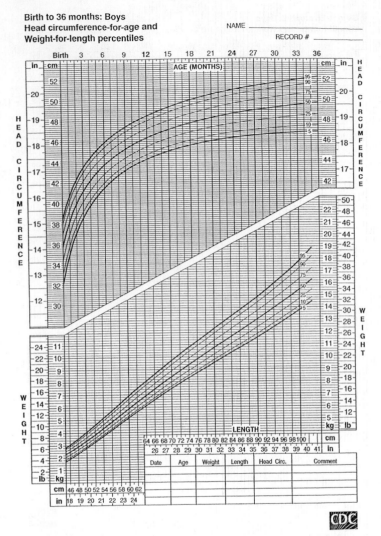

FIGURE **12-4**

Boys from birth to 36 months: head circumference-for-age and weight-for-length percentiles. (Developed by the National Center for Health Statistics in collaboration with the National Center for Chronic Disease Prevention and Health Promotion [2000]. http://www.cdc.gov/growthcharts)

Table **12-2**	Recommended Dietary Allowances for Infants and Toddlers		
	0-0.5 yr	**0.5-1.0 yr**	**1-3 yr**
Calories	108 kcal/kg	98 kcal/kg	102 kcal/kg
Protein	2.2 g/kg	1.6 g/kg	1.2 g/kg
Vitamins			
A	1250 IU/day	1250 IU/day	1330 IU/day
D	300 IU/day	400 IU/day	400 IU/day
E	3 IU/day	4 IU/day	6 IU/day
K	5 µg/day	10 µg/day	15 µg/day
C	30 mg/day	35 mg/day	40 mg/day
Thiamine	200 µg/day	400 µg/day	700 µg/day
Riboflavin	400 µg/day	500 µg/day	800 µg/day
B_6	300 µg/day	600 µg/day	1000 µg/day
B_{12}	0.3 µg/day	0.5 µg/day	1.7 µg/day
Niacin	5 mg/day	6 mg/day	9 mg/day
Folic acid	25 µg/day	35 µg/day	50 µg/day
Pantothenic acid*	2 mg/day*	3 mg/day*	3 mg/day*
Biotin*	10 µg/day*	15 µg/day*	20 µg/day*
Minerals			
Magnesium	40 mg/day	60 mg/day	80 mg/day
Iron	6 mg/day	10 mg/day	10 mg/day
Iodine	40 µg/day	50 µg/day	70 µg/day
Zinc	5 mg/day	5 mg/day	10 mg/day
Copper*	400-600 µg/day*[†]	600-700 µg/day*[†]	700-1000 µg/day*[†]
Manganese*	300-600 µg/day*[†]	600-1000 µg/day*[†]	1000-1500 µg/day*[†]
Chloride	180 mg/day[‡]	300 mg/day[‡]	350-500 mg/day[‡]
Sodium	120 mg/day[‡]	200 mg/day[‡]	225-300 mg/day[‡]
Potassium	500 mg/day[‡]	700 mg/day[‡]	1000-1400 mg/day[‡]
Calcium	400 mg/day	600 mg/day	800 mg/day
Phosphorus	300 mg/day	500 mg/day	800 mg/day

From Kalhan SC, Price PT (2001). Nutrition and selected disorders of the gastrointestinal tract. In Klaus MH, Fanaroff AA, editors. Care of the high-risk neonate, ed 5, Philadelphia: WB Saunders, p. 163.
*Safe range.
[†]Safe and adequate range.
[‡]Estimated minimum requirements for sodium, potassium, and chloride.

Table 12-3	Enteral Intake for Premature Infants
	Advisable Intake
Calories	110-150 kcal/kg
Protein	3-4 g/kg
Fat	5-7 g/kg
Carbohydrate	10-15 g/kg
Osmolality	≤300 (mOsm/kg H_2O)
Vitamins	
A	1400-2500 IU/day
D	400-600 IU/day
K	15 µg/kg/day
E	25 IU/day (5 IU/day after 2-4 wk)
C	609 mg/day
Thiamine	200-400 µg/day
Riboflavin	400-500 µg/day
B_6	250-400 µg/day
B_{12}	0.15 µg/kg
Niacin	6 mg/day
Folic acid	50 µg/day if <2 kg
	15 µg/kg
Pantothenic acid	1.0-4 mg/kg
Biotin	0.6-2.3 µg/kg
Minerals	
Magnesium	20 mg/kg
Iron	2-4 mg/kg (begin 2-3 wk to 2 mo)
Iodine	1-7 µg/kg
Zinc	0.8-1.2 µg/kg
Copper	100-200 µg/kg
Chromium	2-4 µg/kg
Molybdenum	2-3 µg/kg
Selenium	1.5-2.5 µg/kg
Manganese	10 µg/kg (800-1200 g BW)
	8.5 µg/kg (1200-1800 g BW)
Chloride	110 mg/kg (800-1200 g BW)
	89 mg/kg (1200-1800 g BW)
Sodium	80 mg/kg (800-1800 g BW)
	69 mg/kg/(1200-1800 g BW)
Potassium	98 mg/kg (800-1200 g BW)
	90 mg/kg (1200-1800 g BW)
Calcium (Ca)	210 mg/kg (800-1200 g BW)
	185 mg/kg (1200-1800 g BW)
Phosphorus (P)	140 mg/kg (800-1200 g BW)
	123 mg/kg (1200-1800 g BW)
Ca/P ratio	1.7-2

From Kalhan SC, Price PT (2001). Nutrition and selected disorders of the gastrointestinal tract. In Klaus MH, Fanaroff AA, editors. Care of the high-risk neonate, ed 5, Philadelphia: WB Saunders, p. 162.
BW, Body weight.

MINIMAL ENTERAL FEEDINGS

Trophic or minimal enteral feedings (MEFs) are feedings that are administered by tube that are subnutritional and whose intent is to prime the gut for future feedings. These feedings are usually small (a few cc's), dilute (often one-half strength formula), and frequent (every 2 to 3 hours) and are provided by gravity via a gavage tube. Results from research are varied; however, there seems to be greater evidence from both retrospective analysis and controlled trials of increased feeding tolerance, fewer residuals, and fewer numbers of days to full feeding, with a decreased incidence of necrotizing enterocolitis (NEC). More research is needed in the area of MEFs and minimal enteral nutrient delivery in relationship to the development of NEC and also to the development of biliary cholestasis, a complication of long-term total parenteral nutrition (TPN) (Mason-Wyckoff et al., 2003).

FEEDINGS*

General Information

- The feeding instructions may be found on the Kardex in the bedside chart. On this sheet can be found the infant's name, the type and dilution of the formula to be used, the route of feeding, the schedule and the time the feeding is to be initiated.
- Unless otherwise ordered by physician/certified nurse practitioner (CNP), level III/II infants are placed on their side or abdomen after the feeding.
- Formula may remain at room temperature for 12 hours and breast milk for 4 hours. When infants are taking solid foods, do not feed the infant directly from the jar. Open jars may be kept in the refrigerator for 24 hours and then discarded. Jars should be initialed and timed when opened.
- Infant feedings/formula may not be thawed or warmed in microwave. May be warmed in H_2O bath and tested before giving.
- Regular, preemie, and low-flow nipples are available. The type used depends on the infant's needs. Never enlarge or slit nipples, except for thickened feeding. Disposable bottles and nipples are to be routinely used. In special cases, other acceptable methods of formula preparation may be utilized.
- All infants are to be held in a sitting position for nipple feedings and never laid flat on mattress, except for infants with myelomeningocele, who are fed prone until otherwise ordered.

---

*From Altimier L, Brown B, Tedeschi L (2000). Tri-Health's manual of neonatal nursing policies, procedures, competencies, & clinical pathways, Glenview, Ill: National Association of Neonatal Nurses.

Nipple Feedings
Initial nipple feedings
1. Include parents in the plan of care when feedings are being initiated.
2. Physician/CNP order is required for initial nipple feeding:
   a. Nursing assessment findings regarding readiness to feed may be discussed with physician/CNP and the order obtained.
   b. Verbal or written order should reflect one nipple feeding with reassessment of how infant tolerated it.
3. Infant should remain on present monitors (heart rate [HR]/respiratory, oximeter) during feeding.

Progression of nipple feeding
1. Increasing the number of nipple feeds per day requires a physician/CNP order:
   a. Increasing feeds should be discussed by the multidisciplinary team during rounds and appropriate orders written.
   b. Orders may be written for a specific number of feeds per day or "as tolerated." An "as tolerated" order gives the registered nurse (RN) latitude to progress based on nursing judgment and plan of care.

Parental involvement in nipple feedings
1. First nipple feeds are generally administered by nurses. In some circumstances (i.e., >37 weeks) if the infant is without complications and stable on room air based on assessment, parents may administer first nipple feeding.
2. RN/occupational therapist (OT) must establish infant's ability to coordinate suck/swallow/breathe before coaching parents through a nipple feeding.

GENERAL GUIDELINES

- Breast milk (BM) is preferred for infant feeding and should be encouraged if no contraindications exist (i.e., positive human immunodeficiency virus [HIV], hepatitis C, or hepatitis B antigen; certain maternal medications). Inform and counsel parents regarding hepatitis C. Check resource material for specifics.
- Any cow's milk–based, commercially available formula may be used in full-term infants. Parental and private physician preferences should be respected unless medical indications exist for special formulas.
- Premature infants (<1800 g) need specially designed preterm formulas or breast milk (BM). Infants with birth weights below 1500 g on BM may need fortifiers to meet their increased mineral/caloric needs. These should be added to BM after infant is tolerating feeds and must be ordered by the physician.

- In general, formulas of 20 cal/oz are used. If fluid restriction or increased caloric needs are present then feedings of 22 or 24 (rarely 27) cal/oz may be used. Start with 20 cal/oz, and increase the concentration over time as tolerated by the infant.
- Most infants require 120 cal/kg/day (range 100 to 140) to maintain growth at 15 to 20 g/kg/day. This corresponds to approximately 180 cc/kg/day of 20 cal/oz feedings and 150 cc/kg/day of 24 cal/oz feedings.
- Actual weight is used to calculate fluid and caloric requirements in most cases.
- Nipple feeds may be attempted per physician/CNP order if the infant is 32 to 34 weeks' estimated gestational age and over 1250 g. Intermittent gavage feedings are used in infants who are immature or unable to nipple feed. Continuous drip feedings may be indicated.
- Infants with umbilical lines may be fed orally on a physician/CNP order after discussion with the neonatologist.
- It is recommended to make one change at a time to ensure the infant is tolerating the change, (e.g., do not add fortifier or change concentration and increase volume at the same feed).
- Premature infants may need special arrangements for going-home formula. Before discharge, the multidisciplinary team will determine identification of formula type.

Starting Feeds
The following recommendations are for routine situations. For individual infants requiring modifications, check with neonatologist.
1. Several sips of sterile water should be given to establish esophageal patency before initial BM/formula feed.
2. Feeding strengths
   a. Above 1000 g: full-strength BM or formula unless otherwise ordered
   b. Below 1000 g: start with diluted formula/BM and work up slowly, check with neonatologist
3. Feeding intervals
   a. Above 1800 g to term infant: every 3 to 4 hours
   b. 1500 to 1800 g: every 2 to 3 hours
   c. Below 1500 g: every 2 hours
   d. Breast-feeding on demand every 2 to 3 hours minimum

Guidelines for Advancing Feeding Volumes
1. Term infants may be advanced ad lib, with physician/CNP order.
2. Advancement of premature infants must be individualized and should be discussed with neonatologist/team (often an increase of 20 to 30 cc/kg/day is used).
3. Interval adjustments
   a. Advance to every–3 hour feeds when infant taking 20 cc every 2 hours.

b. Advance to every–4 hour feeds when infant taking 60 cc every 3 hours.
4. Breast-fed infants 35 weeks or older may be given 15 to 20 cc of formula as mom's expressed breast milk (EBM) volume is increasing. Adjust to baby's feeding volume proportionately.

Vitamin Supplementation

Generally, full-term infants on full-volume feeds or infants on premature formulas (on full feeds) do not require additional vitamins.

Breast-Feeding/Collection/Storage of Breast Milk
Guidelines for initiating breast-feeding

- Infant tolerates feeds (if receiving orogastric [OG] feed).
- Infant maintains stable temperature with skin-to-skin or close body contact with mother.
- Infant shows signs of readiness to feed, such as rooting, sucking, and an active gag reflex.
- An infant of at least 35 weeks may breast feed at initial feeding.
- BM may remain at room temperature 4 hours when infant is receiving continuous feeds (Table 12-4).
- "Nuzzling" is skin-to-skin contact between infant and mother to familiarize infant with smell and texture of mother's breast. Initiate nuzzling as soon as infant can be held outside Isolette. Time should be limited according to infant's tolerance. Infant should remain on monitors as appropriate. Nuzzling may be initiated with the ventilated infant, but sucking is not permitted.
- Tolerance of feeds by artificial nipple should *not* be a determinant of readiness to breast feed. Breast-feeding is natural and physiologic. Studies repeatedly show that breast-feeding is less stressful than feeding with an artificial nipple, which requires a different mechanism of sucking.
- Infants requiring oxygen for bottle or gavage feeds may breast feed with a nasal cannula (NC). Oximetry should be employed if there is a question of tolerance.

Table **12-4**	Storage Guidelines for Breast Milk in the NICU/SCN
Fresh	2-5 days in refrigerator
Thawed	24 hr in refrigerator
Frozen (home freezer unit)	3-6 mo
Frozen (deep freeze –0° F)	6-12 mo

- Length of actual nursing time should be limited only by infant's tolerance. If infant nurses effectively, allow infant to self-detach in order to obtain hindmilk (higher in fat and calories).
- If there is any question regarding infant's ability to tolerate feeding or mother's ability to recognize changes in tone or color, RN supervises feedings (as with initial bottle feeds).
- Individuals with special problems or concerns should be referred to a member of the breast feeding resource team/lactation consultant for further counseling.

Documentation of breast-feeding
- Infant too sleepy or reluctant to achieve latch; *or*
- Latch achieved with tongue down, lips flanged, and rhythmic sucking
- Swallowing heard and actual length of sucking time
- Mom's nipple inverted, flat, or everted after stimulation?
- Comfort level of mom's breasts and nipples during nursing
- Position of baby during breast-feeding and amount of help required by staff
- Nursing observed by staff or reported by the mom?
- Any teaching done or referrals made

Collection and storage of breast milk
- Notify physician/CNP if mother has any illness or is taking any medications other than prenatal vitamins.
- Mothers should be given a double pump adapter kit available from mother/baby unit (MBU) or neonatal intensive care unit/special care nursery (NICU/SCN). Pump setup and usage will be demonstrated to the mom. Printed information on pumping procedures, cleaning, and EBM storage is provided.
- Milk should be collected in sterile plastic containers provided by the NICU/SCN.
- Each container should be labeled with mother's full name, date, and time pumped.
- Always use fresh milk first before going to frozen milk supply. Baby's primary and associate nurses should work closely with mother to determine amount of milk baby can use daily. Amounts in excess of a 48-hour supply should be frozen for future use.
- Do not thaw or heat milk in microwave (use warm water bath).

Insertion of Nasogastric or Orogastric Tube/Gavage Feeds for Bolus Gavage Feeds
Purpose   Orogastric/nasogastric tubes are inserted for feeding by way of gravity or infusion pump (never pushed). Orogastric/nasogastric tubes may also be inserted for abdominal decompression in a variety of situations. They are inserted when hand bagging is taking place to

prevent the stomach from filling with air. They are also used for this same purpose when nasal prong continuous positive airway pressure (CPAP) is in use based on clinical assessment. In these situations, the orogastric/nasogastric tube may be placed without a physician/CNP order.

Equipment needed
- No. 5 or 8 polyvinyl chloride (PVC) tube *or*
- No. 6 or 8 polyurethane enteral feeding tube (for indwelling use)
- Commercial reservoir
- Syringe to measure desired volume of formula
- Tape
- Stethoscope
- If continuous: also a syringe pump, 60-cc syringe, and enteral extension tubing

General guidelines
- Feedings on all infants are initiated on physician/CNP orders only. Formula dilution, route of feeding, amount, and schedule are prescribed by the physician/CNP. The plan of care should also include type of tube and whether it is indwelling vs. inter-mittent.
- Gavage feedings are done by RNs.
- Before initiating gavage feedings, assess the infant for abdominal distention and/or bowel loops. Abdominal girth should be checked and documented every shift. Wrap paper measuring tape around abdomen over umbilicus. Infants with umbilical arterial catheters (UACs)/umbilical venous catheters (UVCs) should have girth measured directly above the umbilicus. Notify physician/CNP of significant changes and/or if abdomen is distended or bowel loops, guaiac-positive stools, or large (>20% of feed) aspirates are present. Record girth on nursing flow sheet.
- Choose the appropriate size tube; for indwelling tubes: no. 6 if 1500 g or less, no. 8 if 1500 g to 3 kg.
- Measure from tip of nose to earlobe and then from earlobe to midway between the xyphoid and umbilicus. Mark length by tape or pen to ensure insertion to the proper distance.
- You may offer the infant a pacifier during insertion. Do not obstruct nares in a nonventilated infant without assessing mouth-breathing capability because infants are obligate nose breathers.
- Insert the tube gently via the mouth or nare, allowing the infant to swallow the tube to the predetermined length. Hold the tube securely in place or tape in place. Inject 1 to 2 cc of air, and listen over stomach with stethoscope. Aspirate the 1 to 2 cc of air and check for residual gastric content. Document tube placement by air and aspirate on the feeding section of the nursing flow sheet. If there are any signs of respiratory distress, withdraw the tube. Confirm nasogastric position by inserting 1 to 2 cc of air

and then auscultation over the stomach and aspiration of gastric contents. Confirmation by x-ray is usually only indicated when duodenal/jejunal placement is desired.

- Secure tube with Tegaderm after proper placement is confirmed. After proper position is confirmed, record the centimeter marking at the mouth or nare on the Kardex and on the nursing flow sheet. Tube position should be checked every shift (b.i.d.) to evaluate for migration of the tube. Infants exhibiting signs of improper tube placement (i.e., apnea and bradycardia, desaturations, bile-stained aspirates, formula in the mouth) should have this distance checked more frequently. X-ray confirmation of proper placement of the nasogastric (NG)/orogastric (OG) tube may be ascertained with a physician/CNP order.

- Pour measured formula into the syringe. Allow formula to infuse by gravity or, if ordered, by infusion pump, and observe infant for any signs of respiratory distress or abdominal distention. Discontinue feeding if either occurs.

- When feeding is complete, pinch off gavage tube tightly and quickly withdraw if tube is not indwelling. PVC nasogastric tube may be left in place up to 72 hours. The polyurethane tubes may be left in 30 days. Label tubing and record on Kardex and the nursing flow sheet, the date and time of insertion. Place infant on side or abdomen to prevent aspiration in the event of emesis.

- Refeed aspirate unless otherwise ordered. If large amount of aspirate (>20% of feed) found, check with physician/CNP before refeeding or discarding and document.

- Increases are by 1- to 5-cc increments according to infant's condition and physician order. If nipple/gavage is ordered for a given feeding, the infant is allowed to nipple feed; unless ordered otherwise, the balance of the feeding may be given by gavage 15 to 20 minutes after nipple feeding.

- Infants are to be offered a nipple to suck whenever gavage fed. All infants are to be kept on the monitor during gavage feeds.

- During continuous feeds formula should be changed every 12 hours and breast milk should be changed every 4 hours. Aspirates must be checked before each feed or every 4 hours if feeding is continuous. Document all feeding and tube changes plus aspirate checks. Tubing should be changed every 4 hours when using breast milk and can be changed every 24 hours when using formula. When using formula, flush tubing with sterile H_2O before adding new formula.

- After administration of feeding, indwelling tubes must be flushed with 0.5 to 1 cc of sterile water if needed. Document amount of sterile water flush used on the intake record.

- Tube should be reinserted if unable to verify position or every 4 weeks per manufacturer's recommendations for polyurethane indwelling tubes.

- On nursing flow sheet, document time, amount, and type of feeding; tube changes; and tube position at nare or mouth.

Insertion of Nasojejunal Tube by Peristalsis

Purpose   The purpose of a nasojejunal tube is to facilitate adequate nutrition.

Personnel
- When passed directly in the jejunum using fluoroscopy, physicians only perform the placement.
- When polyurethane feeding tube is used and the tube is initially placed in the duodenum and allowed to pass into the jejunum by peristalsis, it may be inserted by a physician, CNP, or RN with a physician's order.

Implementation
1. Equipment
   a. Polyurethane feeding tube; nonweighted tubes preferred for initial attempt
   b. Tape
   c. Water
   d. 5-cc syringe
   e. Stethoscope
2. Preparation
   a. Position patient with head elevated and right side down.
   b. If weighted tube is used, check the feeding tube to ensure the wire stylet is not coming through any of the holes near the end of the feeding tube.

   Note: If the stylet is poking through one of the holes, adjust the stylet to correct the position.

Procedure
- Measure tube from tip of the nose to earlobe and then from earlobe to the umbilicus, and mark this location with a piece of tape or pen.
- Lubricate the tube by dipping in sterile water.
- Slowly insert the tube through the nares to the desired length marked on the tube.
- Observe the patient for dusky color and/or respiratory difficulty while inserting feeding tube. If either occurs, remove the tube immediately. When color is pink, begin procedure again.
- When the tube is at the desired length, tape the tube to the patient's cheek.
- Check the position of the tube by placing a stethoscope over the stomach and quickly inserting 2 to 3 cc of air into the tube, listening for a "whooshing" to confirm the tube is in the stomach.

- If weighted tube with stylet is used, hold the feeding tube with one hand at the patient's nose and gently remove the stylet from the tube by withdrawing the stylet with your free hand. **Note:** Leave stylet at bedside in case it is needed to be used for reinsertion. Store stylet in plastic feeding tube bag.
- Remove the tape securing the tube from the infant's nose. Retape the tube leaving a loop 2 to 3 inches in a manner that will prevent dislodgment of the tube but will allow the tube to slowly migrate into the jejunum via peristalsis.
- Try to position patient on right side.
- A physician/CNP's order may be obtained to administer feedings through the tube, while waiting for the tube to pass in jejunum.
- A physician/CNP's order must be obtained to confirm placement of the tube by x-ray.
- After placement is verified, begin feedings per physician/CNP's order.
- After proper position is confirmed, record the centimeter marking at the mouth or nare on the Kardex and nursing flow sheet. Tube position should be checked at least once every shift (b.i.d.) to evaluate for migration of the tube. Infants exhibiting signs of improper tube placement (i.e., apnea and bradycardia, desaturations, formula in the mouth) should have this distance checked more frequently.
- When feeding through a duodenal/jejunal tube, aspirates do not need to be checked.

Documentation   Document the type/size of tube, confirmation of tube placement, taping of tube to allow for passage, and place of insertion on the Kardex and nursing flow sheet.

Comments
- Never reinsert stylet when tube is in patient.
- To maintain optimum tube performance in long-term enteral feeding, the feeding tube should be considered for replacement every 4 weeks.

UNIVERSITY OF ILLINOIS MEDICAL CENTER AT CHICAGO CLINICAL CARE GUIDELINE

Subject: Breast-Feeding for the Newborn Infant in the NICU/ICN*

Objective

To establish the nurse's role for the promotion and support of breast-feeding mothers and their infants who require specialized care in the NICU or intermediate care nursery (ICN).

*From University of Illinois Medical Center at Chicago Women's and Children's Nursing Services. Used with permission by Dharmapuri Vidyasagar, MD; Catherine Theorell, RNC, MSN, NNP; Beena Peters, RN, MS.

Position Statements

The University of Illinois and Chicago Medical Center supports breast-feeding/breast milk as the feeding method of choice for all newborns, but especially for those who are compromised by acute illness or prematurity as long as the mother does not have one of the very few situations for which breast-feeding is contraindicated.

All mothers should have adequate information antenatally concerning breast-feeding to make an informed choice. Frequently the premature birth or illness of a term infant is unexpected, and breast-feeding should be discussed with the mother again in light of its benefits to an already compromised infant. Expressing milk for a limited time while the child is ill should be presented as a viable option and will be facilitated if the mother chooses it.

The ideal is to have the baby feed directly from the breast. Because of varying situations in the NICU/ICN that may not be possible. A mother may choose to only pump milk for the baby and never put the baby to breast. Ultimately our goal is to provide the mother with as much information as possible concerning her different options and facilitate and support whatever decision she makes.

Standards

1. Every mother whose infant is admitted to the NICU/ICN will be assessed by the RN or lactation consultant for willingness to pump milk during the infant's hospital stay, even if her long-term plan is to formula feed.
2. When maternal breast-feeding problems requiring medical consultation are noticed, the mother will be referred back to her obstetrician (OB) care provider for consultation as needed. If the mother has no OB care provider and needs to be seen urgently she can be seen by the attending OB on call in labor and delivery (L&D) in a triage visit.
3. The mother will be assisted in getting baby to breast, when possible, if mother chooses to do so. Getting the baby to actually latch on at the breast may be a slow process requiring a number of attempts. In many cases, the mother will be encouraged to continue to pump milk with an electric pump, even though baby is doing some feedings at breast, so she does not lose her milk supply, since it reflects the amount of stimulation provided.

Procedures

Milk expression and collection

1. Instruct the mother to always wash hands thoroughly with soap and water before handling the breast, pump, and attachments.
2. Instruct the mother how to set up the pump equipment properly.

3. Instruct the mother to wash all breast pump equipment that has contact with the breast or breast milk. They should be washed thoroughly with hot, soapy water, rinsed to ensure all soap is removed, and let to air dry on clean towel. Instruct her once per day to boil equipment (everything but the tubing) for 10 minutes and then let air dry (or may use dishwasher cycle).

4. Instruct mother to begin milk expression as soon as possible after birth, ideally in the first few hours.

5. Instruct the mother to pump, with a hospital-grade electric pump, using a double-collection kit every 2½ hours for 10 to 15 minutes or until milk stops flowing, in order to initiate lactation. Encourage mother to keep a log of the time of day that she pumped and volume expressed (Table 12-5).

6. Instruct mother to use lowest pump setting for pumping; the highest setting can injure breast tissue. It is possible that the mother may see no or very little breast milk for the first 4 days of pumping, but she should continue to pump to initiate lactation; without pumping she will be limiting milk production. It is possible that the mother will make more breast milk than the baby needs initially; excess should be frozen. If the mother delays beginning pumping, it is possible that she will go on to not develop a full milk supply.

7. Reassure the mother that uterine cramping during pumping is a normal physiologic response from the release of oxytocin and expected in the early days of milk expression. It is safe to take ibuprofen for pain relief without harming the infant, as long as the mother has not been prohibited from taking it.

8. Mothers receiving magnesium sulfate and most intravenous (IV) antibiotics while on the postpartum unit are not prohibited from beginning pumping breast milk.
   a. For premature infants who are physiologically stable and at least 28 weeks post conceptual age (PCA), encourage nonnutritive sucking (after the mother has pumped during kangaroo care).
   b. Encourage nutritive sucking at the breast when infant is tolerating nonnutritive sucking well, shows some oral-motor coordination and with physician's approval/support.
   c. Instruct the mother on different positions that may assist the small premature infant to latch on.

Estimating intake
Prefeeding and postfeeding weights may be used to estimate intake.
- Use the electronic infant scale, and make sure that it is balanced and nothing is touching the edges.
- Weigh the baby before breast-feeding. It is best to disconnect baby from monitor, but have the monitor lead wires fully on the scale.

Table 12-5	Guidelines for Storing/Thawing Mother's Milk for Feeding Preterm Infants*		
Milk Type	**To Be Fed Within**	**Warming/Thawing**	**Special Considerations**
Fresh, unrefrigerated	1 hr	Not necessary	Extra milk can be refrigerated or frozen after 1 hr at room temperature.
Fresh, refrigerated	48 hr	1. Warm slowly over 30 min to approximately body temperature. *Do not overheat.* 2. *Do not microwave.*	1. Literature indicates milk is suitable for 48 hr with refrigeration ≤4° C. 2. "Cream" layer separates with refrigeration, so milk should be shaken vigorously before use. 3. Milk remaining after 48 hr should be discarded, not frozen.
Frozen	24 hr after thawing	1. Thaw gradually (over 1 hr) to approximately body temperature. Do not overheat. 2. Do not microwave. 3. Take care not to contaminate milk if warm water bath is used.	1. Do not refreeze milk. 2. Do not add fresh milk to bottles of frozen milk; use separate containers. The exception would be with colostrums. 3. Discard unused milk after 24 hr of refrigeration. 4. Frozen milk will keep 3-4 mo in freezer compartment of refrigerator and 6 mo in deep freeze (0° F or less).

From University of Illinois Medical Center at Chicago Women's and Children's Nursing Services. Used with permission by Dharmapuri Vidyasagar, MD; Catherine Theorell, RNC, MSN, NNP; Beena Peters, RN, MS.

*Breast milk fortifier should be added to fresh or thawed frozen milk in amounts that will be used in less than 24 hr. Milk that is already fortified should be discarded after 24 hr if not used. **Labeling of milk:** Containers of milk should be labeled by mother or nurse with infant's name, mother's room number, and date/time expressed. Fresh milk should be labeled as such. Colostrum should have an additional label with "Colostrum" written on it. Date and time of thawing should be written on frozen milk.

- After feeding, weigh baby again in exactly the same condition (i.e., same diaper, T-shirt, blanket).

Documentation

Reassessment of the mother's willingness to pump milk and instructions on how to pump milk will be documented in Gemini (computer system) under patient education. Periodic assessment of the mother's adequacy of pumping will also be documented in Gemini (computer system).

On the NICU/ICN flow sheet:
- When double-checking breast milk, the RN checking will initial on the flow sheet on the page documenting intake volumes.
- The type of milk being given will be indicated on the intake page: colostrum, fresh or previously frozen milk, and fortified milk. (Appropriate abbreviations will be Co, FBRM, fresh BRM.)
- When the infant goes to the breast, document if baby latched on to breast, duration of breast-feeding one or both breasts, behavioral response of the infant.
- If prefeeding and postfeeding weights are done, the estimate will be recorded in the "volume" space with an*, which will be defined as meaning "estimated by scale."

Unit equipment logs:
- Temperature of the refrigerator and freezers used for breast milk will be recorded daily on a log by the equipment technician.
- Equipment technician will be responsible for periodic cleansing of refrigerator and freezers and cleaning the electric breast pumps daily with topical disinfectant.

In addition to its nutritional properties (Table 12-6), breast milk confers some passive immunity for the infant (Table 12-7). Table 12-8 compares various formulas when bottle-feeding is necessary.

Tables 12-9 to 12-13* and Figure 12-5 include present guidelines for trophic and nutritional feedings for various weight levels of very low-birth-weight infants. All of these are evidence based.

*From Premji SS, et al. (2002). Evidence-based feeding guidelines for very low-birth-weight infants. Advances in neonatal care, 2(1), 5-18.

Table 12-6	Distribution of Secretory Products in Human Colostrum and Milk (Water 86%-87.5%; Total Solids 11.5 g)*

Nutritional Components

Lactose	6.9-7.2 g
Fat	3.0-4.4 g
Protein	0.9-1.03 g
Alpha-lactalbumin	150-170 mg
Beta-lactoglobulin	Trace
Serum albumin	50 mg

Electrolytes, Minerals, Trace Metals

Sodium	14-17.5 mg
Potassium	51-55 mg
Calcium	32-43 mg
Phosphorus	14-15 mg
Chloride	38-40 mg
Magnesium	3 mg
Iron	0.03 mg
Zinc	0.17 mg
Copper	15-105 µg
Iodine	4.5 µg
Manganese	1.4-2.4 µg
Fluoride	4-25 µg
Selenium	1.9-3.2 µg
Boron	−10 µg

Nitrogen Products (Total 0.15-2 g)

Whey protein nitrogen	75-78 mg
Casein protein nitrogen	38-41 mg
Nonprotein nitrogen	25% of total nitrogen
Urea	0.027 g
Creatinine	0.021 g
Glucosamine	0.112 g

Table **12-6**	Distribution of Secretory Products in Human Colostrum and Milk (Water 86%-87.5%; Total Solids 11.5 g)*—cont'd

Vitamins

C	4.5-5.5 mg
Thiamine (B_1)	12-15 µg
Niacin	183.7 µg
Biotin	0.5-0.9 µg
Folic acid	4.1-5.2 µg
Choline	8-9 mg
Inositol	40-46 mg
Pantothenic acid	200-240 µg
A (retinol)	54-56 µg
D	<0.42 IU
E	0.56 µg
K	1.5 µg

From Rassin DK, Garofalo RP, Ogra PL (2001). Human milk. In Remington JS, Klein JO, editors. Infectious diseases of the fetus and newborn infant, Philadelphia: WB Saunders, p. 172.
*Estimates based on amount per deciliter.

Table **12-7**	Level of Immunoglobulins in Colostrum and Milk and Estimates of Delivery of Lactational Immunoglobulins to the Breast-Feeding Neonate*

Day Postpartum	Percentage of Total Proteins Represented by Immunoglobulin (Ig)			Output of Immunoglobulin (mg/24 hr)		
	IgG	IgM	IgA	IgG	IgM	IgA
1	7	3	80	80	120	11,000
3	10	45	45	50	40	2000
7	1-2	4	20	25	10	1000
7-28	1-2	2	10-15	10	10	1000
<50	1-2	0.5-1	10-15	10	10	1000

From Rassin DK, Garofalo RP, Ogra PL (2001). Human milk. In Remington JS, Klein JO, editors. Infectious diseases of the fetus and newborn infant, Philadelphia: WB Saunders, p. 177.
*Estimates based on the available data for total immunoglobulin and daily protein synthesis.

Table 12-8 Bottle-Feeding: Comparison of Formulas

	Formula Type		
	Premature	Standard	Soy
Energy*	24 kcal/oz	20 kcal/oz	20 kcal/oz
Protein	Whey/casein (60:40), 22-24 g protein/L	Whey/casein (60:40 or 18:82), 18 g protein/L	Soy protein isolate, 18 g protein/L
Fat	MCT, LCT	LCT	LCT
Carbohydrate	Glucose polymers Lactose polymers	Lactose	Sucrose and/or glucose
Calcium (Ca) and phosphorus (P)	Fortified to meet needs of preterm infant Ca/P ratio 1:8-2:1	Not fortified to meet needs of preterm infant Ca/P ratio 1:3-1:5:1	Not fortified to meet needs of preterm infant Ca/P ratio 1:3-1:4:1
Iron	Available with or without iron fortification	Available with or without iron fortification	Available with iron fortification only

From Kalhan SC, Price PT (2001). *Nutrition and selected disorders of the gastrointestinal tract.* In Klaus MH, Fanaroff AA, editors. *Care of the high-risk neonate,* ed 5, Philadelphia: WB Saunders, p. 169.

MCT, Medium-chain triglycerides; *LCT,* long-chain triglycerides.

*Premature formula is available as ready-to-feed 20 kcal/oz or 24 kcal/oz. Standard cow's milk–based formulas are available commercially as ready-to-feed, powdered, or liquid concentrate. The powdered and liquid concentrates are less expensive and can be prepared with less water to increase the caloric concentration not to exceed 30 kcal/oz.

Table **12-9**	Guide to Trophic Feedings for Infants Below 750 g
Initiation of feeding	Start at 48 hr of life and continue for 48-72 hr
Feeding method	Indwelling nasogastric tube
Type of feeding	Full-strength expressed breast milk or 24 kcal/oz preterm formula
Amount and frequency	1 ml every 4 hr (equals approximately 12 ml/kg/day for a 500-g infant)
Feeding advances	None

From Premji SS, et al. (2002). Evidence-based feeding guidelines for very low-birth-weight infants. Advances in neonatal care, 2(1), 5-18.

Table **12-10**	Guide to Nutritional Feedings for Infants Below 750 g
Initiation of feeding	Initiate after trophic feedings on day 5 or 6 of life
Feeding method	Indwelling nasogastric tube
Type of feeding	Full-strength expressed breast milk or 24 kcal/oz preterm formula
Amount and frequency	1 ml every 2 hr (equals an increase, from trophic feeds, of 12 ml/kg/day for a 500-g infant)
Feeding advances	1 ml per feeding every 24 hr; continue same increase until at full feeds (equals approximately 24 ml/kg/day increase for a 500-g infant)

From Premji SS, et al. (2002). Evidence-based feeding guidelines for very low-birth-weight infants. Advances in neonatal care, 2(1), 5-18.

Table **12-11**	Guide to Trophic Feedings for Infants 750-1000 g
Initiation of feeding	Start at 48 hr and continue for 48-72 hr
Feeding method	Indwelling nasogastric tube
Type of feeding	Full-strength expressed breast milk or 24 kcal/oz preterm formula
Amount and frequency	1 ml every 2 hr (equals approximately 16 ml/kg/day for a 750-g infant)
Feeding advance	None

From Premji SS, et al. (2002). Evidence-based feeding guidelines for very low-birth-weight infants. Advances in neonatal care, 2(1), 5-18.

Table 12-12	Guide to Nutritional Feedings for Infants 750-1000 g
Initiation of feeding	Initiate after trophic feedings on day 5 or 6 of life
Feeding method	Indwelling nasogastric tube
Type of feeding	Full-strength expressed breast milk or 24 kcal/oz preterm formula
Amount and frequency	2 ml every 2 hr (equals an increase, from trophic feeds, of 16 ml/kg/day for a 750-g infant)
Feeding advance	If tolerates this for 48 hr, then increase 1 ml every 12 hr (equals approximately 32 ml/kg/day increase for a 750-g infant)

From Premji SS, et al. (2002). Evidence-based feeding guidelines for very low-birth-weight infants. Advances in neonatal care, 2(1), 5-18.

Table 12-13	Guide to Nutritional Feedings for Infants 1000-1500 g
Initiation of feeding	Start at 48 hr of life
Feeding method	Indwelling nasogastric tube
Type of feeding	Full-strength expressed breast milk or 24 kcal/oz preterm formula
Amount and frequency	1 ml every 2 hr (equals approximately 12 ml/kg/day for a 1000-g infant)
Feeding advance	1 ml every 12 hr (equals an increase of 18 ml/kg/day for a 1000-g infant)

From Premji SS, et al. (2002). Evidence-based feeding guidelines for very low-birth-weight infants. Advances in neonatal care, 2(1), 5-18.

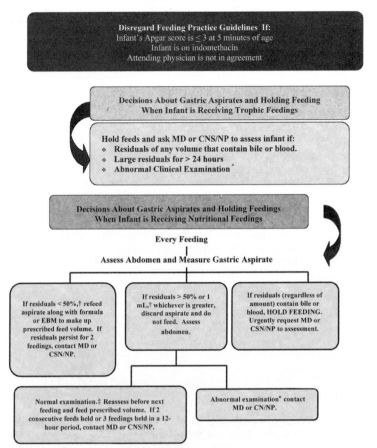

FIGURE 12-5

Guidelines for trophic and nutritional feedings for various weight levels of very low-birth-weight infants. Parameters for nurses to follow for decisions regarding management of gastric aspirates and holding feedings. In a 24-hour period, if emesis more than 50% of previous feeding (based on your best estimate) occurs on more than two occasions, contact physician or CNS/NP to assess the infant. *EBM*, Expressed breast milk. *Abnormal examination includes tense, distended, and/or discolored abdomen, clinically enlarged bowel loops, and/or no bowel sounds. †Mucus contains essential factors, hence, include in residual volume. ‡Normal examination includes distended abdomen but it is soft and nontender and may have visible bowel loops. If in doubt, consult physician or CSN/NP. (From Premji SS, et al. [2002]. Evidence-based feeding guidelines for very low-birth-weight infants. *Advances in neonatal care*, 2[1], 5-18.)

BIBLIOGRAPHY

Aguayo J (2001). Maternal lactation for preterm newborn infants. *Early human development*, 65(Suppl), S19-S29.

Haninger NC, Farley CL (2001). Screening for hypoglycemia in healthy term neonates: effects on breastfeeding. *Journal of midwifery & women's health*, 46(5), 292-301.

Jewell VC, et al. (2001). Nutritional factors and visual function in premature infants. *Proceedings of the Nutritional Society*, 60(2), 171-178.

Kennedy KA, Tyson JE, Chamnanvanikij S (2002). Early versus delayed initiation of progressive enteral feedings for parenterally fed low birth weight or preterm infants. *Cochrane review*. http://www.cochrane.org/cochrane/revabstr/ab001970.htm

Kuschel CA, Harding JE (2002). Calcium and phosphorus supplementation of human milk for preterm infants. *Cochrane review, the Cochrane library*, 1. http://www.cochrane.org/cochrane/revabstr/ab003310.htm

Kuschel CA, Harding JE (2002). Carbohydrate supplementation of human milk to promote growth in preterm infants. *Cochrane review, the Cochrane library*, 1. http://www.cochrane.org/cochrane/revabstr/ab000280.htm

Kuschel CA, Harding JE (2002). Protein supplementation of human milk for promoting growth in preterm infants. *Cochrane review, the Cochrane Library*, 1. http://www.cochrane.org/cochrane/revabstr/ab000433.htm

Mason-Wyckoff M, et al. (2003). Nutrition: physiologic basis of metabolism and management of enteral and parenteral nutrition. In Kenner C, Lott JW, editors. *Comprehensive neonatal nursing: a physiologic perspective*, ed 3, St Louis: WB Saunders.

McGuire W, Anthony MY (2001). Formula milk versus preterm human milk for feeding preterm or low birth weight infants (Cochrane Review). *Cochrane database systematic reviews*, 3.

McGuire W, Anthony MY (2001). Formula milk versus term human milk for feeding preterm or low birth weight infants (Cochrane Review). *Cochrane database systematic reviews*, 4.

Nankervis CA, Reber KM, Nowicki PT (2001). Age-dependent changes in the postnatal intestinal microcirculation. *Microcirculation*, 8(6), 377-387.

Nogami K, et al. (2001). Intravenous low-dose erythromycin administration for infants with feeding intolerance. *Pediatrics international*, 43(6), 605-610.

Ohlsson VA, Lacy JB, Horsley A (2002). Massage for promoting growth and development of preterm and/or low birth-weight infants. *Cochrane review, the Cochrane library*, 1. http://www.cochrane.org/cochrane/revabstr/ab000390.htm

Premji S, Chessell L (2002). Continuous nasogastric milk feeding versus intermittent bolus milk feeding for premature infants less than 1500 grams. *Cochrane review*. http://www.cochrane.org/cochrane/revabstr/ab001819.htm

Steward DK, Pridham KF (2002). Growth patterns of extremely low-birth-weight hospitalized preterm infants. *Journal of obstetrics, gynecology, & neonatal nursing*, 31(1), 57-65.

Tubman TR, Thompson SW (2001). Glutamine supplementation for prevention of morbidity in preterm infants (Cochrane Review). *Cochrane database systematic reviews*, 4.

Tyson JE, Kennedy KA (2002). Minimal enteral nutrition for promoting feeding tolerance and preventing morbidity in parenterally fed infants (Cochrane Review). *The Cochrane library*, 1. http://www.cochrane.org/cochrane/revabstr/ab000504.htm

RENAL CARE

The kidneys function to regulate fluid and electrolyte balance, arterial blood pressure, and toxin levels in the body. Renal blood flow not only provides oxygen and nutrients to the kidneys, but also affects the rate of solute and water reabsorption by the proximal tubule, participates in the concentration and dilution of the urine, and delivers substrates for excretion in the urine.

Glomerular filtration rate (GFR) is the rate at which fluid is filtered through the glomerulus. Because it is equal to the sum of all filtration rates of all nephrons in both kidneys, the GFR is a reflection of kidney function, with a decrease in GFR signaling renal disease. GFR is therefore affected by changes in arterial blood pressure, vascular resistance, concentration of plasma proteins, and glomerular capillary permeability. Alteration in the permeability of the glomerular capillaries may result from inherent damage to the capillary, thus altering the pore size or changing the electrical charge within the membrane. GFR is also affected by urinary system obstruction. Assessment of GFR is important in evaluating renal function.

One method of assessing GFR is by measuring the renal clearance of a substance (Sweetwyne-Thomas, 2003). Measurement of serum creatinine levels is clinically the most useful method of estimating renal function in neonates. When renal blood flow is diminished as the result of a decrease in arterial pressure, the sympathetic nervous system, at the level of the kidney, responds to maintain homeostasis. As the result of the decrease in GFR, there is a decrease in the concentration of sodium and chloride ions, and renin secretion is stimulated. Renin then leads to the production of angiotensin I that is then converted to angiotensin II in the lungs. Angiotensin II then stimulates secretion of aldosterone by the adrenal cortex. Aldosterone in turn triggers the reabsorption of sodium and water, thereby increasing extracellular fluid volume and renal perfusion (Sweetwyne-Thomas, 2003).

NURSING ASSESSMENT

Many urogenital problems have an inheritance pattern that suggests genetic predisposition. The history should focus on any family members who have renal transplants or undergone dialysis, those with a history of renal failure, and those with cystic kidney disease or anomalies of the genitourinary (GU) system.

Prenatal histories should be reviewed for antepartal factors that may predispose the infant to renal problems. Was there polyhydramnios, oligohydramnios, or an increased fetal abdominal area on ultrasonography?

Neonatal history should include the following questions:

1. Has micturition taken place? If so, at what age? (The first voiding may occur in the delivery room or by 24 hours of life.)
2. Has the infant undergone any hypoxic episodes that may result in delayed voiding?
3. Is the infant receiving enteral or parenteral nutrition? If so, is the fluid intake sufficient relative to clinical status, gestational age, and immediate environment (radiant warmer or humidified Isolette)? The radiant warmer increases insensible water loss.
4. Is the infant under treatment for jaundice? (Phototherapy increases fluid losses.)
5. Is the infant experiencing any frank blood loss or increased gastrointestinal (GI) losses such as are caused by nasogastric suctioning, vomiting, diarrhea, or increased ostomy losses?
6. What is the specific gravity of urine? (Normal range is 1.003 to 1.015.)
7. How old is the infant?

Observe the abdomen for any abdominal distention and for signs of poor muscle tone as seen in Eagle-Barrett (prune-belly) syndrome. Observe genitals for urinary meatus, any discoloration of the area indicating possibly a breech delivery, and in the male the position of the meatus on the shaft of the penis. Also look at the scrotal sac for the appearance of testicles—have they descended? Palpate kidneys using the ballottement technique.

Observe for other signs that indicate renal problems, such as Potter's facies (flattened, beaklike nose, wide-set eyes, micrognathia, disproportionately large ears, short neck), accompanied by abnormal positioning of the hands and feet and pulmonary hypoplasia; all these signs are associated with oligohydramnios or a single umbilical artery.

DIAGNOSIS

The diagnosis of a renal problem is usually made based on the following:

- Urine culture
- Urinalysis
- Urine osmolality
- Serum electrolytes including blood urea nitrogen (BUN), creatinine
- Urine chemistries
- Androcorticosteroid levels
- Renal ultrasound
- Renal scan using isotopes

- Voiding cystoureterogram
- Computed tomography

NURSING MANAGEMENT

Nursing care is aimed at maintaining fluid and electrolyte balance. Box 13-1 gives the formula for calculating renal solute load and an example of the calculation.

ACUTE RENAL FAILURE

Acute renal failure may be defined as an abrupt severe decrease or complete halt of kidney function. Neonatal renal failure is suspected when urinary output falls below 1 ml/kg/hr accompanied by serum creatinine levels greater than 1.5 mg/dl and BUN greater than 20 mg/dl. Since the placenta functioned as the major excretory organ in utero, symptoms of renal failure in the newborn may take several days to manifest.

*Causes of Acute Renal Failure in the Neonate**
Prerenal
- Dehydration
- Hemorrhage
- Sepsis
- Necrotizing enterocolitis
- Congestive heart failure
- Drugs: angiotensin-converting enzyme inhibitors, nonsteroidal antiinflammatories, amphotericin, tolazoline

Intrinsic
- Acute tubular necrosis
- Renal dysplasia
- Polycystic kidney disease
- Renal venous thrombosis
- Uric acid nephropathy
- Transient acute renal insufficiency of the newborn

Postrenal
- Posterior urethral valves
- Bilateral ureteropelvic junction obstruction
- Bilateral ureterovesical junction obstruction
- Neurogenic bladder
- Obstructive nephrolithiasis

---

*From Vogt BA, Davis ID, Avner ED (2001). The kidney. In Klaus MH, Fanaroff AA, editors. Care of the high-risk neonate, ed 5, Philadelphia: WB Saunders, p. 434.

Box 13-1

Renal Solute Load Calculation

PRSL (mOsm/L)* = (protein/L) + Potassium (mEq/L) + Chloride (mEq/L)

Example
Preterm formula$_{24}$ (PT$_{24}$) contains the following:

Protein, 22 g/L × 4	= 88
Sodium, 15.2 mEq/L × 1	= 15.2
Potassium, 26.9 mEq/L × 1	= 26.9
Chloride, 18.6 mEq/L × 1	= 18.6
PRSL	= 148.7 mOsm/L

Baby A is a 2-week-old former 32-week AGA infant weighing 1400 g and now receiving PT$_{24}$, 150 ml/kg/day
Estimated fluid losses are as follows:

Stool	10 ml/kg/day
Insensible water loss	70 ml/kg/day
Total water loss	80 ml/kg/day

150 ml/kg/day intake–80 ml/kg/day output = 70 ml/kg/day available for urine output

The PRSL of PT$_{24}$ is 148.7 mOsm/L:

$$\frac{148.7 \text{ mOsm}}{1000\text{ml}} = \frac{X \text{ mOsm}}{150\text{ml}}$$

X = 22.3 mOsm

$$\frac{22.3 \text{ mOsm}}{70\text{ml}} \times 1000 = \text{mOsm/L}$$

318.6 mOsm = X

Therefore the estimated osmolality of the urine is 319 mOsm/L

From Kalhan SC, Price PT (2001). Nutrition and selected disorders of the gastrointestinal tract. In Klaus MH, Fanaroff AA, editors. Care of the high-risk neonate, ed 5, Philadelphia: WB Saunders, p. 149.
PRSL, Potential renal solute load; AGA, appropriate for gestational age.

Risk Factors

Treatments such as mechanical ventilation and umbilical and femoral vessel catheterization may predispose the infant to renal failure because of renal vein and artery thrombosis. Birth injury, hypovolemia, and hypoxemia may compromise renal blood flow. Congenital causes of intrinsic renal failure include aplastic kidney, polycystic renal disease, necrosis, and maternal ingestion of nephrotoxic agents (Sweetwyne-Thomas, 2003).

Diagnosis
The diagnosis of acute renal failure is aimed at the cause and not the symptoms.

Clinical Manifestations
Decreased urine output, edema, lethargy, oliguria, edema, hematuria, and proteinuria are the common clinical signs of renal failure. Urine output should be at least 1 ml/kg/hr.

Nursing Management
Symptomatic treatment is carried out until a definitive cause is determined and treated. Once absence of a urinary obstruction is established, a fluid challenge, intravenous (IV) isotonic solution, 10 to 20 ml/kg given over 1 hour, may be helpful in differentiating prerenal from intrinsic failure. If urine output is at least 1 ml/kg/hr within 2 hours of the fluid infusion, then the cause of the renal failure is probably related to hypoperfusion. Use of a diuretic following the fluid challenge may be necessary if urine output does not increase immediately following the fluid challenge. To treat prerenal renal failure, low-dose dopamine may also be tried in an attempt to increase renal perfusion.

Fluid replacement depends on the type of renal failure the infant is exhibiting. If intrinsic failure exists, fluid replacement is limited to insensible loss and replacement of renal output. If the infant is acidotic, sodium acetate may be used instead of sodium chloride in IV solutions. Sodium bicarbonate should be used with caution because it is hypertonic and has been found to cause increases in intracranial pressure and resultant intraventricular hemorrhage and may also cause a transient hypercarbia.

Peritoneal dialysis or hemodialysis should be used only in infants with severe congestive heart failure, fluid overload, or uremia (Sweetwyne-Thomas, 2003).

NEONATAL CIRCUMCISION

Circumcision is no longer advocated for any medical reasons. It may be culturally acceptable to families to have their male offspring circumcised. If the procedure is done, the infant should be given pain medication before and after the procedure.

Drugs with high sodium levels, such as carbenicillin, penicillin G, ampicillin, and cephalothin, or drugs diluted in sodium chloride should be used with caution. Other medications are cleared through the kidney. These include aminoglycosides, penicillins, cephalosporins, theophylline, indomethacin, tolazoline, and magnesium; they should all be used with caution.

Hypertension that is secondary to fluid overload may be treated by sodium and fluid restriction. Antihypertensive agents may also be effective in management. These infants are prone to infections. The infant should be monitored for signs of infection and any abnormality reported so that treatment is begun immediately.

POTTER'S ASSOCIATION (SYNDROME)

Potter's association (syndrome) refers to a congenital association of clinical manifestations, such as Potter's facies and bilateral renal agenesis. The failure to produce much if any fetal urine leads to oligohydramnios and compression of the developing facial structures. This infant will not survive, and the care is supportive in nature.

POLYCYSTIC KIDNEY DISEASE

Polycystic kidney disease is an autosomal recessive condition.

Nursing Assessment

The infant with polycystic kidney disease may present with abdominal distention. A mass may be felt on palpation. This condition can be unilateral or bilateral.

Clinical Manifestations

Abdominal distention, a palpable mass, and albuminuria are the clinical signs of polycystic kidney disease.

Diagnosis

Polycystic kidney disease must be differentiated from hydronephrosis. This can be done by renal ultrasound, a pyleogram, or a voiding cystoureterogram.

Nursing Management

The treatment for polycystic kidney disease is usually a partial or full nephrectomy. The nursing care is aimed at maintaining fluid and electrolyte balance and protection against infection. Check urine for presence of albumin and blood. Watch the infant's blood pressure because hypertension is a possibility. Postoperative care is aimed at watching for bleeding, comfort measures, and prevention of fluid imbalances and infection.

PRUNE-BELLY (EAGLE-BARRETT) SYNDROME

Prune-belly syndrome is a lack of abdominal muscle tone. In the male, the testicles may be undescended. The infant may have hypoplastic kidneys.

Nursing Assessment

The assessment is based on a thorough physical examination to determine if other anomalies are present.

Clinical Manifestations

Abdominal distention, a wrinkled appearance to the abdomen, and lack of muscle tone in this area are clinical signs of prune-belly syndrome. Other manifestations may include cryptorchidism (undescended testicles), prostatic urethral dilation, bladder distention, patent urachus, abdominal distention or protuberance, malrotation of the intestines, cardiac defects, congenital hip dysplasia and associated "click," and clubfoot (talipes equinovarus).

Diagnosis

The diagnosis of prune-belly syndrome is usually made on observation of poor abdominal musculature. However, there may be an underlying GI problem so palpation of the abdomen is needed to determine if bowel loops are present.

Nursing Management

Most infants with prune-belly syndrome require abdominal supports to keep the internal organs safe and to assist with mobility as the children grow. Reconstructive surgery is generally done at an older age. However, the renal condition must be dealt with during the neonatal period if permanent damage is to be avoided. The condition of the kidney can range from normal kidney mass to complete atresia. The lack of muscle in the ureters leads to their elongation and distention. If obstruction occurs as a result of the tortuous nature of the ureters, surgical intervention may be necessary. Reimplantation or diversion may be necessary to prevent urine stasis and renal failure. If there is a ureteral obstruction it will need to be relieved, but there may still be bladder atonia. For undescended testicles an orchiopexy is done.

Bladder decompression is necessary for the prevention of stasis. To prevent trauma to the distorted urethra and bladder a skilled practitioner should perform catheterization. Any severe abdominal distention and insufficient urinary output in the first day of life observed by the nurse should be evaluated by other members of the health care team to rule out the possibility of this syndrome. A large amount of urine may have accumulated in the fetal period, resulting in a greatly distended bladder. Renal dysplasia may be present.

A nephrostomy or ureterostomy diversion should be considered if urine drainage is compromised. Long-term use of antimicrobial therapy may be necessary to prevent sepsis. In the presence of a patent urachus, closure may not be necessary in the neonatal period if adequate drainage and prevention of infection can be maintained. If the bladder is distended, reduction cystoplasty is performed in order to relieve the tension on the bladder and to promote emptying (Sweet-wyne-Thomas, 2003).

Before- and after-surgery skin care is important. Turning every 2 hours is recommended. Before surgery, bladder decompression can be done via intermittent catheterization or Credé's maneuver of the bladder.

HYDRONEPHROSIS

Hydronephrosis is the accumulation of urine within the renal pelvis and calices to the point of overdistention. Hydronephrosis often follows obstruction of urine flow at the junction of the ureteropelvis, the ureterovesical valve, or the urethrovesical valve. It can occur when there is no obstruction.

Nursing Assessment
The maternal history will reveal oligohydramnios. Usually if this condition is present prenatally it can be detected on ultrasound.

Clinical Manifestations
A large, solid, palpable smooth mass at the region of the kidney can be found. Urine output may be decreased or normal, depending on the amount of functioning kidney mass. Urinary tract infection often accompanies hydronephrosis, making fever and discomfort observable signs. Gross hematuria may be present and must be differentiated from the hematuria associated with Wilms' tumor and renal vein thrombosis (Sweetwyne-Thomas, 2003).

Diagnosis
Renal ultrasound or computed tomography is usually used. Hydronephrosis must be differentiated from other conditions, such as cystic disease, renal vein thrombosis, or Wilms' tumor.

Nursing Management
Decompression and drainage of the urine can be accomplished with a pyeloplasty and nephrostomy tube insertion. If there is apparent renal damage a nephrectomy may be needed.

The presence of cyanosis, grunting, nasal flaring, and retractions is important because the lungs may not have fully developed. The chest should be observed for any alterations in the anteroposterior diameter or asymmetry. Vital signs, including blood pressure, must be monitored at least every 4 hours and more frequently if they are unstable. The blood pressure is especially important because hypertension is common in the infant with hydronephrosis. If hypertension is severe, antihypertensives may be given. Some institutions use IV hydralazine, IV diazoxide, or methyldopa. Use of any of these drugs requires extremely close monitoring of the cardiorespiratory system.

Fluid and electrolyte status also must be carefully watched. Fluid intake and output should be recorded at least every 2 to 4 hours. Specific gravity may be checked every 4 to 8 hours. A urine dipstick assessment may be useful for determining the presence of protein or blood in the urine. Assessment of hydration status is important. The fontanels should be observed to determine if they are sunken or bulging. Skin turgor should demonstrate instant recoil.

Assessment for the presence of any dependent or pitting edema should be performed and recorded. The nurse often detects the early cues that an infant has hydronephrosis. If hydronephrosis is even suspected, the medical team must be notified so that early intervention and prevention of long-term complications can occur. Palpation of the abdomen is also helpful to determine if a mass is present.

After surgery, a nephrostomy or a urinary stent may be placed. These are connected to a closed drainage system (Sweetwyne-Thomas, 2003).

URETHRAL OBSTRUCTION

The obstruction of the urethra usually occurs at the level of the ureter and pelvis. The obstruction causes a backflow of urine into the bladder often leading to an infection.

Nursing Assessment
The infant with a urethral obstruction may be asymptomatic unless the obstruction is severe. Delayed voiding or failure to void may be a presenting sign.

Clinical Manifestations
The clinical sign of a urethral obstruction is delayed voiding or a failure to void. The infant may or may not have signs of a urinary tract infection

Diagnosis
The diagnosis of urethral obstruction is made by renal ultrasound or computed tomography.

Nursing Management
Surgery to remove the obstruction may be needed. Otherwise, the infant is observed and serum and urine chemistries are followed. If there is diminished renal output observe for signs of edema. Also watch for signs of infection.

HYDROCELE

Hydrocele is a condition that reflects a collection of fluid in the scrotal sac.

Nursing Assessment

Nursing assessment of hydrocele consists of physical examination of the scrotal sac.

Clinical Manifestations

Clinical signs of hydrocele are an enlarged scrotum with no palpable masses.

Diagnosis

Transillumination of the sac will demonstrate the presence of fluid. Hydrocele must be differentiated from an incarcerated inguinal hernia, which is a surgical emergency.

Nursing Management

Keep the infant with a hydrocele comfortable. Reassure the parents that this condition is not dangerous. To relieve the pressure, a physician can aspirate fluid from the sac. Surgical repair will be done later so parents must be taught the signs of increased pressure and the possibility of inguinal hernia with incarceration.

INGUINAL HERNIA

Inguinal hernia is especially common in premature infants. It reflects that the small intestine and gonads pass through the open processus vaginalis. If the intestines become trapped and tissue ischemia occurs, an incarceration is present and constitutes a medical/surgical emergency.

Nursing Assessment

The infant is observed for the presence of a hernia. The following signs of incarceration are considered: vomiting, abdominal distention, and increasing irritability.

Clinical Manifestations

The clinical sign of an inguinal hernia is a palpable mass in the groin that usually worsens with crying.

Diagnosis

Inguinal hernia must be differentiated from a hydrocele. It is usually diagnosed on observation and palpation. Some hernias are reducible and easily pop back into place with pressure.

Nursing Management

Surgery is performed on those hernias that are not easily reduced, but if the infant is stable the surgery will not be done in the immediate neonatal period. The exception is with an incarceration that requires immediate surgery. Teach parents signs and symptoms of incarceration; some parents will also feel comfortable in being taught how to reduce the hernia (not an incarcerated one) manually. Comfort measures are important because crying only increases the presence of the hernia.

TORSION OF THE TESTICLES

Torsion of the testicle occurs when the testicle or sperm cord twists, restricting circulation to the testicle.

Nursing Assessment

Nursing assessment of torsion of the testicle consists of physical examination of the scrotal sac for swelling and discoloration.

Clinical Manifestations

Scrotal swelling and discoloration of the scrotum may or may not be present.

Diagnosis

Transillumination is negative, and the diagnosis is made on physical examination

Nursing Management

Surgical correction of the torsion is needed. The focus of nursing care is on keeping the infant comfortable and as quiet as possible. The abdominal girth is measured every 4 hours for any signs of distention. The scrotum must be inspected for edema, discoloration, and skin temperature. If the infant is experiencing vomiting because of abdominal distention, the use of a nasogastric tube attached to intermittent low suction may be necessary. The tube should be irrigated every 2 to 4 hours with 2 ml of saline or air to maintain patency. Positioning of the infant should be only on the back with head turned to the side or in a side-lying position because otherwise too much pressure may be placed on the abdominal and scrotal areas (Sweetwyne-Thomas, 2003).

After surgery, the nursing care centers on stability of the vital signs and prevention of infection. Respiratory status must be carefully assessed because abdominal distention may compromise respiratory function. Nasopharyngeal suctioning may be necessary. The suture line is generally small but still requires aseptic technique. The site should be assessed for the presence of edema, drainage, or discoloration. A urinary drainage bag may be necessary to protect the skin and to prevent infection if excessive drainage is present (Sweetwyne-Thomas, 2003).

NEPHROBLASTOMA

Nephroblastoma (Wilms' tumor) is a neonatal malignancy.

Nursing Assessment

The physical examination must be undertaken with caution. If abdominal distention is present and a tumor is suspected it should not be palpated because this can seed the tumor to other areas of the body.

Clinical Manifestations

The clinical sign of nephroblastoma is a smooth, solid abdominal or flank mass that is actually a renal mass. Hypertension and fever may also be present.

Diagnosis

The diagnosis of nephroblastoma is confirmed by pyelogram and renal ultrasound. A chest x-ray is needed because the tumor may have seeded to this area.

Nursing Management

Supportive care is given during the neonatal period. Parents must be helped to understand the infant's condition and what to expect following the discharge home.

BIBLIOGRAPHY

Blews DE (1999). Sonography of the neonatal genitourinary tract. *Radiology clinics of North America*, 37(6), 1199-1208, vii.

Cromie WJ (2001). Implications of antenatal ultrasound screening in the incidence of major genitourinary malformations. *Seminars in pediatric surgery*, 10(4), 204-211.

Cromie WJ, et al. (2001). Implications of prenatal ultrasound screening in the incidence of major genitourinary malformations. *Journal of urology*, 165(5), 1677-1680.

Fasolato V, et al. (1998). Feto-neonatal ultrasonography to detect renal abnormalities: evaluation of 1-year screening program. *American journal of perinatology*, 15(3), 161-164.

Fonck C, et al. (2001). Autosomal recessive polycystic kidney disease in adulthood. *Nephrology & dialysis transplant*, 16(8), 1648-1652.

Gouyon JB, Guignard JP (2000). Management of acute renal failure in newborns. *Pediatric nephrology*, 14(10-11), 1037-1044.

Kemper MJ, et al. (2001). Antenatal oligohydramnios of renal origin: postnatal therapeutic and prognostic challenges. *Clinical nephrology*, 56(6), S9-12.

Picca S, et al. (2001). Extracorporeal dialysis in neonatal hyperammonemia: modalities and prognostic indicators. *Pediatric nephrology*, 16(11), 862-867.

Qvist E, et al. (2002). Neurodevelopmental outcome in high-risk patients after renal transplantation in early childhood. *Pediatric transplant*, 6(1), 53-62.

Schaefer F, et al. (1999). Dialysis in neonates with inborn errors of metabolism. *Nephrology & dialysis transplant*, 14(4), 910-918.

Summar M (2001). Current strategies for the management of neonatal urea cycle disorders. *Journal of pediatrics*, 138(1 Suppl), S30-S39.

Sweetwyne-Thomas K (2003). Assessment and management of the genitourinary system. In Kenner C, Lott JW, editors. *Comprehensive neonatal nursing: a physiologic perspective*, ed 3, St Louis: WB Saunders.

Toth-Heyn P, Drukker A, Guignard JP (2000). The stressed neonatal kidney: from pathophysiology to clinical management of neonatal vasomotor nephropathy. *Pediatric nephrology*, 14(3), 227-239.

CHAPTER 14

ENDOCRINE CARE

The endocrine system is considered by many to be the master system that regulates all body processes. It comprises the hypothalamus; the pituitary, pineal, thyroid, parathyroid, and adrenal glands; the gonads; and the pancreatic islet cells. Some of the problems that arise in the newborn are related to the metabolism of glucose, calcium, phosphorus, and magnesium that are regulated by the endocrine system.

NURSING ASSESSMENT

The nursing assessment is based on physical examination and serum chemistry levels. The infant may be premature or, in the case of hypothyroidism, postterm. The infant may be small for gestational age or, in the case of an infant of a diabetic mother, large for gestational age. Maternal history is an important factor.

CLINICAL MANIFESTATIONS

Clinical manifestations will vary according to the condition; but the more common symptoms are high-pitched or weak crying, tremors, mottled coloring, episodes of apnea and/or bradycardia, feeding difficulties, and poor weight gain.

DIAGNOSIS

The diagnosis is made based on the serum chemistry levels coupled with the physical examination.

NURSING MANAGEMENT

Nursing management consists of monitoring serum chemistry levels closely; maintaining fluid and electrolyte balance; observing for changes in serum levels of a substance, such as glucose; and observing for changes in the infant's condition, such as increasing lethargy or irritability and increasing or decreasing episodes of apnea and bradycardia.

HYPOGLYCEMIA

Hypoglycemia is defined as a blood sugar level of less than 30 mg/dl in a full-term infant or less than 20 mg/dl in a premature infant.

Treatment goal is to maintain a blood sugar level greater than 40 mg/dl.

Risk Factors
- Infant of a diabetic mother (IDM)
- Prematurity
- Birth asphyxia
- Postmaturity
- Infant small for gestational age
- Intrauterine growth restriction (IUGR)
- Sepsis
- Rh incompatibility
- Congenital metabolic syndromes

Clinical Manifestations
- Poor feeding
- Lethargy
- Hypotonia
- Tremors and/or seizures
- Apnea and/or bradycardia with or without cyanosis

Diagnosis
- Blood glucose: below 30 mg/dl in term infants and below 20 mg/dl in preterm infants indicate hypoglycemia; maintain level above 40 mg/dl in all infants
- Insulin
- Ketones: serum and urine
- Cortisol
- Growth hormone
- Lactate
- Pyruvate
- Serum electrolytes
- Based on blood sugar level

Treatment*
Asymptomatic infants
1. Oral feedings can be tried with 10% dextrose in water or other formulas.
2. If oral feedings are not accepted, start an intravenous (IV) infusion of maintenance dextrose as below.

Symptomatic infants
1. Give an IV bolus of 10% dextrose in water, 2 ml/kg (50% is too concentrated for an infant).
2. Infuse IV dextrose at a rate sufficient to support the blood sugar. Start with a maintenance rate of 5 to 7 mg/kg/min. Adjust the rate

---

*From Goetzman BW, Wennberg RP (1999). Neonatal intensive care handbook, ed 3, St Louis: Mosby, pp. 190-191.

upward or downward to keep blood sugar in the range of 60 to 120 mg/dl.

3. Do not abruptly decrease dextrose infusion, or rebound hypo-glycemia might occur.

4. Monitor blood sugar frequently using glucose oxidase strips, and confirm abnormal values with a true blood sugar test.

5. When the infant is stabilized and if no persistent diagnosis is apparent, slowly decrease the dextrose infusion rate with careful monitoring of blood glucose. Aim to discontinue the infusion only if the blood glucose remains in the acceptable range.

6. After dextrose infusion is discontinued, monitor the blood sugar for at least 24 hours.

Other treatment

1. Glucagon in doses of 300 μg/kg up to 1 mg/kg by intramuscular (IM) injection can be used in conditions with adequate glycogen stores, such as hyperinsulinism. This is an emergency treatment.

2. Glucocorticoids are used as replacement therapy in hypoadrenal infants and can be used temporarily as pharmacologic therapy in other conditions.

3. Growth hormone is used in those infants with growth hormone deficiency.

4. Diazoxide in a dose of 5 to 20 mg/kg/day can be used in hyperinsu-linemic states and may serve as a diagnostic technique; patients with insulinomas are far less likely to respond than functional hyperinsulinemic patients.

5. Somatostin analogues, such as octreotide, are used to suppress insulin secretion. They work better on different beta-cell recep-tors than does diazoxide.

6. Pancreatectomy is reserved for intractable hypoglycemia caused by hyperinsulinism. If an isolated tumor is found, it is removed. An 85% to 90% pancreatectomy may be performed if a tumor is not visualized.

7. Specific diets are necessary for the metabolic diseases listed above.

*Classification**

Neonatal hypoglycemia can be classified as transient or persistent. Box 14-1 lists the various causes of neonatal hypoglycemia.

---

*From Kliegman RM (2001). Problems in metabolism adaptation: glucose, calcium, and magnesium. In Klaus MH, Fanaroff AA, editors. Care of the high-risk neonate, ed 5, St Louis: Mosby, p. 307. Modified from Sperling M, Chernausek S (1990). Endocrine disorders. In Behrman R, Kliegman R, editors. Nelson essentials of pediatrics, Philadelphia: WB Saunders.

Box 14-1

Etiology of Neonatal Hypocalcemia

Hypoparathyroidism
  Transient early neonatal
  Transient late neonatal
  Maternal hyperparathyroidism
  Maternal hypercalcemic hypocalciuria
DiGeorge syndrome: permanent gland hypoplasia or aplasia
  With maternal ^{131}I treatment and congenital hypothyroidism
  Familial X linked
  Familial autosomal dominant
  Inactive hormone (pseudoidiopathic)
  Hormone unresponsiveness (pseudohypoparathyroidism)
Vitamin D deficiency (rickets)
  Diet
    Decreased hepatic synthesis
    Increased renal synthesis
  Malabsorption
  Anticonvulsant drugs
  End-organ resistance (vitamin D dependent)
  Transient resistance to 1,25-dihydroxyvitamin D (infants <1250 g
    birth weight)
  Hypomagnesemia
  Hyperphosphatemia

From Kliegman RM (2001). Problems in metabolic adaptation: glucose, calcium, and magnesium. In Klaus MH, Fanaroff AA, editors. Care of the high-risk neonate, ed 5, Philadelphia: WB Saunders, p. 312.

Neonatal Transient Hypoglycemia
Associated with inadequate substrate or enzyme function
- Prematurity
- Asphyxia
- Small for gestational age
- Smaller of twins
- Infants with severe respiratory distress
- Infants of toxemic mothers

Associated with hyperinsulinemia
- Infants of diabetic mothers (Table 14-1)
- Infants with erythroblastosis fetalis

Table 14-1	Infant of Diabetic Mother (IDM): Pathophysiology of Morbidity and Mortality
Problem	**Pathophysiology**
Fetal demise	Acute placental failure?
	Hyperglycemia, lactic acidosis, hypoxia?
Macrosomia	Hyperinsulinism
Respiratory distress syndrome	Insulin antagonism of cortisol
	Variant surfactant biochemical pathways
Wet lung syndrome	Cesarean delivery
Hypoglycemia	Decreased glucose and fat mobilization
Polycythemia	Erythropoietic "macrosomia"
	Mild fetal hypoxia?
	Decreased O_2 delivery to fetus—HbA_{1c}
Hypocalcemia	Decreased neonatal parathyroid hormone
	Increased calcitonin?
	Decreased magnesium
Hyperbilirubinemia	Increased erythropoietic mass
	Increased bilirubin production
	Immature hepatic conjugation?
	Oxytocin induction
Congential malformation (central nervous system, heart, skeletal)	Hyperglycemia
	Genetic linkage?
	Insulin as teratogen?
	Vascular accident?
Renal vein thrombosis	Polycythemia
	Dehydration
Neonatal small left colon syndrome	Immature gastrointestinal motility?
Cardiomyopathy	Reversible septal hypertrophy
	Increased glycogen
	Increased muscle?
Family psychologic stress	High-risk pregnancy
	Fear of diabetes in infant
Subsequent development	Genetic HLA markers; risk is greater for insulin-dependent infant of diabetic father (type) diabetes
Diabetes	

Modified from Kliegman RM, Fanaroff AA (1983). Developmental metabolism and nutrition. In Gregory GA, editor: Pediatric anesthesiology, New York: Churchill Livingstone. In Kliegman RM (2001). Problems in metabolic adaptation: glucose, calcium, and magnesium. In Klaus MH, Fanaroff AA, editors. Care of the high-risk neonate, ed 5, Philadelphia: WB Saunders, p. 312.

Hb, Hemoglobin; HLA, human leukocyte antigen.

- Infants with intrauterine growth restriction
- Infants with improper position of umbilical artery catheter infusions
- Infants exposed to maternal beta-mimetic agents
- Infants exposed to maternal oral hypoglycemic agents

Neonatal-Infantile Persistent Hypoglycemia

1. Hyperinsulinemic states
   a. Familial hyperinsulinemia
   b. Hyperammonemic hyperinsulinism
   c. Beta-cell adenoma
   d. Leucine sensitivity
   e. Beckwith-Wiedemann syndrome
2. Hormone deficiencies
   a. Panhypopituitarism
   b. Isolated growth hormone deficiency
   c. Adrenocorticotropic hormone deficiency
   d. Adrenal insufficiency
   e. Glucagon deficiency
   f. Epinephrine deficiency
3. Glycogen storage diseases
   a. Glucose-6-phosphatase deficiency
   b. Amylo-1,6-glucosidase deficiency
   c. Liver phosphorylase deficiency
   d. Glycogen synthetase deficiency
4. Disorders of gluconeogenesis
   a. Hyperglycinemia
   b. Fructose-1,6-diphosphatase deficiency
   c. Pyruvate carboxylase deficiency
   d. Phosphoenolypyruvate carboxykinase deficiency
5. Other enzyme defects
   a. Galactosemia: galactose-1-phosphate uridyl transferase deficiency
   b. Fructose intolerance: fructose-1-phosphate aldolase deficiency
6. Disorders of fat (alternate fuel) metabolism
   a. Primary carnitine deficiency
   b. Secondary carnitine deficiency
   c. Carnitine palmityltransferase deficiency
   d. Long-, medium-, short-chain fatty acid acyl-CoA dehydrogenase deficiency
   e. Amino acid and organic acid disorders
   f. Maple syrup urine disease
   g. Propionic acidemia
   h. Methylmalonic acidemia
   i. Tyrosinosis

j. Glutaric aciduria
k. 3-Hydroxy-3-methylglutaric aciduria
7. Systemic disorders
    a. Sepsis
    b. Hepatic failure
    c. Heart failure
    d. Hyperviscosity-polycythemia

Clinical Manifestations

Clinical signs of hypoglycemia include labile blood glucose, large for gestational age, asphyxia, respiratory distress, hypoglycemia, macrosomatia, congenital anomalies, hypocalcemia, hypomagnesemia, hyperbilirubinemia, and polycythemia.

Nursing Management

Although this infant may have problems secondary to a traumatic birth, the major concern is with the stability of the blood glucose level. Emphasis on the care is treating for hypoglycemia and maintaining fluid and electrolyte balance. Follow the prior protocols for hypoglycemia and hyperglycemia treatment.

Other symptoms include jitteriness, extreme hunger (sucking vigorously on hands and fingers), diaphoresis, cyanosis, tachypnea, lethargy, seizures, and apnea. Serum glucose levels must be monitored frequently until they are stable at 80 to 120 mg/dl. After delivery, the glucose level must be monitored at least every hour until it has stabilized. Hypoglycemia is glucose levels less than 30 mg/dl for the term infant, less than 20 mg/dl for the preterm infant, and less than 40 mg/dl for any infant who is showing signs and symptoms of hypoglycemia. If the infant's condition is stable, early feedings should be given. IV fluids of 10% dextrose in water at 6 to 8 mg/kg/min should be started for the infant unable to take oral feedings. If the glucose levels remain low, administering an IV bolus of dextrose may be necessary with a concentration no greater than $D_{10}W$. Administration of more concentrated dextrose solutions may cause rebound hypoglycemia. Failure to achieve stable glucose levels may require pharmacologic and/or surgical intervention.

Diazoxide has become a first-line drug for treatment of hyperinsulinemia. The drug inhibits secretion of insulin and promotes mobilization of glycogen stores. Diazoxide has met with high clinical success with stabilization of serum glucose levels achieved within 24 to 48 hours. Dosage is started at 10 to 15 mg/kg/day in two or three divided doses and then titrated to achieve the desired serum level of glucose (Gamblian et al., 2003).

The infant should be monitored for any signs of birth trauma, such as brachial plexus damage or a fractured clavicle, especially in the macrosomic infant. A spun hematocrit should be carried out to assess

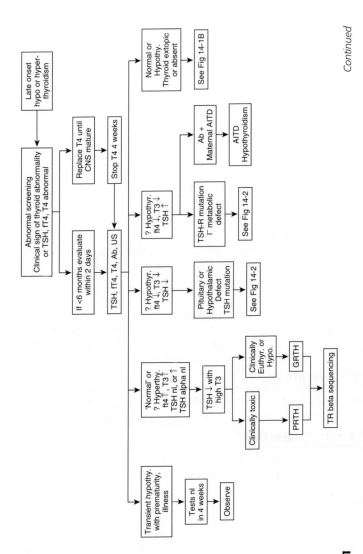

Continued

FIGURE **14-1**

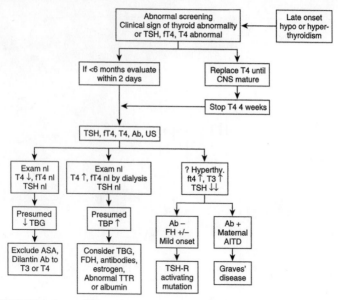

FIGURE **14-1, cont'd**

Neonatal thyroid dysfunction. (From www.thyroidmanager.org © Endocrine Education, Inc.)

for polycythemia. A partial exchange transfusion may need to be performed for a central hematocrit greater than 65%. The infant may need to be given phototherapy for treatment of hyperbilirubinemia (Gamblian et al., 2003).

HYPOTHYROIDISM

Figure 14-1 illustrates neonatal thyroid dysfunction, and Figure 14-2 shows congenital hypothyroidism.

AMBIGUOUS GENITALS

Ambiguous genitals are usually the result of an endocrine problem. The most common cause is congenital adrenal hyperplasia (CAH).

Clinical Manifestations

Salt wasting occurs and creates high urinary sodium levels. Serum sodium levels drop while serum potassium levels rise. Because of the effect on the renin-angiotensin cycle the blood pressure drops and the infant experiences hyponatremic shock.

Diagnosis

A comprehensive diagnostic evaluation involves three areas of testing: (1) measurement of the circulating hormones, (2) analysis of the

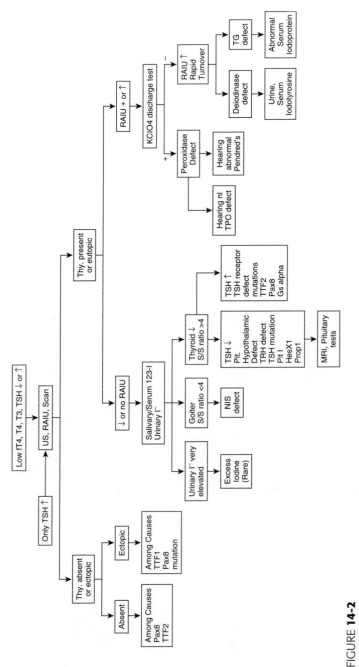

FIGURE **14-2**
Congenital hypothyroidism. (From www.thyroidmanager.org © Endocrine Education, Inc.)

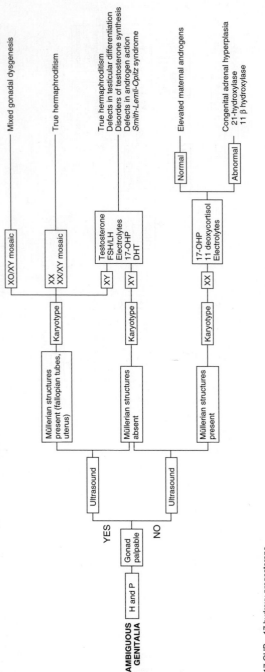

17-OHP = 17 hydroxy progesterone
DHT = Dihydrotestosterone

FIGURE 14-3

Nursing assessment includes taking a thorough history or reviewing one on the chart and conducting a physical examination (head to toe as can be tolerated). If you are a nurse practitioner you may order the tests listed; otherwise, you may wish to make sure these tests are ordered. Follow the results so that you may help the family to understand what is being done. (From Pomeranz AJ, et al., editors [2002]. *Pediatric decision-making strategies to accompany Nelson textbook of pediatrics*, ed 16, Philadelphia: WB Saunders, p. 273.)

chromosomes, and (3) visualization of the internal organs (Gamblian et al., 2003).

Nursing Management

Treatment involves replacing deficient cortisol with hydrocortisone or a similar synthetic substitute, such as dexamethasone. In addition, mineralocorticoid replacement is necessary in the salt-wasting form. The goal of hormone replacement therapy is to prevent adrenal crisis, achieve normal growth and development, and suppress excessive androgen production. Supplemental medication must be taken for the duration of the patient's life. Surgical repair of ambiguous genitals may also be indicated (Gamblian et al., 2003). Figure 14-3 illustrates the nursing assessment process.

BIBLIOGRAPHY

De Zegher F, et al. (2002). High-dose growth hormone (GH) treatment in non-GH-deficient children born small for gestational age induces growth responses related to pretreatment GH secretions and associated with a reversible decrease in insulin sensitivity. *Journal of clinical endocrinology & metabolism*, 87(1), 148-151.

Gamblian V, Weiland J, Parks N (2003). Assessment and management of the endocrine system. In Kenner C, Lott JW, editors. *Comprehensive neonatal nursing: a physiologic perspective*, ed 3, St Louis: WB Saunders.

Larsson A (2001). Neonatal screening for metabolic, endocrine, infectious, and genetic disorders: current and future directions. *Clinics in perinatology*, 28(2), 449-461.

Leger J, et al. (2002). Thyroid developmental anomalies in first degree relatives of children with congenital hypothyroidism. *Journal of clinical endocrinology & metabolism*, 87(2), 575-580.

Woelfle J, et al. (2002). Complete virilization in congenital adrenal hyperplasia: clinical course, medical management and disease-related complications. *Clinics in endocrinology (Oxf)*, 56(2), 231-238.

CHAPTER 15

HEMATOLOGIC CARE

Hematology encompasses immunologic factors as well as blood products that contribute to coagulation. Since neonatal infection and immune function are so important to neonatal nursing care, these topics can be found in Chapter 9, Neonatal Infections. The focus of this chapter is on coagulation problems and on hyperbilirubinemia.

NURSING ASSESSMENT

The first step in the nursing assessment is a thorough history of the maternal perinatal period. This history may give indications of risk factors for coagulopathy problems. A history of intrauterine infection; a positive family history of bleeding disorders, especially hemophilia; a traumatic birth that lends itself to hyperbilirubinemia; and maternal cancer are some of the *"red flags"* for hematologic problems in the newborn.

CLINICAL MANIFESTATIONS

- Lethargy
- Poor feeding
- Excessive bruising
- Blueberry muffin rash or petechiae
- Mottling or pale pink color
- Oozing around umbilical cord
- Apnea and/or bradycardia
- Tachypnea and/or tachycardia
- Anemia

DIAGNOSIS

Laboratory tests help with the diagnosis of these problems. These include prothrombin time (PT); partial thromboplastin time (PTT); complete blood count (CBC) with differential; platelet count, fibrinogen and fibrin degradation products, and microscopic examination of the blood itself. Specific assays may be run to determine discrete factors in the coagulation cascade that may be altered.

NURSING MANAGEMENT

Nursing management is aimed at prevention of further bleeding, protection against infection, and close monitoring of serum chemistry levels (Tables 15-1 to 15-4).

Table 15-1   Effect of Gestational Age of Fetuses in Utero and Newborn Infants on Their Hematocrit, Hemoglobin, Mean Corpuscular Volume, and Reticulocytes

Gestational Age (wk)	Hematocrit (%)*	Hemoglobin (g/dl)	MCV (fL)	Reticulocytes (%)
18-20†	36 ± 3	11.5 ± 0.8	134 ± 9	NR
21-22†	38 ± 3	12.3 ± 0.9	130 ± 6	NR
22-23†	38 ± 1	12.4 ± 0.2	125 ± 1	NR
24-25	63 ± 4	19.4 ± 1.5	135 ± 0	6.0 ± 0.5
26-27	62 ± 8	19.0 ± 2.5	132 ± 14	9.6 ± 3.2
28-29	60 ± 7	19.3 ± 1.8	131 ± 14	7.5 ± 2.5
30-31	60 ± 8	19.1 ± 2.2	127 ± 13	5.8 ± 2.0
32-33	60 ± 8	18.5 ± 2.0	123 ± 16	5.0 ± 1.9
34-35	61 ± 7	19.6 ± 2.1	122 ± 10	3.9 ± 1.6
36-37	64 ± 7	19.2 ± 1.7	121 ± 12	4.2 ± 1.8
Term	61 ± 7	19.3 ± 2.2	119 ± 9	32. ±1.4

From Christensen RD (2000). *Expected hematologic values for term and preterm neonates. In Christensen RD, editor: Hematologic problems of the neonate, Philadelphia: WB Saunders, p. 120. Data from Zaizov R, Matoth R (1976). Red cell values on the first postnatal day during the last 16 weeks of gestation. American journal of hematology, 1, 275; Forestier F, et al. (1986). Hematologic values of 163 normal fetuses between 18 and 30 weeks of gestation. Pediatric research, 20, 342; McIntosh N, Kempson C, Tyler RM (1988). Blood counts in extremely low birth weight infants. Archives of disease in children, 63, 74.*

MCV, Mean corpuscular volume; NR, not reported.
*Values reported as the mean ± SD (standard deviation).
†Fetuses in utero.

Table 15-2	Mean Erythrocyte Values over the First Weeks of Life in Healthy Term Infants				
Test	**Cord Blood**	**Day 1**	**Day 3**	**Day 7**	**Day 14**
Hemoglobin (g/dl)	16.8	18.4	17.8	17.0	16.8
Hematocrit (%)	53	58	55	54	52
Red blood cells ($10^6/\mu L$)	5.2	5.8	5.6	5.2	5.1
MCV (fL)	108	108	99	98	96
MCH (pg)	34	35	33	33	32
MCHC (g/d)	31.7	32.5	33.0	33.0	33.0
Reticulocytes (per μL)	300,000	300,000	50,000	0	0
Nucleated RBCs (per μL)	500	200	0	0	0

From Christensen RD (2000). Expected hematologic values for term and preterm neonates. In Christensen RD, editor. Hematologic problems of the neonate, Philadelphia: WB Saunders, p. 122.
MCV, Mean corpuscular volume; MCH, mean corpuscular hemoglobin; MCHC, mean corpuscular hemoglobin concentration; RBCs, red blood cells.

Table 15-3 Normal Platelet Values for Term and Preterm Neonates

Neonate	Platelets (per µL)*	MPV (fL)	Reticulated Plt (%)	Circulating Platelet Progenitors		
				BFU-MK (per 10^3 circulating mononuclear cells)	CFU-MK (per 10^3 circulating mononuclear cells)	Megakaryocytes (per 10^3 circulating mononuclear cells)
Term infant	310,000 ± 68,000	8.7 ± 1.0	4.0 ± 2.4	663 ± 174	3267 ± 530	37 ± 8
LBW infant	290,000 ± 70,000	8.9 ± 1.1	4.6 ± 1.7		NR	
VLBW infant	275,000 ± 60,000	NR	8.8 ± 5.1		NR	

From Christensen RD (2000). *Expected hematologic values for term and preterm neonates. In Christensen RD, editor. Hematologic problems of the neonate. Philadelphia: WB Saunders, p. 132. Modified from Hathaway WE, Bonnar J (1978). Perinatal coagulation, New York: Grune & Stratton; Arad ID, et al. (1986). The mean platelet volume in the neonatal period. American journal of perinatology, 3, 1; Murray NA, Roberts IA (1995). Circulating megakaryocytes and their progenitors (BFU-MK and CFU-MK) in term and preterm neonates. British journal of haematology, 89, 41; Murray NA, Roberts IA (1996). Circulating megakaryocytes and their progenitors in early thrombocytopenia in preterm neonates. Pediatric research, 40, 112; Peterec SM, et al. (1996). Reticulated platelet values in normal and thrombocytopenic neonates. Journal of pediatrics, 129, 269.*

MPV, Mean platelet volume in femtoliters (1 fL = 10^{-15}L); plt, platelets; BFU-MK, burst-forming unit–megakaryocyte; CFU-MK, colony-forming unit–megakaryocyte; LBW, low birth weight (<2500 g); NR, not reported; VLBW, very low birth weight (<1500 g).
All values are reported as the mean ± SD (standard deviation).

Table 15-4 Expected Hemoglobin Values (g/dl)* in Low–Birth Weight Infants

Birth Weight (g)	>Age (wk)				
	2	4	6	8	10
800-1000	16.0 (14.8-17.2)	10.0 (6.8-13.2)	8.7 (7.0-10.2)	8.0 (7.1-9.8)	8.0 (6.9-10.2)
1001-1200	16.4 (14.1-18.7)	12.8 (7.8-15.3)	10.5 (7.2-12.3)	9.1 (7.8-10.4)	8.5 (7.0-10.0)
1201-1400	16.2 (13.5-18.0)	13.4 (8.8-16.2)	10.9 (8.5-13.3)	9.9 (8.0-11.8)	9.8 (8.4-11.3)
1401-1500	15.6 (13.5-17.8)	11.7 (9.7-13.7)	10.5 (9.1-11.9)	9.8 (8.4-12.0)	9.9 (8.4-11.4)
1501-2000	15.6 (13.5-17.7)	11.0 (9.6-14.0)	9.6 (8.8-11.5)	9.8 (8.4-12.1)	10.1 (8.6-11.8)

From Ohls RK (2000). Evaluation and treatment of anemia in the neonate. In Christensen RD, editor. Hematologic problems of the neonate, Philadelphia: WB Saunders, p. 138. From Stockman JA, Oski FA (1980). Red blood cell values in low birth weight infants during the first seven weeks of life. American journal of disease in children, 134, 945.
*Range given in parentheses.

ANEMIA IN THE NEONATE

Anemia in the neonate can occur for a variety of reasons. It may be physiologic immaturity; caused by increased hemolysis; or secondary to iatrogenic causes, such as excessive blood draws.

Nursing Assessment

The cornerstone of the nursing assessment is the evaluation of risk factors that lead to anemia. Physical examination followed by laboratory tests will help shape a care plan.

Clinical Manifestations

Tables 15-5 and 15-6 differentiate hematologic clinical signs in the newborn.

Diagnosis

The diagnosis is based on the history and laboratory values.

Causes of Hemolysis in the Newborn Period*

1. Immune mediated
   a. Rh incompatibility (anti-D antibody)
   b. ABO incompatibility
   c. Minor blood group incompatibility: c, C, e, G, Fgya, (Duffy), Kell group, jKa, MNS, Vw
   d. Drug induced (penicillin, alpha-methyldopa, cephalothin)
   e. Maternal autoimmune hemolytic anemia
2. Infection
   a. Bacterial sepsis (*Escherichia coli*, group B *Streptococcus*)
   b. Parvovirus B19 (can present with hydrops fetalis)
   c. Congenital syphilis
   d. Congenital malaria
   e. Congenital TORCH infections (toxoplasmosis, other agents, rubella, cytomegalovirus, disseminated herpes)
   f. Other congenital viral infections
3. Disseminated intravascular coagulation (DIC)
4. Hereditary erythrocyte membrane disorders
   a. Spherocytosis
   b. Elliptocytosis
   c. Stomatocytosis
   d. Pyropoikilocytosis
   e. Other membrane disorders

---

*From Ohls RK (2000). *Evaluation and treatment of anemia in the neonate.* In Christensen RD, editor. *Hematologic problems of the neonate,* Philadelphia: WB Saunders, p. 147.

Table 15-5	Differentiation of Acute from Chronic Blood Loss in the Newborn	
Characteristic	**Acute Blood Loss**	**Chronic Blood Loss**
General appearance	Pale, hyper alert, "stunned" gaze	Pale, normal neurologic examination
Cardiovascular system	Tachycardic, weak pulses, low blood pressure	Normal; rarely may have congestive heart failure with hepatomegaly; normal or increased blood pressure
Respiratory system	Tachypneic, no supplemental oxygen requirement	Normal; rarely may be tachypneic with a supplemental oxygen requirement if congestive heart failure is present
Hematologic system Hemoglobin	May be normal; drops over 24 hr	Low at birth
Morphology	Macrocytic normochromic (normal)	Microcytic hypochromic
Iron	Normal	Low
Course	Promptly treat hypovolemia; may need rapid volume expansion to prevent shock, DIC, and death	Usually uneventful hospital course; may need treatment for congestive heart failure and hydrops
Treatment	Volume expansion with isotonic fluid and PRBCs, FFP, and platelets; iron therapy later; EPO therapy may be appropriate to enhance erythropoiesis	Initiate iron therapy; PRBC transfusion rarely needed; EOP therapy may be appropriate to enhance erythropoiesis

From Ohls RK (2000). *Evaluation and treatment of anemia in the neonate*.
In Christensen RD, editor. *Hematologic problems of the neonate*,
Philadelphia: WB Saunders, p. 146.
DIC, *Disseminated intravascular coagulation*; PRBCs, *packed red blood cells*; FFP, *fresh frozen plasma*; EPO, *erythropoietin*.

Table 15-6   Differentiation of Asphyxia, Hemorrhage, and Hemolysis in a Pale Newborn Infant

Affected Organ System	Asphyxia	Severe Acute Hemorrhage	Hemolysis
Neurologic	Abnormal transition period; hypotonic, decreased arousal state; seizures in first day of life	Normal or hyperalert or hyperirritable ("catecholamine response")	Normal
Respiratory	Respiratory distress, oxygen requirements	Tachypnea; no oxygen requirement	Normal (respiratory distress with hydrops)
Cardiovascular	Normal to bradycardia	Tachycardia; hypotension	May vary from normal to presence of congestive heart failure and hydrops, depending on degree of anemia
Hematologic	Hematocrit and hemoglobin levels remain stable over time; may develop thrombocytopenia and disseminated intravascular coagulation from hypoxic injury to marrow	Drop in hematocrit or hemoglobin level	Anemic from birth; hepatosplenomegaly; jaundice; positive Coombs' test

From Ohls RK (2000). Evaluation and treatment of anemia in the neonate. In Christensen RD, editor. Hematologic problems of the neonate, Philadelphia: WB Saunders, p. 141.

5. Congenital erythrocyte enzyme defects
   a. Glucose-6-phosphate dehydrogenase (G6PD) deficiency
   b. Pyruvate kinase (PK) deficiency
   c. Hexokinase deficiency
   d. Glucose phosphate isomerase deficiency
   e. Pyrimidine-5'-nucleotidase deficiency
6. Hemoglobin defects
   a. Alpha-thalassemia syndrome
   b. Gamma-thalassemia syndromes
   c. Alpha- and gamma-chain structural anomalies
7. Macroangiopathic and microangiopathic hemolysis
   a. Cavernous hemangiomas
   b. Arteriovenous malformations
   c. Renal artery stenosis or thrombosis
   d. Other large vessel thrombi
   e. Severe coarctation of the aorta
   f. Severe valvular stenoses
8. Other causes
   a. Galactosemia
   b. Lysosomal storage diseases
   c. Prolonged metabolic acidosis from metabolic disease (amino acid and organic acid disorders)
   d. Transfusion reactions
   e. TAR syndrome (thrombocytopenia with absent radii)
   f. Drug-induced hemolysis (valproic acid)

Nursing Management
Treatment is aimed at correcting the anemia. In many instances this requires blood transfusions (Table 15-7 and Box 15-1).

POLYCYTHEMIA

Polycythemia, or an increased number of red blood cells (RBCs), can occur secondary to many disorders. Most are due to perinatal hypoxemia, congenital adrenal hyperplasia, small for gestational age, intrauterine growth restriction, maternal diabetes, chromosomal abnormalities, delayed cord clamping, twin-to-twin transfusion, and dehydration.

Nursing Assessment
The nursing assessment is based on physical examination, maternal and neonatal history, and laboratory values.

Table 15-7	Transfusion Guidelines for Preterm Infants	
Hematocrit/ Hemoglobin*	**Ventilator Requirement and/or Symptoms**	**Transfusion Volume**
HCT ≤35; Hgb ≤11	Infants requiring moderate or significant mechanical ventilation (MAP >8 cm; H_2O; and FiO_2 >40%)	PRBCs, 15 ml/kg over 2-4 hr
HCT ≤30; Hgb ≤10	Infants requiring minimal mechanical ventilation (any mechanical ventilation, or CPAP >6 cm H_2O; and FiO_2 ≤40%)	PRBCs, 15 ml/kg over 2-4 hr
HCT ≤25; Hgb ≤8	Infants receiving supplemental oxygen who do not require mechanical ventilation and one or more of the following is present: • ≤24 hr of tachycardia (HR >180) or tachypnea (RR >80) • An increased oxygen requirement from the previous 48 hr, defined as less than or equal to fourfold increase in nasal cannula flow (i.e., ¼ L/min to 1 L/min) or an increase in nasal CPAP ≤20% from the previous 48 hr (i.e., 10-12 cm H_2O) • An elevated lactated concentration (≤2.5 mEq/L) • Weight gain <10 g/kg/day over the previous 4 days ≤100 kcal/kg/day	PRBCs, 20 ml/kg over 2-4 hr (divided into two 10 ml/kg volumes if fluid sensitive)

Continued

Table 15-7	Transfusion Guidelines for Preterm Infants—cont'd	
Hematocrit/ Hemoglobin*	Ventilator Requirement and/or Symptoms	Transfusion Volume
	• An increase in the episodes of apnea and bradycardia (>9 episodes in 24 hr or ≤2 episodes in 24 hr requiring bag and mask ventilation) while receiving therapeutic doses of methylxanthines • Undergoing surgery	
HCT ≤20; Hgb ≤7	Infant without any symptoms and an absolute reticulocyte count <100,000 cells/μL (RBCs × % uncorrected reticulocyte count)	PRBCs, 20 ml/kg over 2-4 hr (divided into two 10 ml/kg volumes if fluid sensitive)

From Ohls RK (2000). Evaluation and treatment of anemia in the neonate. In Christensen RD, editor. Hematologic problems of the neonate, Philadelphia: WB Saunders, p. 161.

HCT, Hematocrit; Hgb, hemoglobin; MAP, mean airway pressure; FiO₂, fractional inspired oxygen; PRBCs, packed red blood cells; CPAP, continuous positive airway pressure; HR, heart rate; RR, respiratory rate; RBCs, red blood cells.

*Hematocrit values are percentages; hemoglobin values are given in grams per deciliter.

Clinical Manifestations, Diagnosis and Laboratory Abnormalities of Neonatal Polycythemia*
Clinical symptoms
• Weak suck (i.e., feeding difficulties)
• Plethora
• Lethargy

---

*From Lindemann R, Haga P (2000). Evaluation and treatment of polycythemia in the neonate. In Christensen RD, editor. Hematologic problems of the neonate, Philadelphia: WB Saunders, p. 178.

Box **15-1**

Guidelines for Neonatal Blood Component Transfusion

Red Blood Cells
Hemoglobin <130 g/L (HCT <40%) with severe* cardiopulmonary disease
Hemoglobin <100 g/L (HCT <30%) with moderate cardiopulmonary disease
Hemoglobin <100 g/L (HCT <30%) with major surgery
Hemoglobin <80 g/L (HCT <24%) with symptomatic anemia
Bleeding with >25% loss of circulating blood volume

Platelets
Platelets <100 × 10^9/L and bleeding
Platelets <50 × 10^9/L and invasive procedure
Platelets <20 × 10^9/L and no bleeding but clinically stable
Platelets <1000 × 10^9/L and no bleeding but clinically unstable

Fresh Frozen Plasma
Severe clotting factor deficiency with bleeding
Severe clotting factor deficiency and invasive procedure
Vitamin K deficiency with bleeding
Dilutional coagulopathy with bleeding
Severe anticoagulant protein deficiency

Neutrophils
Neutrophils <3 × 10^9/L and fulminant sepsis during first week of life
Neutrophils <1 × 10^9/L and fulminant sepsis after first week

From Strauss RG (2000). Blood banking and transfusion issues in perinatal medicine [supported in part by NIH Program Project Grant P01 HL46925]. In Christensen RD, editor. Hematologic problems of the neonate, Philadelphia: WB Saunders, p. 407.
HCT, Hematocrit.

- Rubeosis-like cyanosis
- Tachypnea (i.e., respiratory distress)
- Jitteriness or tremulousness
- Difficult to arouse
- Irritable when aroused
- Hypotonia
- Easily startled

- Myoclonic jerks
- Vomiting
- Cardiomegaly (heart murmur)
- Hepatomegaly
- Jaundice

Laboratory abnormalities
- Hypoglycemia
- Hypocalcemia
- Thrombocytopenia

Nursing Management

Management is aimed at reducing the viscosity of the blood to about 60% hematocrit. Usual treatment includes partial exchange transfusion during which plasma, albumin, or other products may be used, and increased fluid volume.

COAGULOPATHY PROBLEMS IN THE NEONATE

Tables 15-8 and 15-9 cover coagulopathy problems in the newborn, and Table 15-10 gives normal values for coagulation screening tests. Figure 15-1 illustrates an overview of the coagulation proteins.

Disseminated Intravascular Coagulation

One of the most serious conditions in the newborn that involves bleeding is disseminated intravascular coagulation (DIC). This condition is usually secondary to neonatal sepsis, an immune reaction, purpura, or liver disease. Ironically this condition results in microsized blood clots that disseminate or circulate throughout the body in the vascular space. The bleeding is due to the system's loss of clotting factors and platelets.

Nursing assessment The assessment starts with the history that indicates sepsis or a maternal history of abruptio placentae or severe trauma that may have resulted in an antibody reaction and bleeding on the part of the mother.

Clinical manifestations Clinical signs include pale color, bruising, petechiae, bleeding or oozing from intravenous (IV) or heel sticks, apnea/bradycardia or tachypnea/tachycardia, hypotension, and decreasing arterial oxygen saturations.

Diagnosis The diagnosis is confirmed based on the history and on thrombocytopenia, increased PT and PTT times, decreased fibrinogen and increased fibrin split products, and blood smears that show red cell fragments.

Table 15-8   Conditions Associated with Bleeding and Thrombocytopenia

Diagnosis	Appearance	Prothrombin Time	Partial Thromboplastin Time	Other Useful Tests
Disseminated intravascular coagulation	Sick	Increased	Increased	Fibrinogen; fibrin degradation products
TORCH (toxoplasmosis, other agents, rubella, cytomegalovirus, herpes simplex)	Sick	Normal or increased	Normal or increased	Liver function tests; fibrinogen; fibrin degradation products
Leukemia	Sick	Normal	Normal	Bone marrow
Maternal immune thrombocytopenic purpura	Well	Normal	Normal	Maternal platelet count
Alloimmune thrombocytopenia	Well	Normal	Normal	Maternal platelet count and platelet antigen typing (PAI-1)
Giant hemangioma	Well	Normal or increased	Normal or increased	Fibrinogen; fibrin degradation products
Defective platelet production	Well	Normal	Normal	Bone marrow examination

From Clapp DW, Shannon KM, Phibbs RH (2001). In Klaus MH, Fanaroff AA, editors. Care of the high-risk neonate, ed 5, Philadelphia: WB Saunders, p. 449.

Table 15-9 Conditions Associated with Bleeding and Normal Platelet Count

Diagnosis	Appearance	Prothrombin Time	Partial Thromboplastin Time	Other Useful Tests
Hemorrhagic disease of the newborn (vitamin K deficiency)	Well	Increased	Increased	Fibrinogen; fibrin degradation products
Hepatic disease	Sick	Increased	Increased	Albumin; fibrinogen; fibrin degradation products; liver function tests
von Willebrand's disease*	Well	Normal	Normal or increased	Bleeding time
Hemophilia	Well	Normal	Increased	Mixing tests; factor VIII and IX assays
Factor XIII deficiency	Well	Normal	Normal	Urea clot solubility
Afibrinogenemia	Well	Increased	Increased	Fibrinogen; fibrin degradation products; thrombin time
Disorders of platelet function*	Well	Normal	Normal	Bleeding time; platelet aggregometry

From Clapp DW, Shannon KM, Phibbs RH (2001). In Klaus MH, Fanaroff AA, editors. Care of the high-risk neonate, ed 5, Philadelphia: WB Saunders, p. 454.
*Some patients with these disorders show mild to moderate thrombocytopenia.

Table 15-10	Normal Values for Coagulation Screening Tests		
Test	Older Child	Full-Term Newborn	Healthy Growing Premature Infant
Platelets (per mm³)	150,000-410,000	150,000-400,000	150,000-400,000
Prothrombin time(s)	10-14	11-15	11-16
Partial thromboplastin time(s)	25-35	30-40	35-80
Fibrinogen (mg/dl)	175-400	165-400	150-325
Fibrin degradation products (μg/ml)	<10	<10	<10

From Buchanan GR (1987). Neonatal hemorrhagic diseases. In Nathan DG, Oski FA, editors. Hematology of infancy and childhood, ed 3, Philadelphia: WB Saunders. As cited in Clapp DW, Shannon KM, Phibbs RH (2001). In Klaus MH, Fanaroff AA, editors. Care of the high-risk neonate, ed 5, Philadelphia: WB Saunders, p. 448.

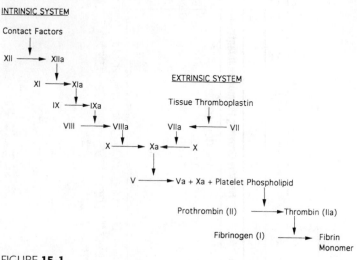

FIGURE **15-1**
Overview of the coagulant proteins of the intrinsic system (*upper left*) and extrinsic system (*upper right*), which both feed into the common pathway (*bottom*). (From Clapp DW, Shannon KM, Phibbs RH [2001]. Hematologic problems. In Klaus MH, Fanaroff AA, editors. *Care of the high-risk neonate*, ed 5, Philadelphia: WB Saunders, p. 448.)

Nursing management The first line of treatment is aimed at the causative agent. If it is infection, then treatment with appropriate antimicrobial therapy is in order. The next step is the replacement of platelets and clotting factors to restore normal levels. Cryoprecipitate is used along with fresh frozen plasma and platelets. The platelet count, PT, and PTT are checked every 4 to 6 hours until the infant is stable. Anticoagulant therapy is only used as a last resort.

HYPERBILIRUBINEMIA

Hyperbilirubinemia is defined as elevated bilirubin levels. If these occur within the first 24 hours of life or if levels exceed 12 mg/dl, they are not considered physiologic and deserve investigation. Many conditions other than blood group incompatibilities can cause jaundice in the newborn. The majority of commonly seen problems result in elevated unconjugated rather than conjugated bilirubin levels. These pathologic conditions can be classified as (1) problems causing increased RBC breakdown, such as sepsis, drug reactions, and extravascular blood; (2) problems that interfere with bilirubin conjugation, such as breast milk, jaundice, drug interactions, hypothyroidism, hypoxia, and asphyxia; or (3) problems causing abnormal bilirubin excretion, such as bowel obstruction. The single factor most implicated in hyperbilirubinemia is prematurity, with the severity of jaundice directly correlated to decreasing gestational age. The premature infant is theorized to be subject to a combination of increased RBC breakdown secondary to decreased RBC life span and impaired bilirubin conjugation because of liver immaturity (Shaw, 2003).

Risk Factors
- Prematurity
- Sepsis
- ABO incompatibility
- Rh incompatibility
- Certain medications, such as synthetic analogues of vitamin K or large doses of natural vitamin K
- Accumulation of blood, as seen in cephalohematoma
- Hepatic metabolic disease
- Complication of total parenteral nutrition
- Physiologic adaptation to extrauterine life (after 24 hours of age and before the end of the first week of life)

Diseases That May be Seen as Conjugated Hyperbilirubinemia in Neonatal Period
1. Hepatocellular disturbances in bilirubin excretion
   a. Primary hepatitis
      (1) Neonatal idiopathic hepatitis (giant cell hepatitis)
      (2) Hepatitis caused by identified infectious agents
         (a) Hepatitis B
         (b) Rubella
         (c) Cytomegalovirus
         (d) *Toxoplasma* organisms
         (e) Coxsackievirus
         (f) Echovirus 14 and 19
         (g) Herpes simplex and varicella zoster
         (h) Syphilis
         (i) *Listeria* organisms
         (j) Tubercle bacillus
   b. "Toxic hepatitis"
      (1) Systemic infectious diseases
         (a) *Escherichia coli* (sepsis or urinary tract)
         (b) Pneumococci
         (c) *Proteus* organisms
         (d) *Salmonella* organisms
         (e) Idiopathic diarrhea
      (2) Intestinal obstruction
      (3) Parenteral alimentation
      (4) Ischemic necrosis
   c. Hematologic disorders
      (1) Erythroblastosis fetalis (severe forms)
      (2) Congenital erythropoietic porphyria

    d. Metabolic disorders
        (1) Alpha$_1$-antitrypsin deficiency
        (2) Galactosemia
        (3) Tyrosinemia
        (4) Fructosemia
        (5) Glycogen storage disease type IV
        (6) Lipid storage diseases
           (a) Niemann-Pick disease
           (b) Gaucher's disease
           (c) Wolman's disease
        (7) Cerebrohepatorenal syndrome (Zellweger syndrome)
        (8) Trisomy 18
        (9) Cystic fibrosis
        (10) Familial idiopathic cholestasis: Byler's disease
        (11) Hemochromatosis
        (12) Idiopathic hypopituitarism
2. Ductal disturbances in bilirubin excretion
    a. Extrahepatic biliary atresia
        (1) Isolated
        (2) Trisomy 18
        (3) Polysplenia-heterotaxia syndrome
    b. Intrahepatic biliary atresia (nonsyndromatic paucity of bile ducts)
    c. Alagille syndrome (arteriohepatic dysplasia)
    d. Intrahepatic atresia associated with lymphedema
    e. Extrahepatic stenosis and choledochal cyst
    f. Bile plug syndrome
    g. Cystic disease
    h. Tumors of the liver and biliary tract
    i. Periductal lymphadenopathy

Signs and Symptoms
- Increasing jaundice of skin and/or sclera
- Increasing lethargy if allowed to continue
- Irritability

Laboratory Tests
The following laboratory tests are recommended for evaluation of neonatal conjugated hyperbilirubinemia*:
1. Liver function tests
    a. Total and direct-reacting serum bilirubin, total serum protein, and serum protein electrophoresis

---

*From Halamek LP, Stevenson DK (2002). Neonatal jaundice and liver disease. In Fanaroff AA, Martin RJ, editors. Neonatal-perinatal medicine: diseases of the fetus and infant, ed 7, St Louis: Mosby, pp. 1338-1340.

    b. Serum glutamic-oxaloacetic transaminase (SGOT; aspartate transaminase [AST]), serum glutamate pyruvate transaminase (SGPT; alanine transaminase [ALT]), alkaline phosphatase (5'-nucleotidase if alkaline phosphatase [elevated]), and gamma-glutamyl transpeptidase (GGTP)

    c. Cholesterol

    d. Serum and urine bile acid concentrations if available

    e. Alpha$_1$-antitrypsin

    f. Technetium-99m iminodiscetic acid (^{99m}Tc-IDA) scan

    g. Alpha-fetoprotein

2. Hematologic tests

    a. Complete blood count, smear, and reticulocyte count

    b. Direct Coombs' test and erythrocyte glucose-6-phosphate dehydrogenase

    c. Platelet count

    d. Prothrombin time and partial thromboplastin time

3. Tests for infectious disease

    a. Cord blood immunoglobulin M (IgM)

    b. Venereal Disease Research Laboratory (VDRL), fluorescent treponemal antibody absorption test, complement fixation titers for rubella, cytomegalovirus, and herpes virus, and Sabin-Feldman dye test titer for toxoplasmosis

    c. Hepatitis B surface antigen (HbsAg) in both infant and mother

    d. Viral cultures from nose, pharynx, blood, stool, urine, and cerebrospinal fluid

4. Urine tests

    a. Routine urinalysis, including protein and reducing substances

    b. Urine culture

    c. Bilirubin and urobilinogen

    d. Amino acid screening

5. Liver biopsy

    a. Light microscopy

    b. Specific enzyme assay (if indicated)

6. Radiologic/ultrasound studies as indicated

7. Additional specific diagnostic studies for metabolic disorders to be performed as indicated or suspected

    Table 15-11 gives guidelines for the management of hyperbilirubinemia in the healthy term newborn.

*Phototherapy**

Purpose

The purpose of phototherapy is to reduce the level of bilirubin in infants with hyperbilirubinemia.

---

*From Altimier L, Brown B, Tedeschi L (2000). Tri-Health's manual of neonatal nursing policies, procedures, competencies, & clinical pathways, Glenview, Ill: National Association of Neonatal Nurses.

| Table 15-11 | American Academy of Pediatrics Guidelines for Management of Hyperbilirubinemia in the Healthy Term Newborn |

Total Serum Bilirubin Level in mg/dl (mmol/L)

Age (hr)	Consider Photo- therapy	Phototherapy	Exchange Transfusion if Intensive* Photo- therapy Fails†	Exchange Transfusion and Intensive* Photo- therapy
25-48	≥12 (170)	≥15 (260)	≥20 (340)	≥25 (430)
49-72	≥15 (260)	≥18 (310)	≥25 (430)	≥30 (510)
>72	≥17 (290)	≥20 (340)	≥25 (430)	≥30 (510)

From Halamek LP, Stevenson DK (2002). Neonatal jaundice and liver disease. In Fanaroff AA, Martin RJ, editors. Neonatal-perinatal medicine: diseases of the fetus and infant, ed 7, St Louis: Mosby, p. 1335. From Provisional Committee for Quality Improvement and Subcommmittee on Hyperbilirubinemia, American Academy of Pediatrics (1994). Pediatrics 94, 558.

*Intensive phototherapy includes using more than one bank of lamps, employing units containing "special blue" lamps, maximizing the surface area illuminated by the use of a phototherapy blanket or other means, and delivery on a continuous, noninterrupted schedule.

†Intensive phototherapy failure is defined as (1) an inability to produce a decline of total serum bilirubin of 1 to 2 mg/dl within 4 to 6 hours after initiation or (2) subsequent failure to produce a steady decrease in total serum bilirubin to levels remaining below the exchange transfusion threshold.

Equipment for spotlight/bank light phototherapy
- Phototherapy light
- Eye patches
- Phototherapy light meter

Equipment for fiberoptic phototherapy (bili blanket)
- Phototherapy system/illuminator
- Fiberoptic pad
- Disposable cover/vest
- Eye patches, when needed

General procedure
1. Phototherapy requires a physician's/certified nurse practitioner's (CNP's) order to initiate and discontinue treatment. The order should specify phototherapy per spotlight, phototherapy per bank

light, phototherapy per bili blanket, or a combination of both types of therapy.

2. Obtain serum bilirubin as ordered per physician/CNP before initiation of treatment and then total serum bilirubin levels as ordered.

3. Document initiation and discontinuance of phototherapy. Observe and record clinical signs of increase or decrease of jaundice in the notes. Document the removal of eye patches and skin integrity.

4. When a bilirubin level is being drawn, turn the phototherapy unit off.

5. Check with physician/CNP regarding removal from phototherapy for feeds and treatments.

6. While the infant is receiving phototherapy, the registered nurse (RN) should assess and document observations and interventions to prevent or alleviate the following possible complications of phototherapy:
   a. Increased insensible water loss leading to dehydration
   b. Loose stools
   c. Poor feeding
   d. Skin rash
   e. Ocular damage
   f. Hypothermia or hyperthermia

7. Bulbs will be changed by the Biomedical Engineering Department.

Procedure for overhead phototherapy

1. To begin treatment, place infant in Isolette/radiant warmer undressed with genitals covered. Monitor temperature at least every 3 to 4 hours.

2. Before turning on phototherapy light, cover infant's eyes securely with eye patches.
   a. Be sure lids are closed to prevent corneal scarring.
   b. Cleanse eyes daily at bath time.
   c. Remove eye patches for 5 to 10 minutes every 4 hours to observe for irritation or drainage.
   d. Remove eye patches for short periods during parent visitation to encourage bonding.

3. Change the infant's position every 2 to 4 hours to allow maximum skin exposure. On a large infant, two phototherapy lights may be necessary to allow maximum skin exposure.

4. Measure light intensity with phototherapy light meter at the initiation of treatment and as needed until treatment is discontinued. The minimum reading should be 6 to 8 $\mu W/cm^2/nm$ for spotlights and bank lights. The readings for blankets should be 18 to 20 $\mu W/cm^2/nm$ (minimum). Document light level on nursing assessment sheet.

Procedure for fiberoptic phototherapy (bili blanket)

1. Insert the fiberoptic pad into a new disposable cover or vest. The white side of the disposable vest goes over the clear illuminating side of the pad. Secure the cover or vest around the pad cable with the self-adhesive tabs.

2. Firmly place the fiberoptic cable connector into the illuminator port.

3. Lay the covered light pad on the mattress or other flat surface with the white illuminating side facing up. Place the infant's back or chest directly on the white side of the pad with the tip of the pad at the baby's shoulders and the pad's cable at the infant's feet.

4. Ensure the following:
   a. As much of the infant's skin is in direct contact with the lighted sections of the pad as possible—diapers may be worn.
   b. There is nothing between the infant's skin and the light pad other than the disposable cover—clothing may be worn over the pad, or the infant may be bundled in a blanket.

5. If the baby is positioned on his/her abdomen, the eye patches should be worn. If the baby is positioned supine or is dressed, and the eyes are not exposed to the light, then eye patches do not need to be worn. (Refer to procedure above for overhead phototherapy regarding eye care when patches are used.)

6. When using the vest, wrap the strap section snugly around the infant's mid-section to hold the pad in position, and secure it with the tape tabs. The vest should only be worn on term infants that are wrapped or being held by parents.

7. Set the brightness selector switch on the front panel to the high level. (High level is indicated by the largest dot.)

UNIVERSITY OF ILLINOIS MEDICAL CENTER AT CHICAGO CLINICAL CARE GUIDELINE

Subject: Care of an Infant Receiving Phototherapy*

Objective

To establish standards for the care of all newborn infants receiving phototherapy for the treatment of unconjugated hyperbilirubinemia.

Definitions

For the purpose of this guideline the following definitions apply:

Hyperbilirubinemia—An elevation of serum bilirubin in the newborn. Bilirubin may exist as either a conjugated or an unconjugated molecule. Excessive levels of unconjugated bilirubin may be toxic to the newborn.

*From University of Illinois Medical Center at Chicago Women's and Children's Nursing Services. Used with permission by Dharmapuri Vidyasagar, MD; Catherine Theorell, RNC, MSN, NNP; Beena Peters, RN, MS.

Phototherapy—Light therapy that provides energy to exposed skin in order to convert unconjugated bilirubin to a water-soluble form to enhance its excretion. The effectiveness of phototherapy depends on the area of exposed skin surface and the amount of luminescence from the light source. Phototherapy may be provided by overhead units or light-emitting blankets.

Irradiance—The amount of light energy emitted from the phototherapy unit.

Position Statements

The initiation and discontinuation of phototherapy require a written order by a physician.

The effectiveness of phototherapy energy (irradiance) shall be evaluated with a radiometer at the beginning of each shift.

The phototherapy unit shall be exchanged with another if the irradiance level is subtherapeutic.

The nurse shall ensure that blood specimens for bilirubin are drawn as ordered and results are reported to the physician.

Infants exposed to phototherapy light shall have their eyes shielded by opaque patches.

Procedures

1. The irradiance level of the phototherapy unit shall be checked when beginning therapy and at the start of every shift.
2. The irradiance levels of phototherapy lights shall be 4 uw/ca^2/nm.
3. The infant's eyes will be covered with a phototherapy mask while under phototherapy lights.
4. The infant's eyes will be assessed at least every 4 hours and cleaned with sterile water as needed.
5. Accurate intake and output will be maintained.
6. The infant will be weighed daily.
7. For infants being fed:
   a. Breast-feeding infants will be fed every 2 to 3 hours.
   b. Bottle-feeding infants will be fed every 3 to 4 hours.
8. The infant's temperature will be monitored at least every 4 hours.
9. Measures will be taken to maintain infant's temperature at 97.8° F or greater.
10. The infant will be repositioned at least every 4 hours to expose more of infant's skin surface to the light.
11. The infant will be undressed while under phototherapy lights.
12. The infant's gonads will be shielded with mask (for infants <1500 g) or diaper while under phototherapy.
13. Phototherapy may be interrupted for feedings and parental visits.
14. Parent(s) will be provided an explanation of hyperbilirubinemia and phototherapy.

15. The nurse will document the following in the medical record:
   a. Irradiance level measured and corrective action completed when levels are subtherapeutic
   b. Condition of infant's eyes and eye care provided
   c. Hydration status of infant and measures taken to ensure adequate fluid intake
   d. Temperature status and measures taken to ensure adequate temperature
   e. Frequency of repositioning
   f. Education provided to parent(s)
   g. Bilirubin levels, as ordered by physician

UNIVERSITY OF ILLINOIS MEDICAL CENTER AT CHICAGO CLINICAL CARE GUIDELINE

Subject: Exchange Transfusions in the Newborn*

Objectives

• To establish written guidelines for the performance of complete and partial exchange transfusions.
• To monitor and maintain hemodynamic homeostasis throughout the procedure.

Definitions

For the purpose of this guideline the following definitions apply:

Total or Complete Exchange Transfusion—A procedure that removes whole blood from an infant for the purpose of removal of toxic substances, such as bilirubin, and the simultaneous replacement of an equal volume of whole blood lacking the toxins.

Partial or Reduction Exchange Transfusion—An exchange transfusion that removes a volume of whole blood from an infant while replacing an equal volume of blood expander, such as saline. A partial exchange transfusion is performed on infants who are polycythemic experiencing symptoms of hyperviscosity.

Position Statements

University of Illinois Medical Center at Chicago recognizes that newborn infants may require therapeutic interventions, such as complete or reduction exchange transfusions, to remove toxins from blood, such as in hyperbilirubinemia, or to reduce the concentration of circulating red blood cells, such as in polycythemia.

These procedures require the insertion of vascular catheters under strict aseptic technique. Informed consent for the procedure and for

*From University of Illinois Medical Center at Chicago Women's and Children's Nursing Services. Used with permission by Dharmapuri Vidyasagar, MD; Catherine Theorell, RNC, MSN, NNP; Beena Peters, RN, MS.

the administration of blood should be obtained by the physician as needed.

The removal of whole blood and the volume of fluid that is replaced must be carefully monitored to avoid imbalances.

The hemodynamic status of infants undergoing such procedures must be carefully and continuously monitored. Pain should be assessed and managed through the administration of medication or nonpharmacologic comfort measures.

Preprocedural and postprocedural laboratory values are ordered to evaluate the efficacy of the therapeutic intervention.

Procedures

1. Preexchange activities
   a. Verify that the consent has been obtained for the procedure and for the administration of blood products as needed.
   b. The events of the exchange transfusion are monitored and recorded.
   c. The clinical status of the infant is continuously monitored and recorded during and after the procedure.
   d. All equipment is assembled and ready for the procedure:
      (1) Sterile gloves, gowns, and drapes; obtain surgical masks
      (2) Umbilical catheter insertion tray
      (3) Povidone-iodine solution
      (4) Exchange transfusion tray
      (5) Blood component, as ordered
      (6) Blood warmer
      (7) Two additional 5-cc syringes
      (8) Two lavender Vacutainers
      (9) Two Microtainers
      (10) Chemstrips
   e. Aseptic technique (including sterile gown, gloves, and mask) will be used during insertion of umbilical venous line and during procedure.
   f. Standard Precautions are utilized according to Infection Control and Isolation Procedure Manual.
   g. The infant may be restrained during insertion of umbilical venous line to prevent contamination of the sterile field.
2. Exchange activities
   a. The infant will be kept NPO (nothing by mouth) for 3 to 4 hours before the procedure, or the stomach contents will be aspirated with an NG (nasogastric) tube before the procedure.
   b. The infant will have a peripheral IV line infusing with appropriate solution as ordered by the physician.
   c. The infant will be continuously monitored for cardiorespiratory status throughout the procedure.

    d. The infant will be maintained in a radiant warmer throughout the procedure.

    e. The blood or blood component as ordered by the physician will be obtained and checked per medical center management policy.

    f. The amount required for a double-volume exchange is as follows:

        (1) Term—160 cc/kg

        (2) Preterm—200 cc/kg

    g. The temperature of the blood will be maintained at 98.6° F (37.0° C), not to exceed 100.4° F (38.0° C).

    h. The infant's vital signs including blood pressure will be monitored and recorded as follows:

        (1) Immediately before initiating procedure

        (2) Every 5 minutes for the first 15 minutes

        (3) Then every 15 minutes for the remainder of the procedure

    i. Preexchange lab work may include the following:

        (1) Electrolytes

        (2) Bilirubin

        (3) Serum glucose

        (4) Hematocrit/CBC

    j. The specimen for this lab work will be obtained from the first aliquot removed from the infant.

    k. Blood will be removed and replaced at aliquots of 5 ml/kg. The removal/infusion rates will not exceed 5 ml/kg/min.

    l. The donor blood bag will be gently massaged periodically throughout the procedure to prevent settling of the RBCs.

    m. Calcium gluconate may be administered by the physician at each 100 cc of whole blood replaced.

3. Postexchange activities

    a. When exchange is complete, obtain the blood specimens for the following:

        (1) Electrolytes

        (2) Bilirubin

        (3) CBC

        (4) Serum glucose

    b. Blood glucose will be monitored every hour for 2 hours after the exchange and then every 2 hours × 1.

    c. Vital signs including blood pressure will be monitored every 15 minutes for the first hour, then every 30 minutes for 1 hour, and then every hour for 2 hours. Preexchange schedule may be resumed, if the infant is stable.

    d. The infant will be assessed for signs of hypocalcemia.

    e. The umbilical venous line may be removed at the discretion of the physician.

    f. The discarded blood will be disposed of according to the biohazardous waste disposal guidelines in Environmental Health & Safety Standards Manual.

4. Documentation: the RN will document the following on the exchange transfusion record:
   a. The time the exchange began and ended
   b. Vital signs as required
   c. Time, volume of blood in and out and total volume exchanged
   d. Medications given, if appropriate

While in these protocols the orders are done by a physician, in many institutions these are done by neonatal nurse practitioners. Policies may vary slightly among institutions but the general guideline parameters remain the same. Figure 15-2 gives you a nursing assessment of jaundice in the newborn.

KERNICTERUS

Kernicterus is a serious complication of high bilirubin levels.

Differential Diagnosis

The diagnosis is based on history, age of the infant, and laboratory findings.

Treatment and Evaluation

Guidelines for the management of hyperbilirubinemia are based on the gestational age and relative health of the newborn (Table 15-12).

The Joint Commission on Accreditation of Healthcare Organizations (JCAHO) has been concerned about adverse newborn outcomes of kernicterus. The commission has done a root cause analysis and developed suggested recommendations for avoiding this condition (Box 15-2).

Table **15-12**	Total Serum Bilirubin Level (mg/dl)			
	Healthy		**Sick**	
Gestational Age/Birth Weight (g)	**Photo-therapy**	**Exchange Transfusion**	**Photo-therapy**	**Exchange Transfusion**
Premature				
<1000	5-7	Variable	4-6	Variable
1001-1500	7-10	Variable	6-8	Variable
1501-2000	10-12	Variable	8-10	Variable
2001-2500	12-15	Variable	10-12	Variable
Term				
>2500	15-18	20-25	12-15	18-20

From Halamek LP, Stevenson DK (2002). Neonatal jaundice and liver disease. In Fanaroff AA, Martin RJ, editors. Neonatal-perinatal medicine: diseases of the fetus and infant, ed 7, St Louis: Mosby, p. 1335.

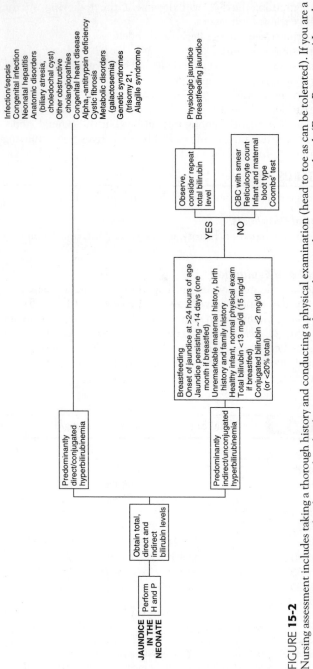

FIGURE 15-2

Nursing assessment includes taking a thorough history and conducting a physical examination (head to toe as can be tolerated). If you are a nurse practitioner you may order the tests listed; otherwise, you may wish to make sure these tests are ordered. (From Pomeranz AJ, et al., editors. [2002]. *Pediatric decision-making strategies to accompany Nelson textbook of pediatrics*, ed 16, Philadelphia: WB Saunders, p. 105.)

Box 15-2

Kernicterus

Root Causes Identified
Examination of the recent cases has identified a pattern of root causes related to four patient care processes:
1. Patient assessment
   a. The unreliability of the visual assessment of jaundice in newborns with dark skin
   b. Failure to recognize jaundice in an infant—or its severity—based on visual assessment, and measure a bilirubin level before the infant's discharge from the hospital or during a follow-up visit
   c. Failure to measure the bilirubin level in an infant who is jaundiced in the first 24 hours
2. Continuum of care
   a. Early discharge (before 48 hours) with no follow-up within 1 to 2 days of discharge. This is particularly important for infants less than 38 weeks of gestation.
   b. Failure to provide early follow-up with physical assessment for infants who are jaundiced before discharge
   c. Failure to provide ongoing lactation support to ensure adequacy of intake for breast-fed newborns
3. Patient and family education
   a. Failure to provide appropriate information to parents about jaundice and failure to respond appropriately to parental concerns about a jaundiced newborn, poor feeding, lactation difficulties, and change in newborn behavior and activity
4. Treatment
   a. Failure to recognize, address, or treat rapidly rising bilirubin
   b. Failure to aggressively treat severe hyperbilirubinemia in a timely manner with intensive phototherapy or exchange transfusion

Available Risk Reduction Strategies
AAP Practice Guidelines for Management of Hyperbilirubinemia in the Healthy Term Newborn, which are based on available data and expert consensus, provide guidelines for identifying at-risk newborns, their diagnosis, and their treatment. These guidelines include specific recommendations to evaluate all cases of jaundice appearing in the first 24 hours, appropriate assessment of maternal and infant blood types, and detailed treatment strategies for specific levels of bilirubin at different ages. Other strategies to consider include the following:
1. Predischarge bilirubin measurement with use of a percentile-based nomogram to predict the risk of hyperbilirubinemia in newborns and to guide follow-up.

Continued

Box 15-2

Kernicterus—cont'd

Available Risk Reduction Strategies—cont'd

2. Policies and procedures or standing orders allowing nurses to order TSB (total serum bilirubin) or TcB (transcutaneous bilirubin) tests for jaundiced newborns and to provide for proper documentation of bilirubin values and a report to the pediatrician.

3. Policies for assessing the risk of severe hyperbilirubinemia in all infants by history, clinical evaluation, and, if necessary, by laboratory measurement. (Because clinical assessment is imprecise, if there is any doubt about the presence or severity of jaundice, a serum or transcutaneous bilirubin measurement should be obtained.)

4. Procedures for follow-up of all newborns within 24 to 48 hours by a physician or pediatric nurse. *If this cannot be achieved*, decisions regarding timing of discharge or other follow-up must be based on risk assessment.

5. Policies and procedures on jaundice management that specifically cover the nurse's role, documentation, charting requirements, and monitoring of jaundice before discharge.

6. Provide parents with adequate educational materials about newborn infants that includes information about jaundice.

7. Provide adequate equipment—bilirubin lights and blankets, and noninvasive TcB measurement device or lab services for timely TSB test.

Recommendations

The Joint Commission recommends that organizations (1) take steps to raise awareness among neonatal caregivers of the potential for kernicterus and its risk factors; (2) review their current patient care processes with regard to the identification and management of hyperbilirubinemia in newborns; and (3) identify strategies from the above list of available risk reduction strategies that could enhance the effectiveness of these processes.

From JCAHO (2001). Kernicterus threatens healthy newborns, April, Issue 18, Chicago: JCAHO.

BIBLIOGRAPHY

Agrawal R, et al. (2001). Jaundice in the newborn. *Indian journal of pediatrics*, 68(10), 977-980.

Kohli-Kumar M (2001). Screening for anemia in children: AAP recommendations—a critique. *Pediatrics*, 108(3), E56.

Latini G, Rosati E, Del Vecchio A (2001). Low doses of recombinant erythropoietin in the treatment of anemia of prematurity. *Acta paediatrics*, 90(7), 825-826.

Mercer JS (2001). Current best evidence: a review of the literature on umbilical cord clamping. *Journal of midwifery & women's health*, 46(6), 402-414.

Ohls RK, et al. (2001). Effects of early erythropoietin therapy on the transfusion requirements of preterm infants below 1250 grams birth weight: a multicenter, randomized, controlled trial. *Pediatrics*, 108(4), 934-942.

Puckett RM, Offringa M (2002). Prophylactic vitamin K for vitamin K deficiency bleeding in neonates. *Cochrane review, the Cochrane Library*, 1, http://www.update-software.com/abstracts/ab002776.htm, retrieved February 24, 2002.

Shaw N (2003). Assessment and management of the hematologic system. In Kenner C, Lott JW, editors. *Comprehensive neonatal nursing care: a physiologic perspective*, ed 3, St Louis: WB Saunders.

Stevenson DK, et al. (2001). Prediction of hyperbilirubinemia in near-term and term infants. *Journal of perinatology*, 21 Suppl 1, S63-S72; discussion S83-S87.

Strauss RG (2000). Data-driven blood banking practices for neonatal RBC transfusions. *Transfusion*, 40(12), 1528-1540.

Strauss RG (2001). Managing the anemia of prematurity: red blood cell transfusions versus recombinant erythropoietin. *Transfusion medicine reviews*, 15(3), 213-223.

Zhou X, et al. (2001). Successful mismatched sibling cord blood transplant in Hb Bart's disease. *Bone marrow transplant*, 28(1), 105-107.

SURGICAL CARE

The surgical neonate is a challenge to most nurses. The care requires excellent nursing assessment preoperatively and postoperatively. The following guidelines will assist you in the stabilization of the infant as well as the surgical wound care.

SURGICAL NEONATE STABILIZATION

Purpose
- To stabilize infant for transport to a medical center for surgery
- To notify surgeon and neonatal intensive care unit (NICU)/special care nursery (SCN) transport team as soon as possible, so that an optimum work-up may be planned

In all cases, these guidelines need to be observed, with directions and equipment needed for specific surgical anomalies given later in this chapter.

General Guidelines
1. Obtain parents' consent to transport.
2. Maintain sterile technique.
3. Position infant side-lying (possibly supine) to prevent organ angulation and circulatory compromise.
4. Place gauze dressing (moistened in warm normal saline [NS]) loosely around herniated tissue. Cover defect completely with sterile drawstring plastic bag. This is usually done in delivery/cesarean delivery room. Get warm NS from labor and delivery warmer. Prevent wrapping and rewrapping for inspection.
5. Start intravenous (IV)/umbilical lines if required, starting IV infusion. Obtain x-rays if required.
6. Start antibiotics as ordered after blood cultures are obtained. Other blood work may include complete blood count (CBC), renal indices, hematocrit (HCT), and glucose.
7. Monitor saturation and vital signs.
8. Keep urine and stool away from affected area with urine bags.
9. Obtain initial neurologic baseline, and continually assess for any changes. Assess wink response, motor function, bladder emptying, reflexes, and sensory response. If defect becomes dusky, notify neonatologist/resident/certified nurse practitioner (CNP).

10. Assess and manage bowel and urologic systems: monitor for consistency of stool/avoid constipation; monitor intake and output (I&O; observe for bladder distention).

11. Assess and manage orthopedic status:
    a. Use sheepskin/other behavioral support interventions (maintain extremities, hips in neutral position).
    b. Neurologic function may be lost at or below the lesion level as in spinal cord injuries; also movement may decrease after surgery.
    c. Assess extremities for temperature, mottling, and cyanosis.

12. Postsurgical care:
    a. Surgery is usually done within 24 to 48 hours after birth to prevent further damage and/or infection.
    b. Postoperative site care is done.
    c. Usually primary suture line with collodion coating is used—no suture line care is needed.
    d. Observe for edema, erythema, and drainage.
       (1) Protect site from contamination by urine or stool.
    e. Urologic consult may be done.
       (1) Continue to check for bladder distention (Credé's method of bladder expression or catheterization may be warranted).
       (2) Maintain position and orthopedic support; monitor extremity movement.

OMPHALOCELES/GASTROSCHISES

Equipment
- Sterile 4 × 4 gauze/Telfa pad
- IV supplies
- One bottle NS, warmed
- 10 Fr. Double-lumen orogastric (OG) or nasogastric (NG) (replogle) tube
- Sterile plastic bags/bowel bags

Guidelines
- Follow general guidelines.
- Place replogle tube to continuous low wall suction at 20 cm, and monitor I&O every hour.

MYELOMENINGOCELE

Equipment
- Sterile 4 × 4 gauze
- One bottle NS, warmed
- IV equipment

Guidelines
1. Position infant prone or side-lying.

2. Place roll under abdomen to decrease stress on sac.
3. Perform neurologic assessment preoperatively and postoperatively.
   a. Continue to assess for signs of increased intracranial pressure (ICP). Some infants will have increasing hydrocephalus after closure of defect. Observe head circumference; assess fontanel, neurologic status, and changes in behavior.
4. Maintain lower extremities in a neutral position. Observe for signs of movement. Usually infant is kept prone for 5 to 7 days, depending on healing time. Infant may nipple feed prone.
5. For teaching and support, refer to myelomeningocele clinic if available.

DIAPHRAGMATIC HERNIA

- Position infant supine with head of bed (HOB) elevated.
- Bag and mask ventilation should be avoided if possible. Ventilation through an endotracheal tube is preferred.
- A replogle tube should be inserted at the time of diagnosis and placed to wall suction as ordered.
- Have equipment available for umbilical lines. Umbilical lines should be attempted as soon as possible.
- Confirm diagnosis by x-rays.
- Obtain lab work as ordered.
- Have available equipment for needle aspiration/chest tube set-ups.
- Monitor vital signs closely.

TRACHEOESOPHAGEAL FISTULA

- Tracheoesophageal fistula should be suspected in infant with excessive secretions or infant where NG tube cannot pass.
- Insert appropriate-sized replogle tube to end of blind pouch, and maintain with suction as ordered.
- Obtain chest x-ray (CXR) and abdominal x-ray as ordered. The injection of 5 to 10 cc of air into the NG tube followed by clamping of the tube may aid in the diagnosis. Check with physician/CNP.
- Visualize blind esophageal pouch. Air in the stomach with an esophageal pouch will confirm a fistula. The aim of treatment is to keep airway/lungs and pouch clear of secretions and gastric contents from any fistulas that may be present.
- Keep infant prone or side-lying with HOB raised—to prevent reflux and to puddle secretions in pouch.
- Assess respiratory status.
- Administer antibiotics as ordered.

CYANOTIC CONGENITAL HEART DISEASE

- Assess respiratory status and maintain ventilation.

- Prostaglandin drip must be available on transport.
- Maintain IV fluids with filter in line to prevent foreign matter and bacteria from shunting through defects.
- Obtain lab work, electrocardiogram (ECG), echocardiogram, and CXR as ordered.

VENTRICULOPERITONEAL (V/P) SHUNT

Supplies
- Donut for head
- Razor
- 4 × 4's
- Keflin
- Gentamycin
- Sterile H_2O
- 5-cc syringes
- 1-cc syringe
- Alcohol sponges
- Eye retractors
- Spray benzoin
- Steri-strips
- Collodion
- Paper tape

Guidelines
- Follow general guidelines.
- The surgeon routinely notifies operating room (OR), but verification with OR should also be done by the charge nurse.
- Preoperative preparation should be done (to be ordered).
- CXR, CBC, and type and crossmatch of blood should be done.
- Assist with intubating infant—x-ray placement and arterial blood gases (ABGs).
- Place monitors—heart rate (HR), respiratory rate (RR), blood pressure (BP), and oximeter.
- Restrain extremities.

LASER SURGERY FOR RETINOPATHY OF PREMATURITY*

Purpose
This section describes care of infants requiring laser surgery after a diagnosis of retinopathy of prematurity (ROP).

---

*From Altimier L, Brown B, Tedeschi L (2000). Tri-Health's manual of neonatal nursing policies, procedures, competencies, & clinical pathways. Glenview, Ill: National Association of Neonatal Nurses.

Guidelines/Responsibilities

1. It is the responsibility of the NICU registered nurse (RN) to get patient, room, and medications ready for procedure.
2. It is the responsibility of the eye surgeon to contact family, call consent to the admitting department, arrange for laser to be available, and notify the attending neonatologist of the procedure (for anesthesia).
3. It is the responsibility of the attending neonatologist/fellow to provide anesthesia coverage or delegate that responsibility to another neonatologist/fellow.
4. It is the responsibility of resident/CNP to write IV fluid orders when infant is NPO (nothing by mouth).
5. The following staff shall be in attendance for laser surgery:
   a. Eye surgeon to perform surgery with assistant
   b. Designee (physician) or CNP to monitor baby and administer anesthesia
   c. NICU RN to prepare baby for procedure and stabilize baby's head for procedure
   d. Second NICU RN (OR nurse) to record procedure and vital signs

Procedures

1. Reserve procedure room for time designated by eye surgeon.
2. Set up procedure room (set-up time approximately 1 hour) with the following:
   a. Open warmer with temperature probe
   b. Cardiac monitor and pulse oximeter
   c. O_2 bag and mask
   d. Emergency drug card for baby's current weight
   e. Crash cart and intubation supplies in room
   f. Ventilator outside
   g. Necessary medications
      (1) Tetracaine (local anesthetic)
      (2) Balanced salt solution available in main pharmacy—two bottles
      (3) Cyclomydril or other dilating drops as ordered by eye surgeon
      (4) Atropine (minimizes bradycardic response to procedure) for IV use
      (5) Versed
      (6) Morphine sulfate
      (7) Narcan
3. Check that windows or doors are covered with dark paper or curtain.
4. Check for goggles (provided with laser equipment).
5. Check for laser (will be brought up from surgery).

Preoperatively

- Make infant NPO as ordered by eye surgeon for 4 to 6 hours.
- Administer Cyclomydril as ordered by eye surgeon.
- Start peripheral IV and administer fluids as ordered.
- Ensure physician administering anesthesia writes orders for medications 3 to 4 hours earlier.
- If infant needs intubation before surgery, confirm tube placement with CXR.
- Prepare anesthetic medications in syringes for administration 1 to 2 hours before procedure.
- Set up procedure room.
- Transport infant to procedure room (swaddled with IV accessible for medications); place neck roll to help maintain airway during procedure.

Intraoperatively

- Monitor infant continuously with oximeter and cardiac/apnea monitor.
- Record HR, RR, and saturations every 5 minutes.
- Record BP every 5 minutes after morphine administration and then at least every 10 minutes.
- Administer medications as ordered.
- Notify eye surgeon of bradycardia or desaturation.

Postoperatively

- Assess RR and saturations; observe for respiratory depression from anesthetic medications.
- Check vital signs every 15 minutes × 2, then every 30 minutes × 4 or until stable, and then every 1 to 2 hours as ordered.
- Maintain on oximeter for 24 hours after procedure and then as ordered by physician.
- Assess eyes for drainage; they will be red and puffy.
- Administer medications as ordered (may order Cyclomydril and Pred-Forte postoperatively).

Documentation

- Document any pertinent observations that occurred during the procedure or after: color change, apnea/bradycardia, tolerance of procedure (need for intubation/ventilation), swelling/redness/drainage from eyes.
- Document medications administered.

Follow-up

- Arrange follow-up (determined by ophthalmologist) to assess/reassess retina for 2 to 3 months after surgery.
- First postoperative visit is usually in 7 to 10 days.

- Long-term pediatric ophthalmology follow-up should be stressed to parents as an expected need for infants with ROP requiring laser surgery.
- Infant will be monitored for lazy eye or the need for glasses from early infancy.
- Possible complications include retinal detachment, cataracts, and infection (rare).

SKIN CARE OF THE NEONATE

Purpose

This section provides standard guidelines for skin care of the premature and term infant. The skin is a protective organ, and any break in integrity may create an opportunity for infection. Neonatal skin is more fragile than adult skin because fewer fibers connect the epidermis and dermis. In addition, the stratum corneum is thinner in the newborn. Increased skin permeability in the premature infant also increases the risk of infection and the susceptibilities to quickly absorb topical agents.

Nursing Care Guidelines

1. Clean skin with water.
   a. Clean after using adhesive remover/alcohol/iodine solutions/benzoin, because increased permeability may allow absorption of these products.
   b. Mild nonalkaline soap may be used at bath time.
2. Avoid perfumed creams/lotions. Perfumes may irritate skin, and chemical may be absorbed. Any creams/ointments require a physician's or CNP's order.
3. Do not use creams, ointments, or lotions on infants while under phototherapy.
4. Change diapers when wet or soiled or as infant's condition permits.
5. Reposition infant at least every 4 hours.
6. Minimize use of adhesives. Remove gently; loosen with water to avoid tearing skin. Use baby tape (Hydrogel) whenever possible.
7. May use Stomahesive® (Hollister, Libertyville, Ill.) under tape to protect skin (i.e., on face where oral tracheal tube is taped on skin) when indicated in infants needing long-term intubation or indwelling tubes.
8. May use Tegaderm® (3M, St Paul, Minn.) or Duoderm (Bristol-Myers Squibb Co., Princeton, NJ) on bony prominences when indicated.
9. Use semipermeable dressings (Tegaderm® or Opsite® [Smith & Nephew, Andover, Mass.]) to heal skin breakdown/protect IV sites.

10. Handle gently to avoid any trauma to skin.
11. In very low–birth weight infants, use warm mist to decrease insensible water loss and maintain temperature.

Assessment

The skin should be assessed on admission and at least every 4 hours for the following:
- Turgor
- Color
- Perfusion
- Edema
- Pressure areas on bony prominences
- Bruises or abrasions
- Dry, peeling, or scaly skin
- Postoperative wounds (see policy for specific surgery)
- IV sites (should be assessed every hour)
- Congenital abnormalities of the skin
- Temperature
- Diaphoresis

Skin Breakdown

- Vigilon® (Bard Medical Div., Covington, Ga.) may be used over areas of breakdown to protect the skin.
- When Vigilon® is impractical, i.e., oozing off when there is high humidity, an increased Isolette temperature, and the Vigilon® will roll off the skin or skin is sloughling off, bacteriocidal/antifungal cream or ointment and Adaptic® (Johnson & Johnson, New Brunswich, NJ) may be applied to affected area per physician's or CNP's order. Wrap area with gauze twice daily. When applying Bacitracin® (Pharmacia: Upjohn Co, Kalamazoo, Mich.) and Adaptic®, only cover open area without overlapping healed areas, since this may cause maceration.

Use of Vigilon Wound Dressing*

1. Hydrogel composition is 96% H_2O and 4% polyethylene oxide. It is permeable to oxygen, is occlusive, and can absorb its own weight in wound exudates.
2. Use in conjunction with topical medications or skin preparations if desired. Use with skin breakdown and/or to prevent skin breakdown.

---

*From Altimier L, Brown B, Tedeschi L (2000). *Tri-Health's manual of neonatal nursing policies, procedures, competencies, & clinical pathways*. Glenview, Ill: National Association of Neonatal Nurses.

3. Equipment needed
   a. Vigilon wound dressing
   b. One pair of sterile gloves
   c. Betadine scrub
   d. 2 × 2's
   e. Sterile H$_2$O
   f. Suture set
4. Procedure
   a. Wash hands.
   b. Position patient to expose the area involved.
   c. Apply gloves.
   d. Remove drainage (which may appear on the wound) with a gauze pad and lukewarm water.
   e. Gently cleanse area with Betadine scrub, rinse with sterile water, and pat the area dry with 2 × 2.
   f. Using suture set, cut Vigilon® to size of wound.
   g. Remove film on the side of dressing to be placed on wound. Apply Vigilon®, gel side down.
   h. Remove the film on top. Keep area open to air, and allow to dry.
   i. Allow Vigilon® to remain intact. It will peel off skin as skin underneath heals.
   j. If drainage continues, assess for signs of infection: odorous drainage, fever, increased redness, warmth. Report signs to physician/CNP, and document in the nursing notes. Culture may be indicated.
   k. Document the use of Vigilon® in the nursing notes.

UNIVERSITY OF ILLINOIS MEDICAL CENTER AT CHICAGO CLINICAL CARE GUIDELINE

Subject: Meningomyelocele (MM) Wound Care and Dressing Changes*

Objective

To prevent infection of the meningomyelocele and its surgical repair from potential contamination from stool or other foreign substances.

Definition

For the purposes of this care guideline, the following definition will apply:

Meningomyelocele—A congenital defect of the formation of the spinal cord and vertebrae that results in failed closure of the embryonic neural tube and absence of skin and malformed vertebrae over the defect. The defect may develop anywhere along

*From University of Illinois Medical Center at Chicago Women's and Children's Nursing Services. Used with permission by Dharmapuri Vidyasagar, MD; Catherine Theorell, RNC, MSN, NNP; Beena Peters, RN, MS.

the length of the neural tube from the cervical to lumbosacral vertebrae.

Position Statements

Strict aseptic technique will be utilized when applying and changing MM wound dressings. This minimally includes head covering, face mask/shield, and sterile gloves.

Postoperatively, the MM dressing will be covered with occlusive dressing (Tegaderm®).

Medical adhesive will be applied to the lower edge of the occlusive dressing. Medical adhesive spray will be applied to the skin just below the occlusive dressing.

A Duoderm® flap may be placed beneath the lower edge of the occlusive dressing and above the opening.

All internal and external supplies used on these infants shall be free from latex.

Procedures

1. Preoperatively
   a. After delivery, the open spinal defect is covered with a sterile, warm, moist saline dressing using strict aseptic technique.
   b. The sterile, warm, moist dressing is subsequently wrapped in plastic covering to prevent heat and fluid loss through the defect.
   c. The infant is positioned prone or side-lying. Supine position is avoided.
2. Postoperatively
   a. The neurosurgical physician will inspect the MM surgical wound and change the dressing daily or as deemed necessary.
   b. The RN assigned to care for the infant with MM repair or her designee will assist the neurosurgical physician in dressing changes.
   c. The RN may change the MM wound dressing if the dressing becomes inadvertently soiled and the neurosurgical physician is not available to change the dressing.
   d. Assemble the necessary clean and sterile supplies.
      (1) Sterile 4 × 4 dressings
      (2) Cloth tape
      (3) Sterile suture removal kit
      (4) Sterile gloves
      (5) Surgical mask
      (6) Duoderm® Extra Thin and Steri Drape 1000® (3M, St Paul, Minn.)
      (7) Medical Adhesive Spray (no. 99-08-0550)
      (8) Occlusive dressing (Tegaderm)®
   e. Postoperatively, the surgical wound is covered by sterile gauze that lies beneath a clear occlusive Tegaderm® barrier.

f. Medical adhesive is applied to the skin just below the edge of the Tegaderm® and above the anal opening.

g. Duoderm® film is attached to the medical adhesive, providing a protective barrier for the skin. Steri Drape 1000® is secured to the Duoderm® as a barrier against stool and urine contamination of the surgical site.

h. Medical adhesive application and Duoderm® barrier may be replaced by nursing when soiled.

OSTOMY CARE*

Objective

The objective of ostomy care is to apply a pouch to contain fecal drainage from an ostomy.

Equipment

- Pouch
- Barrier

Procedures

1. Remove pouch.
   a. Gently lift adhesive edges of pouch from skin. Press skin with one finger, and pull adhesive with other hand.
   b. To remove Stomahesive® gently press damp cloth against skin and pull skin barrier off with other hand.
   c. Wash skin with tap water; may wash with plain soap. Bits of Stomahesive will wash off with water.
2. Apply pouch.
   a. Measure stoma with guide provided. Trace stoma size onto the white backing paper of Stomahesive®; cut out opening. Opening should fit so that $1/16$ to $1/8$ inch of skin is showing after banner is applied over stoma, to prevent seepage that could lead to skin breakdown.
   b. Prepare and apply pouch. For adhesive-backed pouch, apply with Stomahesive® only. Draw and cut opening as described above; attach shiny side of Stomahesive to adhesive pouch. Pouch is ready to apply. Remove white paper from Stomahesive®, and apply over stoma to dry skin. Close bottom of bag with closure by turning pouch several times and bending closure over it.

---

*From Altimier L, Brown B, Tedeschi L (2000). Tri-Health's manual of neonatal nursing policies, procedures, competencies, & clinical pathways. Glenview, Ill: National Association of Neonatal Nurses.

Documentation

Record pouch change in the nursing notes. Record color and condition of stoma (i.e., edematous, red, bluish tinged, bleeds easily) and condition of skin under abdominal assessment. Record description of output under stool output.

Comments

Plan to empty pouch before meals or 2 to 3 hours after a meal. Eating will stimulate stool and makes changing the pouch more difficult. To empty, open clamp and press stool out of pouch; wipe bottom of pouch, and close.

BIBLIOGRAPHY

Abrahamov D, et al. (2002). Plasma vascular endothelial growth factor level is a predictor of the severity of postoperative capillary leak syndrome in neonates undergoing cardiopulmonary bypass. *Pediatric surgery international*, 18(1), 54-59.

Bellotti M, et al. (2002). Different acute-phase response in newborns and infants undergoing surgery. *Pediatric research*, 51(3), 333-338.

Cass DL, Wesson DE (2002). Advances in fetal and neonatal surgery for gastrointestinal anomalies and disease. *Clinics in perinatology*, 29(1), 1-21.

Clancy J, McVicar A, Boyd S (2001). The surgical neonate. *British journal of perioperative nursing*, 11(1), 21-27.

Hamdan AH, et al. (2002). Gestational age at intrauterine myelomeningocele repair does not influence the risk of prematurity. *Fetal diagnosis & therapy*, 17(2), 66-68.

Henderson-Smart DJ, Steer P (2001). Prophylactic caffeine to prevent postoperative apnea following general anesthesia in preterm infants. *Cochrane review, Cochrane database systematic reviews*, 4.

Kuwano H (2001). Results of bowel plication in addition to primary anastomosis in patients with jejunal atresia. *Journal of pediatric surgery*, 36(12), 1752-1756.

NEUROLOGIC CARE

Neurologic care is concerned with assessing the infant for signs of central nervous system (CNS) problems. Some of the more common problems are problems with neurulation, such as neural tube defects. Meningomyleocele is the best-known dysfunction. It is discussed in Chapter 16, because it requires surgical intervention. Congenital hydrocephalus may accompany a neural tube defect. It also is discussed in Chapter 16.

NURSING ASSESSMENT

The nursing assessment focuses on knowledge of risk factors. Obstetric risk factors include prematurity; postmaturity; placental problems, such as abruptio placentae and placenta previa; analgesia; anesthesia; and maternal problems, such as infection, hypertension, and substance abuse. Large–for–gestational age infants, prolonged or precipitate labor, forceps delivery, and abnormal presentation increase the risk of birth trauma and hemorrhage. Alterations in intrauterine growth and polyhydramnios may be present with an infant who has a CNS malformation. Fetal distress, perinatal asphyxia, and low Apgar scores are associated with intracranial hemorrhage and hypoxic ischemic encephalopathy (HIE) (Blackburn, 2003). Postnatally the history should be examined for periods of hypoxemia, trauma during delivery, low Apgar scores, or other conditions that result in decreased perfusion.

The physical examination should focus on signs of birth trauma, such as petechiae, ecchymosis, excessive bruising, edema, lacerations, and fractures. The infant should be observed for signs of infection including chorioretinitis since this may lead to hypoxia. If there is neurologic damage the infant is often irritable with either a weak or high-pitched cry and there may be tremors, excessive jitteriness, or even seizures. Observation of the head for asymmetry, premature closure of suture lines, or bulging fontanels is important. The quality and symmetry of activity with spontaneous and elicited movement are assessed. Alterations in symmetry of the trunk, face, and extremities at rest or with spontaneous movement suggest congenital anomalies, birth injury, or neurologic insult. Tight fisting is an abnormal sign. A cortical thumb (inside thumb on closure of the hand) may be normal, but it is abnormal if it is persistent. Opisthotonos and decerebrate or decorticate posturing may be present (Blackburn, 2003). Primitive reflexes may be diminished or absent.

CLINICAL MANIFESTATIONS

Clinical manifestations are those listed in the Nursing Assessment section.

DIAGNOSIS

The diagnosis is made using radiographic tests, computed tomography (CT), magnetic resonance imaging (MRI), radionucleotide tests, cerebral angiogram, brain-stem–evoked response, electroencephalogram, cerebral blood flow via Doppler ultrasound, measurement of intracranial pressure (ICP), and lumbar puncture.

Laboratory examination should include blood cultures and cerebrospinal fluid culture, as well as examination for increased red blood cells and protein and decreased glucose levels. Serum glucose, electrolytes, and complete blood count (CBC) with differential are important too.

NURSING MANAGEMENT

Management is aimed at alleviating the symptoms that the infant is exhibiting and preventing complications. Blackburn (2003) suggests the following general interventions:

1. Alteration in level of consciousness
   a. Monitor infant state, activity, responsiveness, eye movements, head circumference, vital signs, seizure activity, and signs of increased ICP.
   b. Position to promote skin integrity, prevent contractures, and reduce ICP (head in midline and slightly elevated).
   c. Monitor fluid and electrolyte status.
   d. Maintain adequate ventilation and perfusion.
   e. Implement comfort measures.
   f. Maintain an appropriate thermal environment.
   g. Reduce environmental stressors.
   h. Promote neurobehavioral stability.
2. Potential for injury related to trauma or infection
   a. Maintain use of aseptic techniques.
   b. Use sterile technique when appropriate.
   c. Position to prevent contamination of defects or operative sites.
   d. Monitor for signs of localized infection or neonatal sepsis.
   e. Handle gently.
   f. Position to reduce potential of trauma or contamination.
3. Impairment of skin integrity
   a. Position in alignment, and change position.
   b. Use foam, sheepskin, lambskin, or waterbeds.

    c. Massage skin gently to stimulate circulation.
    d. Use appropriate skin care measures.
4. Alteration in comfort
5. Impaired mobility
    a. Position in alignment, and change position.
    b. Promote skin integrity.
    c. Use gentle range-of-motion exercises.
6. Alteration in thermoregulation
7. Alteration in nutrition
8. Promotion of neurobehavioral organization and development

    Nursing assessment is detailed in Figure 17-1. Table 17-1 gives the main causes of generalized hypotonia in newborns, and Table 17-2 lists nonneurologic findings associated with neurologic diagnoses.

UNIVERSITY OF ILLINOIS MEDICAL CENTER AT CHICAGO CLINICAL CARE GUIDELINE

Subject: Arteriovenous Malformation (AVM) Management*

Objective

To establish clinical care guidelines for the complex, multidisciplinary care for seriously ill infants presenting with AVMs.

Definition

For the purposes of this care guideline, the following definition will apply:

    Arteriovenous Malformation (AVM)—a malformation of the developing peripheral vascular system that results in abnormal connections of arteries, arterioles, and capillaries to the venous system. This abnormality creates a large shunt and can involve vessels of any size and in any location. Surgical treatment of these lesions may involve ligation or coil embolization.

Position Statements

Infants with AVMs may be diagnosed antenatally or after birth. The clinical presentation, management, and prognosis for these infants depend on the size and location of the involved vessels.

    If the AVM lesion is suspected before birth, the parents should be referred to high-risk perinatologists if possible. The perinatologists will meet with the family, review the results of diagnostic scans, and discuss the findings with the neonatology staff to collaboratively plan the management.

*From University of Illinois Medical Center at Chicago Women's and Children's Nursing Services. Used with permission by Dharmapuri Vidyasagar, MD; Catherine Theorell, RNC, MSN, NNP; Beena Peters, RN, MS.

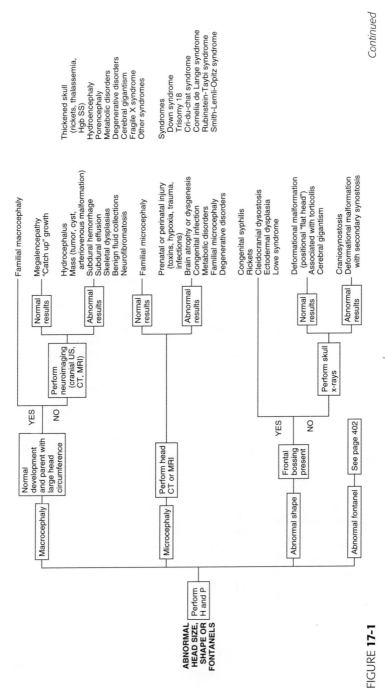

FIGURE **17-1**

Continued

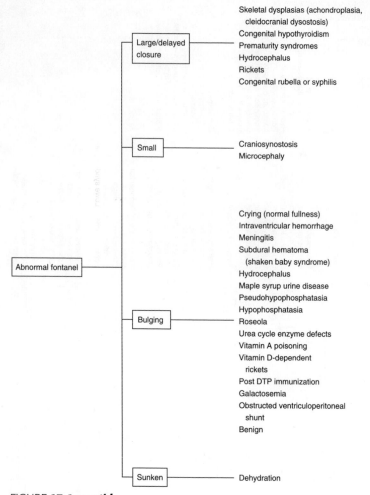

FIGURE **17-1, cont'd**
Nursing assessment includes taking a thorough history or reviewing one on the chart and conducting a physical examination (head to toe as can be tolerated). If you are a nurse practitioner you may order the tests listed; otherwise, you may wish to make sure these tests are ordered. Follow the results so that you may help the family to understand what is being done. (From Pomeranz AJ, et al., editors. [2002]. *Pediatric decision-making strategies to accompany Nelson textbook of pediatrics,* ed 16, Philadelphia: WB Saunders, pp. 13-15.)

Table **17-1**	Main Causes of Generalized Hypotonia in the Newborn Infant

Site of Major Pathologic Condition	Disorder
Anterior horn cell	Spinal muscular atrophy
	Other anterior horn cell disease (in association with cerebellar atrophy)
Peripheral nerves or roots	Congenital polyneuropathies (several types)
Muscle	Congenital muscular dystrophy (several types, including Fukuyama type and "occidental" types with and without merosine deficiency)
	Congenital myotonic dystrophy
	Congenital myopathies
	Central core disease
	Centronuclear myopathy
	Nemaline myopathy
	Congenital fiber type disproportion
	Other structural myopathies
	Glycogen storage diseases, types II and III
	Mitochondrial myopathies (deficit in cytochrome-*c* oxidase)
	Severe type
	Transient type
Neuromuscular junction	Neonatal myasthenia (infants of myasthenic mothers)
	Congenital myasthenia and myasthenic syndromes (several types)
	Infantile botulism
Central nervous system	Hypoxic-ischemic encephalopathy
	Brain malformations (including trisomy 21)
	Hemorrhagic and other brain damage
	Drug intoxication
Mixed origin (mainly central nervous system)	Zellweger syndrome and related peroxisomal disorders
Connective tissue abnormality	Marfan syndrome
	Ehlers-Danolos syndrome

In Scher MS (2001). Brain disorders of the fetus and neonate. In Klaus MH, Fanaroff AA, editors. Care of the high-risk neonate, ed 5, Philadelphia: WB Saunders, p. 498; Aicardi J, et al. (1998). Diseases of the nervous system in childhood. Clinics in developmental medicine, ed 2, New York: MacKeith Press.

Table 17-2	Nonneurologic Findings Associated with Neurologic Diagnoses
Nonneurologic Finding	**Neurologic Diagnosis**
Cardiac rhabdomyoma	Tuberous sclerosis
Hypoplastic left heart syndrome	Brain malformations (e.g., microgyria, agenesis of corpus callosum)
Multicystic dysplastic kidney	Brain malformations with specific genetic syndromes vs. destructive brain lesions
Diaphragmatic hernia	Brain malformations (e.g., cerebellar hypoplasia)
Polyhydramnios	Brain malformations with genetic syndromes or destructive brain lesions
Hydrops fetalis	Congenital syndromes (e.g., Turner's syndrome) or destructive brain lesions, usually of vascular or infectious origin (e.g., asphyxia, parvovirus, metabolic disorders)
Cleft lip and palate	Midline brain malformations (e.g., holporsecephaly)
Arthrogryposis	Neuromuscular disease or destructive brain lesions (e.g., congenital muscular dystrophies)
Multiple-gestation pregnancy	Destructive brain lesions of white or gray matter (e.g., periventricular leukomalacia)
Omphalocele/gastroschisis	Neural tube defects

From Scher MS (2001). Brain disorders of the fetus and neonate. In Klaus MH, Fanaroff AA, editors. Care of the high-risk neonate, ed 5, Philadelphia: WB Saunders, p. 486.

Before delivery or as soon as feasible, medical and surgical consulting services should be involved as dictated by the location of the lesion and the clinical presentation.

Delivery of a fetus with an AVM is considered a high-risk delivery and to the extent possible, should be attended by the neonatal intensive care unit (NICU) resuscitation team.

Transfers of infants suspected of having an AVM should be routed through the usual transport channels.

Procedures
Preoperative evaluation

1. In addition to the routine admission assessment and evaluation, infants with AVM should have umbilical catheters inserted in the artery and vein in order to administer glucose and fluids, monitor hemodynamic status, evaluate blood gases, and monitor systemic blood pressure.
2. Consultation from the pediatric cardiology service should be considered for the assessment of ventricular function and to evaluate for the presence of other cardiac abnormalities.
3. Consider inotropic support and other measures (digitalization) to control cardiac failure.
4. Elective intubation to provide ventilatory support may be appropriate.
5. Assess nutritional status, and provide adequate calories and maintenance fluids. Usually, infants with AVM need fluids in the range of the lower limits of their overall daily requirements (approximately 60 to 65 ml/kg/day).
6. Obtain baseline laboratory tests, and assess renal function. Closely monitor the urinary output and blood chemistry values.
7. Optimize hematocrit; if necessary, administer blood transfusions.
8. Diagnostic radiologic investigations may include a chest x-ray and preferably an MRI study. If the latter is not feasible because of the infant's status, arrange for CT scan of the head. No contrast is needed for either of these studies.
9. Evaluate and treat other co-existing conditions, such as respiratory distress syndrome (RDS), hypoglycemia, and hyperbilirubinemia.
10. In collaboration with the consulting services, plan the postoperative chain of notification for changes in infant status.

Intraoperative Management

1. Ideally, a pediatric anesthesiologist should be conducting anesthesia for infants with AVM.
2. A respiratory therapist may be needed to evaluate the humidity settings in the neonatal ventilators in the operating room, particularly if the operative procedure is prolonged.
3. During embolization, iodine-containing contrast material, up to 15 ml/kg, may be injected. This contrast material has a high osmolarity and may result in intravascular fluid shifts during the procedure, significantly affecting the cardiac status. Therefore it is extremely critical for both the anesthesiologist and the surgeon to communicate the extent of fluid administered, withdrawn, and lost during the procedure to guide appropriate fluid

therapy during and after the procedure. The anesthesiologist is responsible for monitoring the blood gases and blood glucose levels. As the need arises, furosemide (Lasix) may be administered for the control of pulmonary edema from fluid overload.

4. Appropriate maintenance of temperature during the intraoperative period is critical, as is avoiding hypothermia or hyperthermia.

Postoperative Care

1. Obtain vital signs and reweigh the baby on readmission from the operating room to the NICU.

2. Obtain blood for serum glucose, electrolytes, and blood gases and acid-base status assessment. Notify the neonatal attending physician and/or fellow if abnormal laboratory findings are noted. Notify consulting surgical services as needed.

3. A baseline postoperative chest x-ray may be obtained to evaluate the degree of pulmonary edema. This may aid in planning for ventilatory care and evaluation of fluid therapy.

4. It is important to maintain a normal arterial pH and blood gas status, since infants with AVMs have intracranial hypertension and may develop persistent pulmonary hypertension. Avoiding metabolic acidosis during the postoperative period is therefore critical.

5. Evaluate the cardiac and renal status continually using clinical findings and pertinent laboratory data (urinary output, blood gases, vital signs).

6. Obtain additional diagnostic tests, such as echocardiography and renal function assessments as required. Consider a repeat MRI and/or CT scan if the infant's neurologic or clinical condition deteriorates.

7. Please inform the surgical team of the progress of the infant's postoperative course.

8. Following the first embolization procedure, subsequent sessions can be determined based on cardiac output and the extent of cardiac failure. Delaying subsequent embolization sessions may be appropriate if the infant has made significant recovery and continues to improve.

9. Subsequent embolizations should be considered when, in spite of vigorous cardiovascular support and therapy, the infant continues to demonstrate signs of cardiac decompensation.

10. It may be prudent to leave the peripheral arterial and venous catheters after the initial procedure postoperatively, so that these routes can be used for repeat embolization; however, if the overall condition of the infant has improved and a decision has been made to postpone embolization, these catheters may then be removed.

Summary

Infants with large symptomatic AVMs presenting in the fetal or neonatal period pose particularly challenging situations. They have significant cardiac failure and a complex pathologic condition; these require a multidisciplinary team approach for management.

The initial goals are to make a thorough assessment of the cardio-vascular and respiratory functions and to provide appropriate preoperative fluid management. Preoperative assessments included an MRI, cardiac consultation, and if needed, consultation with the renal service. In lieu of an MRI, a CT scan may be obtained, if the infant cannot tolerate the former; for either of these, there is no need for contrast material.

Intraoperatively, one must pay close attention to the temperature, blood glucose, and fluid status. AVM embolization should be considered a step-wise procedure; each subsequent step is determined based on the infant's progression from the previous clinical status, a change in the overall condition of the infant, and our assessment of the infant's ability to tolerate future procedures.

Long-Term Follow-Up Care

Arrangements must be made for close, long-term follow-up of infants with AVMs treated in the newborn period.

Informing the Referring Physician

The physicians and hospitals referring patients to University of Illinois Medical Center are routinely informed of the progress of the infants by the perinatal or neonatal attending physicians.

Table 17-3 gives information on five types of perinatal brain damage.

HYPOXIC-ISCHEMIC ENCEPHALOPATHY

Hypoxic-ischemic encephalopathy (HIE) is a severe consequence of perinatal hypoxia. It results in developmental delays, mental retardation, seizures, and sometimes cerebral palsy. Much research is ongoing regarding this condition and preventive strategies. Some areas under investigation are listed in Table 17-4. Figures 17-2 and 17-3 detail nursing assessments; and Box 17-1 classifies the four grades of periventricular-intraventricular hemorrhage.

MENINGOMYELOCELE

Although the surgical care for meningomyelocele is found in Chapter 16, it is important to assess the level of function that may be affected in these children (Tables 17-5 and 17-6).

Table 17-3	Clinical Features and Ultimate Outcome in Five Types of Perinatal Brain Damage						
Type of Brain Damage	Gestational Age	Timing	Risk Situations	Anatomic Findings	Acute Clinical Features	Confirmation	Late Outcomes
Hypoxic-Ischemic Encephalo-pathy (Severe)	Full term or after term	Intrapartum or immediate postnatal	Acute birth asphyxia (abruptio placentae, hemorrhage, cord compression, mechanical injury)	Brain edema, massive cellular necrosis (cortex, basal ganglia, brain stem), ± hemorrhage (intraventricular, subdural, or intracerebral)	Major CNS depression, repeated seizures (often subtle in comatose child), ± brainstem signs (no spontaneous respiration, no suck)	EEG findings	Severe sequelae in 50% of survivors, with microcephaly, multiple handicaps, epilepsy
			Prolonged subacute asphyxia (prenatal or intrapartum)		Usually systemic signs of acute hypoxia-ischemia (e.g., acute	Critical and severe interictal abnormalities	Motor handicap always more severe than cognitive

renal tubular necrosis, paralytic ileus)

Inadequate resuscitation

Ultrasound and CT scan findings

Edema ± hemorrhage within first wk

Less severe degree of neuromotor, sensorial, intellectual, or behavioral deficit in others

Normal or subnormal outcome possible

Continued

Table 17-3	Clinical Features and Ultimate Outcome in Four Types of Perinatal Brain Damage—cont'd						
Type of Brain Damage	Gestational Age	Timing	Risk Situations	Anatomic Findings	Acute Clinical Features	Confirmation	Late Outcomes
Hypoxic-Ischemic Encephalopathy (Severe), cont'd						Cerebral necrosis of various degrees and localization but imaging often normal acutely	
Hypoxic-Ischemic Encephalopathy (Moderate to Mild)	Same as above	Same as above	Same circumstances as above but less severe and for shorter duration	Brain edema ± cellular damage ± subarachnoid hemorrhage	In moderate cases, CNS depression ± isolated seizures	EEG moderate or no abnormalities	Any type of permanent deficit including cerebral palsy in about 20% of

In "mild" cases, hyperexcitability and tone abnormalities (no depression, no seizure)	Purely clinical diagnosis based on signs within the first wk of life	moderate cases
		Normalization fast and complete in most mild cases and about 50% of "moderate cases
	Ultrasound usually normal	MBD at school age in about 30% of moderate cases

Continued

Table 17-3		Clinical Features and Ultimate Outcome in Four Types of Perinatal Brain Damage—cont'd					
Type of Brain Damage	Gestational Age	Timing	Risk Situations	Anatomic Findings	Acute Clinical Features	Confirmation	Late Outcomes
Periventricular Leukomalacia	Any age	Any time (prenatal or postnatal)	Chronic fetal distress (± intrauterine growth retardation)	Ischemic necrosis of periventricular white matter (centrum semiovale, corona radiata, occipital and temporal zones)	CNS depression within first wk	Ultrasound findings	Persisting neurologic findings (including typical spastic diplegia) ± sensorial and intellectual deficit of various degrees
			Low CBF	Coagulation necrosis in acute stage ± hemorrhage	Poor visual pursuit and poor axial tone at 40-wk corrected age	Periventricular leukomalacia including echogenicity	

Intraventricular Hemorrhage								
Prematurity (below 34 wk)	Postnatal (first wk of life)	Immaturity + RDS leading to hypoxia, hypercarbia, unstable CBF Chorioamnionitis Acute hypotension (may be associated with apneic spell and bradycardia, cardiac arrest, or hemorrhagic shock)	Hemorrhage in germinal matrix (grade I) Distribution often asymmetric Cavitation and gliosis later	Organization within 1 mo: porencephalic cysts ± ventricular enlargement caused by cerebral atrophy	Major CNS depression ± seizure, onset at birth or later	Ultrasound findings	Usually excellent in grades I and II

Continued

Table 17-3	Clinical Features and Ultimate Outcome in Four Types of Perinatal Brain Damage—cont'd						
Type of Brain Damage	Gestational Age	Timing	Risk Situations	Anatomic Findings	Acute Clinical Features	Confirmation	Late Outcomes
Intraventricular Hemorrhage, cont'd			Pneumothorax	Intraventricular hemorrhage without ventriculomegaly (grade II)	Nonspecific and unexplained deterioration	Resorption of blood in about 10 days	Poor or very poor in grade III, especially when associated with extensive periventricular leukomalacia
				Intraventricular hemorrhage with ventriculomegaly (grade III)	Often silent	Normalization in grades I and II	Possible hydrocephalus (10%-30% risk)

| Cerebral Infarction (Arterial Territory) | Any age (frequently full term) | Mainly prenatal; can occur intrapartum or first 24 hr | Embolization in twin-to-twin transfusion, placental abnormality | Infarction of both white matter and cortex in arterial distribution | Repeated focal seizures within first 3 days | CT scan within 48 hr of birth: wedge-shaped area of low attenuation with irregular margins; may be normal if scan too | Improvement of neuromotor function within first year, with mild residual hemiparesis (usually walk alone) |

Hemorrhagic venous infraction (grade IV)

Organization of periventricular leukomalacia often associated with grade III within 1 mo (see above)

Continued

Table 17-3 Clinical Features and Ultimate Outcome in Four Types of Perinatal Brain Damage—cont'd

Type of Brain Damage	Gestational Age	Timing	Risk Situations	Anatomic Findings	Acute Clinical Features	Confirmation	Late Outcomes
Cerebral Infarction (Arterial Territory), cont'd			Thrombo-philia	Contraction of affected area, multiple cystic degener-ation	No major depression	soon after actual infarction Rescanning a few mo later to evaluate loss of tissue	Mild mental deficit or none

Thrombosis in DIC, sepsis, maternal cocaine	Middle cerebral artery most common (two times more common than other arteries) Left hemisphere mainly (three times more common than right)	Asymmetric findings in case of middle cerebral artery	EEG findings: focal seizures	No speech disorder, usually
Often no predisposing factors				Epilepsy uncommon
Low risk full term				

From Scher MS (2001). Brain disorders of the fetus and neonate. In Klaus MH, Fanaroff AA, editors. Care of the high-risk neonate, ed 5, Philadelphia: WB Saunders, pp. 506-507.

CNS, Central nervous system; EEG, electroencephalogram; CT, computed tomography; MBD, minimal brain dysfunction; CBF, cerebral blood flow; RDS, respiratory distress syndrome; DIC, disseminated intravascular coagulation.

Table 17-4	Investigational Neuroprotective Strategies to Minimize Hypoxic-Ischemic Injury in the Newborn
Strategies	**Interventions**
Decrease cerebral metabolic rate	High-dose barbiturates
	Hypothermia
Block NMDA (*N*-methyl-D-aspartate) receptor channel	MK-801
	Magnesium
Decrease glutamate release	Adenosine or adenosine agonists
	Adenosine uptake inhibitors
Inhibit voltage-sensitive calcium channels	Calcium channel blockers
Terminate free radical reactions	Free radical scavengers: vitamin C, vitamin E, allopurinol
Prevent free radical formation	Iron chelators
	Indomethacin
	Allopurinol
	NOS (nitric oxide synthase) inhibitors
Reduce inflammatory response	Inflammatory antagonists (e.g., interleukin-1, tumor necrosis factor-alpha antagonists)
	Allopurinol
Attenuate apoptosis pathway	Caspase inhibitors

From Marro PJ (2002). Etiology and pharmacologic approach to hypoxic-ischemic encephalopathy in the newborn. NeoReviews, 3(6), 99-107. Available at www.aap.org

---

Box 17-1

Classification of Periventricular-Intraventricular Hemorrhage

GRADE I
Isolated germinal matrix hemorrhage

GRADE II
Intraventricular hemorrhage with normal ventricular size

GRADE III
Intraventricular hemorrhage with acute ventricular dilation

GRADE IV
Intraventricular hemorrhage with parenchymal hemorrhage

In Lowdermilk DL, Perry SE, Bobak IM (2000). Maternity & women's health care, ed 7, St Louis: Mosby, p. 1121; Moe P, Paige P (1998). Neurologic disorders. In Merenstein G, Gardner S, editors. Handbook of neonatal intensive care, ed 4, St Louis: Mosby.

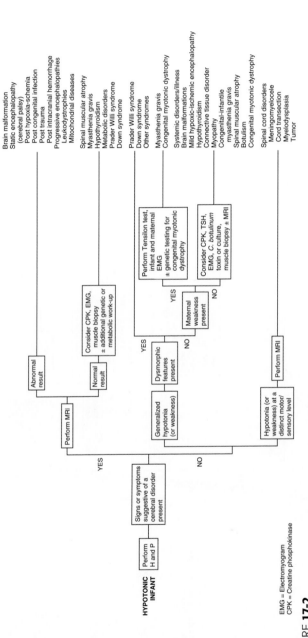

FIGURE 17-2

Nursing assessment includes taking a thorough history or reviewing one on the chart and conducting a physical examination (head to toe as can be tolerated). If you are a nurse practitioner you may order the tests listed; otherwise, you may wish to make sure these tests are ordered. Follow the results so that you may help the family to understand what is being done. (From Pomeranz AJ, et al., editors. [2002]. *Pediatric decision-making strategies to accompany Nelson textbook of pediatrics*, ed 16, Philadelphia: WB Saunders, p. 207.)

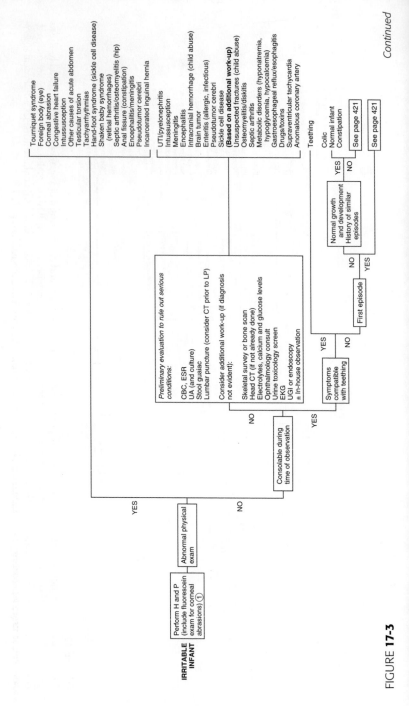

IRRITABLE INFANT

Perform H and P (include fluorescein exam for corneal abrasions) ①

Abnormal physical exam

YES

- Tourniquet syndrome
- Foreign body (eye)
- Corneal abrasion
- Congestive heart failure
- Intussusception
- Other causes of acute abdomen
- Testicular torsion
- Tachyarrhythmias
- Hand-foot syndrome (sickle cell disease)
- Shaken baby syndrome (retinal hemorrhages)
- Septic arthritis/osteomyelitis (hip)
- Anal fissure (constipation)
- Encephalitis/meningitis
- Pseudotumor cerebri
- Incarcerated inguinal hernia

NO

Consolable during time of observation

NO

Preliminary evaluation to rule out serious conditions:

CBC, ESR
UA (and culture)
Stool guaiac
Lumbar puncture (consider CT prior to LP)

Consider additional work-up (if diagnosis not evident):

Skeletal survey or bone scan
Head CT (if not already done)
Electrolytes, calcium and glucose levels
Ophthalmology consult
Urine toxicology screen
EKG
UGI or endoscopy
± In-house observation

- UTI/pyelonephritis
- Intussusception
- Meningitis
- Encephalitis
- Intracranial hemorrhage (child abuse)
- Brain tumor
- Enteritis (allergic, infectious)
- Pseudotumor cerebri
- Sickle cell disease
- **(Based on additional work-up):**
- Unsuspected fractures (child abuse)
- Osteomyelitis/diskitis
- Septic arthritis
- Metabolic disorders (hyponatremia, hypoglycemia, hypocalcemia)
- Gastroesophageal reflux/esophagitis
- Drugs/toxins
- Supraventricular tachycardia
- Anomalous coronary artery

YES

Symptoms compatible with teething

YES

Teething

NO

First episode

NO

Normal growth and development History of similar episodes

YES

- Colic
- Normal infant
- Constipation

YES

See page 421

NO

See page 421

Continued

FIGURE **17-3**

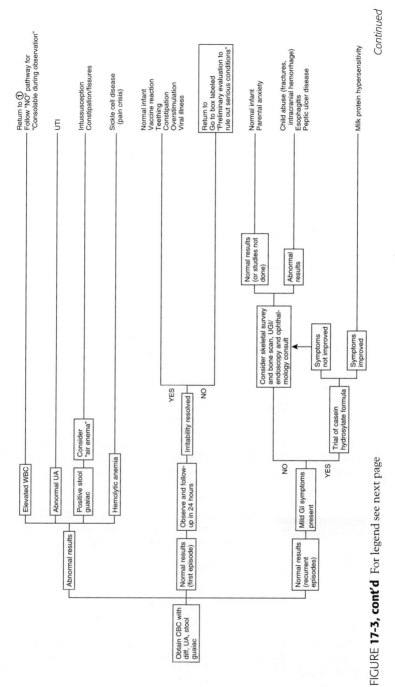

FIGURE **17-3, cont'd** For legend see next page

Continued

FIGURE **17-3, cont'd**

Nursing assessment includes taking a thorough history or reviewing one on the chart and conducting a physical examination (head to toe as can be tolerated). If you are a nurse practitioner you may order the tests listed; otherwise, you may wish to make sure these tests are ordered. Follow the results so that you may help the family to understand what is being done. Some of these conditions may not present during the initial neonatal period, but if you are doing follow-up care in the clinic or home situation you may discover these signs and symptoms. (From Pomeranz AJ, et al., editors. [2002]. *Pediatric decision-making strategies to accompany Nelson textbook of pediatrics*, ed 16, Philadelphia: WB Saunders, pp. 309, 311.)

Table **17-5**	Motor and Sensory Findings in the Myelomeningocele		
Level	**Motor**	**Sensory**	**Reflex**
L1-2	Hip flexion	Inguinal to anterior upper thigh	
L3-4	Knee extension	Anterior lower thigh and knee to medial lower leg	Knee
L5-S1	Ankle flexion, knee extension	Lateral lower leg and medial foot to sole of foot	S1-2
S1-2	Ankle extension	Sole of foot; posterior leg and thigh	
S3-4	Bladder and anal	Perineum and buttocks function	Anal wink

From Ichord RN (1997). The nervous system. In Seidel HM, Rosenstein BJ, Pathak A, editors. Primary care of the newborn, ed 2, St Louis: Mosby-Year Book, p. 162.

Table **17-6**	Functional Prognosis in Myelomeningocele with Optimal Aggressive Management
Motor Level	**Prognosis**
Above L3	Mostly wheelchair bound
L4-S1	Partial ambulation with assistive devices
Below S1	Ambulate without assistance

From Ichord RN (1997). The nervous system. In Seidel HM, Rosenstein BJ, Pathak A, editors. Primary care of the newborn, ed 2, St Louis: Mosby-Year Book, p. 163.

BIBLIOGRAPHY

Amess PN, et al. (1999). Early brain proton magnetic resonance spectroscopy and neonatal neurology related to neurodevelopmental outcome at 1 year in term infants after presumed hypoxic-ischaemic brain injury. *Developmental medicine in child neurology*, 41(7), 436-445.

Amiel-Tison C (1998). Clinical neurology in neonatal units. *Croatian medical journal*, 39(2), 136-146.

Blackburn S (2003). Assessment and management of the neurologic system. In Kenner C, Lott JW, editors. *Comprehensive neonatal nursing: a physiologic perspective*, ed 3, St Louis: WB Saunders.

Krageloh-Mann I, et al. (1999). Brain lesions in preterms: origin, consequences and compensation, *Acta paediatrics*, 88(8), 897-908.

Whitelaw A (2001). Postnatal phenobarbitone for the prevention of intraventricular hemorrhage in preterm infants. *Cochrane database systematic reviews*, 1.

Wildrick D (1997). Intraventricular hemorrhage and long-term outcome in the premature infant. *Journal of neuroscience nursing*, 29(5), 281-289.

CHAPTER 18

DEVELOPMENTAL CARE

Developmental care is an approach that takes into consideration the macroenvironment (the unit) and the microenvironment (the environment in the immediate area of the infant). Much research is focusing on the effects of light, sound, and touch on the neonate.

LIGHTING

Premature infants are photophobic yet will open their eyes in dim lights. Lighting in most neonatal intensive care units (NICUs) is continuous, high level, and fluorescent. NICUs should provide ambient lighting at levels of 10 to 20 foot-candles. Ambient light levels need to be adjustable at each bedside (Altimier, 2003). It is recommended that the level range from 1 to 60 foot-candles (White, 2002). Procedural lighting should be used at the bedside for procedures. Bright lights in the NICU can disrupt sleep/wake states. Cycling of lights to resemble day and night will help infants adjust their sleep/wake patterns and decrease the secretion of stress hormones, such as cortisol. Windows that allow for daylight are helpful to the infant's well being and for staff as well.

SOUND

Excessive noise can damage delicate auditory structures and can have adverse physiologic effects, such as hypoxia, increased intracranial pressure, increased blood pressure, apnea, bradycardia, and color changes (Altimier, 2003). Sound levels in the NICU have ranged up to 120 dB. Ideally noise levels should be less than 65 dB. Use of visual alarms, placing pagers on vibrate, no overhead paging, and use of acoustical ceiling tiles are all strategies for reducing noise.

DEVELOPMENTAL CARE APPROACHES

The approach to the immediate environment of the infant means assessment of potential noxious stimuli. Just as light and sound have been noted to have adverse effects on heart rate, respiratory rate, and arterial saturations, so has the way we approach our care. Taking vital signs off a monitor may reduce the number of times that an infant is touched, allowing more time for sleep. Moving toward cue-based care or increasing our awareness of stress signals will dictate how and when we touch, move, and do certain procedures. Pain medications and comfort measures are important to providing developmentally appropriate care. Cluster procedures and treatments are a good idea as long as the rule of thumb is to assess the infant's response and, when stress signals or vital signs including oxygen saturations begin to drop or change, to recognize that "enough is enough." Use of nonnutritive sucking is another way to soothe an infant and evokes comfort. Use of boundaries in the bed to support positive positioning is another important aspect of developmental care.

Observe the infant for signs of stress, such as excessive crying, irritability, finger splaying, back arching, and "ooh" face. When these appear attempt to alter the environment to increase the infant's comfort and induce calm, less crying, relaxed posture, and a smiling face. Teach parents how to observe for each of these sets of cues. Help them to be a part of the developmentally supportive environment or the environment that promotes positive growth and development.

Some techniques that are associated with developmental care include co-bedding, kangaroo care, and infant massage. These techniques should be used with caution, since they need more evidence to support their incorporation into care, at least with most NICU infants. For example, co-bedding remains controversial and, to some people, even dangerous. It appears to go against some of the "back to sleep" principles. So before undertaking any of these protocols, be sure to review existing studies that have been done and consider institutional policies. Even kangaroo care, which has a long history, is not suggested for all infants. Infant massage has been linked with increased weight gains when used in stable infants, but it also has been linked to drops in heart rates and changes in oxygen saturations. More research is needed before it can be totally embraced in the NICU. Only co-bedding and kangaroo care protocols are included in this chapter.

CO-BEDDING MULTIPLES*

Infant Objectives
- To improve heart/respiratory rate, oxygen requirement, physical growth/development, and motor development in flexor and extensor patterns
- To show co-regulation and appropriate states consistent and/or interactive with each other, environment, care providers

---

*From Altimier L, Brown B, Tedeschi L (2000). Tri-Health's manual of neonatal nursing policies, procedures, competencies, & clinical pathways. Glenview, Ill: National Association of Neonatal Nurses.

Benefits
- Enhance parent/infant bonding
- Ease transition to home
- Consistency of care: same registered nurse (RN) and same physician take care of both babies

Risk
Because this new practice is emerging throughout the United States, there is no documented research to support or negate it. Risks are unknown at this time. A potential risk may be infection.

Protocols
- Infants are stable and free from infection/sepsis before being bedded together.
- Infants do not have an endotracheal tube (ETT) and are not under an oxygen hood.
- Infants are in room air or nasal cannula (NC) oxygen.
- If both infants require NC oxygen, place an emergency oxygen tank on wheels at bedside.
- Infants do not have an indwelling catheter (i.e., C-line, intravenous [IV] Heplock).
- Infants may be on cardiorespiratory monitors and/or pulse oximeters.
- Infants may be gavage feeding.
- Infants may be in cribs or Isolettes.
- If one infant requires servomechanism, put temperature probe on smallest or one with temperature instability.

Procedures
- Infection control: provide complete care for each infant before beginning care for next infant with good hand washing between. Keep equipment/supplies separate (i.e., pacifier, monitor).
- Identification: properly labeled ID bands and all equipment color coded (supplies, papers for monitor, pulse oximeter, flow meters; stethoscope, pacifiers, bulb syringe if necessary; flow sheets; etc.). Ask parent(s) to select color codes for the babies. If infants are dressed, ask parents to select colors and keep them dressed in their respective colored outfits.
- Bed side-by-side, facing each other or one another's back; if able use same position as in utero; ask parents.
- Place boundary and swaddle blanket around both of them, not individually.
- Cluster care and perform vital signs, feeding, etc. on the one that is more alert.
- If necessary to separate (i.e., one becomes unstable) call parents; separate only as long as necessary.

UNIVERSITY OF ILLINOIS MEDICAL CENTER AT CHICAGO CLINICAL CARE GUIDELINE

Subject: Kangaroo Care (Skin-to-Skin Care)*

Objective

To establish criteria and procedure for infants/families who wish to participate in kangaroo or skin-to-skin care.

Position Statements

Skin-to-skin care is a well-established practice that is supportive of both families and the infants. Most infants benefit from the warmth and tactile contact with their parent(s) and frequently demonstrate an improvement in both their behavioral and physiologic responses. This activity is one that the parents can initiate early within the hospitalization period, which thus facilitates the integration of their parental role.

Standards

The RN will ensure that parents are educated about skin-to-skin care as soon after delivery as possible, even if it will not be able to be feasible to implement it at the time because of the infant's condition.

The RN will offer skin-to-skin care to parents as soon as the infant meets the criteria and may request permission from the neonatal fellow or attending physician if the infant does not meet criteria but she/he assesses that the infant or family would benefit.

The RN will monitor the family's and infant's response to skin-to-skin care and document findings.

Because there are insufficient data to support universal skin-to-skin care for all infants, exclusionary criteria have been established in order to ensure the safety of the most fragile infants.

Infants who are **not** eligible for skin-to-skin care are the following:

1. Infants who are receiving supplemental humidity
2. Infants receiving high-frequency oscillating ventilation
3. Infants who have indwelling chest tubes
4. Infants with PPHN (persistent pulmonary hypertension)
5. Infants who are receiving paralytic agents
6. Infants receiving pressors or sedation at high levels where the transfer from the incubator to the parent's body may dangerously counteract the effect of the pressor/sedation
7. Infants with femoral or radial arterial lines
8. Infants under respiratory isolation

*From University of Illinois Medical Center at Chicago Women's and Children's Nursing Services. Used with permission by Dharmapuri Vidyasagar, MD; Catherine Theorell, RNC, MSN, NNP; Beena Peters, RN, MS.

9. Infants who are diagnosed with NEC (necrotizing enterocolitis), have open abdominal wounds, or have suspicious abdominal distention
10. Infants with gastroschisis/omphalocele that has not been fully reduced

Procedures

1. The RN/care coordinator/developmentalist will educate parents about skin-to-skin care in the first days of life.
2. When the infant is physiologically able to be placed skin-to-skin, the RN will offer the experience to the parents, explaining the need for their cooperation in the following: wearing appropriate clothing (shirt that buttons down in front or hospital gown) and staying at least 1 hour with infant.
3. Recliner or rocking chair should be brought to the bedside.
4. Infant is dressed only in a diaper and hat.
5. Infant's temperature is taken before removing from the bed. If below 98° F, measures will be taken to warm the infant before transfer.
6. Infant is moved so that he/she is placed vertically on the parent's chest.
7. After the infant is placed on chest, his/her back is covered with the parent's shirt and one or two blankets.
8. If infant is transferred from the incubator, the temperature control should be set to "air" and the control temperature should be the current incubator ambient temperature. If the infant has a skin temperature probe on, this should remain on, so that the current skin temperature can be easily monitored.
9. If infant is intubated, solicit the help of another nurse or respiratory therapist.
10. One person will be responsible for the patient, IV lines, and monitoring cables; the other is responsible for the ventilator tubing.
11. Infant can be transferred with parent standing or sitting. If standing, one nurse will disconnect the infant from the ventilator and manage the IV lines and cables while the parent lifts the baby to her chest; the other nurse will move the ventilator tubing out of the incubator and bring to the baby. The parent will then be assisted to sit in the chair. If the parent is sitting, one nurse will disconnect the infant from the ventilator, pick up the baby, IV lines, and cables, and carry to the parent, while the other nurse manages the ventilator tubing.
12. When infant is transferred back, two people again will be needed, one to help the parent out of the chair and one to guard the endotracheal tube (ETT) and lines. The parent can help contain the infant in the incubator while the others work to secure the lines, tubing, and cables.

13. Infants should be encouraged to suck at the breast while the mother is performing skin-to-skin care. If the mother is expressing milk, she should be encouraged to pump after skin-to-skin care, because this helps stimulate her milk supply.

14. All mothers who are having trouble establishing or maintaining their milk supply should be encouraged to perform skin-to-skin care every time they are with their baby.

15. The infant's temperature should be taken with the thermometer 1 hour after transfer. If over 99.2° F, remove a blanket. If the temperature has decreased more than 1° F, discontinue skin-to-skin care.

16. The RN should document the following in Gemini (computer system) and daily flow sheets:

    a. The initial education concerning skin-to-skin care in Gemini (computer system)

    b. Who performed skin-to-skin and for what time period on the daily flow sheet

    c. The infant's behavioral responses before, during, and after skin-to-skin care

    d. Any complications or problems encountered during the skin-to-skin care

    e. Parental reaction

Table 18-1 gives categories of kangaroo care.

BIBLIOGRAPHY: FURTHER READINGS ON KANGAROO CARE

Anderson GC, Dombrowski MAS, Swinth JY (2001). Kangaroo care: it's not just for stable preemies anymore. *Reflections on nursing scholarship*, 27, 32-34, 45.

Dombrowski MA, et al. (2001). Kangaroo (skin-to-skin) care with a postpartum woman who felt depressed. MCN. *The American journal of maternal child nursing*, 26(4):214-216.

Dombrowski MA, et al. (2000). Kangaroo (skin-to-skin) for premature twins and their adolescent parents. MCN. *The American journal of maternal child nursing*, 25, 92-94.

POSITIVE TOUCH AND INFANT MASSAGE

The following two guidelines for touch and infant massage were developed by the Infant Massage Interest Group (Northern and Yorkshire Region), United Kingdom. Again, although these are included in this section of the book there is need for more research to determine when infant massage is safely done. The infant's gestational age, severity of illness, and stability must be considered.

Positive Touch and Containment Holds
Aim   This section provides a description and rationale for containment holds. These are designed to be used where massage is not

Table **18-1**	Categories of Kangaroo Care (KC)
Category	**Description**
Late KC (LK)	Begins when the infant is relatively stable, usually breathing room air and almost ready to go home This can be days or weeks after birth. Also included is the infant who has been very ill and continues to require mechanical ventilation.
Intermediate K (IK)	Usually begins 1 wk or more after birth, when the infant has completed the early intensive care phase but usually still needs oxygen and probably has some apnea and bradycardia. Also included are weak preterm infants who are placed at the breast during gavage feedings and infants who are easily stabilized on mechanical ventilation.
Early (EK)	Begins as soon after birth as the infant is stable and breathing room air, usually during the first week and sometimes later during the first day.
Very early K (VEK)	Begins in the delivery room usually between 30 and 40 min after birth. In this category the mother helps to stabilize her infant during the process of adaptation to extrauterine life.
Birth K (BK)	The infant is returned to the mother during the first minute after birth for her assistance with stabilization. If the mother is lying down, the infant is simply placed prone on her abdomen with its face near her breast; if the mother has given birth in a semisquatting position, she sits cross-legged and picks her infant up and holds the infant, again prone on her abdomen and chest with the infant's face near her breasts.

From Dr. Gene Cranston Anderson, Case Western Reserve University, Cleveland, Ohio August 2002.
Note: Infants who require mechanical ventilation can be in LK, IK, or EK, depending on how soon KC begins after birth. Ideally all full-term infants, if reasonably healthy (1-minute Apgar >6), would receive BK or at least VEK; in either category the infant is gently dried, a warm blanket is placed across the infant's back (never between the mother and the infant), and the infant wears a cap that is replaced with a dry one as soon as it becomes damp. Both methods have been done successfully with reasonably healthy 34- to 36-week infants and full-term infants.

Table 18-2	Positive Touch

Action	Rationale
1. Assess the needs of the neonate and family; do not disturb the baby if sleeping.	Touch must be adapted to the individual infant's behavior and physiologic responses and medical condition and also the family's needs.
2. Explain to the parents the indications for "positive touch" and the benefits for baby and parents.	Touch helps reduce stress by calming the infant and promotes sleep and parental attachment and involvement.
3. Wash hands and remove jewelry before beginning positive touch.	This minimizes the risk of infection and reduces the risk of abrasions from jewelry.
4. Consider the environment, and where possible shade the baby's face from the light and turn down alarm settings (decibels).	A beneficial environment helps eliminate stress.
5. Request baby's permission to be touched.	This enables the baby to prepare and become aware of the beginning of positive loving touch.
6. Begin with still touch, one hand on head and one on trunk.	Simple introduction of containment holding assists babies in organizing their behavior.

Continued

Table 18-2	Positive Touch—cont'd
Action	**Rationale**
7. When moving from one hold to the next move one hand at a time and remain in contact with baby throughout. Small, premature, or sensitive babies may need to be kept covered with clothes or a blanket.	This prevents loss of contact and makes the baby feel secure at all times.
8. Continue the hold as long as the baby will allow, observing cues throughout.	Allow the baby to communicate with parents through positive behavior and eye contact. This promotes bonding and empowers parents to be involved in the baby's development.
9. Evaluate containment/positive touch in care plan.	This ensures individualized care has been given and provides a rationale for the way the baby is positioned at that time.

From Wall A (2002). . Agreeing a standard for infant massage: not a soft touch. Journal of neonatal nursing, 8(3), 93-96.

Table 18-3	Infant Massage
Action	**Rationale**
1. Assess the needs of the neonate, talk to parents about relaxation, and practice some simple exercises and visualization.	It is essential that parents understand their role in massage. Infants can sense if someone is feeling tense. Parents are mirrors for their babies, and massage offers parents the opportunity to give themselves some attention.
2. Wash hands and remove jewelry before beginning massage.	Even though you may not be undertaking the massage this sets a good example for parents.
3. Consider the environment, and where possible shade the baby's face from the light and turn down alarm settings (decibels).	A beneficial environment helps eliminate stress.
4. Request baby's permission to begin.	This lets the baby know that a new experience is about to begin and helps the infant to prepare for it. It also communicates respect.
5. Point out various behavioral states to parents (e.g., waking activity, fussing, crying). Ask parents to observe their baby and note sleep/wake cycles.	This helps parents discover the best massage time for their baby. Best stage for massage is the quiet alert state, being mindful of the ward environment.
6. Teach the parent massage strokes by demonstration on soft doll. Demonstrate the series of strokes, instructing verbally as progressing. Teach parents to read cues.	Parents can massage with you or watch first, depending on preference. This empowers parents to massage when they feel ready and makes them feel that they are doing something of value for their baby.

Continued

Table 18-3	Infant Massage—cont'd

Action	Rationale
7. Teach touch relaxation for the parent to condition baby to respond to touch and voice with relaxation.	Touch relaxation is positive reinforcement.
8. Encourage parents to continue to offer massage to baby throughout childhood.	This makes parents aware of techniques that are best for each stage of development.
9. Work within the multidisciplinary team to promote infant massage within a safe environment.	Safety should be maintained at all times, and it is important that your colleagues are aware of what is being done.
10. Provide information of how massage can benefit the individual child.	This provides parents with sound knowledge base of why they are providing massage.
11. Evaluate results of massage, and document in care plan.	This provides continuity of care.

From Wall A (2002). Agreeing on a standard for infant massage: not a soft touch. Journal of neonatal nursing, 8(3), 93-96.

appropriate for whatever reason and are applied with no pressure, with the hands resting on the baby. Although ideally this touch is done by parents, all staff members should be encouraged to use it for settling, for calming, or during procedures.

Objective Positive touch (Table 18-2) is a medium for establishing a working relationship with the family; it is infant led and parent directed and is an integral part of a family-centered developmental care program.

Infant Massage, Preterm and Term

Aim This section introduces massage to parents/caregivers of hospitalized infants. This protocol also acknowledges the existence of appropriate and inappropriate touch.

Objective The objective of infant massage is to reduce stress and the effects of separation. Table 18-3 gives the steps in infant massage and the rationale for each step.

BIBLIOGRAPHY

Altimier L (2001). High-tech, high-touch care. *Nursing management*, 32(7), 40-43.

Altimier L (2003). Managing the NICU environment. In Kenner C, Lott JW, editors. *Comprehensive neonatal nursing: a physiologic perspective*, ed 3, St Louis: WB Saunders.

Altimier L, Lutes L (2000). Changing units for changing times: the evolution of a NICU. *Neonatal intensive care*, 13(6), 23-27.

Altimier L, et al. (1999). Value study. *Neonatal network*, 8(4), 35-38.

American Society of Heating, Refrigerating, and Air-Conditioning Engineers (1995). Sound and vibration control. In *ASHRAE handbook*, Atlanta: American Society of Heating, Refrigerating, and Air-Conditioning Engineers.

American Society for Testing and Materials (1992). *Standard definitions of terms relating to environmental acoustics*. *Publication ASTM C-634*, Philadelphia: American Society for Testing and Materials.

DellaPorta, K, Aforismo D, Butler-O'Hara M (1998). Co-bedding of twins in the neonatal intensive care unit. *Pediatric nursing*, 24(6), 529-531.

Gorga MP, et al. (2000). Identification of neonatal hearing impairment: distortion product otoacoustic emissions during the perinatal period. *Early hearing*, 21(5), 400-424.

Graven SN (2000). Sound and the developing infant in the NICU: conclusions and recommendations for care. *Journal of perinatology*, 20(8 Pt 2), S88-S93.

Gray JE, et al. (2000). Baby CareLink: using the internet and telemedicine to improve care for high-risk infants. *Pediatrics*, 106(6), 1318-1324.

Mishoe SC, et al. (1995). Octave waveband analysis to determine sound frequencies and intensities produced by nebulizers and humidifiers used with hoods. *Respiratory care*, 40(11), 1120-1124.

Norton SJ, et al. (2000). Identification of neonatal hearing impairment: transient evoked otoacoustic emissions during the perinatal period. *Early hearing*, 21(5), 425-442.

Oelberg DG, et al. (1999). Contribution of heating, ventilation, and air conditioning airflow and conversation to the ambient sound in a neonatal intensive care unit. *Journal of perinatology*, 19(5), 362-366.

Simpson D (2000). Transitional care for neonates. *Practical midwife*, 3(2), 13-15.

Sininger YS, et al. (2000). Identification of neonatal hearing impairment: auditory brain stem responses in the perinatal period. *Early hearing*, 21(5), 383-399.

Slevin M, et al. (2000). Altering the NICU and measuring infants' responses. *Acta paediatrica*, 89(5), 577-581.

Stevens B, Gibbins S, Franck LS (2000). Treatment of pain in the neonatal intensive care unit. *Pediatric clinics of North America*, 47(3), 633-650.

Symington A, Pinelli J (2000). Developmental care for promoting development and preventing morbidity in preterm infants. *Cochrane database systematic reviews*, 4.

Symington A, Pinelli J (2001). Developmental care for promoting development and preventing morbidity in preterm infants. *Cochrane review, Cochrane database systematic reviews*, 4.

Thomas KA, Martin PA (2000). NICU sound environment and the potential problems for caregivers. *Journal of perinatology*, 20(8 Pt 2), S94-S99.

Walsh-Sukys M, et al. (2001). Reducing light and sound in the neonatal intensive care unit: an evaluation of patient safety, staff satisfaction and costs. *Journal of perinatology*, 21(4), 230-235.

White R (2002). Recommended standards for newborn ICU design. Report of the Fifth Consensus Conference by the Committee to Establish Recommended Standards for Newborn ICU Design. Hyperlink: http://www.nd.edu/nkkblberg/designstandards.htm

DISCHARGE PLANNING/COORDINATION OF HOME CARE

Discharge planning and coordination of home care services require anticipation of the family and health care needs of the newborn. Depending on their geographic location, financial status, insurance status, and social support network, the discharge can be traumatic. This chapter offers several guidelines and clinical pathways that will assist with this process. We have included a parental stress instrument developed by Dr. Margaret Miles who has worked with parents of neonatal intensive care unit (NICU) graduates for many years. You may want to use this instrument as a guide to consider how to help alleviate parental stress before the infant's discharge. To ease the transition home, parent teaching and preparation are a cornerstone of nursing interventions at this time. We have included a guideline for transitional care in the hospital by parents. Although we espouse that parents are not visitors in the NICU, many parents, until close to discharge, still feel that way. Helping parents take over the primary care responsibilities before discharge is important to successful transition home. Teaching tools are offered that were published in the National Association of Neonatal Nurses (NANN)'s official journal, *Advances in Neonatal Care*. Finally, car seat safety is a "hot topic" when it comes to the trip home. A guideline is included on this topic.

UNIVERSITY OF ILLINOIS MEDICAL CENTER AT CHICAGO CLINICAL CARE GUIDELINE

Subject: Care-by-Parent and Extended/Overnight Stays in the Parent's Room*

Objectives

- To facilitate the transition from the NICU/intermediate care nursery (ICN) to home, parents are encouraged to provide an extended period of care to their child. This period of care-by-parent may also include an overnight stay of the family in the Parent Room.
- To provide support and to reinforce parental knowledge of the home care instructions and equipment while the infant is still hospitalized.

*From University of Illinois Medical Center at Chicago Women's and Children's Nursing Services. Used with permission by Dharmapuri Vidyasagar, MD; Catherine Theorell, RNC, MSN, NNP; Beena Peters, RN, MS.

- To ensure the physical well-being of the infant during the period of time during care-by-parent.

Definitions

For the purposes of this guideline, the following definitions apply:

Care-By-Parent—The period of time when the parent(s) stay in the Parent Room with their infant and provide for their infant's health care needs in preparation for discharge.

Extended or Overnight Stays—Before discharge, parent(s) are encouraged to provide for their infant's care for extended periods of time that may include care throughout the night.

Position Statements

The infant's assigned nurse will monitor the status of the infant and the care provided by the parent(s) during the extended or overnight stays.

The nurse shall oversee the parent(s) administering all medications to ensure proper administration.

Procedure

1. The Parent Room will be reserved for extended or overnight stays by signing out the time period on the calendar placed on the door of the room.
2. The parents will receive a copy of the extended or overnight stay guidelines at the time the appointment is arranged.
3. Before the extended or overnight stay, the parent(s) will do the following:
   a. Be instructed on the use of home equipment and cardiopulmonary resuscitation (CPR) by the respiratory therapist from the equipment vendor
   b. Demonstrate the safe operation of that equipment
4. The nurse shall ensure that the electrical equipment has hospital-grade plugs and has been checked by clinical engineering services for electrical safety.
5. The nurse will discuss the following with parent(s):
   a. Their role in assuming caretaking tasks for the period of time
   b. The role of the nurse and the schedule of nursing checks of the infant and parent throughout the period
   c. The use of the emergency red phone
6. The nurse will fully assess all infants when initially moved into the Parent Room. Subsequent assessments will proceed as follows:
   a. Monitored and/or oxygen-dependent infants will be assessed every 3 to 4 hours.
   b. Infants not requiring special equipment for home will be assessed every 4 to 6 hours.
7. The nurse shall document the following in the medical record:

a. The initial infant assessment and vital signs before the care-by-parent
b. Subsequent infant assessments during the care-by-parent
c. Assessment of parent(s)/infant interaction and parent(s') care-taking abilities
d. Summary of the care provided by the parent(s) throughout the stay
e. Additional teaching or coaching provided to the parent(s)

UNIVERSITY OF ILLINOIS MEDICAL CENTER AT CHICAGO CLINICAL CARE GUIDELINE

Subject: Discharge Planning Guideline for Infants with a History of a Recent Significant Cardiopulmonary Event (SCPE)*

Objective

To provide some guidelines in determining which infants can be safely discharged home, after having a recent history (<2 weeks) of a SCPE.

Definitions

Significant cardiopulmonary event is defined as follows:

1. Documented apnea of 20 seconds or longer as recorded through electronic monitoring
2. Bradycardia of less than 80 beats/min for at least 5 seconds
3. Oxygen desaturation of less than 85% for at least 5 seconds that requires stimulation to bring to baseline

Position Statement

There is no universally accepted standard for a "safe, apnea-free" interval; and practice varies tremendously among neonatologists. The published studies are few, and some of these are not scientifically rigorous and therefore may not stand the test of time. Both the general well-being of the infant and the family's ability to care for the infant are key to appropriate decision making. A thorough assessment of the family's home situation, support systems, and competence in caring for the infant must be done and documented. It is important for parents to be fully informed about the risks. Preterm infants are inherently susceptible to unexpected life-threatening events, and these guidelines cannot guarantee that there will not be adverse outcomes. However, if exceptions are made to these guidelines, the rationale for the exception should be carefully documented.

*From University of Illinois Medical Center at Chicago Women's and Children's Nursing Services. Used with permission by Dharmapuri Vidyasagar, MD; Catherine Theorell, RNC, MSN, NNP; Beena Peters, RN, MS.

Standards

1. Premature infants with a previous history of SCPE and planned to be discharged to home *without* medications or home oxygen:
   a. Infants not currently receiving medications shall wait for an 8-day period and be free from a SCPE.
   b. Infants taking methylxanthines or caffeine that is about to be discontinued shall wait for 2 days after the last dose of the drug for serum levels to drop and then wait an additional 8 days to be monitored for any SCPE.
2. For premature infants with a history of SCPE for whom an earlier discharge is being contemplated:
   a. Arrange for a home monitor, and train the caregiver in infant CPR.
   b. Do not discharge until there has been at least a 48-hour period that has been SCPE-free.
   c. For infants going home on drug therapy, a predischarge serum drug level shall be obtained so that drug therapy may be adjusted if needed. After drug doses or schedules have been adjusted, consider obtaining another serum drug level to ensure that a therapeutic drug level has been achieved. The infant can then be discharged after a period of 48 hours if free from any SCPE.
3. Nursing assessment is key in determining if an SCPE event has occurred, its clinical significance, and the impact this may have on the timing of discharge.
   a. Nursing will record on the apnea/bradycardia flow sheet all events as follows:
      (1) Where there is a breathing pause of at least 20 seconds or shorter pauses that result in bradycardia or desaturation
      (2) Bradycardias of less than 80 beats/min that last longer than 5 seconds or are accompanied by color change, change in muscle tone, or drop in oxygen saturation
      (3) Spontaneous desaturations requiring intervention to relieve
   b. There are many iatrogenic instances of bradycardia/desaturations, for example, during suctioning or during PO (by mouth) feeding in an infant whose feeding skills are still immature. Infants may also have Valsalva responses that cause transient bradycardia but are not clinically significant.
   c. In an effort to make clearer the distinction between SCPEs that are significant in regard to discharge planning and events that are transient or a result of care practices in the NICU, only those events listed in 3.a above should be recorded on the apnea/bradycardia flow record. An overall summary of other events should be provided in a narrative note in the flow sheet, as a behavioral summary of the infant's reactions to care and environment.

4. Parent education. Parents of all infants who have a history of SCPE should receive the following:
   a. Information on the procedure for infant resuscitation
   b. Information on behavioral signs of SCPE: color change, breathing pauses, limpness in tone
   c. Educational information for when and how to call paramedics
   d. Inquiry to ensure that family has access to a telephone

Procedure

1. Shift-to-shift nursing report will indicate if the infant may be discharged in the next 10 days, the current use of methylxanthine therapy or the date of its discontinuation, and the date of last apnea, bradycardia.
2. Nursing will ensure that all clinically significant apnea and bradycardia is recorded on the apnea/bradycardia flow sheet and reports of any changes are made to the primary physician in a timely fashion.
3. Behavioral patterns of the infant that result in apnea/bradycardia/desaturations will also be reported in shift-to-shift report so that appropriate adjustments in nursing care or environment may be tried to help regulate the infant.
4. Nursing will begin to review with parents the emergency interventions for their infants at least 1 week before discharge.

BIBLIOGRAPHY

American Academy of Pediatrics (AAP) (1998). *Hospital discharge of the high-risk neonate: proposed guidelines.* Elk Grove Village, Ill: AAP.

Eichenwald EC, Aina A, Stark AR (1997). Apnea frequently persists beyond term gestation in infants delivered at 24-28 weeks. *Pediatrics,* 100, 354-259.

Eichenwald EC, et al. (2001). Inter-neonatal intensive care unit variation in discharge timing: influence of apnea and feeding management. *Pediatrics,* 108, 928-933.

FAMILY TEACHING TOOLS

Figure 19-1 shows a teaching guide for safe sleep from *Advances in neonatal care* (ANC), Figure 19-2 shows an ANC teaching guide for newborn jaundice, Figure 19-3 is a parent's guide for advocacy and involvement, and Figure 19-4 is a teaching guide for immunizations.

The following are examples of tools that can be used to work with families in planning the infant's discharge and follow up. These tools provide excellent guidelines for nurses to follow with parents and are easy to understand and can be shared with parents.

The ANC teaching tools are a public service of ANC. The information and recommendations appearing on these pages are appropriate in most instances but are not a substitute for individualized health advice and care. For specific information about your infant's medical condition, ANC suggests that you consult your licensed health care provider. This page may be downloaded from www.advancesinneonatalcare.org and reproduced noncommercially by health care providers to share with infant caregivers. Any other reproduction is subject to NANN approval. To purchase bulk reprints contact 215-238-5534.*

A TEACHING GUIDE FOR SAFE SLEEP

Nursing Actions	Teaching Tips for Ensuring Safe Sleep	Demonstrates Understanding	Needs Further Review	Date/ Initial
Initiate Teaching at 30-32 Weeks PCA Target date: Back to sleep initiated: CPR scheduled: CPR complete:	**General Teaching Guidelines** ❏ Place your baby on his or her back to sleep, both at nighttime and naptime. Babies who sleep on their back have the lowest SIDS risk. ❏ Some parents choose to use side sleeping. Side sleeping is not as safe as back sleeping, although it is safer than putting your baby on his or her tummy. ❏ If side sleeping is used, bring the lower arm forward to lessen the likelihood of rolling. ❏ Never place a baby on a waterbed, sofa, soft mattress, or any other soft surfaces for sleep.			
Feet-to-Foot Placement in the Crib FIGURE 1. Infant tucked in "feet-to-foot" style to avoid risk of suffocation or rebreathing. Note the safe crib environment: absence of blankets, pillows, and bumper pads, all showing a safe sleep environment. (Courtesy of The National Institute for Child Health and Development.)	**Crib & Bedding Safety** ❏ Place your baby on a firm mattress that fits firmly into a safety-approved crib. Check with the Consumer Product Safety Commission to be certain a used crib has not been recalled. www.cpsc.gov/CPSCPUB/PUBS/cribsafe.html ❏ Remove all fluffy and loose bedding from the sleep area. No pillows, quilts, comforters, or sheepskins should be placed under or around a sleeping infant. Do not drape quilts over the top of the crib. ❏ Keep all objects out of the infant's sleep environment. Blankets, if used, should be tucked in around the crib mattress so the baby's face is less likely to be covered. ❏ Wedges and positioning devices, sold at many baby stores, have not been tested and are **not recommended**. Polyurethane and foam positioning devices may also contribute to overheating and should be avoided. ❏ Make sure your baby's face and head stay uncovered during sleep. "Feet to foot" refers to having the infant's feet able to touch the foot of the bed with the blankets tucked in around the crib mattress and only reaching the infant's chest. ❏ Another option, to avoid the risk of blankets, is to use sleep clothing with no other covering over the infant.			

FIGURE **19-1**

Nursing Actions	Teaching Tips for Ensuring Safe Sleep	Demonstrates Understanding	Needs Further Review	Date/ Initial
	Babies Should Sleep Alone			
	❑ Babies should not sleep with adults, siblings, or others.			
	❑ Adult beds are not designed for babies. Do not take your baby to bed with you. Adult beds have many risks for suffocation (comforters, pillows, soft mattresses). There is also a risk that your baby could become trapped between the headboard and wall, or under an adult body.			
	❑ A safe alternative is to move your baby's crib into your room.			
	Avoid Overheating			
Supervised Tummy Time	❑ Do not let your baby overheat during sleep. Lightly clothe the infant for sleep. Avoid over-wrapping.			
	Avoid Smoke and Irritants			
	❑ Do not smoke before or after the birth of your baby. Protect your baby from passive smoke from others.			
FIGURE 2. Placing your baby on his/her tummy will help build a strong upper body and encourage crawling. (Courtesy of The National Institute for Child Health and Development.)	❑ Avoid other items that might irritate your baby's air passages, such as candles, incense, or wood-burning stoves.			
	Provide Supervised Tummy Time			
	❑ Supervised tummy time is recommended while your baby is awake. This will help the baby develop upper body muscles and learn to crawl. It will also help prevent head flattening.			
	Tell Others About Back to Sleep			
	❑ Remind friends, grandparents, day care providers, baby-sitters, and anyone who cares for your baby about the importance of Back to Sleep for the entire first year of life.			
	Individualized Teaching Points:			
	❑ ❑ ❑ ❑			
	Local Emergency Numbers			

FIGURE **19-1, cont'd**
Teaching guide for safe sleep. (From Gracey K [2001]. Family teaching toolbox. *Advances in neonatal care*, 1[2], 115-116.)

UNIVERSITY OF ILLINOIS MEDICAL CENTER AT CHICAGO CLINICAL CARE GUIDELINE

Subject: Discharge Planning of Premature Infants—Car Seat Safety*

Objectives

- To comply with Illinois state law, all infants who are transported in motorized vehicles must be secured in a federally approved,

From University of Illinois Medical Center at Chicago Women's and Children's Nursing Services. Used with permission by Dharmapuri Vidyasagar, MD; Catherine Theorell, RNC, MSN, NNP; Beena Peters, RN, MS.

crash-tested infant passenger restraint device that has been properly secured in the vehicle.

- To ensure that any premature infant, who at the time of discharge is less than 37 weeks' corrected gestational age, tolerates being positioned in a car seat without experiencing apnea, bradycardia, and desaturations.

NEWBORN JAUNDICE

Identified Risk Factors:	Basic Facts About Jaundice
_____	• Jaundice is a yellowish or orange color of the skin. Jaundice is very common. It happens in 2 out of 3 newborns.
_____	• Jaundice is caused by the breakdown of red blood cells. Old red blood cells release a chemical called bilirubin. It is the liver's job to remove bilirubin from the blood so the body can get rid of it. Bilirubin is normally removed from the body in the bowel movements. If it is not removed, bilirubin finds its way to the skin and stays there, causing the yellow color called jaundice.
	• Babies are born with extra red blood cells that their bodies don't need anymore. Breaking down all these red blood cells releases a lot of bilirubin. Babies with bruising have extra cells to remove from the body, so they are at higher risk for jaundice.
TcB measurement using the BiliChek.	• It takes a few days for your baby's liver to be ready for the job of removing extra bilirubin from the blood. The liver of a premature baby has an even tougher job of removing bilirubin. Babies born just a few weeks early are more likely to become jaundiced.
Bilirubin level or TcB	• Sometimes a baby's blood type is different from its mother's blood. In this case, the baby's red blood cells are breaking down even faster than usual. Jaundice in these babies often shows up in the first day or two of life.
_____	**Risk Factors for Jaundice**
Follow-up bilirubin scheduled	• Prematurity (babies born 2 weeks or more before their due date)
_____	• A brother or sister who had jaundice
Follow-up appointment	• Breastfeeding
_____	• Babies with bruising from the birth process
Lactation Resources	• Babies born with the help of a vacuum
_____	**Significance of Jaundice**
_____	• Most jaundice in healthy babies is not serious and does not require treatment. It usually gets worse for several days, reaching its peak on the fourth or fifth day of life. After that the yellow color fades a little each day.
	• Jaundice can become harmful if the bilirubin level in the baby's blood is too high. Extremely high levels can harm the brain and cause hearing loss.
	• The only way to know the bilirubin level is to test the baby's blood. Even if one bilirubin test is normal, your baby's jaundice can still worsen after you go home.
	• Parents often ask, "What is a normal bilirubin level?" It depends how old the baby is, and how fast the bilirubin is rising. A level that is considered normal when a baby is 3 days old might be too high at 1 day of age.

ANC
Journal of the National Association of Neonatal Nurses
Patient Copy

FIGURE **19-2**

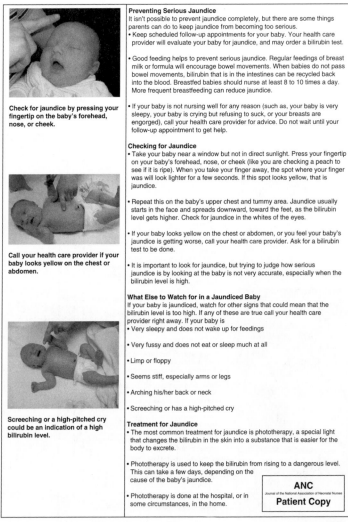

Preventing Serious Jaundice
It isn't possible to prevent jaundice completely, but there are some things parents can do to keep jaundice from becoming too serious.
• Keep scheduled follow-up appointments for your baby. Your health care provider will evaluate your baby for jaundice, and may order a bilirubin test.

• Good feeding helps to prevent serious jaundice. Regular feedings of breast milk or formula will encourage bowel movements. When babies do not pass bowel movements, bilirubin that is in the intestines can be recycled back into the blood. Breastfed babies should nurse at least 8 to 10 times a day. More frequent breastfeeding can reduce jaundice.

• If your baby is not nursing well for any reason (such as, your baby is very sleepy, your baby is crying but refusing to suck, or your breasts are engorged), call your health care provider for advice. Do not wait until your follow-up appointment to get help.

Checking for Jaundice
• Take your baby near a window but not in direct sunlight. Press your fingertip on your baby's forehead, nose, or cheek (like you are checking a peach to see if it is ripe). When you take your finger away, the spot where your finger was will look lighter for a few seconds. If this spot looks yellow, that is jaundice.

• Repeat this on the baby's upper chest and tummy area. Jaundice usually starts in the face and spreads downward, toward the feet, as the bilirubin level gets higher. Check for jaundice in the whites of the eyes.

• If your baby looks yellow on the chest or abdomen, or you feel your baby's jaundice is getting worse, call your health care provider. Ask for a bilirubin test to be done.

• It is important to look for jaundice, but trying to judge how serious jaundice is by looking at the baby is not very accurate, especially when the bilirubin level is high.

What Else to Watch for in a Jaundiced Baby
If your baby is jaundiced, watch for other signs that could mean that the bilirubin level is too high. If any of these are true call your health care provider right away. If your baby is
• Very sleepy and does not wake up for feedings

• Very fussy and does not eat or sleep much at all

• Limp or floppy

• Seems stiff, especially arms or legs

• Arching his/her back or neck

• Screeching or has a high-pitched cry

Treatment for Jaundice
• The most common treatment for jaundice is phototherapy, a special light that changes the bilirubin in the skin into a substance that is easier for the body to excrete.

• Phototherapy is used to keep the bilirubin from rising to a dangerous level. This can take a few days, depending on the cause of the baby's jaundice.

• Phototherapy is done at the hospital, or in some circumstances, in the home.

ANC
Journal of the National Association of Neonatal Nurses
Patient Copy

Photo captions:
Check for jaundice by pressing your fingertip on the baby's forehead, nose, or cheek.

Call your health care provider if your baby looks yellow on the chest or abdomen.

Screeching or a high-pitched cry could be an indication of a high bilirubin level.

FIGURE **19-2, cont'd**
Teaching guide for newborn jaundice. (From Gracey K [2002]. Family teaching toolbox, *Advances in neonatal care*, 2[2],115-116.)

Position Statement

Motor vehicle accidents are a leading cause of injury and fatality for children. Car seats have been very effective in preventing injury, and mandatory restraint laws have contributed to the decline in fatality rates. However, premature infants have special needs because of their size and immature muscle tone development, which place them at higher risk for airway obstruction and respiratory compromise while being in the semiupright position that a car seat demands. The American Academy of Pediatrics has recommended that all premature infants less than 37 weeks' gestational age be tested for tolerance to car seat use.

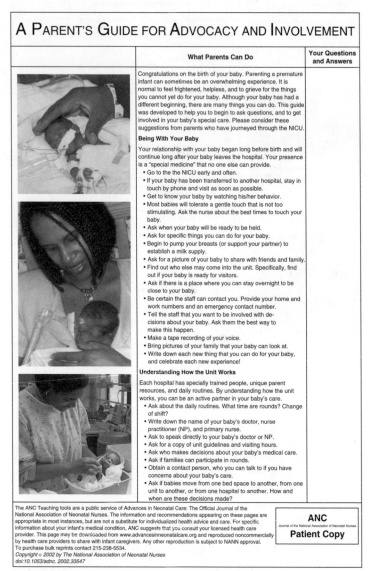

A PARENT'S GUIDE FOR ADVOCACY AND INVOLVEMENT

	What Parents Can Do	Your Questions and Answers
	Congratulations on the birth of your baby. Parenting a premature infant can sometimes be an overwhelming experience. It is normal to feel frightened, helpless, and to grieve for the things you cannot yet do for your baby. Although your baby has had a different beginning, there are many things you can do. This guide was developed to help you to begin to ask questions, and to get involved in your baby's special care. Please consider these suggestions from parents who have journeyed through the NICU.	

Being With Your Baby

Your relationship with your baby began long before birth and will continue long after your baby leaves the hospital. Your presence is a "special medicine" that no one else can provide.
- Go to the the NICU early and often.
- If your baby has been transferred to another hospital, stay in touch by phone and visit as soon as possible.
- Get to know your baby by watching his/her behavior.
- Most babies will tolerate a gentle touch that is not too stimulating. Ask the nurse about the best times to touch your baby.
- Ask when your baby will be ready to be held.
- Ask for specific things you can do for your baby.
- Begin to pump your breasts (or support your partner) to establish a milk supply.
- Ask for a picture of your baby to share with friends and family.
- Find out who else may come into the unit. Specifically, find out if your baby is ready for visitors.
- Ask if there is a place where you can stay overnight to be close to your baby.
- Be certain the staff can contact you. Provide your home and work numbers and an emergency contact number.
- Tell the staff that you want to be involved with decisions about your baby. Ask them the best way to make this happen.
- Make a tape recording of your voice.
- Bring pictures of your family that your baby can look at.
- Write down each new thing that you can do for your baby, and celebrate each new experience!

Understanding How the Unit Works

Each hospital has specially trained people, unique parent resources, and daily routines. By understanding how the unit works, you can be an active partner in your baby's care.
- Ask about the daily routines. What time are rounds? Change of shift?
- Write down the name of your baby's doctor, nurse practitioner (NP), and primary nurse.
- Ask to speak directly to your baby's doctor or NP.
- Ask for a copy of unit guidelines and visiting hours.
- Ask who makes decisions about your baby's medical care.
- Ask if families can participate in rounds.
- Obtain a contact person, who you can talk to if you have concerns about your baby's care.
- Ask if babies move from one bed space to another, from one unit to another, or from one hospital to another. How and when are these decisions made?

ANC
Journal of the National Association of Neonatal Nurses
Patient Copy

FIGURE **19-3**

	What Parents Can Do	Your Questions and Answers

	• Ask what supports are available for my family? Is there any of the following:
	  ✓ Someone to talk to about stresses and coping?
	  ✓ Someone to help with breastfeeding issues?
	  ✓ Someone to help with transportation, food, insurance, and financial assistance?
	  ✓ A place to eat, drink, or nap?
	  ✓ A place for my family to gather?
	  ✓ Someone to provide child care for my other children?
	  ✓ Someone to provide religious support?
	  ✓ Someone to talk to about my baby's development?
	  ✓ Someone to help plan for coming home?
	  ✓ A parent resource library or librarian?
	  ✓ An interpreter to help with talking to staff or reading?
	  ✓ A parent support group?
	  ✓ Someone to talk to if I am feeling depressed?	

Getting and Organizing Information

You will get a great deal of complex information. It can be difficult to keep track of the details. Some days you may feel like you are getting too much information. Other days you may want to know more. Here are some tips that might help.

- Keep a journal. Bring it with you each time you visit. Write down your questions and the answers to the questions every day.
- Ask for a book about premature babies that you can buy or borrow.
- Keep a list of all of the specialists that care for your baby.
- Start a calender and binder.
- Write down important dates (appointments, immunizations, milestones), and file handouts, brochures, and information.
- If you are interested, read your baby's chart. Be certain to ask the staff to help you understand what you are reading.
- Ask to have a care conference with the health care team.
- If staff are using words or phrases that you don't understand, ask for a time out, and ask them to start over.
- Whenever possible, ask staff to write down your baby's diagnosis, medication, or other information that you want to understand better.
- Ask the nurse to review your baby's care plan.
- Ask if you can help write down your baby's likes or dislikes on the care plan.

Coping With Your Emotions and Feelings

This experience can be both the best and some days the worst experience of your life. Often men and women respond very differently, and these different responses may be stressful. You are not alone. There are many people to support you and your family.

- Identify your personal support network, and ask for help with meals, grocery shopping, transportation, child care, or emotional support.
- Spend time with your family every day, and share your feelings and concerns.
- Tell the staff directly, when you have a comment, suggestion, or concern.
- Meet with the social worker or chaplain.
- Share your thoughts, fears, hopes, and dreams with someone you trust.
- Tell the staff if you are having difficulty eating, sleeping, or think that you or your spouse might be depressed.
- If desired, contact a parent support group. There may be groups that meet locally, as well as via the Internet. Some units have "parent partners" available—parents who have had premature children and can provide support by phone or in person.

ANC

Journal of the National Association of Neonatal Nurses

Patient Copy

FIGURE **19-3, cont'd**

Parent's guide for advocacy and involvement. (From Gracey K [2002]. Family teaching toolbox, *Advances in neonatal care,* 2[3],170-171.)

A TEACHING GUIDE FOR IMMUNIZATIONS

Nursing Actions	Teaching Topic	Demonstrates or Verbalizes Understanding	Needs Further Review	Date/Initials
Initiate parent teaching at least 1 week before vaccinations **FIGURE 1.** Parents review the Vaccine Information Sheet produced by the Centers for Disease Control. **Target Date:** _____ **Discuss the need to provide cardiorespiratory monitor after vaccines?** ❑ Yes ❑ No	**Routine Vaccinations** ❑ Review the most recent 'Recommended Childhood Immunization Schedule, US, Jan–Dec of the current year. Available from http://www.cdc.gov/nip ❑ Name the different types of vaccines needed, starting with hepatitis B vaccine at birth ❑ Discuss the reasons why immunizations are important for child health ❑ Review current Vaccine Information Sheets (VIS) for each vaccine • Hepatitis B vaccine • DTaP Vaccine • IPV Vaccine • Pneumococcal Vaccine (PCV-7) • Hib Vaccine Available from http://www.cdc.gov/nip. Additional languages available from http://www.immunize.org ❑ Request more information on vaccines as needed. • Consider AAP information (www.aap.org) 'Why Should I Immunize My Child?'; • supplemental information from the CDC; • www.immunize.org: Questions Parents Ask about Immunizations pamphlet			
FIGURE 2. One strategy for preventing colds and influenza is to use good handwashing.	**Preventing Viruses Using Special Vaccines** ❑ Verbalizes strategies for preventing colds and influenza • Use good handwashing • Avoid crowds • Keep sick people away from your baby • Do not smoke around your baby • Wash toys, clothes and bedding frequently ❑ Influenza Vaccine Check with your primary provider when your baby is at least 6 months of age, at the beginning of flu season (generally in October) for high risk infants. Also recommended for parents and care providers to these infants. Candidate: Yes_____ No_____ Date Due:_____ ❑ Palivizumab (Synagis) Provided to specific high risk premature infants, as a shot given once a month during cold and flu season. • Verbalizes reasons why infant must receive monthly injections for adequate coverage • Additional handouts provided Candidate: Yes_____ No_____ First Date Due:_____ Follow-up Dates:_____			

ANC
Journal of the National Association of Neonatal Nurses
Patient Copy

FIGURE **19-4**

Nursing Actions	Obtaining Vaccines	Demonstrates or Verbalizes Understanding	Needs Further Review	Date/Initials
Verify Immunization Status of siblings Target date: _____	❑ Insurance coverage for vaccines provided by:_____ ❑ Closest health department (location & phone #):_____ ❑ National Immunization Information Hotline (800) 232-2522 for 'Vaccines for Children' Information			
  FIGURE 3. Hold and cuddle infant before and after injections to help deal with pain and discomfort. **Target Date:** **24 Hours Before Immunization** **Individualized Plan for Pain Control:**	**Dealing with Injection Pain and Discomfort** ❑ Demonstrates comforting measures after injection: soothing, holding, cuddling before, during and after injections ❑ Verbalizes and demonstrates understanding of acetaminophen administration for discomfort or fever (consider obtaining 'After the Shots' pamphlet www.immunize.org or other supplemental materials) ❑ Verbalizes strategies for post-injection pain & fever: • Apply a cool washcloth for redness or swelling at injection site • If a low-grade fever is present—clothe lightly, lukewarm sponge bath • Contact your physician or nurse practitioner if your baby is crying that won't stop, has fever of 105° or greater • Provide Tylenol or a sucrose pacifier as follows: Individual Dose:_____			
  FIGURE 4. Providing an oral dose of sucrose can block the pain response in infants.	**Adverse Events Reporting & National Childhood Vaccine Injury Compensation Program** ❑ Adverse Events Reporting System Information provided ❑ Aware of reporting form and events reporting guidelines on the Web site www.vaers.org or by calling VAERS at (800) 822-7967 **Documentation of Vaccines & Vaccine Registry** ❑ Understands the need for documentation of all vaccines ❑ Has a parent held vaccine documentation record ❑ Aware of option to enroll in state/national immunization registry, if available			
  FIGURE 5. Administer acetaminophen before vaccines and for 24 hours after vaccination to minimize discomfort.			**ANC** _{Journal of the National Association of Neonatal Nurses} **Patient Copy**	

FIGURE 19-4, cont'd

Teaching guide for immunizations. (From Gracey K [2002]. Family teaching toolbox, *Advances in neonatal care*, 2[1],53-54.)

Definitions

For purposes of this guideline, the following definitions apply:

Infant Passenger Restraint Seat—used for infants less than 1 year of age and weight less than 20 pounds.

Infant Car Bed—a passenger restraint for an infant who is unable to tolerate a sitting position.

Apnea—A breathing pause greater than 20 seconds as indicated on electronic monitoring.

Bradycardia—Heart rate of less than 80 beats/min sustained for at least 5 seconds.

Desaturation—Oxygen saturation of less than 85% for at least 5 seconds or requiring stimulation to recover to baseline.

Standards

1. The registered nurse (RN)/care coordinator will inform the parents of the need for car seat use for any motor vehicle use.
2. The RN/care coordinator will inform the parents of the special concerns with premature infants and educate them on the proper positioning of a premature infant in the car seat.
3. The RN/care coordinator will inform the family of the requirements of a proper infant seat:
   a. Use of seats is appropriate for infants less than 20 pounds.
   b. The belt has a three-point harness.
   c. The harness does not have a large breast shield.
   d. The distance between back of the seat and buckle should measure 5½ inches.
   e. The distance from the lower back to the lowest harness insertion is .01 inches.
4. The nurse will conduct the car seat trial if indicated and notify the physician of any adverse event.
5. If the infant does not tolerate the infant care seat, the parents will be informed of the need to transport the infant in a car bed and the need to avoid other similar devices (infant swings, carrier seats) until their primary physician has cleared their use.

Procedures

1. At least 3 days before discharge; have parents bring in their infant car seat.
2. If parents do not own a car seat or do not bring it in at timely fashion, the nurse may use the car seat belonging to the unit for the car seat tolerance test.
3. Educate parents on how to properly position baby in car seat (demonstration or video).
4. Car seat tolerance test shall take place for a 90-minute duration between feeding times.
   a. Position baby in the car seat while baby is being monitored by a trending monitor. Baby should not be wrapped in blanket, which prevents secure restraint.
   b. Place car seat on a warmer or large crib. There may be a level on the side of the car seat to indicate the proper angle to recline.
   c. Place blanket rolls around the infant's body to keep it centered and a washcloth or blanket roll between crotch and buckle to ensure the infant does not slide down.

d. Monitor baby for apnea, bradycardia, and desaturation; document; and inform physician.

e. If the infant did not tolerate the car seat, inform the parents of the need for a car bed, and contact the care coordinator to facilitate obtaining one. Further caution parents in placing infant in any similar device (swings, carriers) until primary physician has cleared it.

5. RN documentation of car seat tolerance test in the medical record:

a. Parent education concerning car seat use and safety in Gemini® (Cerner Inc., Kansas City, Mo) (computer system)

b. Parent education on proper positioning of smaller premature infants (under 37 weeks) in Gemini® (computer system)

c. Also in Gemini® (computer system), time, date, and results of car seat tolerance test

d. Physician notification of infants who did not tolerate and what follow-up measures are being taken

BIBLIOGRAPHY

American Academy of Pediatrics (AAP) (1999). *Safe transport of premature and low birth weight infants.* Elk Grove Village, Ill: AAP Committee on Injury and Poison Prevention and Committee on Fetus and Newborn.

Merchant JR, Worwa C, Porter S (2001). Respiratory instability of term and near-term healthy newborn infants in car safety seats. *Pediatrics,* 108, 647-652.

Figure 19-5 gives a critical pathway for discharge of preterm infants.

PARENTAL STRESS SCALE: NEONATAL INTENSIVE CARE UNIT*

Self Report Format

Nurses and others who work in neonatal intensive care units are interested in how the experience of having a sick baby hospitalized in the neonatal care unit (NICU) affects parents. We would like to know what aspects of your experience as a parent are stressful to you. By stressful, we mean that the experience has caused you to feel anxious, upset, or tense.

This questionnaire lists various experiences other parents have reported as stressful. Please indicate how stressful each item listed below has been for you using the following scale:

1 = Not at all stressful: the experience did not cause you to feel upset, tense, or anxious

---

Date			Completion Date
Phase	***ADMISSION THROUGH 33RD WEEK***		
ORDERS	Activate the Preterm Discharge CareMap ***Physician/CRNP*** ***Signature_____***		
CONSULTS	Follow-up consults ☐ N/A Home evaluation referral made, if indicated		
TESTS	Metabolic screening completed as per protocol ☐ N/A		Date:_____
TREATMENTS	Isolette wean to open crib as per protocol		

EDUCATION	Invite parent and support person to D/C class
	(when 30-40 wks corrected gestational age)
	PROVIDE FAMILY FOCUSED CARE TO
	FACILITATE INTEGRATING THE INFANT
	INTO THE FAMILY:
	• Show respect for family's values, preferences & expressed
	  needs
	
	• Provide coordination of care
	
	• Provide information & education
	
	• Address physical comfort needs
	
	• Provide emotional support & alleviate fears
	  and anxiety
	
	• Involve families & friends in care
	
	• Provide continuity in planning care and transition home
			Date
			attended:_____

Date			Comments
Phase	***ADMISSION THROUGH 33RD WEEK***		
EDUCATION CONTINUES	SUPPORT PARENT/CAREGIVER TO BEGIN A RELATIONSHIP WITH THE INFANT BY: • Teaching how the infant communicates with them • Facilitate holding/kangarooing each visit, incorporating them in caregiving activities		
PSYCHOSOCIAL	Discharge family meeting conducted at 34 wks		Date:_____

Date			Completion Date
Phase	***34th WEEK THROUGH DISCHARGE***		
CONSULTS	Follow-up consults		
TESTS	• HUS: at 33-34 wks, if history of any IVH, head growth above curve, asphyxia, or BW less than 1250 g ☐ N/A		Date:_____
	• BAER at 33-34 wks ☐ Pass ☐ Fail		Date:_____
	• OPHTHO EXAM At 4-6 wks of age if 32 wks GA or < 1500 g birth weight; or 34 wks GA and was ventilated or on 0⁻ > 5 days Result:_____		Date:_____
	Resuls:_____		Date:_____

FIGURE **19-5**

	• PNEUMOGRAM: Yes No	
	If < 37 wks gestation at birth, perform when 34-35 wks ☐ Normal ☐ Immature ☐ N/A	Date:_____
	• HOME MONITORING: Yes No	
	• Monitor/CPR training completed ☐ N/A	Date:_____
	• CAR SEAT TEST: < 37 wks gestation at birth, completed prior to discharge day ☐ Pass ☐ Fail	Date:_____ Retest Date:_____

Date		Completion Date
Phase	***34th WEEK THROUGH DISCHARGE***	

MEDICATIONS	• Hepatitis vaccine #1 given, if consented ☐ Immunization Information Sheet provided to parent/caregiver	Date Info Sheet Given:_____
		Edition Date:_____
	Manufacturer:_____	
		Date injection given:_____
	Lot#_____	
	☐ Refusal form (#913) completed	Date injection given:_____
	• Hepatitis vaccine #2 given	
	(Due @ 1 month after #1)	
	Manufacturer:_____	
	Lot#_____	Date Info Sheet Given:_____
	• Synagis given if consented, for infants 32 wks GA or < 34 wks with risk factors, November through April	Edition Date:_____
		Date injection given:_____
	• Age appropriate immunizations if 2 mon of age	Date Info Sheet Given:_____
	DpaT, Hib, IPV & Prevnar	
	Manufacturer:_____	Edition Date:_____
	Lot#_____	Date injection given:_____
	Manufacturer:_____	Date injection given:_____
	Lot#_____	Date injection given:_____
	Manufacturer:_____	Date injection given:_____
	Lot#_____	
	Manufacturer:_____	Date:_____
	Lot#_____	

	• Prescription(s) for discharge medications given to parent/
	   caregiver at least 24 hrs prior to D/C and reviewed and
	   verbalized understanding
	☐ N/A	

	☐ Medication instruction sheets(s) provided	

FIGURE **19-5, cont'd**   *Continued*

	Open crib	Date:_____
ACTIVITY	Circumcision desired:	
	☐ N/A ☐ Yes ☐ No	
	Parents have obtained consent.	Date:_____
	OB physician notified	Date:_____
	Circumcision performed with good hemostasis, no signs of infection: (1-3 days prior to discharge)	Date:_____
	WHEN INDICATED: Identified medical/nursing needs or social work referral for home care:	
	☐ Antibiotic Tx ☐ Labs	
	☐ Bilirubin (repeat) ☐ Repeat PKU	
	☐ Premature ☐ Cardiac F/U	
	☐ Apnea monitor ☐ Oxygen therapy	
	☐ Other (list) ☐ Developmental follow-up	
ACTIVITY CONTINUES	• Primary Care Physician/NP	
	Name:_____	
	Address:_____	
	Telephone no.:_____	Date:_____
	Follow-up appointments scheduled, explained, and parents/caregiver verbalizes understanding	
	Discharge packet provided refer to teaching sheet	Date:_____
	Developmental follow-up plan identified as per standard ☐ N/A	Date:_____
	• Change to NeoSure formula at 33-34 wks, if adequate weight gain, if formula fed ☐ N/A	Date:_____
	If breast feeding: LATCH score > 6 with good weight gain	Date:_____
	WIC form given to parents/caregiver if indicated ☐ N/A	

Date		Completion Date
Phase	*34th WEEK THROUGH DISCHARGE*	
EDUCATION	Invite parent and support person to D/C class (when 30-40 wks corrected GA)	Date attended:_____
	PROVIDE FAMILY FOCUSED CARE TO FACILITATE INTEGRATING THE INFANT INTO THE FAMILY: • Show respect for family's values, preferences & expressed needs	
	• Provide coordination of care	
	• Provide information & education	
	• Address physical comfort needs	
	• Provide emotional support & alleviate fears and anxiety	
	• Involve families & friends in care	
	• Provide continuity in planning care and transition home	
	SUPPORT PARENT/CAREGIVER TO BEGIN A RELATIONSHIP WITH THE INFANT BY: • Teaching how the infant communicates with them	
	• Facilitate holding/kangarooing each visit, incorporating them in caregiving activities	

FIGURE **19-5, cont'd**

	Educational form completed:		Date:_____
PSYCHOSOCIAL	Overnight stay for parents/caregiver: ☐ N/A		Date:_____

Date		Completion Date
Phase	*DAY OF DISCHARGE*	
TESTS	• Hearing evaluation completed: ☐ Pass ☐ Fail ☐ Not done: schedule as out-patient Follow-up needed: ☐ Yes ☐ No Script/slip for out-patient lab work given: ☐ Yes ☐ N/A	Date attended:_____
TREATMENTS	Discharge exam MD/CRNP completed Circumcision site assessed, healing, no signs of infection ☐ N/A	

MEDICATIONS	Immunization card provided, explained, and parent/caregiver verbalizes understanding ☐ N/A Medications documented on discharge instruction sheet and reviewed ☐ N/A	
ACTIVITY	Car seat available Discharge to: ☐ Home with parents ☐ Rehab ☐ Foster care ☐ Adoption ☐ Other_____ Infant identification verified and compared to footprint sheet Home care needs identified and referrals completed: ☐ N/A Primary care physician notified by MD/NP: ☐ N/A Parents/caregiver provided Neonatal D/C instructions sheet	Time of discharge:_____
NUTRITION	Adequate nutritional intake supported q3-4 Bottle feeding: Coordinated suck and swallow Breast feeding: LATCH score > 6	
EDUCATION	Family teaching outcomes completed and documented on teaching record Infant needs reviewed with parent/caregiver	

SIGNATURES	INITIALS	Name & Title

FIGURE **19-5, cont'd**

2 = A little stressful
3 = Moderately stressful
4 = Very stressful
5 = Extremely stressful: the experience upset you and caused a lot of anxiety or tension

DISCHARGE ORDERS

• Discharge to Parents ☐ Other_____

• Diet_____

• CR monitor • Discontinue monitor
if on moitor, check download in_____weeks

• Pediatric check in 1 week ☐ Other_____

• Visiting nurse visit in_____days

• Developmental follow-up at 3 months PCA

• Other follow-up visits_____

• Ophthalmology check_____weeks

• Synagis – Dose on or about_____& repeat monthly through April

• Medications: MVI 1cc po qd_____

_____

_____

| CRNP/resident's signature:_____ Date:_____ |
| Attending physician's signature:_____ Date:_____ |

FIGURE **19-5, cont'd**

Critical pathway for preterm infant's discharge. *CRNP*, Certified registered nurse practitioner; *N/A*, not applicable; *D/C*, discharge; *HUS*, head ultrasound; *IVH*, intraventricular hemorrhage; *BW*, birth weight; *BAER*, brain auditory evoked response; *GA*, gestational age; *CPR*, cardiopulmonary resuscitation; *DpaT*, diphtheria, pertussis, and tetanus; *Hib*, hepatitis B; *IPV*, inactive polio vaccine; *OB*, obstetrician; *Tx*, treatment; *PKU*, phenylketonuria; *F/U*, follow up; *NP*, nurse practitioner; *WIC*, Women, Infants, and Children Program; *MD*, medical doctor; *CR*, cardiorespiratory; *PCA*, postconceptual age; *MVI*, multivitamin. (Courtesy University of Pennsylvania Hospital.)

If you did not have the experience, indicate this by circling NA, meaning that you have "not experienced" this aspect of the NICU.

Now let's take an item for an *example*: The bright lights in the NICU.

If, for example, you feel that the bright lights in the neonatal intensive care unit were extremely stressful to you, you would circle the number 5 below:

NA 1 2 3 4 <u>5</u>

If you feel that the lights were not stressful at all, you would circle the number 1 below:

NA <u>1</u> 2 3 4 5

If the bright lights were not on when you visited (not likely), you would circle NA indicating "not applicable" below:

<u>NA</u> 1 2 3 4 5

Now begin.

The following is a list of the various **SIGHTS AND SOUNDS** commonly experienced in an NICU. We are interested in knowing about your view of how stressful these **SIGHTS AND SOUNDS** are for you. Circle the number that best represents your level of stress.

1. The presence of monitors and equipment	NA	1	2	3	4	5
2. The constant noises of monitors and equipment	NA	1	2	3	4	5
3. The sudden noises of monitor alarms	NA	1	2	3	4	5
4. The other sick babies in the room	NA	1	2	3	4	5
5. The large number of people working in the unit	NA	1	2	3	4	5
6. Having a machine (respirator) breathe for my baby	NA	1	2	3	4	5

Below is a list of items that might describe the way your **BABY LOOKS AND BEHAVES** while you are visiting in the NICU as well as some of the **TREATMENTS** that you have seen done to the baby. Not all babies have these experiences or look this way, so circle the NA, if you have not experienced or seen the listed item. If the item reflects something that you have experienced, then indicate how much the experience was stressful or upsetting to you by circling the appropriate number.

1. Tubes and equipment on or near my baby	NA	1	2	3	4	5
2. Bruises, cuts, or incisions on my baby	NA	1	2	3	4	5
3. The unusual color of my baby (e.g., looking pale or yellow jaundiced)	NA	1	2	3	4	5
4. My baby's unusual or abnormal breathing patterns	NA	1	2	3	4	5
5. The small size of my baby	NA	1	2	3	4	5
6. The wrinkled appearance of my baby	NA	1	2	3	4	5
7. Seeing needles and tubes put in my baby	NA	1	2	3	4	5
8. My baby being fed by an intravenous line or tube	NA	1	2	3	4	5
9. When my baby seemed to be in pain	NA	1	2	3	4	5
10. When my baby looked sad	NA	1	2	3	4	5
11. The limp and weak appearance of my baby	NA	1	2	3	4	5
12. Jerky or restless movements of my baby	NA	1	2	3	4	5
13. My baby not being able to cry like other babies	NA	1	2	3	4	5
14. My baby crying for long periods	NA	1	2	3	4	5
15. When my baby looked afraid	NA	1	2	3	4	5
16. Seeing my baby suddenly change color (e.g., becoming pale or blue)	NA	1	2	3	4	5
17. Seeing my baby stop breathing	NA	1	2	3	4	5

The last area we want to ask you about is how you feel about your own **RELATIONSHIP** with the baby and your **PARENTAL ROLE.** If you have experienced the following situations or feelings, indicate how stressed you have been by them by circling the appropriate number. Again, circle NA if you did not experience the item.

1. Being separated from my baby	NA	1	2	3	4	5
2. Not feeding my baby myself	NA	1	2	3	4	5
3. Not being able to care for my baby myself (e.g., diapering, bathing)	NA	1	2	3	4	5
4. Not being able to hold my baby when I want	NA	1	2	3	4	5

5. Feeling helpless and unable to protect my baby from pain and painful procedures	NA	1	2	3	4	5
6. Feeling helpless about how to help my baby during this time	NA	1	2	3	4	5
7. Not having time to be alone with my baby	NA	1	2	3	4	5
8. Sometimes forgetting what my baby looks like	NA	1	2	3	4	5
9. Not being able to share my baby with other family members	NA	1	2	3	4	5
10. Being afraid of touching or holding my baby	NA	1	2	3	4	5
11. Feeling staff is closer to my baby than I am	NA	1	2	3	4	5

Using the same rating scale, indicate how stressful in general, the experience of having your baby hospitalized in the NICU has been for you.

1 = Not at all stressful: the NICU experience did not cause me to feel upset, tense, or anxious

2 = A little stressful

3 = Moderately stressful

4 = Very stressful

5 = Extremely stressful: the NICU experience upset me and caused a lot of anxiety or tension

Thank you for your help. Now, was there anything else that was stressful for you during the time that your baby has been in the neonatal intensive care unit? Please discuss below.

BACK TO SLEEP

The American Academy of Pediatrics (AAP) instituted a "Back to Sleep" campaign several years ago to decrease the incidence of sudden infant death syndrome (SIDS). Although this program has been successful it requires the infant to be stable to be placed on the back or side-lying position. So it is usual for most infants in an NICU to never be placed on their backs for extended periods before discharge, yet we teach the parents that once home this is the position of choice. Some NICUs are beginning to try the infants on their backs before discharge to make sure this position will be tolerated. TriHealth, Cincinnati is in the process of developing a protocol for this transition.

The AAP recommendations for the "Back to Sleep" program* follow. During the past decade, a variety of strategies have been developed that reduce the risk of SIDS. The following list includes a modification and expansion of the recommendations made by the AAP's task force since 1992. It should be emphasized that the recommendations are intended for sleeping infants and primarily for well

---

*From American Academy of Pediatrics (AAP) (2000). Changing concepts of sudden infant death syndrome: implications for infant sleeping environment and sleep position (RE9946). Pediatrics, 105(3), 650-656.

infants. Individual medical conditions may warrant a physician to recommend otherwise, after weighing the relative risks and benefits.

1. Infants should be placed for sleep in a nonprone position. Supine (wholly on the back) confers the lowest risk and is preferred. However, although side sleeping is not as safe as supine, it also has a significantly lower risk than prone. If the side position is used, caretakers should be advised to bring the dependent arm forward to lessen the likelihood of the infant rolling to the prone position.

2. A crib that conforms to the safety standards of the Consumer Product Safety Commission and the ASTM (formerly the American Society for Testing and Materials) is a desirable sleeping environment for infants. (Although many cradles and bassinets also may provide safe sleeping enclosures, safety standards have not been established for these items.) Sleep surfaces designed for adults often are not free of the aforementioned hazards and may have the additional risk of entrapment between the mattress and the structure of the bed (e.g., the headboard, footboard, side rails, frame), the wall, or adjacent furniture, as well as between railings in the headboard or footboard.

3. Infants should not be put to sleep on waterbeds, sofas, soft mattresses, or other soft surfaces.

4. Avoid soft materials in the infant's sleeping environment.
   a. Soft materials or objects, such as pillows, quilts, comforters, or sheepskins, should not be placed under a sleeping infant.
   b. Soft objects, such as pillows, quilts, comforters, sheepskins, stuffed toys, and other gas-trapping objects, should be kept out of an infant's sleeping environment. Also, loose bedding, such as blankets and sheets, may be hazardous. If blankets are to be used, they should be tucked in around the crib mattress so the infant's face is less likely to become covered by bedding. One strategy is to make up the bedding so that the infant's feet are able to reach the foot of the crib (feet-to-foot), with the blankets tucked in around the crib mattress and reaching only the level of the infant's chest. Another strategy is to use sleep clothing with no other covering over the infant.

5. Bed sharing or co-sleeping may be hazardous under certain conditions.
   a. As an alternative to bed sharing, parents might consider placing the infant's crib near their bed to allow for more convenient breast-feeding and parent contact.
   b. If a mother chooses to have her infant sleep in her bed to breast-feed, care should be taken to observe the aforementioned recommendations (nonprone sleep position, avoidance of soft surfaces or loose covers, avoidance of entrapment by moving the bed away from the wall and other furniture and avoiding beds that present entrapment possibilities).

    c. Adults (other than the parents), children, or other siblings should avoid bed sharing with an infant.

    d. Parents who choose to bed share with their infant should not smoke or use substances, such as alcohol or drugs, that may impair arousal.

6. Overheating should be avoided. The infant should be lightly clothed for sleep, and the bedroom temperature should be kept comfortable for a lightly clothed adult. Overbundling should be avoided, and the infant should not feel hot to the touch.

7. A certain amount of tummy time while the infant is awake and observed is recommended for developmental reasons and to help prevent flat spots on the occiput. Positional plagiocephaly also can be avoided by altering the supine head position during sleep. Techniques for accomplishing this include placing the infant to sleep with the head to one side for 1 week or so and then changing to the other and periodically changing the orientation of the infant to outside activity (e.g., the door of the room).

8. Although various devices have been developed to maintain sleep position or to reduce the risk of rebreathing, such devices are not recommended, because none have been tested sufficiently to show efficacy or safety.

9. Electronic respiratory and cardiac monitors are available to detect cardiorespiratory arrest and may be of value for home monitoring of selected infants who are deemed to have extreme cardiorespiratory instability. However, there is no evidence that home monitoring with such monitors decreases the incidence of SIDS. Further, there is no evidence that infants at increased risk of SIDS can be identified by in-hospital respiratory or cardiac monitoring.

10. There are no new data that would lead to a change in the recommendations made in the 1985 statement of the American Academy of Pediatrics on prolonged infantile apnea or the 1986 National Institutes of Health consensus statement on the value of home monitors.

11. There is concern that the annual rate of SIDS, which has been decreasing steadily since 1992, now appears to be leveling off, as has the percentage of infants sleeping prone. The national campaign for reducing prone sleeping (Back to Sleep) should continue and be expanded to emphasize the safe characteristics of the sleeping environment, including safe bedding practices, and focus on the portion of the population that continues to place their infants prone. Other potentially modifiable risk factors, such as avoidance of maternal smoking, overheating, and certain forms of bed sharing, should be included as important secondary messages.

Task Force on Infant Positioning and SIDS, 1998-1999
John Kattwinkel, MD, Chairperson
John G. Brooks, MD
Maurice E. Keenan, MD
Michael Malloy, MD

HOME CARE

Home care is a growing business. Like other aspects of nursing there is a shortage of health professionals in this area, especially those who have NICU or neonatal experience. Sometimes parents feel that they have to watch and teach the nurse who is sent to provide care because the person has never seen such a small baby. We must empower parents to ask questions of agencies that they employ for home health care. Ask if there are experts who have taken care of NICU graduates with special needs. Some hospitals now have integrated health systems that include home health care agencies and in some instances employ nurses who have worked in NICU or special care nurseries.

The most common forms of home care are home monitoring, oxygen therapy, intravenous (IV) therapy, phototherapy, suctioning, and specialized feedings. Specialized forms of home care include hospice and respite care. In both instances the nurse discharging the infant and family needs to help with the selection of appropriate, licensed agencies to ensure safe care. To qualify for home care there are criteria for the infant, family, and equipment.

Infant Criteria

The infant's home health care needs must be assessed as to technical feasibility and medical requirement. Nutritional support must be evaluated. How does the infant feed and how frequently? How often does the infant require gavage feedings, and which feeding techniques are required? Pharmacologic support assessment must be evaluated. What medication does the infant need and how often? What are the desired and adverse effects of these drugs? Does the infant require supplemental oxygen, respiratory therapy treatments, or chest physical therapy? The assessment of the level of care required must be matched to the ability and skills of the home care providers (Durfor, Ratcliffe, 2003).

Family Criteria

After extensive discharge teaching, skills development, and repetitive occasions of caregiving, the family must want the child at home and under their care. They must be willing and able to devote the time and energy required to meet the physical and emotional needs of the child (Durfor, Ratcliffe, 2003).

NICU personnel must begin teaching parents as soon as the neonate is admitted to the unit. Once the family is confident and capable of meeting the needs of the infant, a home assessment should be completed. Basic facilities such as heat, water, telephone, electricity, and transportation must be available. Appropriate support systems must be set up in the home, including the technology necessary for the delivery of care. The operation of phototherapy lights or blankets, oxygen delivery systems, portable suction equipment, respiratory and cardiac monitoring systems, ventilators, and numerous other devices must be thoroughly understood by the caregivers. Clear instructions need to be given to the family members by the providers of the home care technology. Ideally, the parents should bring the equipment to the hospital, or the equipment company can help transport it to the hospital before discharge. The rationale is that the parents can be taught on their own equipment. If there is a problem, it can usually be identified before the infant's discharge. The parents should spend at least 24 hours providing total care before discharge. This time under a health professional's supervision helps the family gain confidence in their caregiving abilities. They can also be reassured that they have the proper equipment (Durfor, Ratcliffe, 2003).

Home Equipment Criteria

The most common equipment needs for neonates are cardiopulmonary monitoring, oxygen, suction, and feeding implements. The first decision that the family needs help in making, is how to select a home care equipment company. Most hospital discharge planners or the nurse responsible for the discharge has recommendations. Burstein (1995) outlined the criteria for selecting a home care pulmonary equipment company (Box 19-1). These criteria can be used for other types of equipment suppliers as well.

Once the supplier has been selected and the equipment that will be necessary identified, parent education can begin. This education should include neonatal CPR. The parents should be given written instructions to take home and a checklist for the CPR procedure that can be clearly posted. If parents cannot read, visual charts outlining the steps should be made available.

A cardiopulmonary monitor is the most common equipment needed in the home. Infants who should be placed on this type of monitoring are those whose sibling died of SIDS or who are at risk for SIDS. These infants are usually monitored until age 6 to 12 months (Burstein, 1995). An infant receiving home oxygen or one who has neurologic impairment is at risk for apneic or bradycardic episodes. Most of these monitors have built-in impedance pneumography capabilities that allow strips to be watched or viewed by home care nurses. In some instances, these can be sent via computer modems. The parents should be told that when there is an episode of apnea or

Box **19-1**

Criteria for Selecting a Home Care Pulmonary Equipment Company

Accreditation by the Joint Commission on Accreditation of Healthcare Organizations (JCAHO)
Location: within 1 hour's driving radius of home
Availability of equipment and supplies required for care
Experience with equipment required for care
24-Hour on-call service for emergencies
Professional home care clinicians or staff*
Record system available to communicate with physician
Availability of backup equipment on site
Experience with similar clinical situations
Acceptance of assignment on insurance benefits

From Greene D (2003). Home care. In Czervinske MP, Barnhart SL, editors. Perinatal and pediatric respiratory care, ed 2, Philadelphia: WB Saunders, p. 709.
Some areas may require professional services to be contracted. Contracted professionals must be available on a 24-hour on-call basis.

bradycardia, they must mark on the strip the infant's color, activity, and what they had to do, if anything, to stop the episode (Burstein, 1995). Burstein (1995) made two important points about this type of monitor. For infants on mechanical ventilation, chest excursion that is detected by the monitor as breathing does not allow the alarm to sound until the heart rate is affected, as in the NICU. Also, for infants who have tracheostomies, the monitoring is to identify episodes in which breathing may stop as a result of mucous plugs or thickened secretions, yet the survival instinct of the infant, to struggle to breathe, will not allow the respiratory monitor alarm to sound as movement is detected. It is the cardiac portion of the monitor that at a much later stage detects bradycardia. Parents need to understand these delays and how to respond.

Suctioning equipment is needed for patients with tracheostomies. This equipment requires electricity and running water. One type of suctioning equipment must be portable and battery powered for trips to and from the clinic and other excursions out of the home. It should have a regulator valve to adjust the amount of suction. If the valve is not present, negative pressure can be very great and cause mucosal trauma to the nasopharyngeal and tracheal tissues. The battery-powered suction machines can be recharged much like portable phones with a direct A/C adapter into a wall outlet or via a cigarette lighter adapter (Burstein, 1995). Most run about 2 hours without recharging. The recharging process takes about 12 hours. The other type of suctioning equipment can be a stationary setup.

Parents should be taught clean suctioning technique, which is used as long as there is no danger of cross-contamination with other infectious agents in the home, as may be the case when siblings are ill. Nosocomial infections and cross-contamination are very real possibilities when the infant is hospitalized. The parents should also be taught sterile technique, which should be used only when there is illness in the home that may put the infant at risk for cross-contamination.

Suctioning should be taught according to the physician's/practitioner's orders. Usually this is done on an as-needed basis. Signs that indicate the need for suctioning are the same as those used by health professionals in the NICU: restlessness, decreased color, coughing, increased respiratory effort, or sounds of congestion. In general, suctioning is necessary every 2 to 4 hours. Parents should keep a log of the timing of the suctioning and the type of secretions obtained. In addition to the suctioning equipment, parents will need a 50-pound per square inch (psi) portable air compressor and possibly compressed oxygen with portable reservoir.

Portable or stationary oxygen devices vary in size and the amount of time that they will last. They are classified as sizes AA through K; G, H, and K are large and stationary, whereas the others are portable. The oxygen tanks for these devices differ from those of liquid oxygen in that they can be stored and will not leak if the shut-off valve is left on. They are larger and are filled under high pressure so they are more difficult to move. There is slight danger from pressure if they are accidentally dropped or damaged. The liquid oxygen is more portable and smaller in size. It does not require external electricity or battery-powered sources. The cylinder is small and filled under very little pressure. The liquid oxygen must be moved from the base of the chamber to a portable reservoir. It is more costly than gas pressure oxygen cylinders.

These infants often also need an oxygen concentrator. The concentrator resembles the old-fashioned mix-box used in the NICU to mix air and oxygen to achieve the desired oxygen concentration. It separates oxygen from nitrogen in room air and collects oxygen (Burstein, 1995). The concentrations that are possible with these home devices are between 45% and 95% (Burstein, 1995). They cannot deliver very low flow rates such as 0.5 L/min. They are electrically powered. Portable units are needed outside the home. A backup gas oxygen cylinder is necessary for electrical failures and for excursions outside the home (Dufor, Ratcliffe, 2003).

Humidification of the airway is necessary for infants with artificial airways, regardless of whether they are on oxygen. If the airway is not humidified, mucous membranes may dry and crack, creating areas that may become infected. Volume jet nebulizers can provide humid-ification with a 50-psi portable air compressor. Humidification levels of 35% to 100% can generally be achieved (Burstein, 1995). This compressor should be capable of providing high-or low-pressure aerosol. This capability is important if the infant requires a mist tent at night but during the day is connected to a tracheostomy collar or other airway devices. Some companies suggest use of a heat and mois-ture exchanger (HME), which can be used for travel and is used by itself and not in conjunction with other humidifying devices. It can be attached to the airway without intermediate equipment (Burstein, 1995).

Mechanical ventilation is another area of home care. Information on home use of ventilators can be obtained from the National Center for Home Mechanical Ventilation. The physician or practitioner, on the basis of the infant's need, orders the specific type of ventilator. The decision also takes into consideration the family's lifestyle. If the family anticipates movement from home to other areas or other rela-tives' homes, a portable unit may be best. All portable units must have an internal and external battery. An emergency backup unit must be available; whether it is housed in the home or at immediate dispatch from the equipment company does not matter as long as it is available for times when there are equipment failures with the portable device. Battery backup is necessary, too. Usually a 12-volt battery with 74 amp/hr potential is suggested; such a battery can go about 18 to 20 hours without recharge (Durfor, Ratcliffe, 2003).

These areas of home care monitoring are the most common. Specific instructions on which equipment is necessary and how to use it in each situation should be obtained from the home health care agency that is to provide care, the hospital equipment vendors, and the home health care equipment vendors. Nurses who are responsible for discharge should be very familiar with the advantages and disad-vantages of the equipment that the family will need. The family's lifestyle and capabilities also have to be considered when an infant is sent home on equipment (Durfor, Ratcliffe, 2003).

Home care equipment and supplies must fit the patient just as they did in the hospital. The nurse responsible for the discharge must make sure that the child's size is considered when ordering equip-ment. For example, if the infant is now 12 pounds, do you still use a preemie stethoscope? If the child has a tracheostomy, is there a backup one that is of proper size? (Durfor, Ratcliffe, 2003).

Ideally the nurse should make a home visit before the discharge to assess the home environment for safety hazards. For example, is the house/apartment too hot or cold—either condition can lead to apneic spells. Are there exposed wires in the house? Peeling paint? Open flames used for cooking when oxygen is going to be used in the house? Are there any strong or chemical odors that may be harmful to a child with respiratory compromise? Is there an emergency phone? All aspects of the home and the community setting should be considered when discharging the infant and family (Durfor, Ratcliffe, 2003).

If oxygen is to be used in the home the guidelines given in Table 19-1 should be considered.

Table **19-1**	Safe Use of Oxygen at Home
Safety Guidelines	**Rationale**
Secure oxygen tank in upright position. Keep oxygen tanks at least 5 ft from heat source and electrical devices (e.g., space heaters, heating vents, fireplaces, radios, vaporizers, humidifiers).	Oxygen tanks are highly explosive; if a horizontally positioned tank explodes, the rapid release of oxygen can catapult it through animate (e.g., human bodies) and inanimate (e.g., walls) objects.
Ensure that no one smokes in the room or in the area of the oxygen tank.	Smoking increases the risk of fire, which could cause the tank to explode; escaped oxygen would feed the fire.
Use lemon-glycerin swabs to relieve dryness around the child's mouth; avoid oil or alcohol-based substances (e.g., petroleum jelly, vitamin A and D ointment, baby oil).	Both alcohol and oil are flammable and increase the risk of fire.
Have the child wear cotton garments.	Silk, wool, and synthetics can generate static electricity and cause fire.
Keep a fire extinguisher readily available.	It is necessary to put out fire immediately.
Turn off both volume regulator and flow regulator whenever oxygen is not in use.	If the volume regulator is on when oxygen is turned on, the child might receive a rapid, forceful flow of oxygen in the face that could be frightening and uncomfortable.
	Oxygen leakage, which might not be detected because oxygen is odorless, can cause fire.

In Harvey K (2000). Bronchopulmonary dysplasia. In Jackson PL, Vessey JA, editors. Primary care of the child with a chronic condition, St Louis: Mosby, p. 254; Hagedorn MI, Garnder SL (1989). Physiologic sequelae of prematurity: the nurse practitioner's role. I. Respiratory issues. Journal of pediatric health care, 3, 288-297.

BIBLIOGRAPHY

Barrington KJ, Tan K, Rich W (2002). Apnea at discharge and gastro-esophageal reflux in the preterm infant. *Journal of perinatology*, 22(1), 8-11.

Bergius H, et al. (2001). Hospital-managed advanced care of children in their homes. *Journal of telemedicine & telecare*, 7(Suppl 1), 32-34.

Brumfield CG, et al. (2001). Early discharge revisited: problems encountered with the home visit follow-up after the liberalization of eligibility criteria. *Journal of maternal & fetal medicine*, 10(4), 277-282.

Burstein L (1995). Home care. In Barnhart SL, Czervinske MP, editors. *Perinatal and pediatric respiratory care*, Philadelphia: WB Saunders.

Cerny JE, Inouye J (2001). Utilizing the child abuse potential inventory in a community health nursing prevention program for child abuse. *Journal of community health nursing*, 18(4), 199-211.

Contro N, et al. (2002). Family perspectives on the quality of pediatric palliative care. *Archives of pediatric & adolescent medicine*, 156(1), 14-19.

Corkhill MB, Joshua A (2002). Home health nurse's borrowed blessing. *Journal of Christian nursing*, 19(1), 36-37.

Durfor S, Ratcliffe M (2003). Home and community based care. In Kenner C, Lott JW, editors. *Comprehensive neonatal nursing: a physiologic perspective*, ed 3, St Louis: WB Saunders.

Friedewald VE, Pion RJ Jr (2001). Telemedicine/home care: returning home. *Health management technology*, 22(9), 22-24, 26.

Gielen AC, et al. (2002). Effects of improved access to safety counseling, products, and home visits on parents' safety practices: results of a randomized trial. *Archives of pediatric & adolescent medicine*, 156(1), 33-40.

Haffner JC, Schurman SJ (2001). The technology-dependent child. *Pediatric clinics of North America*, 48(3), 751-764.

Koniac-Griffin D, et al. (2002). Public health nursing care for adolescent mothers: impact on infant health and selected maternal outcomes at 1 year postbirth. *Journal of adolescent health*, 30(1), 44-54.

Monterosso L, Kristjanson L, Cole J (2002). Neuromotor development and the physiologic effects of positioning in very low birth weight infants. *Journal of obstetric, gynecologic, and neonatal nursing*, 31(2), 138-146.

Norzila MZ, et al. (2001). Home oxygen therapy for children with chronic lung diseases. *Medical journal of Malaysia*, 56(2), 151-157.

O'Brien ME, Wegner CB (2002). Rearing the child who is technology dependent: perceptions of parents and home care nurses. *Pediatric nursing*, 7(1), 7-16.

Parra MM, Goldsleger F, Chandler S (2001). The ventilator-assisted children home program: supporting families. *Caring*, 20(6), 12-15.

Radmacher P, Massey C, Adamkin D (2002). Hidden morbidity with "successful" early discharge, *Journal of perinatology*, 22(1), 15-20.

Ritchie SK (2002). Primary care of the premature infant discharged from the neonatal intensive care unit. *The American journal of maternal/child nursing, MCN*, 27(2), 76-86.

Zanardo V, Freato F (2001). Home oxygen therapy in infants with bronchopulmonary dysplasia: assessment of parental anxiety. *Early human development*, 65(1), 39-46.

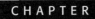
END-OF-LIFE OR PALLIATIVE CARE

End-of-life (EOL) or palliative care is an area of nursing that has belonged to the older or cancer populations. We now recognize that all age-groups are entitled to EOL or palliative care. Some of our patients are born dying. Their families need support during a time that was supposed to be filled with joy. They require special skills to help them face this tough challenge as a parent. EOL care is more than advanced directives or living wills; it is a philosophy of care that provides empathy and support during a crisis. Palliative care is comfort care. This care is not reserved for the dying. It is comfort and support during life-threatening illnesses. Certainly most neonatal intensive care unit (NICU) patients qualify. For us this includes sedation, analgesia, and anesthesia during times of discomfort or painful procedures. It encompasses pharmacologic therapies but nonpharmacologic ones as well. The latter include nonnutritive sucking, gentle touch, skin-to-skin care, music therapy, and positive positioning. To many nurses this opportunity to provide care during one of the most stressful phases of a family's life is a privilege that allows us to do what we do best—provide holistic, family-centered care. We must be fully present to our patients and families, and we must recognize that this type of nursing care is an evolving process and not an event. It requires a shift in our mindset from the curative mode to one of support and comfort. We must also recognize it is stressful for the nurse and health care team as well as the family. This chapter presents tools and guidelines to assist newborn and infant nurses to provide the best possible care, whether it is in the hospital, community, or home setting.

CORE PRINCIPLES FOR CARE OF PATIENTS (NEWBORNS AND INFANTS)

1. Respecting the dignity of both child and caregivers
2. Being sensitive to and respectful of the family's wishes
3. Using the most appropriate measures that are consistent with the family's choices
4. Encompassing alleviation of pain and other physical symptoms
5. Assessing and managing psychologic, social, and spiritual/religious problems
6. Ensuring continuity of care (the child should be able to continue to be cared for, if so desired, by his/her primary care and specialist providers)

7. Providing access to any therapy that may realistically be expected to improve the child's quality of life, including alternative or nontraditional treatments

8. Providing access to palliative care and hospice care

9. Respecting the right to refuse treatment that may prolong suffering of life

10. Respecting the physician's professional responsibility to discontinue some treatments when appropriate, with consideration for both child and family's preferences

11. Promoting clinical evidence-based research on providing care at the end of life*

The overarching philosophy of palliative and hospice care is expressed in seven promises.[†] Although these were created for the adult setting they have applicability to the newborn and infant populations and their families. As neonatal nurses we promise the following:

1. **Good medical treatment:** You will have the best of medical treatment, aiming to prevent exacerbation, improve function and survival, and ensure comfort.

   a. Offer patients proven diagnosis and treatment strategies to prevent exacerbations and enhance quality of life, as well as to delay disease progression and death.

   b. Use medical interventions that are in accord with best available standards of medical practice.

2. **Never overwhelmed by symptoms:** You will never have to endure overwhelming pain, shortness of breath, or other symptoms.

   a. Anticipate and prevent symptoms when possible; evaluate and address symptoms promptly.

   b. Treat severe symptoms, such as shortness of breath, as emergencies.

   c. Use sedation when necessary to relieve intractable symptoms near the end of life.

3. **Continuity, coordination, and comprehensiveness:** Your care will be continuous, comprehensive, and coordinated.

   a. Be sure patients and families can count on having access to health care professionals at all times.

   b. Make sure patients and families can count on an appropriate and timely response to their needs.

---

*Modified from Cassel CK, Foley KM (1999). *Principles of care of patients at the end of life: an emerging consensus among the specialties of medicine.* New York: Milbank Memorial Fund. (www.milbank.or/endoflie/index.html)
[†]Modified from Americans for Better Care of the Dying. *Making promises.* Washington, DC: Americans for Better Care of the Dying.

    c. Try to minimize transitions among services, settings, and personnel; when transitions are necessary, make sure they go smoothly.

4. **Well-prepared, no surprises:** You and your family will be prepared for everything that is likely to happen in the course of your illness.

    a. Let families know what to expect as the illness worsens— and what is expected of them.

    b. Provide families with the supplies and training needed to handle predictable events.

5. **Customized care, reflecting your preferences:** Your family's wishes will be sought and respected and followed whenever possible.

    a. Tell families about the alternatives for services, and encourage them to make choices that matter.

    b. Never give patients treatments that their families refuse.

    c. Help families who want their child to live out the end of life at home to do so.

6. **Consideration for patient and family resources** (financial, emotional, and practical): We will help you to consider your family's personal and financial resources, and we will respect your family's choices about their use.

    a. Inform families about services available in the community and the costs of those services.

    b. Discuss and address the concerns of family caregivers. When appropriate, make respite, volunteer, and home aide care part of the care plan.

7. **Make the best of every day:** We will do all we can to see that you and your family will have the opportunity to make the best of every day.

    a. Treat the patient as a person, not as a disease. What is important to the patient is important to the care team.

    b. Respond to the physical, psychologic, social, and spiritual needs of patients and families.

    c. Support families before, during, and after a loved one's death.

PROFESSIONAL PREPARATION FOR END-OF-LIFE CARE*

Scientific and clinical knowledge and skills include the following:

1. Learning the biologic mechanisms of dying from major illnesses and injuries

---

*Modified from Field MJ, Cassel CK (1997). Approaching death: improving care at the end-of-life. Committee on Care at the End-of-life, Institute of Medicine. Washington, DC: National Academy Press, p. 11.

2. Understanding the pathophysiology of pain and other physical and emotional symptoms

3. Developing appropriate expertise and skill in the pharmacology of symptom management

4. Learning the proper application and limits of life-prolonging interventions

5. Understanding tools for assessing patient symptoms, status, quality of life, and prognosis

6. Interpersonal skills and attitudes, including the following:
   a. Listening to patients, families, and other members of the health care team
   b. Conveying difficult news
   c. Understanding and managing patient and family responses to illness
   d. Providing information and guidance on prognosis and options
   e. Recognizing and understanding one's own feelings and anxieties about dying and death
   f. Cultivating empathy
   g. Developing sensitivity to religious, ethnic, and other differences

Ethical and professional principles include the following:

1. Doing good and avoiding harm
2. Determining and respecting family preferences
3. Being alert to personal and organizational conflicts of interests
4. Understanding societal/population interests and resources
5. Weighing competing objectives or principles
6. Acting as a role model of clinical proficiency, integrity, and compassion

Organizational skills include the following:

1. Developing and sustaining effective professional teamwork
2. Understanding relevant rules and procedures set by health plans, hospitals, and others
3. Learning how to protect patients from harmful rules and procedures
4. Assessing and managing care options, settings, and transitions
5. Mobilizing supportive resources (e.g., palliative care consultants, community-based assistance)
6. Making effective use of existing financial resources and cultivating new funding sources

THE RIGHTS OF THE NEWBORN AND INFANT

I have the right to be listened to as a person with rights and am not property of my parents, medical doctors, nurse practitioners, and society.

I have the right to cry.

I have the right to hope.

I have the right of not being alone.

I have the right to create fantasies.

I have the right to interact with my siblings.

I have the right to have my pain controlled.

I have the right to have my needs taken care of.

I have the right to be at home and not in the hospital if my parents choose to have me there.

I have the right to receive help for my brothers and sisters in dealing with my illness.

I have the right to comfort care.*

The Association of Pediatric Oncology Nurses (APON), National Association of Neonatal Nurses (NANN), and Society of Pediatrics Nurses (SPN) worked together to adapt the last precepts that had been formulated by the "Last Acts" Organization. We felt this adaptation was necessary since death was not a "natural" event in the pediatric population.

PRECEPTS OF PALLIATIVE CARE FOR CHILDREN/ADOLESCENTS AND THEIR FAMILIES†

Palliative care is the comprehensive management of the physical, psychologic, social, spiritual, and existential needs of children/adolescents and their families. It is a suitable approach to care for children/adolescents who are born with incurable, life-limiting conditions as well as children/adolescents with incurable, progressive illnesses.

Palliative care affirms life and regards dying as a process that is a profoundly personal experience for the child/adolescent and family. Palliative care is foremost family-centered with the goal of achieving the best possible quality of life through relief of suffering—physical, psychologic, social, emotional, and spiritual; control of symptoms; and restoration of functional capacity while remaining sensitive to personal, family, cultural, and religious values, beliefs, and practices. On a global level, the death of a child/adolescent may be an expected event for families. However, in the United States, the death of a child/adolescent is not an expected or natural event in the life cycle of most families. Few parents ever expect to outlive their child/adolescent. The death of a child or adolescent is often perceived by a family as a devastating and life-altering event. As a society, we often

---

*Modified from Rights of a child with terminal illness. San Jose, Costa Rica: Palliative Care Foundation. From Palliative Care Center of the North Shore (1999). Care Center for Kids child rights. Evanston, Ill.
†From Association of Pediatric Oncology Nurses, National Association of Neonatal Nurses, Society of Pediatric Nurses (May 2002).

do not know how to respond to the death of a child/adolescent; therefore there are few established social norms to help the family cope.

Palliative care can co-exist with other treatment plans that are available and appropriate to the identified goals of care. The intensity and range of palliative interventions may increase as illness progresses and the complexity of care and needs of the child/adolescent and family increase. The priority of care shifts over time to focus on the dying process with an emphasis on EOL decision making and care that supports physical comfort and a death that is consistent with the values and desires of the child/adolescent and family. The provision of palliative care guides families as they make the transition through the changing goals of care and helps children/adolescents and families address issues of life completion and life closure.

Palliative care requires an interdisciplinary team that includes, among others, physicians, nurses, psychologists, developmental specialists, child life specialists, pharmacists, pastoral caregivers, social workers, ancillary staff, volunteers, and family members. Palliative care has become an area of special expertise within many disciplines. However, advances in palliative care have not yet been integrated effectively into standard pediatric clinical practice. The fundamental precepts of palliation should be a basic component of the attitudes, knowledge base, and practice skills of all health care professionals. Palliative care education must be included in the curricula of nursing and medical schools and other health care professions, with continuing education for health care professionals, as knowledge in the field progresses. The principles of comfort for those who cannot benefit from life-saving treatments should also be routinely reviewed.

The *Last Acts* Palliative Care Task Force believes that acknowledgment and incorporation of the following core precepts into all EOL care can serve as a starting point for needed reform.

Respecting Patient Goals, Preferences, and Choices

Palliative care does the following:

- Incorporates family-centered care and addresses the child's/adolescent's needs within the context of the child's/adolescent's physical condition, developmental stage, family, and community
- Recognizes that the family constellation is defined by the child/adolescent, the family, and their culture and beliefs, and encourages child/adolescent and family involvement in planning and providing care
- Identifies and honors the preferences of the child/adolescent and family through careful attention to their values, goals, and priorities, as well as their cultural and spiritual perspectives
- Assists the child/adolescent and family in establishing goals of care by facilitating their understanding of the diagnosis and

prognosis, clarifying priorities, promoting informed choices, and providing an opportunity for negotiating a care plan with providers; consideration is always given to the child's/adolescent's developmental stage, chronologic age, and the family's wishes

- Strives to meet the child's/adolescent's and family's preferences about care settings, living situations, and services, recognizing the uniqueness of these preferences and assisting the family to work through any barriers
- Encourages advanced care planning, including advance directives, through ongoing dialogue among providers, the child/adolescent, and family
- Recognizes the potential for conflicts among the child/adolescent, family, providers, and payers, and develops processes to work toward resolution

Comprehensive Caring

Palliative care does the following:

- Emphasizes that dying is a poignant period in the life of the child/adolescent and family and responds actively to the associated human suffering
- Appreciates differences among children/adolescents and families regarding the meaning of their experience; for some children/adolescents and families, this experience is considered growth producing whereas others will never view this event in this light
- Places a high priority on physical comfort and functional capacity, including, but not limited to, expert management of pain and other symptoms, diagnosis and treatment of psychologic distress, and assistance in remaining as independent as possible or desired
- Provides physical, psychologic, social, and spiritual support to help the child/adolescent and family adapt to the anticipated decline associated with advanced, progressive, incurable disease
- Alleviates isolation through a commitment to nonabandonment, ongoing communication, and sustaining relationships
- Assists with reaffirmation of the child's/adolescent's life and the parent's role in that life, as well as issues of life review, life completion, and life closure within the context of family culture and values
- Extends support beyond the life span of the child/adolescent to assist the family in their bereavement through ongoing support, guidance, and remembrance

Using the Strengths of Interdisciplinary Resources

Palliative care does the following:

- Requires an interdisciplinary team of knowledgeable, skilled, and experienced pediatric health care professionals, who are

provided the opportunity for ongoing education, professional support, and development
- Includes a clearly identified, accessible, and accountable individual or team responsible for coordinating care to ensure that changing needs and goals are met and to facilitate communication and continuity of care
- Incorporates the full array of interinstitutional and community resources (e.g., schools, hospitals, home care, hospice) and promotes a seamless transition between institutions/settings and services
- Determines if these services are available for the child/adolescent and family and that the staff of hospice or those who provide palliative care are knowledgeable about the unique needs of the terminally ill child/adolescent and the family

Acknowledging and Addressing Caregiver Concerns

Palliative care does the following:
- Appreciates the substantial physical, emotional, and economic demands placed on a family caring for the child/adolescent at home or during prolonged and/or repeated hospitalizations as they attempt to fulfill caregiving responsibilities and meet the entire family's needs
- Provides concrete supportive services to caregivers, such as respite, around-the-clock availability of expert advice and support by telephone, grief counseling, personal care assistance, and referral to community resources
- Anticipates that some family caregivers may be at high risk for fatigue, physical illness, and emotional distress and considers the special needs of these caregivers in planning and delivering services
- Recognizes and addresses the economic costs of caregiving, including loss of income and nonreimbursable expenses

Building Systems and Mechanisms of Support

Palliative care does the following:
- Requires an environment that supports innovation, research, education, and dissemination of best practices and models of care
- Needs an infrastructure that promotes the philosophy and practice of pediatric palliative care
- Relies on the formulation of responsible policies and regulations by institutions and by state and federal governments
- Promotes equitable and timely access to the full array of interdisciplinary services necessary to meet the multidimensional needs of patients and their caregivers
- Demands ongoing evaluation, including the development of evidence-based standards, guidelines, and outcome measures

- Ensures that mechanisms are in place at all levels (e.g., systems, direct care services) to guarantee accountability in provision of care
- Requires appropriate financing, including the development of new methods of reimbursement within the context of a changing health care financing system

BREAKING BAD NEWS: THE NURSE'S ROLE (FOR NEWBORNS AND INFANTS)*

1. Provide a "warning shot" or an introductory sentence before presenting the distress information.
2. Provide an opportunity for supportive friends of family to be present when the information is shared.
3. Tell the news in a private setting, with the physician, nurse, and social worker present. Bring the family to a private room. If appropriate and desired by the parents, assist them in telling their children afterward.
4. Sit down near the family, not across a table. Do not stand. Look the family members in the eye to engender trust. Ask them to tell you about their child and about things that give him or her pleasure (keep consoled). Ask family members to explain what they understood was said. Clarify misconceptions. Then solicit additional questions.
5. Be unhurried. Do not look at your watch. Have the charge nurse or another nurse care for your patients while you sit with the family. Remind the other team members to give their beepers to someone else during the family meeting, when possible; otherwise, switch the beepers to vibrate mode.
6. Ideally members of the multidisciplinary team participate as full members during the family conference. The nurse, chaplain, or social worker can solicit questions, clarify misconceptions during the meeting and after the physician or nurse practitioner leaves, and address other facts of the child's situation that the conversation with the physician or nurse practitioner evokes. Each team member can also give feedback regarding his or her communication with the patient and family, such as words they did not understand, and can help address any unresolved issues at the next meeting.
7. Bring trainees to the family meeting. It keeps trainees informed so that unnecessary and often damaging miscommunications do not occur. However, do not overwhelm the family with white coats—have trainees take turns in attending family meetings.

---

*Modified from Levetown M (2001). Pediatric care: the inpatient/ICU perspective. In Ferrell B, Coyle N, editors. The textbook of palliative nursing. New York: Oxford University Press, pp. 572-573.

8. Be specific. The physician or nurse practitioner should present the options, including a description of life-sustaining treatments, the child's current status, the chance of survival, the probability of full recovery (and the probability of significant disability), and the possible effects of the child's long-term survival on the family. Be sure to explain the benefits and burdens (including prolongation of suffering) of each potential care plan, the potential reversibility or irreversibility of the conditions being treated, the time frame of reevaluation, the projected future quality of life, and the comfort measures available if the ICU interventions are curtailed or discontinued. Give reassurances that, if life-sustaining medical interventions are discontinued, the child will continue to receive attentive care for the relief of symptoms; describe the procedures to be undertaken, including the opportunities to observe important customs and rituals and the visitation allowances.

AMERICAN ACADEMY OF PEDIATRICS GUIDELINES

Each year, 53,000 children in the United States die from trauma, extreme prematurity, hereditary disorders, acquired illness, or other conditions. An infant or child with a terminal or very serious illness, and his or her family, may benefit from palliative care—care designed to relieve or minimize the symptoms of the condition, including the physical, emotional, social, and spiritual.

For children living with life-threatening or terminal illness, medical professionals are obligated to ensure that suffering is minimized and medical technology is used only when the benefit for the child outweighs the burden.

Because children's needs are often significantly different from those of adults, the American Academy of Pediatrics (AAP) has outlined recommendations* for providing palliative care for children.

The recommendations include the following:

- The development of widely available palliative care and respite programs to alleviate suffering and to promote the welfare of children and their families living with life-threatening or terminal conditions
- The implementation of a comprehensive palliative care program from the time a child is diagnosed with a life-threatening or terminal condition to complement life-prolonging care, as well as assist if it becomes clear that the child will not survive
- Changes in the regulation of palliative care to allow broader eligibility criteria, equitable reimbursement of simultaneous life-prolonging and palliative care, as well as respite care and other therapies beyond those currently mandated

---

*From American Academy of Pediatrics (August 7, 2000); www.aap.org

- An effort by all general and subspecialty pediatricians, family physicians, pain specialists, and pediatric surgeons to familiarize themselves with palliative care practices for children, including palliative medicine, communication skills, and grief counseling
- An increase in support for research into effective pediatric palliative care
- Labeling information provided by the pharmaceutical industry for symptom-relief medications applicable to children

HOSPICE CARE

The Hospice Philosophy

Regardless of the setting of care, hospice care embodies the following characteristics*:

- The patient and family are the unit of care (however, the patient defines his or her family).
- An interdisciplinary team cares for the needs of the patient and family.
- Emphasis is on control of pain and other symptoms, as well as relief of suffering.
- The patient and family are recognized as the best judges of their needs, and thus control and choice are afforded them in all decisions regarding their care.

Differences Between Hospice Care for Newborns/Infants and Adults†

Patient issues

- Patient is not legally competent.
- Patient is in developmental process, which affects understanding of life and death, sickness and health, God, and so on.
- Patient has not achieved a "full and complete life."
- Patient lacks verbal skills to describe needs, feelings, and so on.
- Patient is often in a highly technical medical environment.

Family issues

- Family needs to protect the child from information about his/her health.
- Family needs to do everything possible to save the child.
- Family may have difficulty dealing with siblings.
- Family experiences stress about finances.
- Family fears that care at home is not as good as at the hospital.

---

*From Kuebler KK, Berry PH (2002). End-of-life care. In Kuebler KK, Berry PH, Heidrich DE, editors. End-of-life care: clinical practice guidelines, Philadelphia: WB Saunders, p. 25. Used with permission.
†Modified from Children's Hospice International. Website: www.chionline.org. Prepared by Paul R. Brenner.

- Grandparents feel helpless in dealing with their children and grandchildren.
- Family needs relief from burden of care.

Caregiver issues
- Caregivers need to protect children, parents, siblings.
- Caregivers feel a sense of failure in not saving the child.
- Caregivers feel a sense of "ownership" of children, even at expense of parents.
- Caregivers have out-of-date ideas about pain in children, especially infants.
- Caregivers lack knowledge about children's disease processes.
- "Unfinished business" can influence caregivers' style of care.

Institutional/agency issues
- There is less reimbursement or none for children's hospice/home care.
- Intensity is high for staff caring for children at home.
- Ongoing staff support is necessary.
- Children's services have immediate appeal to public.
- Special competencies are needed in pediatric care.
- Assess how admission criteria may screen out children.
- Address unusual bereavement needs of family members.

PALLIATIVE CARE

The World Health Organization (WHO) defines palliative care as "the active total care of patients whose disease is not responsive to curative treatment." Control of pain, of other symptoms, and of psychologic, social, and spiritual problems is paramount. The goal of palliative care is achievement of the best quality of life for patients and their families.

Recommendations for Palliative Care for Children of the AAP Committee on Bioethics and Committee on Hospital Care*

1. Palliative care and respite programs need to be developed and widely available to provide intensive symptom management and promote the welfare of children living with life-threatening or terminal conditions.
2. At diagnosis of a life-threatening or terminal condition, it is important to offer an integrated model of palliative care that continues throughout the course of illness, regardless of the outcome.

---

*From American Academy of Pediatrics Committee on Bioethics and Committee on Hospital Care (2000). Palliative care for children. Pediatrics, 200; 106(2), 351-357.

3. Changes in the regulation and reimbursement of palliative care and hospice services are necessary to improve access for children and families in need of these services. Modifications in current regulations should include (1) broader eligibility criteria concerning the length of expected survival, (2) the allowance of concurrent life-prolonging and palliative care, and (3) the provision of respite care and other therapies beyond those allowed by a narrow definition of "medically indicated." Adequate reimbursement should accompany these regulation changes.

4. All general and subspecialty pediatricians, family physicians, pain specialists, and pediatric surgeons need to become familiar and comfortable with the provision of palliative care to children. Residency, fellowship training, and continuing education programs should include topics such as palliative medicine, communication skills, grief and loss, managing prognostic uncertainty and decisions to forgo life-sustaining medical treatment, spiritual dimensions of life and illness, and alternative medicine. Pediatric board and subboard certifying examinations should include questions on palliative care.

5. An increase in support for research into effective pediatric palliative care programming, regulation and reimbursement, pain and symptom management, and grief and bereavement counseling is necessary. The pharmaceutical industry must provide labeling information about symptom-relieving medications in the pediatric population and provide suitable formulations for use by children.

6. The practice of physician-assisted suicide or euthanasia for children should not be supported.

A part of palliative and hospice care involves consideration of the religious, spiritual, and cultural beliefs of the family. The following sections present guidelines to assist with parents, siblings, and grandparents.

ASSESSMENT TOOLS

Table 20-1 addresses assessment of family concerns. Boxes 20-1 and 20-2 give lists for dealing with the spiritual care of patients and families, and Table 20-2 details the spiritual assessment of parents and families of newborns.

Toolkit of Instruments to Measure End-Of-Life Care by J.M. Teno and colleagues will provide health professionals methods of examining family reactions to EOL care.

Table 20-1	Assessment of Family Concerns
Family Concern	**Family Assessment**
Patient comfort	Are all symptoms optimally managed? Are there simple comfort measures that the caregiver can offer? Are the spiritual issues being attended to?
Information on caregiving	Does the caregiver understand how to give the needed care (e.g., administering medications, feeding, turning, bathing)? Does the caregiver understand the operation of the equipment? Does the caregiver know who to call when concerned about physical caregiving issues?
General information about the patient	Does the caregiver understand the goals of care? Has the caregiver been given information about what to expect as the patient's condition changes? Does the caregiver need help in speaking with others about the patient's condition (e.g., children)?
Care of the dying patient	Has the caregiver been instructed as to the normal processes of dying (e.g., apnea, cool extremities)? Does the caregiver know who to call for support as the patient's condition deteriorates? Is the caregiver alone? Does the caregiver understand the necessary steps once the patient has died?

Continued

Table 20-1	Assessment of Family Concerns—cont'd
Family Concern	**Family Assessment**
Family needs and resources	How is the caregiver adjusting to being the caregiver? Acknowledge that the caregiver is doing a good job. Does the caregiver have a support system? What are the resources available (e.g., home environment, caregiving assistance, financial)? Does the caregiver have a chance to get a break from the caregiving? What are the resources in the patient's community? Is there a hospice? Is there a place for respite care? Is the caregiver coping well physically, emotionally, and spiritually?
Emergency information	Does the caregiver know what to do in the event of an emergency, such as uncontrolled symptoms or the sudden death of the patient? Does the caregiver have access to a health care professional 24 hours per day? This is essential for the caregiver's well-being.

Adapted from Loseth DB (2002). Psychosocial and spiritual care. In Kuebler KK, Berry PH, Heidrich DE, editors. End-of-life care: clinical practice guidelines. Philadelphia: WB Saunders, p. 106, which was modified from Cherny NI, Coyle N, Foley KM (1996). Guidelines in the care of the dying cancer patient. Hematology/oncology clinics of North America, 10(1), 261-286. Used with permission.

Table **20-2**	Spiritual Assessment (of Parents/Family of Newborns)
Key Assessment Areas	**Sample Questions**
Concept of God or deity	Is religion or God significant to you? Can you describe how?
Sources of hope and strength	Who do you turn to when you need help? Are they available?
Important religious practices	Are any religious practices important to you?
Relationship between spiritual beliefs and health	Has having a child who is sick made any difference in your feelings about God or the practice of your faith?

Modified from Highfield MEF (2000). Providing spiritual care to patients with cancer. Clinical journal of oncology nursing, 4(3), 115-120.

Box **20-1**
Model of Spiritual Care for Nurses
Permission **L**imited information **A**ctivating resources **N**onnursing assistance

From Highfield ME (2000). Providing spiritual care to patients with cancer. Clinical journal of oncology nursing, 4(3), 115-120.

Box 20-2

SPIRITual Interview
(of Parents/Family of Newborns)

- Spiritual belief system
  (religious affiliation)

- Personal spirituality
  (beliefs and practices of affiliation that parents/family accepts)

- Integration with a spiritual community
  (role of the religious/spiritual group; individual role in that group)

- Ritualized practices and restrictions
  (health care activities that parents'/family's faith encourages or forbids)

- Implications for medical care
  (beliefs that health care providers should remember during care)

- Terminal events planning
  (impact of beliefs; contacting clergy)

From Highfield MEF (2000). Providing spiritual care to patients with cancer. Clinical journal of oncology nursing, 4(3), 115-120.

GUIDELINES FOR ADDRESSING SPIRITUALITY IN NONRELIGIOUS OR NONTRADITIONAL PERSONS/FAMILIES*

1. What do you believe about the purpose of human life?
2. What is it that establishes the purpose for you?
3. What are the values that have been most important to you as you have lived your life?
4. Is there a reason you do not practice a religion? Tell me about this.
5. What gives you strength and comfort during this emotionally stressful time?
6. What serves as a source of guidance, inspiration, or protection for you?
7. What helps you find meaning and hope regarding your child's life and illness at this time?
8. What do you believe about death?
9. What do you believe will happen to your child if he/she were to die?
10. In what ways has the illness of your child affected your values? Your understanding of the purpose of life? Your own humanity?
11. How can we be helpful to you with this?
12. How does your belief (system) enhance your life?
13. What makes your feel "safe in the world"? In what do you trust for that feeling?

GUIDELINES FOR ADDRESSING THE FAMILY'S RELIGIOUS NEEDS*

1. What is the religious identity of the father and mother? Same? Different? How?
2. Do both parents practice their religion? Does only one? Who? How is it practiced?
3. If the religious identity is different, are the parents in conflict about this? Integrated?
4. In what religion is the child being raised?
5. Tell me about the specific rituals of your faith (e.g., baptism) in which your child has participated.
6. What religious/spiritual activities does the family do together? In the home? Out of the home? Attend services? Grace at meals? Bedtime prayers? Other?

*From Davies B, et al. (2002). *Addressing spirituality in pediatric hospice and palliative care. Journal of palliative care,* 18(1), 59-67.

7. Do the parents (or does one parent) regularly pray with the child? Who? When? For what?
8. What evidence of religious/spiritual devotion is there in the home? Religious pictures or objects? Crosses? Statues? Menorahs? Mezuzah? Candles? Holy books? Prayer books? Other?
9. Is there distinctly religious/spiritual object/material in the child's room? What?
10. Does the family believe in "faith healing"? How is it expressed?
11. How does the family's belief system enhance their life?

RELIGIOUS BELIEFS THAT INFLUENCE HEALTH CARE*

A word of caution must regularly be expressed when one is trying to speak absolutes about any religion. Within each denomination or belief system there are always variations. Geographic location, generation gaps, gender differences, or cultural diversity may impact these convictions. Whenever there are any doubts, the best advice is always to ask questions and seek the assistance of professional clergy. Chaplains or other professional pastoral care providers are a good source for information and resources.

Baptist
• **Birth:** Infant baptism is not practiced. However, many churches present the baby and the parents to the congregation when they attend services for the first time after the birth.
• **Death:** It is not mandatory that clergy are present at death, but families often desire visits from clergy. Scripture reading and prayer are important.
• **Organ donation/transplantation:** There is no formal statement regarding this issue. It is considered a matter of personal conscience. It is commonly regarded as positive (an act of love).
• **Beliefs regarding medical care:** Some may regard their illness as punishment resulting from past sins. Those who believe in predestination may not seek aggressive treatment. Fundamentalist and conservative groups see the Bible as the infallible word of God to be taken literally.

---

*From *Texas Children's Cancer Center–Texas Children's Hospital* (2000). *End-of-life care for children*, Houston: Texas Cancer Council, pp. 78-79.

Buddhist
- **Birth:** Buddhists do not practice infant baptism.
- **Death:** A Buddhist priest is often involved before and after death. Rituals are observed during and after death. If the family does not have a priest, they may request one be contacted.
- **Organ donation/transplantation:** There is no formal statement regarding organ donation/transplantation. This is seen as a matter of individual conscience.
- **Beliefs regarding medical care:** Buddhists believe that illness can be used as a tool to aid in the development of the soul. They may see illness as a result of karmic causes; and they may avoid treatments or procedures on holy days. Cleanliness is important.

Church of Jesus Christ of Latter Day Saints (Mormon)
- **Birth:** Infant baptism is not performed. Children are given a name and a priesthood blessing sometime after the birth, from 1 or 2 weeks to several months. In the event of a critically ill newborn, this might be done in the hospital at the discretion of the parents. Baptism is performed after the child is 8 years old. Church of Jesus Christ of Latter Day Saints feel that a child is not accountable for sins before 8 years of age.
- **Death:** There are no religious rituals performed related to death.
- **Organ donation/transplantation:** There is no official statement regarding this issue. Organ donation/transplantation is left up to the individual or parents.
- **Beliefs regarding medical care:** Administration to the sick involves anointing with consecrated oil and a blessing performed by members of the priesthood. Although this is usually requested by the individual or a member of the family if the individual is unconscious and there is no one to represent him or her, it would be appropriate for anyone to contact the church so that the ordinance may be performed. Refusal of medical treatments would be left up to the individual. There are no restrictions relative to "holy" days.

Episcopal
- **Birth:** Infant baptism is practiced. In emergent situations, request for infant baptism should be given high priority and could be performed by any baptized person, clergy or lay. Often in situations of stillbirths or aborted fetuses, special prayers of commendation may be offered.
- **Death:** Pastoral care of the sick may include prayers, laying on of hands, anointing, and/or Holy Communion. At the time of death, various litanies and special prayers may be offered.

- **Organ donation/transplantation:** Both are permitted.
- **Beliefs regarding medical care:** Respect for the dignity of the whole person is important, including physical, emotional, and spiritual needs.

Friend (Quaker)

- **Birth:** The Friends do not practice infant baptism.
- **Death:** Each person has a divine nature, but an encounter and relationship with Jesus Christ are essential.
- **Organ donation/transplantation:** Quakers have no formal statement on organ donation and transplantation, but generally both are permitted.
- **Beliefs regarding medical care:** Quakers have no special rites or restrictions. Leaders and elders from the church may visit and offer support and encouragement. Quakers believe in plain speech.

Islam (Muslim/Moslem)

- **Birth:** At birth, the first words said to the infant in his/her right ear are "Allah-o-akbar" (Allah is great) and the remainder of the Call for Prayer is recited. An *aqeeqa* (party) to celebrate the birth of the child is arranged by the parents. Circumcision of the male child is practiced.
- **Death:** In Islam, life is meant to be a test for the preparation for the everlasting life in the hereafter. Therefore, according to Islam, death is simply a transition. Islam teaches that God has prescribed the time of death for everyone and only He knows when, where, or how a person is going to die. Islam encourages making the best use of all God's gifts, including the precious gift of life in this world. At the time of death, there are specific rituals (bathing, wrapping the body in cloth, etc.) that must be done. Before moving and handling the body, it is preferable to contact someone from the person's mosque or Islamic society to perform these rituals.
- **Organ donation/transplantation:** Organ donation and transplantation are permitted. However, there are some stipulations depending on the type of transplant/donation and its effect on the donor and recipient. It is advisable to contact the individual's mosque or the local Islamic society for further consultation.
- **Beliefs regarding medical care:** Humans are encouraged in the Koran to seek treatment. It is taught that only Allah cures. However, Muslims are taught not to refuse treatment in the belief that Allah will take care of them because even though he cures, he also chooses at times to work through the efforts of humans.

International Society for Krishna Consciousness

The International Society for Krishna Consciousness is a Hindu movement in North America based on devotion to Lord Krishna.

- **Birth:** Infant baptism is not performed.
- **Death:** The body should not be touched. The family may desire that a local temple be contacted so representatives may visit and chant over the patient. It is believed that in chanting the names of God, one may gain insight and God consciousness.
- **Organ donation/transplantation:** There is no formal statement prohibiting this act. It is an individual decision.
- **Beliefs regarding medical care:** Illness or injury is believed to represent sins committed in this or a previous life. Members accept modern medical treatment. The body is seen as a temporary vehicle used to transport them through this life. The body belongs to God, and members are charged to care for it in the best way possible.

Jehovah's Witness

- **Birth:** Infant baptism is not practiced.
- **Death:** There are no official "rites" that are performed before or after death; however, the faith community is often involved and supportive of the patient and family.
- **Organ donation/transplantation:** There is no official statement related to this issue. Organ donation is not encouraged, but it is believed to be an individual decision. According to the Watchtower (legal corporation for the denomination), all donated organs and tissue must be drained of blood before transplantation.
- **Beliefs regarding medical care:** Adherents are absolutely opposed to transfusions of whole blood, packed red blood cells, platelets, and fresh or frozen plasma. This includes banking of one's own blood. Many accept use of albumin, globulin, factor replacement (hemophilia), vaccines, hemodilution, and cell salvage. There is no opposition to nonblood plasma expanders.

Judaism (Orthodox and Conservative)

- **Birth:** Circumcision of male infants is performed on the eighth day if the infant is healthy. This ritual is performed by a mohel (ritual circumciser familiar with Jewish law and aseptic technique).
- **Death:** It is important that the health care professional facilitates the family's need to comfort and be with the patient at the time of death.
- **Organ donation/transplantation:** Organ donation and transplantation are permitted and are considered mitzvahs (good deeds).

- **Beliefs regarding medical care:** Only emergency surgical procedures should be performed on the sabbath, which extends from sundown Friday to sundown Saturday. Elective surgery should be scheduled for days other than the sabbath. Pregnant women and the seriously ill are exempt from fasting. Serious illness may be grounds for violating dietary laws but only if it is medically necessary.

Lutheran
- **Birth:** Infant baptism is practiced. If the infant's prognosis is poor, the family may request immediate baptism.
- **Death:** Family may desire visitation from clergy. Prayers for the dying, commendation of the dying, and prayers for the bereaved may be offered.
- **Organ donation/transplantation:** There is no formal statement regarding this issue. It is considered a matter of personal conscience.
- **Beliefs regarding medical care:** Illness is not seen as an act of God; rather, it is seen as a condition of humanity's fallen state. Prayers for the sick may be desired.

Methodist
- **Birth:** Infant baptism is practiced but is usually done within the community of the church after counseling and guidance from clergy. However, in emergency situations, a request for baptism would not be seen as inappropriate.
- **Death:** In the case of perinatal death, there are prayers within the *United Methodist Book of Worship* that could be said by anyone. Prayer, scripture, and singing are often seen as appropriate and desirable.
- **Organ donation/transplantation:** Organ donation/transplantation is supported and encouraged. It is considered a part of good stewardship.
- **Beliefs regarding medical care:** In the Methodist tradition, it is believed that every person has the right to death with dignity and has the right to be involved in all medical decisions. Refusal of aggressive treatment is seen as an appropriate option.

Pentecostal
Assembly of God, Church of God, Four Square, and many other faith groups are included under this general heading. Pentecostal is not a denomination but a theologic distinctive (pneumatology).
- **Birth:** No rituals such as baptism are necessary. Many Pentecostals have a ceremony of "dedication," but it is done in the context of the community of faith/believers (church). Children belong to heaven and only become sinners after the age of accountability, which is not clearly defined.

- **Death:** Death is the only way to transcend this life; it is the door to heaven (or hell). Questions about "salvation of the soul" are very common and important. Resurrection is the hope of those who "were saved." Prayer is appropriate, as are singing and scripture reading.
- **Organ donation/transplantation:** Many Pentecostal denominations have no statement concerning this subject, but it is generally seen as positive and well received. Education concerning wholeness of the person and nonliteral aspects such as "heart" and "mind" have to be explained. For example, a Pentecostal may have a problem with donating a heart to a "nonbeliever."
- **Beliefs regarding medical care:** Pentecostals are sometimes labeled as "in denial" because of their theology of healing. Their faith in God for literal healing is generally expressed as intentional unbelief in the prognostic statements. Many Pentecostals do not see sickness as the will of God; thus one must "stand firm" in faith and accept the unseen reality, which many times may mean healing. As difficult as this position may seem, it must be noted that, when death occurs, Pentecostals may leap from miracle expectations to joyful hope and theology of heaven and resurrection without facing issues of anger or frustration because of unfulfilled expectations. Prayer, scriptures, singing, and anointing of the sick (not a sacrament) are appropriate/expected pastoral interventions.

Presbyterian
- **Birth:** Baptism is a sacrament of the church but is not considered necessary for salvation. However, it is seen as an event to take place, when possible, in the context of a worshipping community.
- **Death:** Family may desire visitation from clergy. Prayers for the dying, commendation of the dying, and prayers for the bereaved may be offered.
- **Organ donation/transplantation:** There is no formal statement regarding this issue.
- **Beliefs regarding medical care:** Communion is a sacrament of the church. It is generally celebrated with a patient in the presence of an ordained minister and elder. Presbyterians are free to make their own choices regarding the use of mechanical life-support measures.

Roman Catholic
- **Birth:** Infant baptism is practiced. In medical facilities, baptism is usually performed by a priest or deacon; as ordinary members of the sacrament. However, under extraordinary circumstances, baptism may be administered by a lay person, provided that the intention is

to do as the church does, using the formula, "I baptize you in the name of the Father, the Son, and the Holy Spirit."

- **Death:** Sacrament of the sick is the sacrament of healing and forgiveness. It is to be administered by a priest as early in the illness as possible. It is not a last rite to be administered at the point of death. The Roman Catholic church makes provisions for prayers of commendation of the dying, which may be said by any priest, deacon, sacramental minister, or lay person.
- **Organ donation/transplantation:** Catholics may donate or receive organ transplants.
- **Beliefs regarding medical care:** The sacrament of Holy Communion sustains Catholics in sickness as in health. When the patient's condition deteriorates, the sacrament is given as viaticum ("food for the journey"). Like Holy Communion, viaticum may be administered by a priest, deacon, or sacramental minister. The church makes provisions for prayers for commendation of the dying that may be said by any of those listed above or by a lay person.

GUIDELINES FOR ADDRESSING SPIRITUALITY IN PARENTS

Assess each parent individually with the following questions*:

1. How have your child's diagnosis and illness affected your beliefs about God? The practice of your religion? The practice of your personal faith/spirituality?
2. From the perspective of your faith what has been most difficult to cope with? What helps?
3. Do you believe in such a thing as "divine purpose"? Describe.
4. How have the daily care needs of the child been managed? Who is responsible for what? For the child's spiritual care?
5. Are you supported by a priest, rabbi, minister, guru, holy person, or the like?
6. Would you like to be reconnected to a priest, rabbi, minister, or religious representative?
7. What do you understand a chaplain does? Would the support of a hospice chaplain be of help?
8. Do you pray about the child's illness? For what? How do you feel when you pray?
9. What concerns do you have about the seriousness of your child's illness?
10. Have you ever discussed with each other what might happen if your child were to die? When? What was that like? (If no, why?)

---

*From Davies B, et al. (2002). Addressing spirituality in pediatric hospice and palliative care. Journal of palliative care, 18(1), 59-67.

11. Have you ever discussed this with someone else? With whom? What was that like?

12. How has your child's illness affected your interactions with your spouse/partner?

13. How has your child's illness affected your relationship to your other child/children? Your parents?

14. How has the diagnosis and illness of this child affected his/her grandparents or the extended family? What has this been like for you?

15. What helps you to cope? To keep going on a daily basis?

16. Has anything changed for you in terms of your priorities or values or how you determine what is important in your day-by-day life as a result of your child's illness? What? How?

17. Are there any rituals or keepsakes (e.g., memory box, hand prints of child and family members, recordings) that might be important to you now? Later?

GUIDELINES FOR ADDRESSING SPIRITUALITY IN SIBLINGS

Adapt the following guidelines* to the child's developmental level; use drawing, storytelling, or favorite objects as necessary.

1. What do you understand about your brother's/sister's illness?

2. How has the illness of your brother/sister changed the life of your family?

3. What has that been like for you? What has changed for you specifically?

4. How has it changed the way your mother/father relates to you?

5. What kinds of things do you do to try to help your sister/brother?

6. What is the most difficult thing for you about your brother's/sister's illness?

7. Do you ever think that she/he may die? What is that like?

8. Why do you think your brother/sister got sick?

9. Do you think anything you ever said or did caused her/his illness?

10. Do you pray for your sister/brother? For what? When?

11. What do you think it would be like if your brother/sister were to die?

12. Where do you think he/she would go if he/she dies? What is that like for you?

13. Do you have someone you can talk to about your own feelings?

14. What do you think God is like? (What toy, object, animal does that child have that reminds him/her of God?)

15. How do you think God feels about your sister/brother? You?

---

*From Davies B, et al. (2002). Addressing spirituality in pediatric hospice and palliative care. Journal of palliative care, 18(1), 59-67.

16. What is it about your brother/sister you would most remember about him/her if he/she were to die?
17. Is there anything about your sister's/brother's illness that is hard to talk about with your father/mother? What?
18. What helps you to keep going day by day?
19. Do you have a "secret" place to which you go to feel "safe" or "secure"? Describe.
20. To whom do you turn for support when you need it most?

GUIDELINES FOR ADDRESSING SPIRITUALITY IN GRANDPARENTS*

Identify the grandparents' relationship as paternal or maternal.

1. What has it been like for you to have a grandchild so ill?
2. What concerns you the most?
3. Have you thought about what might happen if your grandchild were to die? What is that like?
4. What kind of support are you able to give to his/her parents? How does that feel?
5. Has your grandchild's illness affected your relationship with her/his parents? If so, how?
6. What concerns you most about them?
7. What concerns you about the rest of the family, such as the child's siblings or your other children and grandchildren?
8. Have there been any religious/spiritual conflicts between you and the child's parent(s) that are unresolved? What? How does that affect you now? Would you like to see if that could be resolved?
9. What do you do to try to find meaning or purpose in this experience?
10. What gives you hope during your grandchild's illness?
11. Are there any rituals or keepsakes (e.g., memory box, hand prints of child and family members, recordings) that might be important to you now? Later?

• • •

Culture (Table 20-3) is another consideration when discussing death and the dying process. It colors the world view of the family and must be valued when providing care.

---

*From Davies B, et al. (2002). Addressing spirituality in pediatric hospice and palliative care. Journal of palliative care, 18(1), 59-67.

Table 20-3	Multicultural Outcomes: Guidelines for Cultural Competence (Summary of the Domains of Culture)*
Domain	**Description**
Ethnic identity	Country of origin, ethnicity/culture with which the group identifies, current residence, reasons for migration, degree of acculturation/assimilation, level of cultural pride
Communication	Dominant language and any dialects, usual volume/tone of speech, willingness to share thoughts/feelings/ideas, meaning of touch, use of eye contact, control of expressions and emotions, spokesperson/decision maker in family
Time and space	Past, present, or future time orientation; preference for personal space and distance
Social organization	Family structure; head of household, gender roles, status/role of older people; roles of children, adolescents, husband/wife, mother/father, extended family; influences on the decision-making process; importance of social organization and network
Workforce issues	Primary wage earner, impact of illness on work, transportation to clinic visits, health insurance, financial impact, importance of work
Health beliefs, practices, and practitioners	Meaning/cause of cancer and illness/health, living with life-threatening illness, expectations and use of Western treatment and health care team, religious/spiritual beliefs and practices, use of traditional healers/practitioners, expectations of practitioners, loss of body part/body image, acceptance of blood transfusions/organ donations, sick role and health-seeking behaviors

Continued

Table 20-3	Multicultural Outcomes: Guidelines for Cultural Competence (Summary of the Domains of Culture)* —cont'd
Domain	**Description**
Nutrition	Meaning of food and mealtimes, preferences and preparation of food, taboos/rituals, religious influences on food preferences and preparation
Biologic variations	Skin/mucous membrane color, physical variations, drug metabolism, laboratory data, and genetic variations—specific risk factors and differences in incidence/survival/mortality of specific cancers
Sexuality and reproductive fears	Beliefs about sexuality and reproductive/childbearing activities, taboos, privacy issues, interaction of cancer diagnosis/treatments with beliefs about sexuality
Religion and spirituality	Dominant religion; religious beliefs, rituals, and ceremonies; use of prayer, meditation, or other symbolic activities; meaning of life; source of strength
Death and dying	Meaning of dying, death, and the afterlife; belief in fatalism; rituals, expectations, and mourning/bereavement practices

From Oncology Nursing Society (1999). Oncology Nursing Society multicultural outcomes: guidelines for cultural competence. Pittsburgh, Pa: Author.

***Note:** To use for developmentally and appropriate child/adolescent and/or parent and family. In the case of newborns and infants these guidelines can be applied to the family unit.*

CULTURAL SELF-ASSESSMENT*

1. Where were you born? If an immigrant, how long have you lived in the United States?
2. How old were you when you came to the United States? Where were your grandparents born?
3. What is your ethnic affiliation, and how strong is your ethnic identity?
4. How does your culture affect decisions regarding medical treatment? Who makes decisions—you, your family, or a designated family member? What are the gender issues in your culture and in your family structure?
5. What are your primary and secondary languages, speaking and reading ability?
6. How would you characterize your nonverbal communication style?
7. What is your religion, its importance in your daily life, and current practices? Is religion an important source of support and comfort?
8. What are your food preferences and prohibitions?
9. What is your economic situation, and is the income adequate to meet the needs of you and your family?
10. What are your health and illness beliefs and practices?
11. What are your customs and beliefs around such transitions as birth, illness, and death? What are your past experiences regarding death and bereavement? How much do you and your family wish to know about the disease and prognosis? What are your beliefs about the afterlife and miracles? What are your beliefs about hope?

CULTURAL INFLUENCES ON HEALTH BELIEFS AND PRACTICES†

Asian Chinese
- A healthy body is viewed as gift from parents and ancestors and must be cared for.
- Health is one of the results of balance between the forces of yin (cold) and yang (hot)—energy forces that rule the world.
- Illness is caused by imbalance.
- Blood is source of life and is not regenerated.
- Chi is innate energy.

---

*Modified from Zoucha R (2000). The keys to culturally sensitive care. American journal of nursing, 200, 24GG-24II. Modified from Davies B, et al. (2002). Addressing spirituality in pediatric hospice and palliative care. Journal of palliative care, 18(1), 59-67.
†Modified from Wong D, et al. (1999). Nursing care of infants and children, ed 6, St Louis: Mosby. From Texas Children's Cancer Center–Texas Children's Hospital (2000). End-of-life care for children, Houston: Texas Cancer Council.

- Lack of chi and blood produces fatigue, poor constitution, and long illness.
- There is wide use of medicinal herbs procured and applied in prescribed ways.
- Folk healers are herbalist, spiritual healer, temple healer, and fortune healer.

Japanese

Japanese health beliefs and practices stem from three major belief systems:

1. Shinto religious influence
   a. Humans are inherently good.
   b. Evil is caused by outside spirits.
   c. Illness is caused by contact with polluting agents (e.g., blood, corpses, skin disease).
2. Chinese and Korean influence
   a. Health is achieved through harmony and balance between self and society.
   b. Disease is caused by disharmony with society and not caring for body.
3. Portuguese influence
   a. Upholds germ theory of disease: evil is removed by purification.
   b. Kampo medicine is use of natural herbs.
   c. Care for disabled is viewed as family's responsibility.
   d. Take pride in child's good health.
   e. Seek preventive care, medical care for illness.

Vietnamese

- Good health is considered to be balance between yin and yang.
- Vietnamese believe person's life has been predisposed toward certain phenomena by cosmic forces.
- Health is believed to be result of harmony with existing universal order; harmony attained by pleasing good spirits and avoiding evil ones.
- There is a belief in *am duc*, the amount of good deeds accumulated by ancestors.
- Many use rituals to prevent illness.
- Vietnamese practice some restrictions to prevent incurring wrath of evil spirits.
- Vietnamese regard health as family responsibility; outside aid is sought when resources run out.

Filipino

- Filipinos believe God's will and supernatural forces govern universe.
- Illness, accident, and other misfortunes are God's punishment for violations of his will.
- Filipinos widely accept "hot" and "cold" balance and imbalance as cause of health and illness.
- Some use amulets as a shield for witchcraft or as good luck pieces.

African American

1. Classification of illness
   a. Natural forces of nature against which there is not adequate protection (e.g., cold air, pollution, food and water)
   b. Unnatural, evil influences (e.g., witchcraft, voodoo, hoodoo, hex fix, root work); symptoms often associated with eating
2. Believe serious illness sent by God as punishment (e.g., parents punished by illness or death of the child)
3. Self-care and folk medicine very prevalent
4. Attempt home remedies first
5. May resist health care because illness is "will of God"
6. Prayer common means for prevention and treatment

Haitian

1. Illnesses have a supernatural or natural origin.
2. Supernatural illnesses are caused by angry voodoo spirits, enemies, or the dead, especially deceased ancestors.
3. Natural illnesses are based on conceptions of natural causation: irregularities of blood volume, flow, purity, viscosity, color, and/or temperature (hot/cold).
   a. Gas (gaz)
   b. Movement and consistency of mother's milk
   c. "Hot/cold" imbalance in the body
   d. Bone displacement
   e. Movement of diseases
4. Health is maintained by good dietary and hygienic habits.
5. Health is a personal responsibility.
6. Foods have properties of hot/cold and light/heavy and must be in harmony with one's life cycle and body states.
7. Supernatural illness is treated by healers: voodoo priest (houngan) or priestess (mambo), midwife (fam saj), and herbalist or leaf doctor (dokte fey).
8. Amulets and prayer are used to protect against illness caused by curses or willed by evil people.

Hispanic/Mexican

- Health beliefs have strong religious association.
- Body imbalance between *caliente* (hot) and *frio* (cold) or "wet" and "dry" is a cause of illness.
- Some maintain good health is a result of good luck.
- Illness prevented by performing properly, through prayer, by wearing religious medals or amulets, and by sleeping with relics at home.
- Illness is a punishment from God for wrongdoing, forces of nature, and the supernatural.
- Seek help from curandero or curandera, especially in rural areas. Curandero(a) receives his/her position by birth, apprenticeship, or a "calling" via dream or vision.
- Practices used for severe illness include making promises, visiting shrines, offering medals and candles, and offering prayers.
- Hispanics/Mexicans adhere to "hot" and "cold" food prescriptions and prohibitions for prevention and treatment of illness.

Puerto Rican

- Puerto Ricans subscribe to the "hot and cold" theory of causation of illness.
- They believe some illness is caused by evil spirits and forces.
- They consult spiritualist medium for mental disorders.
- *Santeria* is system, and practitioners are called *santeros*.

Cuban

- Prevention and good nutrition are related to good health.
- Cubans are diligent users of the medical model.
- Cubans have eclectic health-seeking practices: folk medicine of both religious and nonreligious origins; home remedies; in many instances, seek assistance of santeros and spiritualists to complement medical treatment.

Native American

- Native Americans believe health is state of harmony with nature and universe.
- They respect their bodies through proper management.
- All disorders are believed to have aspects of supernatural.
- Violation of a restriction or prohibition is thought to cause illness.
- Native Americans fear witchcraft.
- They may carry objects believed to guard against witchcraft.
- Theology and medicine are strongly interwoven.

ASSESSMENT FOR DEPRESSION: CRITERIA FOR MAJOR DEPRESSIVE EPISODE

At least five of the following symptoms* have been present most of the day, or almost every day, for at least 2 weeks. At least one of the symptoms must be item 1 or 2.

1. Depressed mood (feeling sad or empty; appears tearful)
2. Markedly decreased interest or pleasure in all, or almost all, activities
3. Significant weight loss
4. Insomnia or hypersomnia
5. Psychomotor agitation or retardation
6. Fatigue or loss of energy
7. Feelings of worthlessness or excessive or inappropriate guilt
8. Diminished ability to think or concentrate or indecisiveness
9. Recurrent thoughts of death (not just fear of dying), recurrent suicidal ideation, or suicide attempt

INTERVENTIONS TO FOSTER HOPE FOR FAMILIES OF NEWBORNS†

Experiential Processes

1. Prevent and manage EOL symptoms.
2. Encourage family to transcend their current situation.
   a. Encourage aesthetic experiences.
   b. Encourage engagement in creative and joyous endeavors.

---

*From Kuebler KK (2002). Depression. In Kuebler KK, Berry PH, Heidrich DE, editors. End-of-life care: clinical practice guidelines, Philadelphia: WB Saunders, p. 270. Modified from American Psychiatric Association (2000). Major depressive disorder. a patient and family guide, Washington, DC: APA; American Psychiatric Association (2000). Practice guidelines for the treatment of patients with major depression, ed 2, Washington, DC: APA. Used with permission.
†Modified from Ersek M (2001). The meaning of hope in the dying. In Ferrell BR, Coyle N, editors. Textbook of palliative nursing, New York: Oxford University Press.

   c. Suggest literature, films, and art that are uplifting and high-light the joys in life.
   d. Encourage reminiscing.
   e. Assist family to focus on present and past joys.
   f. Share positive, hope-inspiring stories.
3. Support family in positive self-talk.
4. Utilize lightheartedness and humor appropriately.
5. Facilitate positive self-esteem for the family.

Spiritual/Transcendental Processes
1. Facilitate participation in religious rituals and spiritual practices.
2. Make necessary referrals to clergy and other spiritual support people.
3. Assist the family in finding meaning in the current situation.
   a. Suggest keeping a journal (family).
   b. Suggest literature, films, and art that explore the meaning of suffering.
   c. Suggest music, imagery, meditation, or other complementary therapies appropriate for the child.

Relational Processes
- Minimize family isolation.
- Establish and maintain an open relationship.
- Affirm the family's sense of self-worth.
- Recognize and reinforce the reciprocal nature of hopefulness between the family and their support system.
- Provide private time for relationships (especially important in institutional settings).
- Assist the family to identify significant family member/other and then to reflect on personal characteristics and experiences that endear the significant family member/other to the family.
- Communicate one's own sense of hopefulness.
- Assist the family in identifying range of hopes.

Rational Thought Processes
- Assist the family to establish, obtain, and revise goals without imposing one's own agenda.
- Assist in identifying available and needed resources to meet goals.
- Assist in procuring needed resources.
- Assist with breaking larger goals into smaller steps to increase feelings of success.
- Provide accurate information regarding child's condition and treatment.
- Help the family identify past successes.
- Increase the family's sense of control when possible.

HELPING PARENTS FACE THE DEATH OF THEIR CHILD*

Communication

- Listen attentively.
- Find out what the family knows and what they want to know.
- Use language that family members can understand.
- Call the child by name.
- Use silence as an ally, but watch for signs that parents need to talk.
- Encourage questions.
- Do not offer platitudes.
- Do not automatically offer tissues.

Facilitating Family Grieving

- Offer a private place for the family to retreat.
- If death occurs, allow the family time with the child after the death.
- Encourage involvement of siblings.
- Preserve memories of the child: last height, weight, lock of hair, hospital name band, plaster of Paris hand print or footprint, picture of the child, child's blanket and clothes in a plastic bag (to preserve scent).
- Help establish links with a social worker, spiritual support person (chaplain, priest, rabbi, healer), funeral director.
- Provide specific information about how the needs of siblings can be met.
- Provide pamphlets for family members and friends to give them tips about how to help the parents.

Anger![†]

Don't tell me that you understand,
Don't tell me that you know.
Don't tell me that I will survive,
How I will surely grow.

Don't tell me this is just a test,
That I am truly blessed,
That I am chosen for this task,
Apart from all the rest.

Don't come at me with answers
That can only come from me,
Don't tell me how my grief will pass . . .
That I will soon be free.

---

*Modified from Bowden V, et al., editors. Children and their families: the continuum of care, Philadelphia: WB Saunders, p. 649.
[†]From Hendel J (1996). Anger! In Gambill A, editor. Food for the soul, Colorado Springs, Colo: Bereavement Publishing, Inc. Reprinted with permission from Bereavement Publishing.

Don't stand in pious judgment
Of the bonds I must untie.
Don't tell me how to suffer,
And don't tell me how to cry.

My life is filled with selfishness,
My pain is all I see,
But I need you, and I need your love...
Unconditionally.

Accept me in my ups and downs.
I need someone to share,
Just hold my hand and let me cry,
And say, "My friend, I care."

GUIDELINES FOR WORKING WITH SIBLINGS OF ILL NEWBORNS AND INFANTS*

Recommendations for Parents

Suggestions that may help parents to assist the siblings of the ill newborn or infant are given below:

1. Treat the children equally by taking into account each child's special needs.
2. Keep in contact with the siblings during the hospital stays with the ill newborn or infant.
3. Spend even limited time alone with the siblings.
4. Permit the siblings to continue with their lives as normally as possible.

Counseling the Sibling

Specific recommendations for the caregiver in counseling the sick child's sibling during the phase of palliative care include the following:

1. Give the sibling a clear and unambiguous concept of the child's illness and its cause.
2. Encourage the sibling to dispense with any erroneous concepts of the cause of the child's illness.
3. Allow the sibling to visit the clinic, meet the staff caring for the child, and witness the child's treatment program.
4. Assign the sibling a helpful task in the child's home care.
5. Reassure the sibling that he or she will not develop the same illness (this is always slightly difficult, since the physician or nurse

---

*Modified from Stevens MM (1999). *Care of the dying child and adolescent: family adjustment and support. In Doyle D, Hanks GWC, MacDonald N, editors. Oxford textbook of palliative medicine, ed 2, Oxford, UK: Oxford University Press.*

practitioner may have had personal experience of a sibling developing the same illness).

6. Provide the sibling with appropriate opportunities for ventilation (verbal and nonverbal) of feelings of resentment toward parents or the patient.

7. Provide an opportunity for the sibling to say good-bye as the child's death approaches.

8. Allow the sibling to attend the funeral along with the rest of the family if he or she wishes to do so. Children should not be forced to attend such events, and they need the freedom to participate to the degree they feel comfortable.

*Sibling Responses**
Psychologic
- Fear of own death and parents' death
- Tearfulness
- Anxiety (over people leaving, with new situations)
- Loneliness
- Angry outbursts or temper tantrums
- Concerns about getting sick
- Attention seeking from parents
- Withdrawn (guarding feelings and thoughts)
- Sadness
- Daydreaming
- Change in school performance (decreased concentration)

Physiologic
- Sleep disturbances (reluctant to go to bed, nightmares)
- Eating disturbances (loss of appetite, lack of interest in food)
- Body complaints (e.g., headaches, stomach aches, generalized aches)
- Increased incidence of colds and influenza episodes
- Frequent infections (urinary tract, respiratory tract)

GUIDELINES FOR THE HEALTH CARE TEAM IN ASSISTING EACH OTHER WITH END-OF-LIFE DECISION MAKING WITH NEWBORNS AND INFANTS†

1. Know the guidelines offered by specific disciplines regarding roles in EOL decision making (i.e., American Nurses Associations, American Academy of Pediatric statements).

---

*Modified from Davies B, Eng BWS (1999). Special issues in bereavement and staff support. In Doyle D, Hands GWC, MacDonald N, editors. The textbook of palliative medicine, Oxford, UK: Oxford University Press.
†Modified from Hinds PS, Oakes L, Furman W (2001). End-of-life decision making in pediatric oncology. In Ferrell B, Coyle N, editors. Textbook of palliative nursing, New York: Oxford University Press, p. 457.

2. Before initiating EOL discussions with families, all members of the health care team should discuss and agree on the following:
   a. The need for discussion
   b. Which options are appropriate and available
   c. Whether outside consultants are needed to identify which options are in the best interest of the patient
   d. Which other team members will participate in the discussion with the parents
   e. A time of the discussion and specific staff members who will participate
   f. Which staff member will document the discussion in the medical record
   g. Availability of the appropriate staff time and resources to address any questions parents may have
3. Be available to team members and to the parents to discuss and rediscuss decision and related concerns.
4. Explore with the team all appropriate options to ensure that all that can be done is being done and being done well.
5. Inform other team members if feedback from or assessment of the parents indicates that any decision needs clarification or reconsideration.

NEONATAL END-OF-LIFE PALLIATIVE CARE PROTOCOL*

The purpose of this protocol of care is to educate professionals and enhance their preparation and support for a peaceful, pain-free, and family-centered death for dying newborns.

Planning for a Palliative Care Environment

Instituting a palliative care program requires planning, training, and commitment from participants. There should be a formal education plan for the staff, including both clinical and ethical training, in the following areas:

1. Alternatives to allowing the newborn to die from his/her condition
2. Long-term outcomes of severely impaired newborns
3. Principles of transition from life-extending care to palliative care
4. Palliative care training from hospice experts, that is, anticipation and ongoing treatment of symptoms, skin care, mouth care, pain medication (Table 20-4), relief of dyspnea, decreased light and noise, use of positioning aids, promotion

---

*Modified from Catlin A, Carter B (2002). Creation of a neonatal end-of-life palliative care protocol. Journal of perinatology, 22(3), 184-195.

Table 20-4	Relevant Medications for Neonatal Palliative Care*			
Drug	**Category**	**Dose (per kg)**	**Route of Administration and Dosing Interval**	**Comments**
Acetaminophen	Analgesic, antipyretic	10-15 mg	PO, PR every 4-6 hr	Inhibits prostaglandin synthesis
Chloral hydrate	Sedative	10-25 mg	PO, PR every 6-8 hr	Gastric irritation
	Hypnotic	25-50 mg	PO, PR × one dose only	
Diazepam	Sedative, anxiolytic, anticonvulsant	0.05-0.3 mg (max. 2 mg/24 hr)	IV every 6-8 hr	Respiratory depression, hypotension
Fentanyl	Analgesic	1-3 μg	IV, IM every 2-4 hr Continuous IV infusion may be given at 1-4 μg/kg/hr	Tachyphylaxis, respiratory depression
Furosemide	Diuretic	1-2 mg	IV, PO, IM every 12 hr	Hypochloremia
Glycopyrrolate	Drying agent	0.01 mg	IV, PO, IM every 4-8 hr	Anticholinergic
Lorazepam	Sedative, anxiolytic, anticonvulsant	0.05-0.10 mg	IV every 4-8 hr	Respiratory depression, hypotension
Metoclopramide	Antiemetic, promotility	0.03-0.1 mg	IV, PO, IM every 8 hr	Controversial benefit for reflux
Midazolam	Sedative, anxiolytic	0.03-0.1 mg (short acting)	IV, IM every 2-4 hr Continuous IV infusion may be given at 0.05 mg/kg/hr	Respiratory depression, hypotension

Continued

Table 20-4	Relevant Medications for Neonatal Palliative Care*—cont'd			
Drug	Category	Dose (per kg)	Route of Administration and Dosing Interval	Comments
Morphine	Analgesic	0.05-0.1 mg	IV, IM, SC every 2-4 hr Continuous IV infusion may be given at 0.01-0.02 mg/kg/hr	Respiratory depression, hypotension
Paregoric (camphorated tincture of opium; contains 45% alcohol)	Sedative Analgesic	0.2-0.5 mg 0.2-0.3 ml/dose	PO every 4-6 hr PO 1-4 times/day	See Morphine; give with feeds; decreases GI motility
Phenobarbital	Anticonvulsant	Loading dose: 20 mg Maintenance: 2.5 mg	IV once IV, IM, PO every 12 hr	CNS depression, sedative effects
Phenytoin	Anticonvulsant	Loading dose: 20 mg Maintenance: 2-4 mg	IV once (slowly) IV, PO every 12 hr	Bradycardia, toxicity: seizures

PO, By mouth; PR, per rectum; IV, intravenously; IM, intramuscularly; SC, subcutaneously; GI, gastrointestinal; CNS, central nervous system.

*See references for sources of information.

of self-regulatory measures such as sucking and grasping if infant is able to do so

5. Familiarization of staff with the various pain assessment tools for use with newborns

6. Staff given information on how to access home care and community resources and how to meet and establish ties with these local services

7. Theories of crisis intervention, grief stages, family dynamics, and stress and coping

8. A plan for conflict mediation

9. Cultural expectations at the time of neonatal death taught by members of ethnic and religious groups in the relevant communities

10. In-service education from the regional organ procurement center that teaches what types of organ and tissue donations are acceptable/desirable in the neonatal population

11. How an ethics consultation may assist the staff and families

Additional considerations when establishing a palliative care service include the following:

- No visiting hour restrictions
- Staff recognition of mother's immediate postpartum needs if she has recently given birth
- Development of a core staff of nurses from obstetrics, neonatal intensive care, pediatric intensive care, and general pediatrics who wish to provide palliative care; these nurses should receive special training and then be allowed palliative care assignments
- Development of a cadre of volunteers who are also interested in this type of care and who can assist the nurses when staffing difficulties preclude one-to-one care
- Trained translation staff available 24 hours per day
- Selection and preparation of an area appropriate for palliative care to take place in, preferably a homelike room with soft lights that is large enough to hold extended family and in which clergy would be able to conduct a service
- Preparation of an information packet to give the parents after the infant dies that presents information about grieving, including local funeral options, memorials, what to expect in themselves and from others, and how to find help with the grieving experience
- If desired, a review of the palliative care protocol by the ethics committee and legal department may be helpful
- A plan in place for staff to review palliative care protocols at the time of annual competency training, neonatal resuscitation protocol (NRP), or pediatric advanced life support (PALS) recertification, or policy and procedure reviews, especially in smaller facilities that do not provide this type of care routinely;

annual review of symptom management, medications, community resources, and home hospice planning

- Inclusion in all new employee orientations and information given to rotating students, residents, fellows, attending physicians, or other medical staff

Prenatal discussion of palliative care It is essential that fetal development and viability be discussed with all families as a part of prenatal care packages and classes and with all families receiving assisted reproductive therapies. As the course of prenatal care progresses, pregnant women should be made aware that newborns in the very early gestational periods of 22 to 24 weeks and birth weights of less than 500 g may not be responsive to resuscitation or applied neonatal intensive care.

Physician considerations

- Physicians presenting these data should include both short- and long-term expectations when such are known or available, including the developmental potential of the infant and the potential impact this may have on the family.
- All high-risk couples should be honestly counseled on their options regarding interventions, timing of delivery, use of tocolytics, transfer to or from a high-risk center, cesarean delivery, keeping the newborn in the local community vs. the high-risk referral center, and the availability of infant hospice support services.
- Early discussion allows time for parents to develop trust in the medical team and tour the neonatal intensive care unit where their newborn may be treated.
- Having a pediatrician at the delivery to confirm the diagnosis is appropriate.
- It is noted that time does not always allow for such discussions, as in the event of rapid preterm delivery, a previously undiscovered problem, or a birth-related incident.

Family considerations

- Families may wish to talk with other parents who have been given the same prenatal diagnosis, and this should be facilitated.
- Encouraging families to make plans for their potentially nonviable infant while in utero is seen as a type of autonomy for the pregnant patient.
- Pregnant mothers and families may need time to notify extended family, arrange for necessary support (family, spiritual, psychologic, emotional), prepare siblings, choose a name for the baby, shop for and bring clothing to the hospital, make funeral and/or memorial service arrangements, and many other tasks of anticipatory grief. This is also a time for the hospital personnel to prepare themselves and for the physicians to decide on a plan of care and whether resuscitation is appropriate at the time of birth.

- Sensitive support for families may include comforting pregnant women and mothers who did not plan the pregnancy and who may be accepting, without grief, that it is ending.

Transport issues   It is best that mothers not be separated from their newborn infants. Transport is considered both traumatic and expensive, and if the newborn's condition is incompatible with prolonged life then arrangement to stay in the local hospital may generally be preferred. It is best to avoid transferring dying newborns to level III NICUs if nothing more can be done there than at the local hospital. The local area is recognized as that location at which parents have their support system, rapport with their established health care providers, a spiritual/religious community, and funeral availability.

Although parents may desire/demand transfer to a level III facility, transport implies that something can be done to help the newborn or change the outcome. There may be cases in which the option of transport should not even be offered. Local protocols and guidelines should be developed between the regional level III referral center and the community hospital.

If a newborn is to remain in the local community hospital, various requirements are needed. These include the availability of specialists, such as a neonatologist, geneticist, or neurologist, to make certain that the diagnosis is correct. The development and use of telemedicine and telehealth technologies between community centers and regional referral centers with subspecialty consultants may assist in this process.

The local hospital must also have in place a palliative care protocol and trained staff as described. Community hospital staff may need to be assisted with providing palliative care by those in the referral centers where it is done more often. A collegial relationship between the referral center and the local providers is essential, since the local staff may require additional education and resources to manage the dying infant and support the family throughout the process.

In addition, if a newborn has been transferred to a level III center and it is determined that no curative treatment is indicated, he/she should be transported back to the local hospital or home with hospice care in order to be together with family in their own community.

Which newborns should receive palliative care?   Whereas many aspects of palliative care should be integrated into the care of all newborns, there are infants born for whom parents and the health care professionals believe that palliative care is the most appropriate form of care. The following list includes categories of newborns that have experienced the transition from life-extending technologic support to palliative care. The individual context of applying palliative care will require that each case, in each family, within each health care center be explored individually. These categories of newborns are provided for educational purposes and may engender discussion at the local institutional level.

1. Newborns at the threshold of viability, with extremely low birth weights and gestational ages, especially those with gestational ages at or under 24 weeks or weighing less than 500 g if no growth retardation exists. Newborns weighing slightly more (<750 g) or who are born slightly older (<27 weeks' gestation) may develop serious complications that become life limiting as additional time passes.

2. Newborns with complex or multiple congenital anomalies incompatible with prolonged life, where neonatal intensive care will not affect long-term outcome, such as the following:

   a. Genetic problems: trisomy 13, 15 or 18; triploidy, thanatophoric dwarfism, or lethal forms of osteogenesis imperfecta; errors of metabolism that are expected to be lethal even with available therapy

   b. Kidney problems: Potter's syndrome/renal agenesis and severe lung hypoplasia; some cases of polycystic kidney disease or renal failure requiring dialysis

   c. Central nervous system abnormalities: anencephaly/acrania, holoprosencephaly, some complex or severe cases of meningomyelocele or large encephaloceles, hydranencephaly; congenital severe hydrocephalus with absent or minimal brain growth; neurodegenerative diseases requiring ventilation (e.g., spinal muscular atrophy)

   d. Heart problems: acardia, inoperable heart anomalies, some cases of hypoplastic left heart syndrome, pentalogy of Cantrell (ectopia cordis)

   e. Structural anomalies: some cases of giant omphalocele, severe congenital diaphragmatic hernia with hypoplastic lungs; inoperable conjoined twins

3. Newborns not responding to intensive care intervention, who are deteriorating despite all appropriate efforts or in combination with a life-threatening acute event:

   a. Nonresponsive to aggressive resuscitation regardless of gestational age

   b. Recipients of repeated cardiopulmonary resuscitations (CPRs)

   c. Severe cases of perinatal brain injury, such as hemorrhages or leukomalacia

   d. Severe asphyxia (pH <7.0, Apgar <3 at 15 minutes)

   e. Hypoxic-ischemic encephalopathy (HIE)

   f. Multiple end-organ disease/failure

   g. Overwhelming sepsis after attempts at support

   h. Necrotizing enterocolitis (NEC) or midgut volvulus without viable intestines or for whom an extremely short gut makes feeding/growth impossible

i. Newborns unable to be weaned off extracorporeal membrane oxygenation (ECMO)

Introducing the palliative care model to parents Speaking to parents about palliative care is difficult. There is heartache from the staff and heartfelt sympathy for the parents. The following points are offered to help physicians and nurse practitioners facilitate the process:

- Let the family members know they will not be abandoned. This will include frequent assessments by the nurse, daily visits by the physician, and the visits of the social worker and the chaplain. "We will be adjusting medications so that your infant is comfortable. What other support can I offer to you?"

- Assist the family in obtaining all of the medical information that they want. Tell them that the entire medical team wishes the situation were different. Let them know you will support them every step of the way and that their infant is a valued and loved member of their family.

- Hold conversations in a quiet, private, and physically comfortable space. Allow a lengthy period of time. Be seated. Give the parents written notes. If indicated, offer to tape record the conversation for their use later. Offer the family the benefit of having a third party present.

- Give them your beeper number or telephone number to call you after they have digested the information and have more questions. Offer the ability to have a second opinion and/or an ethics consultation. One might ask: "Who else do you have to support you? Is there anyone you would like me to call, such as a family member; your rabbi, priest, or minister; or someone important to you that could help you at this time—or would you like to speak to one of the chaplains on staff?"

- Come back later with a statement such as "Many parents in your situation have had similar questions, should I share those questions with you?"

- Provide parents time to consult the local regional center that works with children with special needs or their area pediatrician who can provide information on projected abilities and disabilities.

- Offer to introduce them to parents who have been in a similar situation. Many facilities have parent-counselors as part of the paid or volunteer staff.

- When possible, use lay person language to clarify medical terms and allow a great deal of time for parents to process the information. Strive for nonjudgmental language. Use visual aids to explain the extent of the problem if appropriate.

- The terms *withdrawal of treatment* or *withdrawal of care* should be avoided. Explain that the infant will be continuously cared for by highly trained and dedicated staff and that his/her symptoms will be monitored and discomfort prevented or aggressively treated.

- Communicate and collaborate with parents at all times. Efforts should be made to clarify mutually derived goals of care for the infant. Do not tell parents that they have a choice between technologic support and palliative care if technologic support is no longer an appropriate or beneficial form of care. Given such a choice, parents often mistakenly feel that they would be agents of the infant's death if they do not use all technologic interventions. The team's professional recommendation that the goals of care should be directed toward enhancing comfort rather than trying to unsuccessfully modify the disease process should be clearly stated. Give as many choices as possible about how palliative care should be implemented for their infant. Inform the parents of improved access to the infant for holding, cuddling, kangaroo care, and breast-feeding.

- If the transition in care involves the removal of ventilatory support, explain that the use of ventilators is for the improvement of heart/lung conditions until cure—when cure is a likely outcome. Make clear that using a ventilator to breathe for an infant who is overwhelmed by the underlying disease process and is dying is neither beneficial nor recommended. Affirming this with their spiritual leaders and extended family members is also important, since this is a difficult concept for some families to comprehend and may take recurrent discussion.

- Tell the parents that you cannot change the situation but you can support the infant's short life with comfort and dignity. Explain that discontinuing interventions that cause suffering is a brave and loving action to take for their infant.

- Validate the loss of the dreamed-for healthy infant, but point out the good/memorable features he/she has. Help parents look past any deformities and work to alleviate any blame they may express.

- Encourage parents to be a family as much as possible. Refer to the newborn by name. Assist them to plan what they would like to do while the infant is still alive.

- Encourage them to ask support persons to join them on the unit. Facilitate sibling visitation. Support siblings with child life specialists on staff.

- In daily conversation avoid terms that express improvement such as *good*, *stable*, and *better* in reference to the dying patient so as not to confuse parents. If necessary, use words such as *death*, *die*, and *dying*, and do not speak in euphemisms (e.g., "not doing well" or "passing away"). "There is nothing more we can do" should never be voiced.

- Prepare the family for what may happen as the infant dies. Review what they may see, hear, smell, and feel. Provide information on the estimated length of time it may take until he/she actually dies, from minutes to days, and that palliative care will be continued as long as it is necessary.
- Report to them that not all family members experience grief at the same pace, that differences in coping styles and stages are common, and that each will be supported by staff.
- Introduce families to the chaplain and social worker early in the process. Offer support for extended family. Ask about their desire for infant baptism or other religious services on the unit. Have a hospital chaplain contact their local spiritual advisor in the community.
- Funding palliative care measures remains a concern. When a newborn's care shifts from highly technologic life support to palliative care, it is essential that the written documentation continues to reflect the need for physician management, skilled nursing care, and interdisciplinary support. The physician should note that the infant's condition warrants intensive nursing monitoring and activities. Charting should reflect that the infant is critically ill, and there should be close collaboration with utilization review, coding, and billing staff. Appropriate diagnoses and accurate procedural coding should be used to ensure reimbursement of palliative care measures. Continued advocacy at the federal, state, and local level for hospice/palliative care reimbursement is essential.

Optimal environment for neonatal death   When the decision is made that a newborn infant may be close to death, there are several components to optimizing the care. These include some general principles, such as the following:
- Compassionate, nonjudgmental, consistent staff are available for each infant, including physicians knowledgeable in palliative care. If consistent staff is not an option in a particular unit, then agreement on the plan of care is essential, with proposed revisions to care discussed with the whole team.
- Nurses and other health care staff are educated in providing for the family a meaningful experience while caring for the family's psychosocial needs including a period of time after the death.
- Parents are educated in what to expect and are encouraged to participate in, or even orchestrate, the dying process and environment of their infant in a manner they find meaningful.
- The facility and staff are flexible in responding to parental wishes, such as participation of siblings and other family mem-

bers, and including wishes of parents and families who do not wish to be present.

- Institutional policies allow staff flexibility to respond to parental wishes.
- Time is provided to create memories, such as allowing parents to dress, diaper, and bathe their infant, feed him/her (if it is possible), take photos, and hold the infant in their arms. If they wish to take the infant outdoors to a peaceful and natural setting that should be encouraged.
- Siblings should be made comfortable; they may wish to write letters or draw for the infant. Snacks should be available.
- The family should be allowed to stay with the infant as long as they need to, including after death occurs.
- The process for treating the dying infant is well described in the literature and by the various bereavement programs. Such processes include such things as having one nurse assigned to be with the family, staying with the infant while the parents take breaks, and collecting mementos that families may wish to take home (e.g., pictures or videos, hand prints and footprints, locks of hair).
- Parents should be assisted in making plans for a memorial service, burial, and so on. Some parents might wish to carry or accompany the infant's body to the morgue or take it to the funeral home themselves. Issues such as autopsy, cremation, burial, and who may transport the body should be discussed, especially if the parents are far from home and wish to take the body back to their home area for burial. In some states, hospitals may release a body to parents after notifying the county department of vital statistics. The family must sign a form for removal of the body. The quality assurance department should be notified. Further discussion of autopsy and organ/tissue donation issues is included.

Specific skills are needed by the staff to provide palliative care. These include the following:

- A physician leader of the team who is familiar with family-centered care and the tenets of palliative/hospice care
- A trained nursing staff, clinical social workers, and clergy supportive of this manner of care
- Agreement to cease all invasive care, including taking frequent vital signs, monitoring, medical machinery, and artificial feeding
- Removal of all medications other than those to provide comfort or to prevent or treat a troubling symptom, with continued intravenous (IV) access for pain medication and anxiolytics
- Maintenance of skin care, participation in discussion on the appropriateness of feeding, and prevention of air hunger
- Use of simple blow-by oxygen or suctioning if needed for comfort
- Continuous observation and gentle assessment by nursing staff as individualized by parent wishes

- Physicians' notes describing the need for ongoing physician observation and nursing staff interventions to provide the needed level of care
- Appropriate palliative care orders on the chart

Location for provision of palliative care   Location is not as important as the mindset of persons involved in EOL care. The attitude of staff; their desire to care for dying newborns and their families; their training in observation, support, and symptom management; and their knowledge of how to apply a bereavement protocol are more important than the physical location of the patient. Many agree that an active NICU may not be the optimal place for a dying newborn. Whether the infant is moved to a room off the unit (e.g., a family room), moved onto a general pediatrics ward, or kept on the postpartum floor, the best available physical space with privacy and comfort should be chosen.

In some cases, parents have not wished to leave the NICU where they have bonded with staff and have adjusted to the noise and activity. These families might feel isolated if moved to a private place.

Some families may wish to take their infant home to die. Discharge to home may be a goal for families who are willing and able to do so and have adequate assistance. Significant planning will be necessary to do this, including setting up the provision of home health care or home hospice support.

If families take the infant home, coordination with the emergency medical system (EMS) personnel may be necessary to prevent undesired intervention. Parents need to be instructed not to call 911 because in some places emergency medical technicians (EMTs) are obligated to provide CPR. A letter describing the diagnosis, existence of in-hospital do-not-resuscitate (DNR) order, and hospice care plan for home with the full expectation that the patient will die should be provided to the parents, their primary physician, home health agency/hospice, and perhaps the county EMS coordinator. Generally, hospice nurses are allowed to confirm a patient's death.

Ventilator removal; pain and symptom management   At times, cessation of certain technologic supports accompanies the provision of palliative care. The following information addresses (1) how to prepare the family, staff, and facility for discontinuation of ventilator support and (2) the process of removing the ventilator in a manner that minimizes discomfort for the infant and the family.

Preparation
- The entire focus of ventilator removal must be concern for the comfort of the infant in a setting that allows privacy for the family. Providers should assure parents that every attempt to prevent suffering will be taken and that their infant will be treated with dignity and expertise in comfort measures.

- Parents must be provided time to respond to the critical situation and encouraged to direct how the process should go.
- Medical records should reflect the substance of patient care conferences with parents, and care orders written should be clear to staff members. Orders to cease mechanical ventilation, forgo CPR, or cease monitoring vital signs and drawing blood samples should be written in the chart with appropriate signatures and documentation.
- Parents should be able to gather their significant others and bring in their religious, spiritual, or cultural leader to conduct a ceremony or provide support.
- Once the decision is made, parent education should include that no further resuscitation efforts will occur.
- Consideration for notifying the ethics committee or risk manager about the decision may be appropriate in some facilities.
- Special permission must be obtained by the medical examiner in the instance of coroner's cases.
- The sequence of events should be laid out for parents in advance, and they may express their preferences about the process.
- Parents should be helped to understand that not every newborn dies immediately after the ventilator is removed. A contingency plan should be discussed, specifically including where and by whom the infant will be managed under a palliative care regimen (see below). When available, the hospice team should be notified in advance if it is thought that the infant may not immediately expire or if the family desires to go home if the infant survives after extubation.
- It is appropriate to discuss autopsy and organ/tissue donation concurrently with removal of life-support discussions. Some parents may wish to address how the body will be handled after death and to indicate that they would like to have the infant buried or cremated; others may allow the body to be taken to pathology.

Process

- Parents should decide who will be present at the time of extubation. Staff, including the social worker, neonatologist, spiritual advisor, and primary nurse, should be close by and available on request. Parents can hold a service at the bedside as desired. If parents wish, a nurse or other designee may bless or baptize the baby if no clergy have been invited, or parents may do so themselves.
- Staff should work out in advance who will be doing what part of removal of technologic support, such as removal of invasive lines, monitors, and the endotracheal (ET) tube. The actual turning off of the ventilator has often been seen as a physician responsibility.
- Staff should anticipate and have available medications that may be needed based on the infant's condition. Drugs such as vasopressors and antibiotics should be discontinued. Monitors should be removed and all alarms turned off.

- Neuromuscular blocking agents (paralytics) should never be introduced when the ventilator is being withdrawn. If the newborn has been receiving paralytics, these should ideally have been weaned off hours to days earlier. On rare occasions, the ongoing pharmacologic effect of paralytics might be construed as contributory to patient death following removal of the ventilator. In all cases when paralytics have been recently part of the newborn's care, the medical record should attest to (1) physician and parent discussion, understanding, and consideration of this fact in view of the decision to remove the ventilator; (2) an affirmation of the intent of such decisions being to relieve suffering associated with burdensome and nonbeneficial care; and (3) the disproportionate burden imposed on the patient and family of waiting lengthy hours or days for the paralytic effects to diminish.
- IV access must remain in place to give medication for symptom relief. Infants will need pain relief, relief for labored respirations, or perhaps medication for seizure activity. The pharmacy should assist in preparing proper doses of medications in IV, suppository, or buccal delivery form. Doses of medication should be sufficient to provide comfort and prevent signs of air hunger. Relevant medications include narcotic and nonnarcotic analgesics, medications to relieve air hunger, sedatives, diuretics, hypnotics, anticholinergics, anticonvulsives, and antipyretics.
- Before removal of the ET tube and disconnecting the ventilator, the alarms on the ventilator should be turned off. The ET tube should be gently suctioned when removed and the mouth gently cleaned. Then the ventilator can be shut off. If possible, the baby should be held in the parents' or a staff member's arms when this takes place.
- If possible, any tape on the face or other unnecessary lines should be removed. If not removed, these lines should be tied off and any open areas covered with gauze pads.
- Supplemental oxygen is usually not given when a ventilator is withdrawn. Parents may wish to administer oxygen to provide comfort. It may be more appropriate to administer morphine if an infant exhibits signs of shortness of breath, such as nasal flaring, air hunger, color changes, or grunting, since some clinicians report the possibility of oxygen prolonging the dying process. A suction machine or bulb suction should be available.
- Environmental support should provide for as much of a normal and nurturing environment as possible. Lights can be kept low, especially if color changes are expected. Noise should be kept to a minimum with phones and pagers turned low and staff conversations at a minimum. The infant can be dressed in his/her own clothes, bathed, diapered, and bundled by parents. Parents can bathe the infant, do infant massage, attempt breast-feeding, or engage in

kangaroo care. Availability of music playing and rocking chairs is helpful.

- A nurse should gently describe any physical changes that might be taking place and occasionally check to see if there is no heartbeat. The infant should continue to be observed and treated for any signs of dyspnea, discomfort, agitation, or seizures.
- Parents and family members should be able to hold the infant for as long as they need to, which may be for an extended time after death.
- Mementos can be obtained by nurses, such as a lock of hair, hand prints or footprints in plaster, and photos of family together if this is culturally appropriate. If the infant has serious anomalies, photos of hands, ears, lips, feet, can be provided. Ear prints and lip prints are possible. Some parents have indicated that mementos of a newborn who died are not acceptable in their culture.
- Parents require care after the infant has died. It is helpful to walk parents out to their cars so they do not have to feel so alone when they leave. Parents can be given a memory box or stuffed animal to avoid walking out with empty arms. Cleaning of the bed-space area should not be done until they are gone.
- Occasionally, because of distance or home responsibilities, parents cannot be present or may choose not to participate at all or only in portions of care as described above. The process would be similar, with a staff person holding the infant from the time of extubation until death and a box of keepsakes retained on the unit in case family desires them later.

When death does not occur after cessation of aggressive support A private room somewhere in the hospital is recommended where nurses trained in palliative care are available. If the expected time for expiration passes and death does not take place, the infant could be discharged to home for ongoing palliative care services. The parents, NICU staff, and the hospice staff should meet to make plans for home care, including the investigation of what services are offered and what insurance will cover. Continued palliative care/hospice services with home nursing care are essential, including the possibility of ventilator removal at home.

- If the infant is to go home, a procedure for dispensing outpatient medications should be in place. All needed drugs and directions for use should be sent along with infant so that parents do not have to go to a pharmacy to fill prescriptions. Identifying and communicating with a community health care provider who will continue with the infant's home care needs are essential.
- Some families and health care providers feel dying newborns should be fed and, if unable to suck, should be tube fed. Others feel that artificial feeding is inappropriate. Recent research indicates

that feeding can be burdensome and that an overload of fluids can impede respirations. In all cases, infants should receive care to keep their mouth and lips moist. Drops of sucrose water have been found to be a comfort agent if the infant can swallow, and they may be absorbed through the buccal membrane.

- Parents who feel they cannot take the infant home should be assisted to find hospice care placement.

Discussion of organ and tissue procurement and autopsy   At some point in the course of care, organ and tissue donation and autopsy will need to be discussed. Before discussion with families, the regional organ donation center should be contacted to see if a particular infant qualifies as a potential donor. In some areas only corneas or heart valves are valuable in an infant under 10 pounds; (4540 grams), but in different locations other organs (e.g., heart) or tissues may be appropriate. It is important to know if a newborn has no potential donor use and to communicate this respectfully. Parents often desire the ability to give this gift and may be doubly hurt if they are hoping for the opportunity to help others and are turned down.

The person who discusses organ/tissue procurement must be specially trained. Although the physician usually initiates this, a nurse, chaplain, or representative from the donor services may conduct the conversation with tact and compassion. The provider should be aware of cultural, traditional, or religious values that would preclude organ donation for a specific family, since many cultures and religions would consider this desecration of the dead infant.

It is suggested that this conversation be clearly "uncoupled" from the discussion on treatment goals to avoid any perceived conflict of interest by the caregivers. Conversation regarding autopsy or organ donation should be clearly documented in the chart so all can see that these discussions have already taken place.

Suggestions concerning autopsy   Requests for autopsies are not required in all states but may be considered appropriate in many instances of infant death. If the medical examiner or coroner is involved in the case, law may require autopsy. Some providers feel that asking for an autopsy is important to potentially provide parents with some answers regarding their infant's illness and death. The placenta may also be used for testing to provide information. In the discussion, parents may wish to know all or some of the following:

- Autopsy does not cause any pain or suffering to the infant; it is done only after death.
- The body is handled with the ultimate respect.
- Some insurance companies pay for a physician-ordered autopsy.

- For families who do not wish a complete autopsy, limited-tissue studies can be done on some areas of interest and imaging studies can be done rather than dissection.
- Explanations may include how tissue removed from the body is handled and disposed of and if this tissue can be buried with the infant on request.
- Genetic testing may be done on blood, skin, and certain tissue biopsy specimens.
- If a family desires an open viewing of the infant at the funeral or memorial service, the pathologist must be notified to allow for the least possible disfigurement.
- Preliminary results may be available from the pathologist within 72 hours, with a written report within 7 to 10 days. Conducting an autopsy may slightly delay release of the body to a funeral home for embalming or cremation. There may be cultural issues requiring release of the body for burial within a certain time frame, and these should be observed when possible.
- Final results are returned in approximately 6 to 8 weeks, at which time the primary physician can meet with the parents, conduct a telephone conference, or communicate by letter to discuss the results.
- Informational literature about autopsy is available.

Family care: cultural, spiritual, and practical family needs The hospital social worker is an essential component of supportive palliative care. Families may immediately need the following:
- Meal tickets
- Assistance with parking fees
- A phone card
- Access to transportation
- A place to stay (preferably with the infant)
- Financial assistance as part of their overall care
- Day care for the siblings

Practical considerations
- Parents of multiples in which some lived and one died will need special attention to validate their bereavement as well as to support their love for their living child(ren).
- Time should be permitted for the parents to contact the needed authority in their culture and to plan any necessary ceremony.
- Many ceremonies include the use of incense and/or candles. Special permission may be required from the hospital facility. A specific location in the hospital away from gases and flammable material will be needed.

Cultural sensitivity These support needs should be anticipated and provided as much as possible:

- When using a translator, simple words and phrases should be used so that the translator can convey the message exactly as it is given. It is most appropriate to use hospital-trained and hospital-certified translators to ensure accuracy.
- Whenever possible, written materials should be given in the family's primary language, in an easy-to-read format, culturally and linguistically appropriate for the family.
- For some families eye contact and touch may be expected; for others these may cause them to be uncomfortable and are not appropriate.
- Special cultural practices when an infant is born with malformations should be accommodated.
- Staff may need to model holding the very sick infant. Whereas most families will desire to hold their infant, there are those who will not wish to touch the infant as he/she is dying or after death.
- An autopsy request might be seen as contrary to cultural practices.
- At times there may be difficulty working with families who have a basic fear or distrust of authority figures.
- Culturally sensitive grief counseling and contact with a support group of other parents who have been through this are helpful.

Spiritual support Caregivers should be aware of the tendency of family members to second guess their decisions and feel enormous guilt. It is our job to help families work through this.

Some parents may believe that withholding or withdrawing technologic support is not acceptable in their cultural/religious tradition.

Each family's experience will be unique.

Family follow-up care Families who have experienced a neonatal death will likely leave the facility in a shocked state. Families can be best served by doing the following:

- Establishing contact with a social worker, chaplain, or grief counselor before discharge
- Receiving an information packet as described and a date for a follow-up discussion with the attending physician (which may be in conjunction with autopsy results)
- Notifying the family's obstetrician of the death no matter how long after delivery it occurred
- A home visit by one of the staff or a community health nurse within a few days
- Primary nurse writing a letter about what the baby was like and how it felt to care for the infant
- Phone calls weekly, then monthly, then at 6-month intervals if parents agree; also providing contact on significant days, such as mothers' day, the infant's due date, or anniversary of death

- When making parent contact, remembering to ask how all of the family is doing, including fathers, grandparents, and siblings; each time ask parents, "May I call you again?"
- With parents' permission, posting the family's address in the unit so that staff may send cards
- Providing staff the opportunity to attend services if desired
- If parents desire it, introducing parents to another family who has lost a newborn or young infant
- Facilitating introduction to a support group: some parents prefer to attend a grief group led by someone they have already met in the facility, and others prefer talking with counselors not associated with the hospital
- Inviting family to a group memorial service held by the hospital for those who have lost pregnancies or infants in the past year
- Keeping in mind that subsequent pregnancy may be difficult and offer support at that time; include genetic counseling if indicated
- Keeping snapshots and mementos on the unit if parents do not wish to take them at the time, since some parents may reconsider later

Ongoing staff support The work of providing EOL care for newborns and their families is very intense. Staff needing support must not be limited to the nursing staff and must include physicians and all health care and ancillary personnel who have interacted with the infant or family. Suggested support includes the following:

- Facilitated meetings of the multidisciplinary team during the process are needed, especially if some of the team members are reluctant to change to this mode of care.
- Debriefings after every infant's death and after any critical incident will be helpful for the staff.
- Meetings or counseling sessions should be part of regular work hours and not held on voluntary or unpaid time.
- Planning sessions, allowing for incorporation of lessons learned and for future palliative care cases, may allow staff to have a stake in improving the care and accepting it as they shape the manner in which it is provided.
- It is important to include residents, medical students, and nursing students in the provision of palliative care to model behavior they will incorporate in future actions.
- This type of caregiving should be voluntary, and nurses or physicians who do not wish to be involved should be able to take other assignments.
- Clarity in physician orders is essential for cohesion in the caregiving process. A closely working team allows patient care to go smoothly and lessens individual moral distress.

- Moral support for the nurses and physicians directly caring for the dying newborn is required from peers as well as the unit director, other neonatologists, chaplain, and nursing house supervisor.
- Nursing staff scheduling should be flexible and allow for overtime to continue with the family or orient another nurse to take over.
- If they wish, the primary nurse and physician should be called if not present at the actual time of the infant's dying. With permission by the parents, they should be allowed to attend the funeral if desired and to take time off afterward if needed.

We thank our reviewers, Alex G.M. Campbell, MD, David Clark, MD, Joel Frader, MD, John Lantos, MD, and Bill Silverman, MD; and our Delphi methodology consultant, Dr. Carol Lindemann. The project was funded by the American Nurses Foundation Julia Hardy RN Scholar Award, with travel support from the Lambda Gamma chapter of Sigma Theta Tau. We appreciate support from our institutions, Napa Valley College and Vanderbilt University College of Medicine, and from the Institutional Review Board at Queen of the Valley Medical Center in Napa, California. We sincerely thank our 101 participants for their time, wisdom, and commitment. Readers may contact us for participant names since space did not permit listing: acatlin@napanet.net; bcarter@ghsystem.com

BIBLIOGRAPHY

American Association of Colleges of Nursing (AACN) (1999). *Peaceful death: Recommended competencies and curricular guidelines for end-of-life nursing care: position statement*, Washington, DC: AACN.

Bhungalia S, Kemp C (2002). (Asian) Indian health beliefs and practices related to the end of life. *Journal of hospice & palliative nursing*, 4(1), 54-58.

Ferrell BR, Coyle N, editors (2002). *Textbook of palliative nursing*, New York: Oxford University Press.

Kuebler KK, Berry PH, Heidrich DE (2002). *End-of-life care: clinical practice guidelines*. Philadelphia: WB Saunders.

Sudia-Robinson T (2003). Hospice and palliative care. In Kenner C, Lott JW, editors. *Comprehensive neonatal nursing: a physiologic perspective*, ed 3, St Louis: WB Saunders.

World Health Organization (1990). *Cancer pain relief and palliative care*, (Technical Report Series, 804). Geneva: WHO.

AGENCIES AND CONTACT INFORMATION

National Hospice and Palliative Care Organization (NHPCO)
Alexandria, VA 22314
http://www.nhpco.org

Hospice & Palliative Nurses Association (HPNA)
Penn Center West One, Suite 229
Pittsburgh, PA 15276
Phone: 412-787-9301
Fax: 412-787-9305
hpna@hpna.org

Project on Death in America (PDIA)
http://www.soros.org/death
Phone: 212-548-0600

CHAPTER 21

SAFETY PROTOCOLS

Safety of our health care systems is a "hot topic" today. Emphasis on patient safety, health professional safety, and system safety is driving many health care delivery changes. The Institute of Medicine (IOM) in 2000 issued their report "To Err Is Human," National Academy of Sciences, Washington, D.C. This report pointed out that at least 44,000 Americans die each year in hospitals because of medication errors. This error is usually a systems problem and not just related to a specific health care professional. The IOM made the following recommendations to health care institutions.* They believe that a four-tiered approach is necessary:

1. Establishing a national focus to create leadership, research, tools, and protocols to enhance the knowledge base about safety
2. Identifying and learning from errors through immediate and strong mandatory reporting efforts, as well as the encouragement of voluntary efforts, both with the aim of making sure the system continues to be made safer for patients
3. Raising standards and expectations for improvement in safety through the actions of oversight organizations, group purchasers, and professional groups
4. Creating safety systems inside health care organizations through the implementation of safe practices at the delivery level (This level is the ultimate target of all the recommendations.)

In nursing school we learned the "five rights" of giving medications: right patient, right medication, right dose, right time, and right route. Now the IOM has extended this to suggest a checks and balances system must be at the systems level. Neonatal intensive care units (NICUs) are instituting safeguards to protect patients and ensure that health professionals are giving the right medications to the right patients. Computerized systems are in place that remove the dependence of translating poorly written orders and the "slipping" of decimal points. However, computers will only go so far in these efforts. Quality assurance programs are aimed at determining where

---

*From Institute of Medicine (2000). *To err is human.* Washington, DC: National Academy Press, p. 6.

errors arise. Benchmarking practices and determining "best practices" for health care to ensure quality are "standards for care" in NICUs worldwide. This type of system is one example of the level of concern for patient safety.

TYPES OF MEDICATION ERRORS*

1. Adverse reaction
2. The wrong:
   a. Drug
   b. Patient
   c. Dosing
   d. Time
   e. Route
   f. Documentation
   g. (Medication) not given
3. Pharmacy related
   a. Dispensing error
   b. Change in supplier, labeling confusion, etc.
   c. Education deficit
4. Human related
   a. Zeros and decimal points
   b. Handwriting
   c. Ambiguous or incomplete orders
   d. Phone, verbal order communication
   e. Education deficit
   f. "Single human," confirmation bias, etc.
5. Error reduction
   a. User-friendly, nonpunitive-based, error-reporting system
   b. Access to national reporting database problems and resolutions
   c. Interdisciplinary review process
   d. Identification of causes
   e. Improvement or change in contributing factors
   f. Evaluation of intervention
   g. Planning for intervention when error occurs

INFANT ABDUCTIONS

Another area of patient safety and security that is a concern for NICU care is the rise of infant abductions. A guideline is offered to help prevent these incidents.

---

*From Cohen MR, editor (1999). Medication errors, causes, prevention, and risk management, Sudbury, Mass: Jones & Barlett. Cited in Lefrak L, Lund CH (2001). Nursing practice in the neonatal intensive care unit. In Klaus MH, Fanaroff AA, editors. Care of the high-risk neonate, ed 5, Philadelphia: WB Saunders, p. 238.

UNIVERSITY OF ILLINOIS MEDICAL CENTER AT CHICAGO CLINICAL CARE GUIDELINE

Subject: Prevention of Infant Abduction: NICU/ICN Code Pink Disaster Plan *

Objective

University of Illinois Medical Center at Chicago recognizes that in order to provide for the safety and security of patients, families, and staff, the NICU/intermediate care nursery (ICN) area is a limited access, secured unit.

Definitions

For the purposes of this guideline, the following definitions apply:

Infant Abduction—The unauthorized removal of an infant from a health care facility by persons who are not the infant's parents or guardian.

Code Pink—The comprehensive disaster plan initiated for the prevention of infant abduction.

National Center for Missing and Exploited Children—A national clearinghouse for information related to infant abduction.

Position Statements

University of Illinois Medical Center at Chicago recognizes that newborns and young infants are vulnerable targets for the unauthorized removal from the premises by individuals who are not their parents or guardians (i.e., infant abduction). In order to prevent such occurrences, the University of Illinois Medical Center at Chicago has implemented a plan to prevent infant abduction and to facilitate identity of the perpetrator and the recovery of the infant. The infant abduction prevention plan includes measures of increasing staff awareness of the potential for infant abduction, physical plant alterations that enhance security in and around the vulnerable infants, video surveillance cameras in hallways and stairwells, and improved identification of persons with access to the infants.

Procedures

1. The entire staff of the NICU/ICN participates in periodic review of safety measures implemented to enhance security. Greater staff involvement and vigilance are a prerequisite to all security measures.

   a. Staff will be required to wear proper University of Illinois Medical Center at Chicago identification at all times.

From University of Illinois Medical Center at Chicago Women's and Children's Nursing Services. Used with permission by Dharmapuri Vidyasagar, MD; Catherine Theorell, RNC, MSN, NNP; Beena Peters, RN, MS.

b. Hospital scrubs and or lab coats will be kept in an access-controlled area and are not to be loaned to unauthorized personnel.

c. Staff will ensure that infants are always in direct line-of-sight by parents or hospital staff.

d. An infant is never left anywhere without direct line-of-sight by parents or hospital staff.

e. Parents will be informed of security measures at earliest opportunity after admission of the infant. Nursing staff will document in the patient education notes that they reviewed the security measures with the family.

f. Only authorized NICU staff members are allowed to transport an infant while in the health care facility. Operating room personnel may transport infants undergoing surgical procedures in the operating room.

g. Parents or staff are **not** allowed to carry the infant outside the infant's room or within the facility at any time.

h. NICU staff will transport the infant within the health care facility via wheeled bassinet, incubator, or cart and escort the family to the first floor lobby door at the time of discharge.

i. Staff will immediately report any unidentified individuals, suspicious activity, behavior, or unfamiliar persons to the charge nurse. The charge nurse will in turn contact University of Illinois police.

j. If home visitation services are required after discharge, the discharge coordinator will instruct the families on the specific arrangements (i.e., name of the person or company entering the home and the nature of the visit).

2. Parent and infant identification measures include the following:

a. At delivery or before transport, the parent(s) and each infant will be banded with identically numbered University of Illinois Medical Center at Chicago identification bracelets. In the event of multiple gestation, the parent(s) will be banded with a numbered identification bracelet for each infant. Nursing staff will destroy the unused numbered bands not secured to the parent(s).

b. At all times, the University of Illinois Medical Center at Chicago identification bracelet will be secured to the infant.

c. The parent(s) will be instructed that their University of Illinois Medical Center at Chicago hospital identification bracelet(s) must be worn at all times until the infant is discharged.

d. Should the parents' numbered identification bands become lost or illegible, the parent and infant will be rebanded after confirming the parents' identify documented by picture identification methods, such as a driver's license, passport, or official state identification card.

    e. The parent's numbered identification band must be shown to the NICU/ICN staff when requested.

    f. When the infant's name is changed to that submitted on the state birth certificate, the infant(s) and parent(s) should be rebanded with the infant's actual legal name. The old identification band should be secured to the newborn identification sheet as per policy.

    g. Additional visitors will be required to sign into and out of the visitor's logbook located on the receptionist desk.

    h. A photograph of the infant(s) and parent(s) will be obtained as soon as possible after admission. The photograph(s) will be kept at the infant's bedside for the health care staff to use as additional visual identification of the parent(s).

3. A policy has been established that controls access to the unit.

    a. All NICU/ICN doors have self-closing hardware and are locked at all times.

    b. Doors leading to the NICU/ICN are secured.

    c. An access button located at the front desk electronically unlocks the designated door. The front and back doors are unlocked with their own separate controls.

    d. Signage outside of the unit displays instructions for parents and visitors wishing to enter.

    e. Staff will require all people entering the NICU/ICN to identify themselves and reason for their visit.

4. Video and electronic alarm surveillance monitors traffic flow on the fourth floor hallways and stairwells.

5. A critical-incident-response plan has been developed for a breach of infant security—CODE PINK DISASTER PLAN.

6. Nurse recognizing the breach of security immediately notifies the charge nurse who announces a "Code Pink."

7. All exit doors in the nurseries are immediately observed and blocked by all available staff. All persons are detained from leaving the unit until cleared by the charge nurse and/or the search of the unit has been completed. Staff must immediately search the entire unit if infant abduction is suspected.

8. If a baby is found to be missing, the charge nurse notifies the University of Illinois Medical Center at Chicago police. University of Illinois Medical Center at Chicago police activate hospital "Code Pink" disaster plan.

9. Move the parents of the abducted infant to a private room, and have the nurse assigned to the infant accompany the parents at all times.

10. Locate and secure the infant's medical records.

11. Locate and secure the infant's blood sent for metabolic screen or, if available, other blood samples.

12. Page the patient unit director and the nursing resource office supervisor.
13. Nurse manager or charge nurse briefs all staff on the unit.
14. Nurses should then explain the situation to each mother on the unit while the mother and infant(s) are together.
15. Conduct mandatory group debriefing sessions for personnel.
16. Staff will review video on infant security in health care facilities and participate in yearly mandatory review of procedures.

• • •

Some institutions require a digital infant picture be taken with identification either in or on the picture indicating the infant's name, date of birth, time of birth, delivering physician or nurse-midwife, and identification band number. Two copies are made: one is placed on the chart, and the other is given to the parents.

As our health care delivery is moving away from hospital-based nursing and into community and home settings, safety for nurses in these areas is another concern. A protocol for safe home visits is included.

PROTOCOL FOR PERINATAL HOME VISITS*

Previsit Interventions
1. Contact family to arrange details for home visit.
   a. Identify self, credentials, and agency role.
   b. Review purpose of home visit follow-up.
   c. Schedule convenient time for visit.
   d. Confirm address and route to family home.
2. Review and clarify appropriate data.
   a. Review all available assessment data for mother and fetus or infant (i.e., referral forms, hospital discharge summaries, family-identified learning needs).
   b. Review records of any previous nursing contacts.
   c. Contact other professional caregivers as necessary to clarify data (i.e., obstetrician, nurse-midwife, pediatrician, referring nurse).
3. Identify community resources and teaching materials appropriate to meet needs already identified.
4. Plan the visit, and prepare bag with equipment, supplies, and materials necessary for assessments of mother and fetus or infant, actual care anticipated, and teaching.

---

*From Lowdermilk DL, et al (2000). *Maternity & women's health care*, ed 7, St Louis: Mosby, p. 43.

In-Home Interventions
Establishing a relationship
1. Reintroduce self and establish purpose of visit for mother, infant, and family; offer family members opportunity to clarify their expectations of contact.
2. Spend brief time socially interacting with family to become acquainted and establish trusting relationship.

Working with the family
1. Conduct systematic assessment of mother and fetus or newborn to determine physiologic adjustment and any existing complications.
2. Throughout visit, collect data to assess the emotional adjustment of individual family members to pregnancy or birth and lifestyle changes. Note evidence of family-newborn bonding and sibling rivalry; note relationships among mother, father, children, and grandparents.
3. Determine adequacy of support system.
   a. To what extent does someone help with cooking, cleaning, and other home management tasks?
   b. To what extent is help being provided in caring for the newborn and any other children?
   c. Are support persons encouraging the new mother to care for herself and get adequate rest?
   d. Who is providing helpful information? Emotional support?
4. Throughout the visit, observe home environment for adequacy of resources:
   a. Space: privacy, safe play of children, sleeping
   b. Overall cleanliness and state of repair
   c. Number of steps pregnant woman/new mother must climb
   d. Adequacy of cooking arrangements
   e. Adequacy of refrigeration and other food storage areas
   f. Adequacy of bathing, toilet, and laundry facilities
   g. Arrangements in home for newborn: sleeping, bathing, formula preparation (if needed), layette items, and diapers
5. Throughout the visit, observe home environment for overall state of repair and existence of safety hazards:
   a. Storage of medications, household cleaners, and other substances hazardous to children
   b. Presence of peeling paint on furniture, walls, or pipes
   c. Factors that contribute to falls, such as dim lighting, broken steps, scatter rugs
   d. Presence of vermin
   e. Use of crib or playpen that fails to meet safety guidelines
   f. Existence of emergency plan in case of fire; fire alarm or extinguisher

6. Provide care to mother, newborn, or both as prescribed by their respective primary care provider or in accord with agency protocol.
7. Provide teaching on basis of previously identified needs.
8. Refer family to appropriate community agencies or resources, such as warm lines and support groups.
9. Ascertain that woman knows potential problems to watch for and whom to call if they occur.
10. Ensure that used disposable items have been handled appropriately and that reusable items are cleaned and repacked appropriately in the nurse's bag.

Ending the visit
1. Summarize the activities and main points of the visit.
2. Clarify future expectations, including schedule of next visit.
3. Review teaching plan, and provide major points in writing.
4. Provide information about reaching the nurse or agency if needed before the next scheduled visit.

Postvisit Interventions
1. Document the visit thoroughly, using the necessary agency forms to serve as a legal record of the visit and to allow third-party reimbursement, as possible.
2. Initiate the plan of care on which the next encounter with the woman/family will be based.
3. Communicate appropriately by telephone, letter, progress notes, or referral form with primary care provider, other health professionals, or referral agencies on behalf of woman/family.

BIBLIOGRAPHY

(2001). Infant kidnappings: new approaches; realistic drills; making low-tech and high-tech improvements. *Hospital security & safety management, 22*(2), 5-8.

(2001). New asset tracking systems used for infant abduction prevention. *Hospital security & safety management, 21*(12), 11-2.

Frey B, et al. (2000). Comprehensive critical incident monitoring in a neonatal-pediatric intensive care unit: experience with the system approach. *Intensive care medicine, 26*(1), 69-74.

Geller M (2000). Infant abduction in the hospital setting. *Quality Resource Center (QRC) advisory, 16*(5), 1-4.

Goodwin AB (2001). Striving for a secure environment: a closer look at hospital security issues following the infant abduction at Loyola University Medical Center. *Annals of health law, 10,* 245-287.

Walsh-Sukys M, et al. (2001). Reducing light and sound in the neonatal intensive care unit: an evaluation of patient safety, staff satisfaction and costs. *Journal of perinatology, 21*(4), 230-235.

Widness JA, et al. (2000). Clinical performance of an in-line point-of-care monitor in neonates. *Pediatrics, 106*(3), 497-504.

LIFE BEYOND THE NICU

With advances in technology more infants are surviving to go home. Managed care and insurance agencies are moving these children out quicker and sicker, to the point that many families are setting up mini neonatal intensive care units (NICUs) in the home. Home care is a growing business even for the neonatal population. This population of infants also has special needs that must be considered if positive growth and development are to be fostered. This chapter focuses on special needs in the home and follows concerns.

STRATEGIES FOR PROMOTION OF POSITIVE GROWTH IN NICU GRADUATES*

- Minimize neonatal insult in the NICU by providing developmentally appropriate family-centered nursing care and comprehensive discharge planning.
- Calculate risk scores on children before discharge to guide ongoing planning.
- Inform parents of their children's rights to receive screening and special services.
- Refer children to early intervention programs for screening and follow-up.
- Encourage parents to attend neonatal intensive care follow-up clinics.
- Discuss roles of parent support and advocacy groups with families.
- Counsel parents to carefully screen their children for learning disabilities throughout their school years to obtain prompt, appropriate referrals and services.
- Provide parents with information about Internet resources, community resources, and mandated services for children with special health and education needs.
- Keep abreast of current research about long-term outcomes of prematurity and neonatal illness to provide families with up-to-date information on outcomes.
- Encourage parents to participate in relevant research studies.

---

*From Lindeke LL, et al. (2002). *Neonatal predictors of school-based services used by NICU graduates at school age*. MCN, 27(1), 45.

- Serve on local school boards and early intervention advisory committees to share nursing knowledge and experience with policy makers and interdisciplinary colleagues.
- Subscribe to newsletters of child advocacy groups such as Parent Advocacy Coalition for Educational Rights (PACER) and the Children's Defense Fund to remain current on relevant issues and programs.
- Testify at local, state, and national hearings where policy decisions are made regarding legislation and funding for services for at-risk children and families.
- Communicate across systems with local early intervention and school-based service providers to assist families to obtain appropriate referrals and services.

ASSESSMENT OF MOTHERS FOR USE OF POTENTIALLY HARSH DISCIPLINE*

- Assess mothers prenatally for their perceptions of how their own mothers handled discipline when they were young. Do they recall receiving harsh vs. nurturing responses to their behavior?
- With open-ended questions, discuss with pregnant women their thoughts about future discipline strategies they might use for their own children. Based on their responses, make a clinical decision about a community referral.
- During regular well-baby preventive health care visits, ask whether mother has begun to use discipline. Evaluate the appropriateness of her response.
- When "red flags" for harsh, nonnurturing discipline strategies are seen, support the mother, document findings, and coordinate response with community health nurses and/or other interdisciplinary health team members with expertise in child abuse and neglect prevention.
- Be certain that mothers have a list of local hotlines and community resources to help them should they feel overwhelmed by life's stresses.

NURSERY NEUROBIOLOGIC RISK SCORE†

Overview

Very premature infants are at risk for abnormal neurodevelopmental outcome. The Nursery Neurobiologic Risk Score can be used to predict outcomes at 18 months for very premature infants.

---

*From Gaffney KF, et al. (2002). Early clinical assessment for harsh child discipline strategies. MCN, 27(1), 39.
†From Medical algorithms. www.medal.org

Infants (for Lefebvre, 1998):
- Born at a gestational age of 28 weeks or less
- Includes those that survived until discharge
- Birth weights ranged from 585 to 1450 g

Parameters (Tables 22-1 to 22-3)
1. Ventilation
2. pH
3. Seizures
4. Intraventricular hemorrhage (IVH)
5. Periventricular leukomalacia (PVL)
6. Infection
7. Hypoglycemia (glucose <1.7 mmol/L, or <30 mg/dl)

Table **22-1**	Parameter Finding Points	
Parameter	**Finding**	**Points**
Ventilation	None	0
	≤ 7 days	1
	8-28 days	2
	> 28 days (cumulative)	4
pH	Never < 7.15	0
	< 7.15 for ≤ 1 hr	1
	< 7.15 for ≤ 2 values	1
	< 7.15 (bicarbonate < 16 mmol/L) for > 1 hr	2
	< 7.15 (bicarbonate < 16 mmol/L) for > 2 values	2
	< 7.0 (bicarbonate < 16 mmol/L)	2
	Cardiopulmonary arrest (not at birth)	4
Seizures	None	0
	Controlled on one drug and normal interictal EEG	1
	Not controlled on one drug and/or abnormal interictal EEG	2
	Status epilepticus ≥12 hr with abnormal EEG	4
Intraventricular hemorrhage	None	0
	Subependymal germinal matrix hemorrhage only	1

Continued

Table **22-1**	Parameter Finding Points—cont'd	
Parameter	**Finding**	**Points**
Intraventricular hemorrhage cont'd	Blood in one or both ventricles (grade II or III)	2
	Intraparenchymal blood (grade IV)	4
	Hydrocephalus	4
Periventricular leukomalacia	None	0
	Mild* (questionable changes) that resolves	1
	Moderate* (definite) that resolves	2
	Cyst formation	4
	Cerebral atrophy with large ventricles	4
Infection	None	0
	Possible (negative blood cultures)	0
	Highly suspicious (placed on 10-day course of antibiotics)	1
	Positive blood cultures with normal blood pressure	1
	Septic shock†	2
	Meningitis (positive CSF cultures)	4
Hypoglycemia	None	0
	Asymptomatic and ≤ 6 hr	1
	Asymptomatic and > 6 hr	2
	Asymptomatic and < 24 hr	2
	Symptomatic‡ and ≥ 24 hr	4

References: Lefebvre F, et al. (1998). Nursery Neurobiologic Risk Score and outcome at 18 months. Acta paediatrica, 87, 752; Brazy JE, et al. (1993). Nursery Neurobiologic Risk Score: levels of risk and relationships with nonmedical factors. Developmental and behavioral pediatrics, 14, 376.
Source: Medical Algorithms www.medal.org
EEG, Electroencephalogram; CSF, cerebrospinal fluid.
Neurobiologic risk score = Sum (points for all 7 parameters).
Interpretation: minimum score: 0; maximum score: 28. The higher the score, the worse the outcome at 18 mo.
*Mild or moderate periventricular leukomalacia: increase in echogenicity in periventricular area.
†Septic shock: (1) positive blood cultures and (2) blood pressure <35 mm Hg at ≤750 g or blood pressure <40 at 751-1500 g.
‡Hypoglycemia "symptomatic and <24 hr"

Table **22-2**	Interpretation of Nursery Neurobiologic Risk Score	
Score	**Risk Group**	**Mean Developmental Scores**	**Risk of Developmental Quotient <90 (%)**
0-4	Low	101 +/- 9	12
5-7	Moderate	92 +/-19	24
≥8	High	76 +/- 24	71

Table **22-3**	Correlation of Risk Group with Other Risks		
Risk Group	**Risk of any Disability (%)**	**Risk of Cerebral Palsy (%)**	**Risk of Severe Disability (%)**
Low	16	4	0
Moderate	30	19	24
High	71	41	50

REFERENCES

Brazy JE, et al. (1991). Nursery Neurobiologic Risk Score: important factors in predicting outcome in very low birth weight infants. *Journal of pediatrics*, 118, 783-792.

Brazy JE, et al. (1993). Nursery Neurobiologic Risk Score: levels of risk and relationships with nonmedical factors. *Developmental and behavioral pediatrics*, 14, 375-380.

Lefebvre F, et al. (1998). Nursery Neurobiologic Risk Score and outcome at 18 months. *Acta paediatrica*, 87, 751-757.

BABY CHECK SCORING SYSTEM*

Overview

The Baby Check Scoring System (Tables 22-4 to 22-7) is used to evaluate sick infants less than 6 months of age in developing countries or busy outpatient clinics. It can help separate high-risk infants who need more intensive care from healthy or mildly affected ones.

Instructions

1. Score each item according to the exact wording of the question.
2. Only score an item if it is definitely present.
3. The baby can be rescored at any time to assess changes in the severity of the illness.

*From Medical algorithms. www.medal.org

Table **22-4**	Scoring for Symptoms in the Baby Check Scoring System	
Symptoms in the Past 24 Hr		**Points**
Has the baby vomited at least one half the feed after each of the last three feeds?		4
Has the baby had any bile-stained (green) vomiting?		13
Has the baby taken less fluids than usual in the past 24 hr? If so, score the total amount of fluid taken as follows:		
• Taken only slightly less than usual (more than two thirds of usual intake)		3
• Taken about one half the usual amount (between one third and two thirds of the usual amount)		4
• Taken very little (less than one third of usual intake)		9
(Note: If breast-fed, ask the mother to estimate the amount taken.		
Fluids that have been vomited should still be scored.)		
Has the baby passed less urine than usual?		3
Has there been any frank blood mixed with the baby's stools? **(Note:** Do not score for streaks.)		11
Has the baby been drowsy (less alert than usual) when awake? If so, score for the degree of drowsiness when awake, as follows:		
• Occasionally drowsy (but usually alert)		3
• Drowsy most of the time (occasionally alert)		5
• Drowsy all the time		5
(Note: Ensure that the mother is reporting drowsiness and not just irritability or increased sleeping.)		
Has the baby had an unusual cry (sounds unusual to mother)?		2

REFERENCES

Chandran S, et al. (1998). A trial of baby check scoring system to identify high-risk infants in a polyclinic in Oman. *Journal of tropical pediatrics*, 44, 218-221.

Cole TJ, et al. (1991). A scoring system to quantify illness in babies under 6 months of age. *Journal of the Royal Statistics Society (American)*, 154, 287-304.

Kai J (1994). 'Baby Check' in the inner city—use and value to parents. *Family practice*, 11, 245-250.

Morley CJ, et al. (1991). Baby check: a scoring system to grade the severity of acute systemic illness in babies under 6 months old. *Archives of disease in childhood*, 66, 100-106.

Morley CJ, et al. (1991). Field trials of the Baby Check score card in general practice. *Archives of disease in childhood*, 66, 111-114.

Table **22-5**	Scoring for Examination of the Awake Baby in the Baby Check Scoring System

Examination of the Awake Baby	Points
Is the baby's muscle tone reduced? (Compare tone and head control with normal for baby's age.)	4
Talk to the baby. Is the baby concentrating on you less than you would expect?	4
Is the baby wheezing on expiration? (**Note:** Do not score for snuffles or upper respiratory noises.)	3
Is the baby responding to what is going on less than you would expect?	5

Table **22-6**	Scoring for Examination of the Undressed Baby in the Baby Check Scoring System*

Examination of the Undressed Baby	Points
Is there any in-drawing (recession) of the lower ribs, sternum, or upper abdomen? If so, score as follows:	
• Mild recession (slight in-drawing, just visible)	4
• Moderate recession (obvious in-drawing, clearly visible)	15
• Severe recession (deep in-drawing)	15
Is the baby very pale or does the parent think that the baby has looked very pale in the past 24 hr?	3
Does the baby have peripheral cyanosis?	3
Squeeze the baby's big toe firmly for 2 sec to make it white. Release and observe color return for 3 sec. Score if return is not complete within 3 sec or if toe was completely white to start with.	3
Does the infant have an inguinal hernia? (**Note:** 60% of babies with inguinal hernia develop complications.)	13
Has the baby an obvious generalized truncal rash or a raw or weeping rash covering an area greater than 5 cm × 5 cm?	4
Is the baby's rectal temperature ≥38.3° C?	4
Has the baby cried during the assessment?	3

*Baby check score = (points for symptoms) + (points for examination of the baby awake) + (points for examination of undressed infant).
Interpretation: minimum score: 0; maximum score: 111 points.

Table **22-7**	Interpretation of Scores on Baby Check Scoring System	
Score	**Group**	**Action**
0-7	Well or mildly ill	Infant unlikely to need medical care at the moment
8-12	Unwell but not likely to be seriously ill at the moment	Contact health care provider for advice; monitor the child closely, and reassess if condition worsens
13-19	Moderately to severely ill	Arrange to have child examined by a physician
≥ 20	Seriously ill	Take the infant to see a physician immediately

EMERGENCY TRIAGE, ASSESSMENT, AND TREATMENT (ETAT) GUIDELINES FOR SICK CHILDREN IN DEVELOPING COUNTRIES*

Overview

The ETAT guidelines can be used in developing countries to triage and initially treat sick children (Table 22-8).

Priority Signs

1. Severe wasting
2. Age less than 2 months
3. Irritable or restless
4. Pallor
5. Major burn
6. Edema of both feet
7. Lethargy
8. Any respiratory distress
9. Urgent referral from another health facility

Unconsciousness or coma would be a priority sign, as well as not breathing. A child with one or more priority signs needs urgent assessment.

Emergency Signs and Treatments

1. Airway and breathing (A & B)
2. Circulation (C)
3. Coma (Cm), convulsions (Cn), confusion (Cf)
4. Dehydration in a child with vomiting or diarrhea (D)

---

*Source: Medical Algorithms. www.medal.org

Table 22-8	Emergency Triage, Assessment, and Treatment Guidelines	
Group	**Signs and Symptoms (1 or more Positive)**	**Emergency Treatment**
Airway and breathing (A & B)	Not breathing Central cyanosis Severe respiratory distress Obstructed breathing	Manage airway; give oxygen; remove any foreign body from airway
Circulation (C)	Cold hands Capillary refill >3 sec Pulse weak and fast	Stop bleeding; give oxygen; give IV fluids at 20 ml/kg
Coma (Cm), convulsions (Cn), confusion (Cf)	Unconscious Convulsing now Blood glucose <2 mmol/L	Manage airway; give oxygen; rectal diazepam; give IV dextrose 10%; position child
Dehydration in a child with vomiting or diarrhea (D)	Lethargy Sunken eyes Skin pinch >3 sec	Give IV or nasogastric fluids

IV, Intravenous.

REFERENCES

Robertson MA, Molyneux EM (2001). Description of cause of serious illness and outcome in patients identified using ETAT guidelines in urban Malawi. *Archives of disease in childhood*, 85, 214-217.

Robertson MA, Molyneux EM (2001). Triage in the developing world—can it be done? *Archives of disease in childhood*, 85, 208-213 (Appendix A, p. 212).

CHRONIC LUNG DISEASE (CLD)

Although bronchopulmonary dysplasia (BPD), or chronic lung disease (CLD), is decreasing in incidence, it still is a problem of some NICU graduates. These children have chronic care needs, but they are children first who require primary care if they are to grow to their optimal potential. If you are responsible for follow-up care please consider the following.

SUMMARY OF PRIMARY CARE NEEDS FOR THE CHILD WITH BRONCHOPULMONARY DYSPLASIA*

Health Care Maintenance
Growth and development
- Height and weight are below average in the majority of children— even at 2 years of age. Plot head circumference, height, and length corrected for gestational age with each visit.
- Review caloric intake for adequacy.
- Developmental delay is often seen during the first year of life. Continued delays may be seen in children of very low birth weight or with a history of severe BPD. Learning disabilities are often evident during school years.

Diet
- Adequate caloric intake is important for optimal lung repair and growth and development.
- Difficulties may arise with oral motor function. Oral feedings may need to be supplemented with enteral feedings.
- Early referral to a pediatric nutritionist can prevent long-term problems.

Safety
- Beware of accidental decannulations and disconnections from respiratory support.
- Oxygen should be used with caution in the home.
- Electrical safety requires grounded equipment.
- Establish emergency service contact before a child is discharged from the hospital.

Immunization
- Many children are delayed in receiving immunizations because of prolonged hospitalization. Children should be immunized according to a routine schedule based on chronologic not gestational age.
- Hospital records must be reviewed.
- Pertussis vaccine should only be withheld with just cause because of the high risk of significant morbidity with active disease in children with BPD. Use acellular pertussis if appropriate.
- Inactivated polio vaccine may be administered in the hospital before discharge.
- Influenza vaccine is recommended yearly for children with CLD.
- Pneumococcal vaccines are recommended.

---

*Modified from Harvey K (2000). *Bronchopulmonary dysplasia*. In Jackson PL, Vessey JA, editors. *Primary care of the child with a chronic condition*, St Louis: Mosby, pp. 261-262.

Screening

Vision

- Children should be evaluated by a pediatric ophthalmologist every 2 to 3 months during the first year of life to rule out ROP (retinopathy of prematurity). Cover test should be done and tracking ability screened at each visit.
- Myopia and strabismus are common and must be followed in the primary care office and by a pediatric ophthalmologist.

Hearing

- A brain auditory evoked response (BAER) test should be done before discharge from the hospital.
- There is a risk of hearing loss because of prematurity and medications.
- Age-appropriate screening should be done at each office visit.
- Audiometry screening should be done with recurrent serous otitis media.
- Speech delays are anticipated in children with tracheostomies.

Dental

- Routine screening is recommended.
- Hypoplastic and discolored teeth are common.
- Oral defensiveness may make dental hygiene difficult.

Blood pressure

- Blood pressure should be taken at each visit.
- Children with abnormal blood pressure findings should be referred to a cardiologist.

Hematocrit

- Because of prematurity, iron deficiency anemia is common.
- Hematocrit screening must be done frequently during the first year of life.
- Chronic hypoxia may cause elevated hemoglobin levels.

  Urinalysis   Routine screening is recommended.

  Tuberculosis   Routine screening is recommended.

Condition-specific screening

  Chest radiograph   Radiographic examinations of the lungs should be done at discharge and then annually and as needed per clinical indication.

  Pulmonary function tests   Pulmonary function tests should be done at discharge, annually, and as necessary per clinical indication.

Common Illness Management

Differential diagnosis

  Respiratory distress   Rule out bacterial or viral infection, atelectasis, pneumonia, bronchospasm, pulmonary edema, heart failure, and sinusitis. Consider RSV (respiratory syncytial virus) infections from November to March.

Cough   Rule out sinusitis, GER (gastroesophageal reflux), reactive airway disease, pulmonary edema, pertussis, and RSV.

Fever   Rule out otitis media, sinusitis, upper or lower respiratory tract infection, urinary tract infection, and septicemia. Also rule out respiratory tract infection, otitis media, and viral infection.

Gastrointestinal disturbances   Consider feeding intolerances, bacterial and viral infections, GER, or theophylline toxicity.

Skin   For skin problems around tracheostomy and gastrostomy stomas and diaper areas, consider *Candida* infection and cellulitis.

Drug interactions
- Theophylline interacts with other medications.
- Cough suppressants may mask underlying condition and are not recommended.
- Do not use antihistamines with children with tracheostomy tubes because of the thickening of airway secretions.

Developmental Issues
Sleep patterns
- Attempt to evaluate the child's schedule of care to decrease disturbances and provide for the whole family.
- Evaluate functioning of monitors.

Toileting   Delayed bowel and bladder training may occur as a result of prolonged hospitalization and the use of diuretics and theophylline.

Discipline
- Children should receive discipline appropriate to their developmental level of understanding.
- A consistent plan should be followed.

Child care
- Recommend that children not supported by oxygen and mechanical ventilation attend home or small day care centers to reduce exposure to infection.
- Children with mechanical support may be eligible for nursing support from third-party payers.

Schooling
- Help family with developmental evaluations and planning early intervention programs.
- Assist families with adjustment to developmental delays.

Special Family Concerns

- Financial responsibilities are great even with insurance coverage.
- There may be a lack of privacy in the home because of the need for medical caregivers.
- Developmental outcome is uncertain. The potential for developmental delay and persistent medical problems results in great emotional strain on parents.

CEREBRAL PALSY

Another condition that is found in NICU graduates is cerebral palsy (CP). This condition is actually a group of nonprogressive disorders that affect the actions of the central nervous system. There are four major forms of CP: spastic, in which the muscles are taut and limit movement of extremities; dyskinesic, in which involuntary movements follow intended movements; ataxic, the form that affects muscle tone and coordination (tone can be either hypotonic or hypertonic); and mixed, in which there is a mix of motor problems ranging from spastic to dyskinetic to ataxic.

Problems Associated with Cerebral Palsy*

1. **Cognitive**
   a. Learning disabilities
   b. Mental retardation
2. **Seizure disorders**
3. **Language and speech disorders**
   a. Articulation
   b. Vocal strength and quality
   c. Language processing
4. **Vision**
   a. Refractive errors
   b. Strabismus
   c. Amblyopia
   d. Cataracts
   e. Retinopathy of prematurity
   f. Cortical blindness
   g. Homonymous hemianopsia (hemiplegia)
5. **Hearing**
   a. Conductive
   b. Sensorineural

*From Nehring WM (2000). Cerebral palsy. In Jackson PL, Vessey JA, editors. Primary care of the child with a chronic condition, St Louis: Mosby, p. 314.

6. **Other sensory**
   a. Tactile hypersensitivity or hyposensitivity
   b. Dyspraxia
   c. Balance and movement problems
   d. Proprioception difficulties
   e. Stereognosis
7. **Motor**
   a. Prolonged primitive reflexes
   b. Absence of protective reflexes
   c. Delayed motor milestones
   d. Hip subluxation and dislocation
   e. Scoliosis
   f. Contractures
8. **Feeding and eating problems**
   a. Chewing, sucking, and swallowing deficits
   b. Drooling
   c. Hypoxemia
   d. Fatigue
   e. Underweight and overweight
   f. Gastroesophageal reflux
   g. Aspiration
9. **Bowel**
   a. Constipation
   b. Encopresis
10. **Urinary**
    a. Bladder control
    b. Urinary retention
    c. Urinary tract infections
11. **Dental**
    a. Malocclusions
    b. Enamel defects and caries
    c. Gum hyperplasia (with phenytoin)
12. **Pulmonary**
    a. Respiratory infections
    b. Pneumonia
13. **Skin**
    a. Decubitus
    b. Latex allergy
14. **Behavioral and emotional**
    a. Behavioral disorders
    b. Attention deficit disorder, with and without hyperactivity
    c. Self-injurious behaviors
    d. Depression
    e. Autism
    f. Growth failure
    g. Other

SUMMARY OF PRIMARY CARE NEEDS FOR THE CHILD WITH CEREBRAL PALSY*

Health Care Maintenance
Growth and development
- Undernutrition in infancy often leads to growth retardation.
- Different techniques should be used to get height, arm and leg lengths, and skinfold measurements.
- Weights may be attained via standing or sitting scales or recumbent lifts.
- Overweight conditions may occur in adolescence if mobility decreases.
- Delayed development in motor and communication skills is common.
- Developmental strengths and weaknesses must be assessed and recorded.
- Mental retardation and seizure disorders inhibit intellectual development.

Diet
- Infants can have difficulty with sucking, swallowing, and chewing; so assessment should be done early.
- Drooling and aspiration can also be problems.
- Nutritional concerns may be lifelong, and placement of a gastrostomy tube may be warranted in severe cases.
- Referral to a nutritionist is needed.

Safety
- Children are at risk for injury as a result of spasticity, muscle control problems, delayed protective reflexes, and potential seizures.
- Positioning and adaptive equipment are often required.

Immunizations
- If the etiology for seizure activity is unknown, the pertussis vaccine may be deferred or an acellular vaccine used when age appropriate.
- The measles vaccine should be given as scheduled.
- *Haemophilus influenzae* type B (Hib) vaccine and other immunizations should be given as scheduled.
- Children with cerebral palsy are at risk for complications of influenza and varicella.
- Fever management is necessary to decrease the possibility of febrile seizures.

---

*From Nehring WM (2000). Cerebral palsy. In Jackson PL, Vessey JA, editors. Primary care of the child with a chronic condition, St Louis: Mosby, pp. 326-328.

Screening

Vision

- A pediatric ophthalmologist should be seen during infancy because of the likelihood of vision problems.
- Vision should be checked for acuity, refractive errors, strabismus, retinopathy of prematurity, and cataracts.

Hearing

- Referral to a pediatric audiologist may be necessary during infancy to check for hearing problems and loss.
- Both sensorineural and conductive hearing loss is possible.
- Routine screening for conductive hearing problems and loss should be done.

Dental

- Children should be evaluated by a dentist experienced with children with motor problems every 6 months.
- Proper dental hygiene is needed.
- Administration of phenytoin may cause hyperplasia of the gums; proper preventive care and early treatment of this condition are important.

Blood pressure Routine screening is recommended.

Urinalysis

- Routine screening is recommended.
- A referral to a pediatric urologist may be needed if the child has chronic urinary tract infections.

Hematocrit Routine screening is recommended.

Tuberculosis Routine screening is recommended.

Condition-specific screening A motor assessment, including assessment for scoliosis, hip dislocation, and contractures, should be done at every well-child visit.

Common Illness Management

Differential diagnosis

Fever Management of fever is routine.

Respiratory tract infections Respiratory infections should be promptly treated. Pneumonia may be life threatening to children with severe cerebral palsy. Follow-up is important.

Urinary tract infection Treatment for urinary tract infections should be prompt, and follow-up is essential. Urinary tract abnormalities may also be present.

Gastrointestinal problems Constipation is a chronic problem for many children. A bowel management program may be needed.

Drug interactions No medications are routinely prescribed, except if a seizure disorder is also present.

Developmental Issues

Sleep pattern   Correct positioning is needed during sleep because sleep apnea can occur.

Toileting

- Adaptive equipment is often needed for correct positioning on the toilet.
- Bladder and bowel training may be delayed.

Discipline   It is important that consistent and age-appropriate discipline measures be taken.

Child care   Careful planning must be undertaken in choosing the best child care arrangements, especially regarding issues of safety, accessibility, health care needs, and increased rates of infection.

Special Family Concerns

- Respite care meets a family's needs.
- Effects on individual family members must be assessed and addressed. Special support groups are available for fathers and siblings.
- Family stigmas may be perceived.

BIBLIOGRAPHY

Eichenwald EC, et al. (2001). Inter-neonatal intensive care unit variation in discharge timing: influence of apnea and feeding management. *Pediatrics*, 108(4), 928-933.

Harrold J, Schmidt B (2002). Evidence-based neonatology: making a difference beyond discharge from the neonatal nursery. *Current opinion in pediatrics*, 14(2), 165-169.

Hurst I (2001). Vigilant watching over: mothers' actions to safeguard their premature babies in the newborn intensive care nursery. *Journal of perinatal & neonatal nursing*, 15(3), 39-57.

Leach CE, et al. (1999). Epidemiology of SIDS and explained sudden infant deaths. CESDI SUDI Research Group. *Pediatrics*, 104(4), e43.

Lemons J, et al. (2002). Newborn hearing screening: costs of establishing a program. *Journal of perinatology*, 22(2), 120-124.

Lockridge T, Taquino LT, Knight A (1999). Back to sleep: is there room in that crib for both AAP recommendations and developmentally supportive care? *Neonatal network*, 18(5), 29-33.

Madlon-Kay DJ (2002). Maternal assessment of neonatal jaundice after hospital discharge. *Journal of family practice*, 51(5), 445-448.

Ooi CT (2002). Post-kernicteric syndrome. *Australian family physician*, 31(3), 255-257.

Slack MH, Thwaites RJ (2000). Timing of immunisation of premature infants on the neonatal unit and after discharge to the community. *Community district public health*, 3(4), 303-304.

Watkin PM (2001). Neonatal screening for hearing impairment. *Seminars in neonatology*, 6(6), 501-509.

Worrell LA, et al. (2002). The effects of the introduction of a high-nutrient transitional formula on growth and development of very-low-birth-weight infants. *Journal of perinatology*, 22(2), 112-119.

CHAPTER 23

PROCEDURES

This chapter includes some of the more common procedures done in the neonatal intensive care unit (NICU).

BLOOD COLLECTION*

Heel Stick

Purpose   The preferred method of blood collection during an infant's first 2 years of life is by heel stick. One of the most common heel stick problems is heel or bone injury caused by punctures that are too deep. Infant heel punctures bleed from the vasculature at or near the subcutaneous tissue (fat) at a depth of approximately 1 mm.

Equipment needed
- Lance (only lances with preset stop points)
- Betadine and sterile H_2O swabs
- Sterile gauze pad 2×2
- Blood collection container: capillary tube or filter paper
- Blades are not considered safe for blood sampling
- Heel warmer
- Band-Aid
- Gloves

Procedures
1. Determine safe area to use for neonatal heel stick. This area is "marked" by a line extending posteriorly from a point between the fourth and fifth toes and running parallel to the lateral aspect of heel, and a line extending posteriorly from middle of great toe running parallel to medial aspect of heel.
   a. Warm infant's heel by way of heel warmer 10 to 15 minutes before blood sampling.
2. Infant should be in supine position for foot to hang lower than torso, improving blood flow.
3. Wash hands, and wear gloves.

---

*From Altimier L, Brown B, Tedeschi L (2000). *Tri-Health's manual of neonatal nursing policies, procedures, competencies, & clinical pathways*, Glenview, Ill: National Association of Neonatal Nurses.

4. Clean the incision area of the heel with a Betadine swab. Allow heel to air dry. Remove Betadine with sterile H_2O wipe.
5. Raise foot above baby's heart level, and carefully select safe incision site. Place blade surface of lance flush against heel so its center point is vertically aligned with the desired incision site.
6. Depress the trigger of the lance, and after triggering, immediately remove the instrument from the infant's heel. Move the infant's heel to a position level with or below the baby.
7. Using dry, sterile gauze pad, gently wipe away first droplet of blood that appears at wound site.
8. Fill collection container to desired specimen volume. Squeezing foot is contraindicated because it causes hemolysis and contaminates the specimen with interstitial fluid, thromboplastin, and wound debris. It also causes bruising.
9. Gently press dry, sterile gauze pad to incision site until bleeding ceases. This helps prevent hematoma from forming. Monitor incision for bleeding and inflammation.
10. The amount of blood drawn should be documented with results of the blood tests.

Limitations of the procedure
- Heel edema and inflammation may occur.
- Poor vascularization may cause inadequate blood flow.

Central Hematocrit
Purpose Central hematocrit evaluates hematocrit level in newborn when heel stick hematocrit levels are elevated.

Equipment needed
- Gloves
- Betadine and sterile H_2O swabs
- No. 25 or no. 23 gauge butterfly needle or no. 23 gauge 1-inch needle or syringe
- 5-cc syringe
- Hematocrit tubes
- Band-aid or gauze 2×2
- Rubber gloves
- Tourniquet if needed

Procedures
1. Position infant so site is easily accessible.
2. Follow Standard Precautions guidelines. Prepare area with antiseptic.
3. Occlude vein proximally using the following:
   a. Tourniquet/rubber band
   b. Direct pressure

4. Check syringe function, and attach to needle.
5. Penetrate skin first, and position for entry of vein:
   a. Angle of entry 25 to 45 degrees
   b. Bevel up preferred for optimal blood flow (less chance of needle occlusion by vein wall)
   c. Direction of entry may be with or against direction of blood flow
6. Collect sample by gentle suction:
   a. To prevent occlusion by vein wall
   b. To avoid hemolysis
7. Release tourniquet.
8. Remove needle, apply local pressure with dry gauze for 3 minutes (or until complete hemostasis).
9. Fill hematocrit tubes, and seal.
10. Properly identify sample, and obtain test results.
11. Document results.
12. Notify physician/certified nurse practitioner (CNP) if hematocrit is equal to or great than 65.

UNIVERSITY OF ILLINOIS MEDICAL CENTER AT CHICAGO CLINICAL CARE GUIDELINE

Subject: Capillary Blood Sampling*

Objective

To establish standards for capillary blood sampling that would provide for patient safety and minimize the risk of infection or injury. Registered nurses (RNs), registered nurses license pending (RNLPs), licenses practical nurses (LPNs), and nursing students under the direct supervision of the nursing instructor may obtain capillary blood samples.

Definitions

For the purposes of this guideline the following definitions shall apply:

Heel Sticks—Superficial punctures of the skin of the lateral heel (avoiding the plantar surface) in order to collect small volumes of blood for diagnostic laboratory studies. Heel sticks shall be the preferred site for collecting capillary blood samples in all neonates and infants up to 1 year of age.

Finger Sticks—Superficial puncture of the skin of the lateral aspects of the finger (avoiding the finger pad) to collect small volumes of blood for diagnostic laboratory studies. Finger sticks

*From University of Illinois Medical Center at Chicago Women's and Children's Nursing Services. Used with permission by Dharmapuri Vidyasagar, MD; Catherine Theorell, RNC, MSN, NNP; Beena Peters, RN, MS.

shall be the preferred site for collecting capillary blood samples in children over 1 year of age.

Lancet—A sterile, spring-loaded, single-use puncture device that controls the depth of skin penetration. Different depths of lancet penetration are available depending on the gestation age of the infant.

Procedures

1. Aseptic technique shall be maintained when collecting capillary blood samples.
2. Follow standard blood and body fluid precautions as established.
3. The nurse shall warm the site for 5 to 10 minutes before obtaining the capillary sample.
4. The puncture device blade shall not exceed 2.4 mm in length for newborn babies in the NICU/intermediate care nursery (ICN).
5. Heel stick capillary blood samples shall be obtained from the sites indicated in Figure 23-1.
6. Fingerstick capillary blood samples shall be obtained from the lateral aspect of the finger and not the pad of the finger.

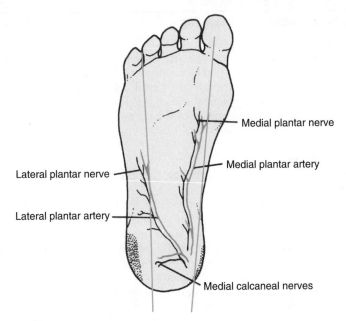

Medial plantar nerve

Medial plantar artery

Lateral plantar nerve

Lateral plantar artery

Medial calcaneal nerves

FIGURE **23-1**
Heel stick sites (*shaded areas*) on infant's foot for obtaining samples of capillary blood. (From Lowdermilk DL, et al. [2000]. *Maternity and women's health care*, ed 7, St Louis: Mosby.)

7. The nurse shall assess the patient to determine an appropriate site to avoid repeated trauma to one area.
8. The first drop of blood shall be removed with gauze before obtaining the specimen.
9. Gentle milking of the extremity above the puncture site may be used to encourage increased blood flow.
10. Application of pressure with sterile gauze may be used for hemostasis.
11. Documentation shall include the following:
    a. Condition of puncture site
    b. Data and time when specimen collected
    c. Laboratory test(s) for which the specimen was collected
    d. Volume of blood obtained
    e. Patient's tolerance

INSTRUCTIONS FOR COLLECTING A BLEEDING TIME TEST IN NEONATE*

Equipment Needed

1. Neonatal blood pressure cuff, appropriate size for forearm (if the thumb is to be used), the upper arm (if the volar surface is to be used), or the lower leg (if the toe is to be used).
2. Betadine and alcohol wipes
3. Filter paper
4. Device for producing the standardized incision
    a. Autolet® (Tenderfoot) (International Technidyne Corp., Edison, NJ)
    b. Surgicutt Newborn® (International Technidyne Corp.)
    c. Simplate Paediatric® (Organon Teknika, Sweden)
5. Stopwatch
6. When it is important to keep track of the "blood out," it is useful to have a scale for weighing the filter paper before and after completion of the test to estimate the blood loss.

Procedures

1. Measure blood pressure in the extremity to be tested.
2. Apply a constant "holding pressure" to the blood pressure cuff equal to the diastolic pressure.
3. Clean the site to be tested with Betadine, and then wipe clean with alcohol and air dry. (If the Autolet is to be used, select the thumb or large toe. If the Surgicutt or Simplate device is to be used, select the volar surface of the forearm.)

---

*From Sola MC, Christensen RD (2000). Developmental aspects of platelets and disorders of platelets in the neonatal period. In Christensen RD, editor. Hematologic problems of the neonate, Philadelphia: WB Saunders, p. 276.

4. Produce the standard puncture (Autolet)® or incision (Surgicutt® or Simplate).
5. Immediately start the stopwatch.
6. Blot the blood from the incision, using filter paper, every 15 seconds until the bleeding stops, and then stop the stopwatch.
7. The time taken for the bleeding to stop is the *bleeding time*.

Interpretation of Results

1. Normal infants (97%) have bleeding times of less than 3.5 minutes. A prolonged bleeding time in a neonate with a normal platelet count indicates an abnormality in one of four functions:
   a. Platelet adhesion
   b. Platelet activation
   c. Platelet aggregation
   d. Vascular defectiveness (Marfan or Ehlers-Danlos syndrome)
2. Blood loss from a bleeding time test in a neonate is usually only 0.1 to 0.3 ml; in cases with very prolonged bleeding time exceeding 10 minutes, we generally stop the test and apply a small bandage.

UNIVERSITY OF ILLINOIS MEDICAL CENTER AT CHICAGO CLINICAL CARE GUIDELINE

Subject: Maintenance of Capped Catheters in Neonates*

Objectives

- To maintain the patency of the catheter lumen for vascular access as indicated.
- To prevent fluid overload and heparinization in neonatal practice.

Definitions

Capped Catheter—A vascular catheter that has been previously inserted under aseptic technique and is no longer required for the provision of a continuous infusion of parenteral fluids. The end of the catheter is thus capped with a needleless connection device that maintains sterility of the line.

Percutaneous Central Venous Catheter (PCVC)—A narrow-gauge, single-lumen, central vascular cathether percutaneously inserted for the prolonged infusion of continuous parenteral fluids or pharmacologic therapy.

Broviac Catheter—A surgically placed central catheter inserted for the prolonged provision of parenteral fluids. These catheters may have a single lumen or multiple lumens.

*From University of Illinois Medical Center at Chicago Women's and Children's Nursing Services. Used with permission by Dharmapuri Vidyasagar, MD; Catherine Theorell, RNC, MSN, NNP; Beena Peters, RN, MS.

Peripheral Catheter—A percutaneously placed angiocatheter with catheter tip in the peripheral vascular system.

Heparin Lock—A central or peripherally located vascular access device that is not used for continuous infusions and has heparinized (10 units per cc) solution in-dwelling within the lumen to prevent thrombus formation.

Position Statements

Catheters that have been capped and are no longer required for continuous infusion of parenteral fluids must be flushed regularly to avoid occlusion of the lumen by a thrombus.

RNs and RNs license pending shall be responsible for flushing capped catheters.

Capped catheters shall be flushed at a flush frequency of at least every 8 hours for peripheral lines and every 24 hours for central lines.

Strict aseptic technique is used when flushing capped central catheters.

Heparin flush solution (10 units per cubic centimeter) shall not contain benzyl alcohol (i.e., preservative free).

Procedures

1. Peripheral lines shall be capped by flushing the line with D5W or normal saline (NS). Central line shall be heparin locked by flushing the line with D5W or NS followed by heparin solution flush.
2. When administering more than one medication in immediate succession, the line shall be flushed with D5W or NS following each medication. After the administration of the last medication, peripheral line shall be flushed with D5W or NS followed by the heparin lock solution.
3. The flush solution for neonates weighing 750 g or less shall be D5W.
4. The flush solution for neonates weighing more than 750 g may be D5W or normal saline as indicated by the physician.
5. The amount of time between heparin flushes shall not exceed the minimal acceptable time interval as established in this guideline.
6. The nurse shall consult the physician regarding where the established flush amounts represent a volume overload.
7. Peripheral venous catheters, Broviac catheters, and PCVCs may be heparin locked with the order of the attending physician/neonatal fellow.
8. Neonatal nurses shall follow the NICU clinical care guideline regarding the maintenance for percutaneous central venous catheter lines (PCVCs).
9. **Documentation:** The nurse shall document all heparin flushes given in the medication administration record (MAR).

10. **Documentation:** The nurse shall record the volume of all D5W, NS, and/or heparin flushes given to neonatal patients on the nursing flow sheet.

UNIVERSITY OF ILLINOIS MEDICAL CENTER AT CHICAGO CLINICAL CARE GUIDELINE

Subject: Percutaneous Central Venous Catheter (PCVC) Use in the Neonate*

Objective

To provide standards for the safe use and care of percutaneous central venous catheters (PCVCs) in the neonate.

Definition

For the purpose of this guideline, the following definition shall apply:

Experienced neonatal RNs who have demonstrated clinical competence in the general care of the PCVC may care for an infant with this medical device.

Position Statements

The neonatal attending physician or fellow will insert the PCVC per manufacturer's recommendations, using aseptic technique, after informed consent is obtained from parent or guardian. The infant should be given medication to relieve pain during insertion of PCVC.

Before insertion, peripherally placed central venous catheters should be trimmed to the desired length (from skin insertion point to the placement in the vena cava). The length of the catheter that remains outside the skin to the catheter hub should be measured and recorded. The nurses will assess the length of the catheter in order to detect inward migration.

After insertion, the location of catheter tip must be verified by x-ray. The physician is responsible for radiographic interpretation of catheter tip location. The optimal location for a central catheter tip is in the superior vena cava. Any infant in whom a PCVC is placed should have the tip location reviewed on all subsequent chest radiographs.

The neonatal attending physician or fellow may do the following:

1. Obtain blood from line for culture.
2. Repair damaged lines.

RNs, RNs license pending supervised by RN preceptor, and nursing students supervised by nursing faculty or staff RN shall do the following:

*From University of Illinois Medical Center at Chicago Women's and Children's Nursing Services. Used with permission by Dharmapuri Vidyasagar, MD; Catherine Theorell, RNC, MSN, NNP; Beena Peters, RN, MS.

1. Change infusion line–related components.
2. Maintain the sterility of the line.
3. Care for insertion site and change dressing as needed.
4. Determine patency when pump occlusion alarm is present.

Aseptic technique (including cap, sterile gloves, mask) is used for dressing changes, change of solutions, or any situation that requires accessing or opening the line. Before disconnecting infusion line, the connection should be cleansed with povidone-iodine solution and allowed to dry.

Procedures: Assessment and Functional Use of PCVC

1. The nurse caring for an infant with a PCVC shall assess the insertion site every hour for evidence of the following:
   a. Leaking of fluids
   b. Bleeding
   c. Drainage
   d. Edema
   e. Venous tracking or palpable vein along the path of the catheter
2. PCVC dressing will be assessed at least every 8 hours, checking that the dressing is intact.
3. The maximum rate of infusion is as follows:
   a. Through 24-gauge PCVC: 26 cc/hr
   b. Through 28-gauge PCVC: 12 cc/hr
4. Intravenous (IV) fluids must be heparinized when administered through PCVC. The routine concentration of heparin is 1 unit per milliliter of parenteral fluid. The concentration of heparin may need to be individualized based on the infant's condition and rate of infusion.
5. Heparin flush solutions will contain 10 units/ml.
6. Stopcocks shall not be used on PCVCs.
7. Blood products must not be infused through PCVC.
8. Medications may be administered through a PCVC, at physician's discretion. Medications administered through a PCVC are not to be given IV push.
9. Blood shall not be drawn from PCVC for routine sampling. When catheter-related sepsis is suspected, blood for cultures can be obtained from PCVC by a physician.
10. Blood pressures will not be obtained from extremity with PCVC.
11. At time of removal, the catheter tip may be sent to the lab for culture.

Procedures: Changing Infusion Fluids and Infusion Tubing

1. Aseptic technique (including cap, sterile gloves, mask) is used for dressing changes, change of solutions, or any situation that requires accessing or opening the line. Before disconnecting

infusion line, the connection should be cleansed with povidone-iodine solution and allowed to dry.

2. Assemble appropriate equipment, sterile supplies, tubing, and solutions.
3. Place needed equipment on sterile field.
4. Don hair covering and mask.
5. Wash and dry hands, don sterile gloves.
6. Draw up at least two (5-cc) syringes with heparinized flush (0.5 cc in each).
7. Connect new infusion solution to new infusion tubing, and flush tubing with clamp.
8. Wipe the connection to be opened with povidone-iodine swab. Allow to dry.
9. Open the system at the end of tubing. Cover the end of PCVC hub to prevent contamination.
10. Fill dead space of PCVCA hub with 3 or 4 drops of flush solution.
11. Connect new infusion tubing to PCVC hub. Place infusion tubing into infusion pump as directed. Release tubing clamp.
12. Set infusion pump rate as ordered. Double check infusion pump rate and volume with additional RN.
13. Document the activities performed on the nursing flow sheet.

Procedures: PCVC Dressing Change

1. Aseptic technique (including cap, sterile gloves, mask) is used for dressing changes, change of solutions, or any situation that requires accessing or opening the line. Before disconnecting infusion line, the connection should be cleansed with povidone-iodine solution and allowed to dry.
2. Two RNs are required when performing PCVC dressing changes. **RNs may remove the PCVC on order from physician.**
3. PCVC dressing will be changed only if the following occur:
   a. The transparent dressing becomes loosened from the skin.
   b. Blood or exudate accumulates under the dressing.
4. Assemble appropriate equipment and sterile supplies including sterile Steri-strips, sterile transparent dressing, povidone-iodine solution, sterile barriers, several 5-cc syringes, heparin flush, and gauze.
5. Position infant appropriately; restrain temporarily or have assistant hold the infant to avoid contamination of the sterile field.
6. Place needed equipment on sterile field.
7. Don head covering and mask.
8. Wash hands, and don clean gloves.
9. Loosen all four corners of adhesive dressing with one hand, while holding forefinger of other hand on top of dressing at center.
10. Remove clean gloves. Don sterile gloves.

11. Draw up at least three (5-cc) syringes with heparinized fluid, 0.5 cc in each.
12. Cut Steri-strips as follows:
    a. 1 × 1 cm
    b. 2 × 3 cm
    c. 3 × 4 cm
13. Drape appropriately.
14. Working with sterile underside of dressing, gently pull away dressing from catheter coils and Steri-strips using forceps if needed.
15. Assess catheter insertion site.
16. Determine if Steri-strips need to be replaced. **Caution:** Attempting to remove Steri-strips stuck to catheter may result in catheter tear. Remove adherent Steri-strips only if necessary.
17. With one sterile, gloved hand, stabilize external portion of catheter. With the other sterile gloved hand, use povidone-iodine–soaked gauze to cleanse from insertion site out. Allow to dry completely.
18. Remove povidone-iodine with alcohol swab, starting from insertion site outward.
19. Replace Steri-strips if removed.
    a. Use 1-cm Steri-strip over catheter insertion site.
    b. Use 3-cm Steri-strip in Y loop around catheter or over catheter distal to insertion site.
    c. Use 3-cm Steri-strip over Y to secure.
20. Wrap external portion of catheter in concentric coils around insertion site and secure with 4-cm Steri-strip. Secure hub with 4-cm Steri-strip.
21. Place occlusive, transparent dressing over all external portions of catheter and one half of hub.
22. Document on nursing flow sheet:
    a. Procedure
    b. Assessment of site
    c. Patient's tolerance

Procedures: Assessing Patency for IVs
1. If the IV pump reads occlusion, reset the pump and immediately investigate the reason for the alarm.
2. Assess the infusion system:
    a. If tubing is kinked or clamped, unkink or unclamp the tubing.
    b. If blood is backed up in PCVC, increase IV rate to maximum infusion rate for the catheter for 1 to 2 minutes to clear blood from line and look for loose connections or leaks in the system.
    c. If filter is filled with air and occluding the flow, change the filter.

3. If the pump alarm continues, assess the PCVC for patency.
   a. Obtain two (5-cc) syringes with (10 units/cc) heparin flush (0.5 cc in each).
   b. Don mask and sterile gloves.
   c. Wipe the connection to be opened with povidone-iodine swab.
   d. Open the system at the end of T connector. Cover the end of T connector to prevent contamination.
   e. Fill dead space with 3 or 4 drops of heparinized flush solution.
   f. Connect 5-cc syringe, and gently attempt to aspirate (excessive pressure could collapse catheter).
   g. If prompt blood return is seen in PCVC, then gently flush to clear the line. Reconnect IV tubing to catheter. Continue infusion.
   h. If no blood return is seen, immediately contact neonatal fellow or attending physician.
4. Document on the nursing flow sheet the activities needed to check patency.

Procedures: PCVC Removal

1. Physicians remove PCVC catheters. Verify order for catheter removal.
2. Ascertain the length of catheter originally inserted in infant.
3. Loosen sterile dressing by pulling back on all four corners.
4. Loosen all adhesives, including Steri-strips, away from skin.
5. Open suture removal kit.
6. Don mask and sterile gloves.
7. With sterile forceps, gently pull catheter back 1 to 2 cm.
8. Cleanse with povidone-iodine solution, beginning with insertion site and moving outward.
9. Continue to remove catheter centimeter by centimeter with sterile forceps.
10. When PCVC is out, if a culture is desired, cut the catheter 1 to 2 cm from the tip with sterile scissors and let fall into sterile specimen container.
11. Clean insertion site with povidone-iodine scrub solution. Let dry completely. Remove povidone-iodine solution from skin with an alcohol prep pad. Dress with Band-aid.
12. Extend and measure the catheter from point of insertion to end. Add amount of catheter sent for culture. Compare the measurement with amount known to have been inserted. Report any differences to physician.
13. Document on nursing flow sheet:
    a. Procedure activities
    b. Condition of insertion site
    c. Length of catheter retrieved

Procedures: Obtaining Blood from PCVC for Blood Culture

1. Assemble equipment and appropriate sterile supplies including povidone-iodine solution; sterile 2 × 2's, sterile drape, sterile gloves and mask; two tuberculin syringes (for drawing blood), 5-cc syringe (for flushing), heparinized flush (10 units/cc), specimen bottle for blood culture.
2. The nurse shall temporarily restrain or have another assistant hold the infant.
3. Assemble equipment on sterile field.
4. Don cap, mask, and sterile gloves.
5. Draw up heparinized flush (0.5 cc) in TB syringe and 5-cc syringe.
6. Clean PCVC hub and T-connector junction carefully with povidone-iodine solution.
7. Place 2 × 2's between PCVC hub and skin, then disconnect the IV solution. Cap IV line with sterile needle to prevent contamination.
8. Attach half-filled heparinized TNl syringe; gently aspirate 0.3 cc of solution from the line. Discard.
9. Attach empty TB syringe, and gently aspirate volume of blood needed for culture.
10. Remove TB syringe filled with blood specimen.
11. Attach 5-cc syringe with flush, and gently flush line until residual blood is cleared (0.6 cc).
12. Reconnect IV line to PCVC.
13. Prepare the identified, labeled specimen for transport.
14. Document on nursing flow sheet:
    a. Blood specimen obtained for suspected catheter-related sepsis
    b. Condition of line after blood drawn

Documentation Procedures: Catheter Insertion and Maintenance

1. For all PCVC insertions, the nurse shall document the following on nursing flow sheet:
    a. Date and time of insertion
    b. Pain medications used during procedure
    c. Location of catheter tip (after physician has verified by x-ray)
    d. Infant's tolerance to procedure
2. Document the following in patient care plan/bedside information card:
    a. Date of insertion
    b. Location of catheter tip after x-ray confirmation by physician
3. The nurse shall document the following for assessment of catheter maintenance:
    a. Assessment of insertion site every hour
    b. Assessment of extremity every hour

c. Solution(s) infusing through PCVC with heparin concentration every shift and with changes
d. Amount of solution infused every hour
e. Assessment of catheter condition every hour

UNIVERSITY OF ILLINOIS MEDICAL CENTER AT CHICAGO CLINICAL CARE GUIDELINE

Subject: Transitioning Preterm Infants from Incubators to Open Cribs*

Objective

To establish standards for the care of preterm infants as they are transitioned from incubator to open crib.

Definitions

For the purpose of this guideline, the following definitions will apply:

Preterm Infant—A newborn infant born before the completion of 37 weeks of gestation.

Neutral Thermal Temperature—An environmental temperature that minimizes the premature infant's oxygen consumption. Standardized graphs of these temperatures are based on the gestational and postnatal ages of the infant.

Incubator—A warming device used to control heat loss via radiation, convection, and evaporation.

Open Crib—Refers to a bassinet or infant crib that provides no external sources of heat.

Position Statements

The University of Illinois Medical Center at Chicago recognizes that in order to sustain a normal, neutral thermal temperature, premature infants require equipment, temperature probes, and beds that provide an external source of heat.

Infants have immature thermoregulatory responses and can be easily heat or cold stressed. Cold stress is a significant and constant threat to preterm infants.

Thermal stress may result in growth failure and increased morbidity.

In collaboration with the physician, the nurse, using best judgment based on infant status and established criteria, shall determine when a preterm infant is able to be dressed in a shirt and hat while in the incubator and when to begin the process of transitioning to an open crib.

From University of Illinois Medical Center at Chicago Women's and Children's Nursing Services. Used with permission by Dharmapuri Vidyasagar, MD; Catherine Theorell, RNC, MSN, NNP; Beena Peters, RN, MS.

Procedures

1. Preparatory phase
   a. Preterm infants will be dressed in cloth shirt and hat while in the incubator. Infants will be dressed as soon as they are medically stable.
   b. Infant's axillary temperature will be maintained between 36.5° and 37.0° C.
   c. Once the infant is dressed, the incubator temperature will be adjusted by 0.5° C increments while maintaining the infant's temperature within the expected range.
2. Criteria for transitioning from incubator
   a. The premature infant may be considered for transitioning from the incubator when the following criteria are met:
      (1) Weight is approximately 1500 g.
      (2) Infant is medically stable per the physician.
      (3) Consistent weight gain has been demonstrated over the past 5 days.
      (4) Infant has been dressed in hat and shirt for a minimum of 5 days.
      (5) Nutrition is being provided exclusively by enteral source.
      (6) Infant's axillary temperature is within the expected range with incubator temperature between 31.0° and 32.0° C.
3. Transitioning process
   a. Infants will remain clothed in hat and shirt throughout thermal challenge and transitioning process.
   b. Infant's axillary temperature will be assessed immediately before and 30 minutes and 60 minutes after thermal challenge or move to open crib.
   c. Infant's axillary temperature will be assessed at 30 minutes and at 60 minutes after an intervention is completed in an effort to warm the infant (i.e., additional blankets, move back into incubator).
   d. Infant's axillary temperature will be maintained between 36.5° and 37.0° C.
4. Thermal challenge
   a. Once it has been determined the infant is to begin the transitioning process, decrease incubator temperature by 1° C and cover infant with two receiving blankets.
   b. Continue to adjust incubator temperature until infant's temperature is within the expected range.
   c. Downward adjustments of the incubator temperature can be continued until reaching 28.0° C as long as infant's temperature is within the expected range.
   d. Once the infant's temperature stabilizes within the expected range, maintain the 28.0° C incubator temperature for a minimum of 8 hours.

e. If the incubator temperature is greater than 28.0° C, then decrease the incubator temperature by 0.5° to 1° C, and then repeat steps b and c as appropriate.

f. If the incubator temperature is less than or equal to 28.0° C, then move infant into open crib, swaddle with one receiving blanket, and cover with two receiving blankets.

g. If the infant's temperature does not remain in the desired range in the open crib, add one more receiving blanket.

h. If the infant's temperature is not within the expected range in the open crib with the addition of the blanket, place the infant back into the 28.0° C incubator covered with two receiving blankets for 24 hours, and then repeat steps e, f, or g as appropriate.

i. Transition to an open crib shall be determined successful if the infant's temperature is maintained while rate of growth is not altered.

5. Nursing shall document the following in the bedside flow sheet:

a. All incubator and infant temperatures assessed

b. Infant's responses to the thermal challenge and transitioning process

c. Interventions provided to keep infant's temperature within the expected range while transitioning

• • •

Although in these protocols the orders are done by a physician, in many institutions these are done by neonatal nurse practitioners. Policies may vary slightly among institutions, but the general guideline parameters remain the same. The other difference that may be noted in some institutional policies is the use of weight as a criterion for weaning from an incubator. Some institutions will use stability of the newborn as the major criterion with less emphasis on an exact weight. Use of 1500 g as one criterion for weaning, however, as a low level is a fairly common practice.

URINARY CATHETERIZATION*

Purpose
The purpose of urinary catheterization is to obtain sterile urine specimen when a "clean catch" specimen or suprapubic bladder tap is not desired.

---

*From Altimier L, Brown B, Tedeschi L (2000). Tri-Health's manual of neonatal nursing policies, procedures, competencies, & clinical pathways, Glenview, Ill: National Association of Neonatal Nurses.

Equipment Needed

- No. 5 Fr. or no. 8 Fr. feeding tube
- Indwelling urinary catheter
- Water-soluble lubricant
- Betadine swabs (3)
- Sterile barrier (2)
- Sterile gloves
- Sterile container
- Catheter size:

	<1000 g	Premature	Newborn
Male	3.5 Fr.	5 Fr.	5 Fr.
Female	3.5 Fr.	5 Fr.	5 or 8 Fr.

Procedures

1. Wash hands, and assemble equipment.
2. Place child supine, female: knees bent—legs fall apart; males: legs straight. Restrain as necessary.
3. Open sterile barriers, place one under buttocks and the other on clean, dry area for infant's genital area.
4. Open catheter package, and drop catheter onto sterile barrier; squeeze lubricant onto sterile barrier.
5. Put on sterile gloves, open sterile container, and generously lubricate catheter tip with water-soluble lubricant.
6. Female: Separate labia with thumb and index finger, cleanse urethral meatus with Betadine swabs front to back. Wipe once downward over meatus and then once on either side of meatus with each swab. Do not wipe over same area more than once with each swab.
7. Male: Hold penis upward with one hand, cleanse glans with Betadine with other hand. Partially retract foreskin on uncircumcised male to visualize meatus (do not force). Wipe in circular fashion over glans beginning over the meatus and ending at the proximal penile shaft.
8. Place distal end of catheter in sterile container to collect urine.
9. Insert catheter into meatus 6 cm plus 1 to 2 cm for male, 1.5 to 2 cm for female. Do not force catheter against resistance. If baby cries or strains, pause and attempt to calm before continuing.
10. Insert catheter (not >10 cm) until urine flow begins. When performing straight intermittent catheterization, remove catheter when urine flow ceases.
11. Collect specimen for culture: if adequate use first 2 to 3 cc for urinalysis (UA) and second specimen for culture.

UMBILICAL ARTERIAL CATHETERIZATION*

Indications

1. Monitoring blood pressure
2. Monitoring arterial blood gases when infant is in supplemental oxygen
3. May be considered as an access and infusion site in all neonates with birth weight below 1.0 kg in whom other access sites carry substantial risk
4. May be used as an alternative site of fluid administration when attempts at venous access are unsuccessful

Contraindications

1. Anomalies of the umbilicus and abdominal wall: relative contraindications
2. Vascular impairments in the lower extremities and buttocks

Equipment

1. Sterile drapes
2. Sterile gown, cap, mask, and gloves
3. Tape measure
4. Betadine solution
5. Umbilical tie tape
6. Scalpel
7. Two Kelly clamps
8. Two iris forceps with teeth
9. Two straight forceps
10. Flush solution
11. Three-way stopcock
12. Two 3-ml syringes
13. Polyvinyl chloride or Silastic catheters in various sizes appropriate to birth weight (birth weight <750 g, 2.5 Fr.; 750 to 1750 g, 3 Fr.; >1750 g, 5 Fr.)
14. Needle driver
15. Absorbable suture
16. Strong light source
17. Graphs to determine appropriate depth of insertion

Technique

1. Determine the appropriate depth of line insertion, using either the total body length or the birth weight.
2. Prepare the catheter with a sterile saline or heparin flush solution (1 unit/ml).

From Walsh-Sukys MC, Krug SE (1997). Procedures in infants and children, Philadelphia: WB Saunders, pp. 124-133.

3. Tie the base of the umbilicus with umbilical tie tape, taking care to avoid the abdominal wall skin.

4. Place a cloth or disposable diaper over the neonate's thighs, and restrain the baby by placing tape across the baby's legs and the bed.

5. Prepare the umbilicus and abdominal wall with Betadine, using sterile technique.

6. Don sterile gown and gloves, and drape the baby's trunk and legs leaving the umbilicus exposed. Ensure that the baby's head and endotracheal tube are visible to an observer during the procedure to avoid endotracheal tube occlusion or dislodgment.

7. Sever the umbilical cord with the scalpel at a 90-degree angle about 1 cm above the abdominal wall.

8. Identify two thick-walled arteries and a single thin-walled vein.

9. Stabilize the umbilical stump by grasping the Wharton's jelly with two Kelly clamps.

10. Gently dilate the artery with the curved iris forceps. Insert the closed forceps into the artery, and then gently open them. Repeat this maneuver three or four times.

11. When the lumen is opened, the assistant gently grasps the arterial wall with two curved forceps on opposite sides of the vessel. This will stabilize the artery and prevent it from sliding away from the catheter during insertion.

12. Grasp the catheter approximately 0.5 cm above the tip with the straight forceps, and gently insert the tip into the vessel lumen.

13. Move the forceps back up the catheter in 1-cm increments, and gently advance the catheter forward.

14. If resistance is met at any point, gentle pressure may be held on the catheter at that point, but no attempt should be made to advance beyond the resistance unless the resistance resolves. Resistance may be produced by vasospasm, which may spontaneously resolve. Alternatively, it may be encountered when the catheter has been introduced to the 3- to 5-cm mark at the point where the umbilical artery enters the iliac artery and the catheter must negotiate an acute turn. Vigorous attempts to advance the catheter past resistance at this point may result in perforation. If the resistance does not spontaneously resolve, it is most prudent to abandon the attempt at placement and try again in the other artery.

15. Advance the catheter to the predetermined appropriate depth to result in either a "high" line (thoracic vertebrae 8 to 11) or a "low" line (lumbar vertebrae 3 to 5). These positions avoid the major vascular branches from the aorta.

16. Suture catheter in place securely to the umbilical stump. One technique to prevent catheter movement is to use a self-retaining suture, that is, one that becomes tighter whenever any traction is

placed on the catheter. Begin the self-retaining stitch by securing the suture to the umbilical stump near the exit site of the catheter. Some surgeons place a purse-string suture around the umbilicus to function as a secondary means to achieve hemostasis, whereas others prefer to begin with a single through-and-through stitch. Secure the stitch with a square knot, and remove the needle leaving long segments of suture on either side of the knot (tails). Grasp one tail and encircle the tip of the needle driver two times, moving toward the catheter. Place the needle driver and the free end of the same tail on opposite sides of the catheter, and pull the free end through the loops. Repeat this same movement on the opposite side using the other tail. Repeat both steps again, which will yield four loops on the catheter. Complete the stitch by tying a square knot with the two suture ends.

17. Ensure correct catheter position by radiograph. On an anteroposterior radiograph a catheter placed in the umbilical artery will descend before turning cephalad, whereas a venous catheter will go immediately cephalad. These two can be further distinguished on a lateral radiograph. The aorta lies just anterior to the vertebrae, whereas the vein tracks in the anterior abdominal wall.

18. One may wish to secure the catheter further by forming a bridge with tape. In very low–birth weight neonates, the skin can be protected from the tape with Stomahesive material and the tape applied to this.

19. A final useful marker is to place a piece of tape across the catheter immediately above the umbilicus. This ensures that catheter movement can be detected readily.

20. A catheter should *never* be advanced once the sterile drape is removed.

Complications

1. The vast majority of complications arise from failure to use adequate caution and time to dilate the umbilical artery at the beginning of catheter insertion. This can lead to vessel perforation, dissection of the tunica intima (false tracking), or avulsion of the tunica intima (false tracking). All these may be suspected during catheter placement when resistance is encountered within 1 to 3 cm of catheter placement or if a "pop" is felt. If any of these are encountered the safest course of action is to remove the catheter from the affected artery and try again in the opposite vessel.

2. Vessel perforation posterior to the bladder: The umbilical artery follows an inferior course, descends behind the bladder, and then turns nearly 180 degrees to join the iliac artery and then the abdominal aorta. At the point at which the umbilical artery turns, the catheter must negotiate an acute angle. Resistance may be

encountered at this point, which is approximately 5-cm catheter depth. Vigorous attempts to advance the catheter may result in perforation of the posterior wall of the umbilical artery and retroperitoneal hematoma formation. Bleeding into this concealed space may be life threatening and requires surgical exploration to correct. Ultrasound may be used to confirm the diagnosis.

3. Complications resulting from malposition of an intraluminal catheter:

   a. The catheter may turn and track inferiorly down the iliac artery, occluding circulation to the leg. Alternatively, the vessel may be in spasm. Immediately following catheter placement, perfusion to the toes of both legs must be assessed. If any evidence of cyanosis is visible, the catheter must be pulled back to a more central position immediately. If one extremity is dusky, vasospasm may be diagnosed and treated by warming the contralateral extremity (wrapping the other extremity with a diaper warmed with tap water works well for this). Warming of the well-perfused extremity induces reflex vasodilation in the affected extremity. If cyanosis persists for more than 5 minutes, the catheter should be removed.

   b. Occlusion to the gluteal artery can lead to necrosis of the buttocks; involvement of the gluteus maximus can lead to major impairment of ambulation later in life. Radiographs will identify malposition in this vessel.

   c. Occlusion of a spinal artery may occur when an otherwise well-placed catheter errantly enters any of the spinal arteries arising from the aorta. Again, radiographs will identify any malposition.

   d. Occlusion of the renal arteries or celiac trunk: Catheters positioned between thoracic vertebra 11 and lumbar vertebra 2 may impinge on the flow of blood into these major vessels. Malposition may be detected radiographically.

   e. Placement at the patent ductus arteriosus (PDA): A catheter placed at thoracic vertebra 4 may be positioned at the PDA, which may contribute to ductal patency.

   f. Placement of the catheter too far superiorly will lead it to advance up the aorta into the left ventricle or vessels serving the arms, neck, or head. Left ventricular placement may precipitate arrhythmias, whereas positioning in more distal vessels may lead to vascular occlusion. These can be prevented by predetermining the depth of catheter insertion and can be detected radiographically.

4. Emboli-related catheters

   a. Air or debris may be introduced whenever the catheter is infused or flushed. Meticulous attention is needed to ensure that air is not introduced. Emboli may be seen in any distal circulatory bed. The most severe consequences of emboli are seen when they involve the coronary circulation, (which may lead to myocardial infarction), the cerebral circulation (which may produce stroke), the renal circulation (with infarction and hypertension), or the gut circulation (leading to necrotizing enterocolitis).

b. High catheters are more frequently associated with embolic events producing seizures, whereas low catheters more frequently are associated with embolic events involving the lower extremity. Necrotizing enterocolitis is equally common in both groups.

UMBILICAL VENOUS CATHETERIZATION*

Indications
1. Emergency vascular access for resuscitation in a neonate
2. Access for exchange transfusion in a neonate
3. Central venous pressure monitoring in a neonate

Contraindication
1. Anomalies of the umbilicus and abdominal wall: relative contraindications

Equipment
1. Sterile drapes
2. Sterile gown, cap, mask, and gloves
3. Tape measure
4. Betadine solution
5. Umbilical tie tape
6. Scalpel
7. Two Kelly clamps
8. Two iris forceps with teeth
9. Two straight forceps
10. Flush solution
11. Three-way stopcock
12. Two 3-ml syringes
13. Polyvinyl chloride or Silastic catheters in various appropriate sizes (preterm, 5 Fr.; term, 8 Fr.)
14. Needle driver
15. Absorbable suture
16. Strong light source
17. Graph to determine appropriate depth of insertion

---

*From Walsh-Sukys MC, Krug SE (1997). Procedures in infants and children, Philadelphia: WB Saunders, pp. 116-123.

Technique

1. Determine the appropriate depth of line insertion using either the total body length or birth weight. In an emergency, the line is inserted until blood return is obtained. Another rule of thumb is to insert approximately 5 cm in a preterm baby and 10 cm in a term baby. The desired location of the catheter tip is in the inferior vena cava (IVC) either below the portal system or at the IVC and right atrial junction.

2. Prepare the catheter by placing a three-way stopcock on the end of the catheter and filling the catheter with a sterile saline or heparin flush solution (1 unit/ml).

3. Tie the base of the umbilicus with umbilical tape, taking care to avoid the abdominal wall skin.

4. Place a cloth or disposable diaper over the neonate's thighs, and restrain the baby by placing tape across the baby's legs and the bed.

5. Prepare the umbilicus and abdominal wall with Betadine using sterile technique.

6. Don sterile gown and gloves, and drape the baby's trunk and legs, leaving the umbilicus exposed. Ensure that the baby's head and endotracheal tube are visible to an observer during the procedure to avoid endotracheal tube occlusion or dislodgment.

7. Sever the umbilical cord with the scalpel at a 90-degree angle about 1 cm above the abdominal wall.

8. Identify two thick-walled arteries and a single thin-walled vein.

9. Stabilize the umbilical stump by grasping the Wharton's jelly with two Kelly clamps.

10. Gently dilate the vein with the curved iris forceps. Insert the closed forceps into the vein, and then gently open them. Repeat this maneuver three or four times. Remove any blood clots found.

11. When the lumen is opened, the assistant gently grasps the venous wall with two curved forceps on opposite sides of the vessel. This will stabilize the artery and prevent it from sliding away from the catheter during insertion.

12. Grasp the catheter approximately 0.5 cm above the tip with the straight forceps, and gently insert the tip into the vessel lumen.

13. Move the forceps back up to the catheter in 1-cm increments, and gently advance the catheter forward.

14. Suture the catheter in place securely to the umbilical stump. One technique to prevent catheter movement is to use a self-retaining suture; that is, one that becomes tighter whenever any traction is placed on the catheter. Begin the self-retaining stitch by securing the suture to the umbilical stump near the exit site of the catheter. Some operators like to place a purse-string suture around the umbilicus to function as a secondary means to

achieve hemostasis, whereas others prefer to begin with a single through-and-through stitch. Secure the stitch with a square knot, and remove the needle, leaving long segments of suture on either side of the knot (tails). Grasp one tail, and encircle the tip of the needle driver two times, moving toward the catheter. Place the needle driver and the free end of the same tail on opposite sides of the catheter, and pull the free end through the loops. Repeat this same movement on the opposite side using the other tail. Repeat both steps again; this will yield four loops on the catheter. Complete the stitch by tying a square knot with the two suture ends.

15. Ensure correct catheter position by radiograph. On an antero-posterior radiograph a catheter placed in the umbilical artery will descend before turning cephalad, whereas a venous catheter will go immediately cephalad. These two can be further distinguished on a lateral radiograph; the aorta lies just anterior to the vertebrae, whereas the vein tracks in the anterior abdominal wall.

16. One may wish to secure the catheter further by forming a bridge with tape. In very low–birth weight neonates, the skin can be protected from the tape with Stomahesive material and the tape applied to this.

17. A final useful marker is to place a piece of tape across the catheter immediately above the umbilicus. This ensures that catheter movement can be detected readily.

18. A catheter should *never* be advanced once the sterile drape is removed.

Complications

1. Complications resulting from malposition of an intraluminal catheter
   a. Heart: Cardiac arrhythmias may be produced by catheters malpositioned in the heart. In addition, catheters that extend into the right atrium may erode, producing pericardial effusion and/or cardiac tamponade.
   b. Great vessels: Umbilical venous catheter may be advanced too vigorously and may pass out of the right atrium and into the superior vena cava or across the foramen ovale and into the left atrium.
   c. Portal system: Thrombosis of the hepatic veins has been associated with infusion of hypertonic solutions into the portal system. This may lead to hepatic infarction and/or later portal hypertension.
2. Thromboembolic events
3. Infection

NICU/SPECIAL CARE NURSING INTRAOSSEOUS INFUSION*

Indications

Intraosseous access allows administration of drugs, fluids, and blood products directly into the bone marrow. It is recommended for neonates in shock who require emergent vascular access when other methods of vascular access have been attempted or failed.

Relative Contraindications

Relative contraindications include recent fracture of the bone considered for access, osteogenesis imperfecta, or an infectious process at the access site. An insertion should not be attempted on the same leg two times.

Equipment Needed

1. Betadine solution
2. Intraosseous or lumbar puncture aspiration needle
3. 5- or 10-cc syringe
4. Normal saline
5. Gloves
6. Sterile towel
7. Adhesive tape
8. Infusion tubing
9. IV fluid
10. 4 × 4 gauze

Procedures

1. The proximal tibia is the preferred site. This site is easily identified, and a large marrow cavity exists with no adjacent structures that are likely to be damaged. The site of insertion is on the flat medial surface of the anterior tibia, one or two finger breadths below and medial to the tibial tuberosity (Figure 23-2).
2. Immobilize the lower leg by holding the leg securely.
3. Place a small towel behind the knee for support.
4. Select the area in the midline of the flat surface of the anterior tibia, 1 to 3 cm below the tibial tuberosity.
5. Clean the area with Betadine solution. Sterile drapes can be placed around the area.

---

*From University of Illinois Medical Center at Chicago Women's and Children's Nursing Services. Used with permission by Dharmapuri Vidyasagar, MD; Catherine Theorell, RNC, MSN, NNP; Beena Peters, RN, MS

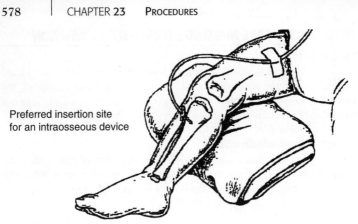

Preferred insertion site for an intraosseous device

FIGURE **23-2**
Site of insertion on medial surface of anterior tibia.

6. Insert the needle at an angle of 10 to 15 degrees toward the foot to avoid the growth plate. Advance the needle by a downward "to and fro" rotary motion. Advance the needle until lack of resistance is felt (usually no more than 1 cm is necessary), at which point of entry into the marrow space should have occurred.

7. Remove stylet from the needle (Figure 23-3).

8. Connect a syringe to the hub of the needle.

9. Check placement:
   a. Placement may be checked by aspirating marrow and then flushing. You may see blood return during aspiration.
   b. Flush with 1 to 2 cc of normal saline, and observe for extravasation (the fluid should flush easily—if no extravasation occurs, placement is confirmed).

10. If placement cannot be confirmed, remove needle, apply pressure for 5 minutes, and cover the insertion site with a sterile dressing. Do not attempt to reinsert the needle on the same site. This will cause leakage of fluids from the insertion site into the surrounding tissues.

11. If placement is confirmed, attach the needle to IV fluids. Place extension tubing directly into the needle, and then attach IV tubing to the extension tubing. Secure the needle and tubing to leg with tape to prevent dislodgment. If the needle is properly inserted, it will stand without support.

12. The needle should not be left in place for more than 12 hours. When it is possible to establish other IV access, then the IO line should be discontinued.

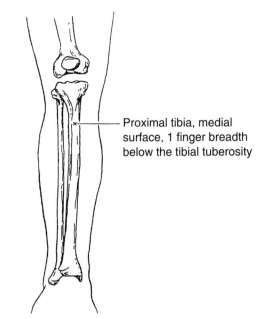

Proximal tibia, medial surface, 1 finger breadth below the tibial tuberosity

FIGURE **23-3**
Removal of stylet from needle.

13. When removing the needle, withdraw needle, and apply pressure over the puncture site. Apply dry, sterile dressing.

Potential Complications
1. Fluid infiltration of subcutaneous tissues
2. Compartment syndrome
3. Skin infection
4. Localized cellulitis
5. Osteomyelitis
6. Fracture

Documentation
1. The date and time the IO line was inserted should be documented on the nursing Kardex and nursing flow sheet.
2. The fluid and the administration site should be checked and documented every hour.
3. The type of fluid administered should be recorded on the IV section of the nursing flow sheet.
4. Document the date and time the IO line was discontinued on the nursing Kardex and nursing flow sheet.

REFERENCES

Altimier L, Brown B, Tedeschi L (2000). *Tri-Health's manual of neonatal nursing policies, procedures, competencies, & clinical pathways*, Glenview, Ill: National Association of Neonatal Nurses.

Kenner C, Lott JW, editors. *Comprehensive neonatal nursing: a physiologic perspective*, ed 3, St Louis: WB Saunders.

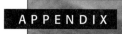
DIAGNOSTIC TESTS AND LABORATORY VALUES

Table A-1	Types of Diagnostic Imaging				
	Diagnostic Imaging Indications	Limitations of Diagnostic Imaging	Potential Risks of Procedure	Preparation of Infant	Cost
Roentgenologic imaging: radiographic	Most common initial diagnostic screening mode	Detects only four different levels of photon absorption (air, fat, water, mineral); two-dimensional projection of three-dimensional structures	Ionizing radiation; thermal stress of cool film plate	Proper positioning essential; must be monitored during procedure	$
Xeroradiographic	Used to evaluate soft tissue structures	Tissue structures defined by relative amounts of air, fat, water, minerals; seldom used with advent of newer diagnostic imaging	Ionizing radiation exposure higher than routine radiographs	Proper positioning essential; must be monitored during procedure	$$
Fluoroscopic	Used to evaluate motion or function of cardiovascular, gastrointestinal, genitourinary systems; may be	Images rely on greater radiation and/or movement of contrast material; improper diagnostic sequencing	Ionizing radiation much higher than routine radiographs; thermal stress of cool radiology environment	Proper positioning essential; must be monitored during procedure	$$-$$$$

	used to guide therapeutic or diagnostic procedures	may delay informational yield; contrast material may have physiologic consequences			
Computerized tomography (CT)	Used to provide detailed, superior characterization of various soft tissue densities that cannot be detected by conventional radiographs	Motion artifact may cause blurring of scans; radiation dose depends on scan time; contrast material may have physiologic consequences	Ionizing radiation; thermal stress of cool environment	Proper positioning essential; must be monitored during procedure	$$$
Ultrasound	Uses sound waves to depict anatomic and functional motion of tissue; sound waves can be directed in a beam in a variety of planes; portable; different graphic displays available	Ultrasound technique is operator dependent; does not provide as much information on organ function as urography; reveals less anatomic detail than does CT; scan adversely affected by presence of bone and air	Does not use ionizing radiation; thermal stress may occur with application of cool scanning gel to infant's skin; no known deleterious effects from clinical application of ultrasound	Proper positioning essential; must be monitored during procedure	$

Continued

Table A-1	Types of Diagnostic Imaging—cont'd				
	Diagnostic Imaging Indications	Limitations of Diagnostic Imaging	Potential Risks of Procedure	Preparation of Infant	Cost
Radionucleotide	Used to trace anatomic proportions and a wide range of physiologic functions in virtually every organ in the body	Diagnostic yield depends on uptake of radionucleotide by different organs; limited anatomic resolution; radionucleotides are rarely organ specific	Ionizing radiation emitted from injected agent is significantly smaller than that for corresponding radiograph; thermal stress during nucleotide scanning	Proper positioning essential; maximum radiation not always the organ of interest; must be monitored during procedure	$$
Positron emission tomography (PET)/single photon emission computed tomography (SPECT)	Have greater sensitivity and qualifications of distribution and density of radioactivity to depict "metabolic" function of tissue; three-dimensional imaging possible with computer reconstruction; dose of nucleotide is the same; artifactual	PET scanning requires access to a cyclotron to produce positrons used in scans	Ionizing radiation emitted from injected agents (carbon 11, oxygen 15, nitrogen 13) significantly smaller than that for corresponding radiograph; thermal stress during nucleotide scanning	Proper positioning essential; must be monitored during procedure	$$$$$

	lesions can be eliminated			
Magnetic resonance	Uses magnetic fields and radio waves to produce images; region of body scanned can be controlled electronically and is not limited by hardware; free of high-intensity artifacts; newer scanning techniques able to quantify many pathologic conditions	Limited by availability and cost; limited use in unstable infants on life support; monitoring equipment must be free from interference with magnetic field	Does not use ionizing radiation to produce images; limited access to infant during procedure	Proper positioning essential; must be monitored during procedure	$$$$$

From Theorell C, Montrowl S (2003). Diagnostic processes. In Kenner C, Lott JW, editors. Comprehensive neonatal nursing: a physiologic perspective, St Louis: WB Saunders.
$, cost.

Table A-2	Radiographic Interpretation
Technical Evaluation	**Characteristics**
Film density and contrast	Intravertebral disk spaces should be visible through the cardiothymic silhouette. Underexposed films appear "whitish" with progressive loss of spaces; overexposed films have a "burned out" appearance with loss of pulmonary vascular markings.
Phase of respiration	Respiratory phase affects appearance of lung fields. In expiration, cardiothymic silhouette appears larger and lung fields appear more opaque; usually hemidiaphragms are at level of seventh rib in expiration. During inspiration, cardiothymic silhouette is normal, pulmonary vascularity is seen, and lung fields are clear. Adequate inspiration results in right hemidiaphragm at level of posterior eighth rib; right hemidiaphragm is usually slightly higher than left during basal breathing.
Motion	Check for motion at the time film was taken. Motion is detected by blurring of hemidiaphragms and cardiothymic silhouette. Motion obscures all fine pulmonary vascular detail making films unsatisfactory for evaluating lung fields.
Tube angulation and patient positioning	Anteroposterior (AP) films of newborn appear lordotic with medial ends of clavicles projecting on or above second dorsal vertebra. If tube has been angled cephalad, lordosis is exaggerated with anterior arcs of ribs positioned superiorly to posterior arcs. Cardiothymic silhouette appears larger as you are viewing through transverse diameter of the heart. This occurs if infant arches during the film or if beam has been centered over abdomen. Caudad angulation of beam over the head results in distortion of chest with anterior rib arcs angled sharply downward in relation to posterior arcs.
Rotation of patient	Assessment of rotation is critical to determine if mediastinal shift is present. Lateral rotation may lead to the false impression of a mediastinal shift. Trachea shifts toward side of rotation, and contours of the heart are altered. Direction and degree of rotation are estimated by comparing lengths of posterior arcs of ribs on both sides. Side with the greatest posterior arc length is the side to which patient is

Heart size/ pulmonary vascularity	rotated. Rotation also results in unequal lengths of clavicles when measured from medial aspects to center of vertebral body at the same level. Patient is rotated to side with the longer clavicle. Difficult to determine in newborn within first 24 hr because of dynamic cardiovascular alterations occurring during this period. Changes of the transitional circulation are associated with increased pulmonary blood flow and increased blood return to left atrium, a decrease in blood return and lower pressure in the right atrium, and changes in systemic and pulmonary arterial pressures. Newborn heart size is relatively increased in first 48-72 hr because of these rapid changes. Accurate assessment of heart size is performed only during basal breathing because size is significantly altered during phases of cardiac cycle and during hyperexpansion of lung. After first 24 hr, a cardiothoracic ratio >0.60 is the upper limit of normal. Fetal lung fluid is reabsorbed, and air spaces are filled with air with inspiration. Reabsorption of lung fluid increases the appearance of pulmonary lymphatics, causing an apparent increase in vascularity at birth. Transient tachypnea of the newborn is characterized by perihilar streaky infiltrates with increased pulmonary vascularity and good lung inflation.
Cardiothymic silhouette	Cardiac configuration is difficult to determine in the newborn largely because of variation in size and shape of thymus. Aortic knob and main pulmonary artery are obscured by thymus, which frequently has a wavy border. There may be a tuck in left lobe of thymus at lateral margin of right ventricle called a *sail sign*. Apex of heart has a more cephalic position, assuming a more caudal position over time. Elevation of apex is due to relative right ventricular hypertrophy of fetus. After birth, as left ventricle becomes more prominent, cardiac apex descends. Thymus involutes rapidly under stress of delivery and, over next 2 wk of life, may increase slightly.
Aeration of lungs	Satisfactory inspiration results in hemidiaphragms positioned at posterior arcs of eighth rib. Expansion and radiolucency of right and left sides are equal. If sides are not comparable, right and left lateral decubitus films should be obtained to evaluate for fluid levels or air. Lungs may slightly bulge through

Continued

Table **A-2**	Radiographic Interpretation—cont'd

Technical Evaluation	Characteristics
Aeration of lungs, cont'd	ribs. On lateral projection, hemidiaphragms should be smoothly domed. AP and transverse diameters of chest vary with age and disease. In normal newborn, AP and transverse diameters are equal. Over time, transverse diameter increases, resulting in an oblong appearance to chest cavity. Air trapping diseases results in a more rounded configuration, whereas hypoaeration results in a more flattened AP diameter. Hypoaeration occurs when right hemidiaphragm is located at seventh rib, posterior arcs have a more downward slope, and transverse diameter of chest is decreased. Laterally, hypoaeration results in increased doming of diaphragm. Hyperaeration is indicated when hemidiaphragm is located below level of ninth rib, diaphragm is flattened, and posterior rib arcs are horizontal. Hyperaeration also results in greater bulging of lungs through intercostal spaces and an increased diameter of upper thorax.
Pulmonary infiltrates	Evaluate for areas of increased pulmonary lucencies or densities. Characteristics of densities and their distribution may lead to a diagnosis. Infiltrates should be described as to their distribution (unilateral or bilateral) and nature (alveolar, reticulated, diffuse, nondiffuse, patchy, or streaky).
Mediastinal shift	Evaluate for mediastinal shift by determining if trachea, heart, and mediastinum are in normal position. In general, the shift occurs toward the side with decreased lung volume or away from hemithorax with increased lung volume. Rotation of patient must be first excluded.
Liver size	Liver edges should be clearly defined and correlate well to size on palpation, especially when intestines are filled with air. If insufficient gas is found in abdomen, liver size is unable to be determined. If atelectasis is present, upper margin of liver is obscured. Radiographically, size of liver is not altered by phase of respiration as it is during palpation. Liver size may vary with progression of right-sided heart failure. Position of liver may be altered by congenital malformations, such as situs inversus.

Abdominal gas pattern	Gas is present in stomach as a result of swallowing air. Gas pattern must be interpreted in light of infant's history. In newborn, stomach air is present with progression of air through small bowel at 3 hr of life and rectal air by 6 hr. In bowel obstructions, there is progressive gaseous distention to the point of obstruction, beyond which is a paucity of air or a gasless bowel. Lack of haustra in colon makes it difficult to distinguish small and large bowels on radiograph. A gasless abdomen may be seen with prolonged gastrointestinal decompression, severe dehydration, acidosis, oversedation, brain injuries, diaphragmatic hernia, midgut volvulus, and esophageal atresia. Marked aerophagia may be due to mechanical ventilation, tracheoesophageal fistula, necrotizing enterocolitis, and mesenteric vascular occlusion. Free peritoneal air will rise to highest level, and outline of superior structures thus is best demonstrated on a left lateral decubitus film.
Catheter and tube positions	All catheter and tube positions should be evaluated and reported each time. Position of these devices may provide clues to underlying disease, and malpositioning of tubes and catheters may be life threatening. Trachea is positioned to the right in mid-mediastinum, anterior and slightly to the right of esophagus. Carina is located at T4. In a right aortic arch, trachea is found slightly to the left of vertebral column. Endotracheal tubes are optimally placed in mid-trachea. If tip is too low (below T4) or too high (above thoracic inlet), ventilation is suboptimal. Inadvertent esophageal intubation is determined when tip of the tube is below T4 but is still in the midline or trachea can be visualized apart from tube. Nasogastric (NG) tube placements should be reported. NG tubes may be too short (in distal esophagus), too long (in duodenum or jejunum), or coiled in esophagus (tracheo-esophageal atresia). Vascular catheter location requires evaluation. Central catheters should be placed with tip in superior inferior cava. Umbilical arterial catheters ideally should have their location in high (T6-9) or low (L3-5) position away from major arterial branches. Umbilical venous catheters should be positioned with tip in inferior vena cava and not a hepatic branch.

Continued

Table A-2	Radiographic Interpretation—cont'd
Technical Evaluation	**Characteristics**
Bony structures	Visually evaluate skeleton noting general configuration of thoracic cage. Normally, cephalic portion of thoracic cage becomes rounded, and over time, transverse diameter will increase. Hyperaeration exaggerates cephalic rounding and horizontal position of rib arcs. Hypoaeration decreases diameter of upper thorax and increases inferior slope of rib arcs (bell-shaped thorax). Evaluate for fractures, dislocations, hypodensities, or other lucencies. Persistent elevation of scapula and ipsilateral elevated diaphragm secondary to phrenic nerve injury may accompany Erb's palsy. Scan for vertebral, rib, and other bony anomalies. Rib aplasia is associated with hemivertebrae, and complete or partial aplasia of clavicles can be a manifestation of chromosomal abnormality. Proximal humeri can yield information related to congenital infections such as in congenital rubella, congenital syphilis, and cytomegalovirus. Bone density should be evaluated in relation to film penetration.

From Theorell C, Montrowl S (2003). Diagnostic processes. In Kenner C, Lott JW, editors. Comprehensive neonatal nursing: a physiologic perspective, St Louis: WB Saunders.

Table A-3	Common Electrolyte and Chemistry Values
Test	**Normal Value**
Serum Electrolytes	
Sodium (Na)	135-145 mEq/L
Potassium (K)	4.5-6.8 mEq/L
Chloride (Cl)	95-110 mEq/L
Carbon dioxide (CO_2)	20-25 mmol/L
Serum Chemistries	
Blood urea nitrogen (BUN)	6.0-30.0 mg/dl
Calcium (Ca)	7-10 mg/dl
Creatinine (Cr)	0.2-0.9 mg/dl
Glucose (G)	40-97 mg/dl
Magnesium (Mg)	1.5-2.5 mg/dl
Phosphorus (P)	5.4-10.9 mg/dl

Data from Fanaroff A, Martin R (1987). Neonatal-perinatal medicine: diseases of the fetus and infant, ed 4, St Louis: Mosby; Cohen S, Kenner C, Hollingsworth A (1991). Maternal, neonatal and women's health nursing, Springhouse, Pa: Springhouse; Kenner C, Harjo J, Brueggemer A (1988). Neonatal surgery: a nursing perspective, Orlando: Grune & Stratton; Streeter NS (1986). High risk neonatal care, Rockville, Md: Aspen Publishers.

Table A-4   Normal Hematologic Values

	Gestational Age (wk)		Full-Term Cord Blood	Day 1	Day 3	Day 7	Day 14
	28	34					
Hb (g/dl)	14.5	15.0	16.8	18.4	17.8	17.0	16.8
Hematocrit (%)	45	47	53	58	55	54	52
Red cells (mm^3)	4.0	4.4	5.25	5.8	5.6	5.2	5.1
MCV (μm^3)	120	118	107	108	99	98	96
MCH (pg)	40	38	34	35	33	32.5	31.5
MCHC (%)	31	32	31.7	32.5	33	33	33
Reticulocytes (%)	5-10	3-10	3-7	3-7	1-3	0-1	0-1
Platelets (1000s/mm^3)			290	192	213	248	252

From Klaus MH, Fanaroff AA (2001). *Care of the high-risk neonate*, ed 5, Philadelphia: WB Saunders, p. 574.
Hb, Hemoglobin; MCV, mean corpuscular volume; MCH, mean corpuscular hemoglobin; MCHC, mean corpuscular hemoglobin concentration.

Table A-5   White Cell and Differential Counts in Premature Infants

	Birth Weight						
	1500 g				1500-2500 g		
Age (wk)	1	2	4	1	2	4	
Total Count (x 103/mm3)							
Mean	16.8	15.4	12.1	13.0	10.0	8.4	
Range	6.1-32.8	10.4-21.3	8.7-17.2	6.7-14.7	7.0-14.1	5.8-12.4	
Percent of Total							
Polymorphs							
Segmented	54	45	40	55	43	41	
Unsegmented	7	6	5	8	8	6	
Eosinophils	2	3	3	2	3	3	
Basophils	1	1	1	1	1	1	
Monocytes	6	10	10	5	9	11	
Lymphocytes	30	35	41	9	36	38	

From Klaus MH, Fanaroff AA (2001). *Care of the high-risk neonate*, ed 5, Philadelphia: WB Saunders, p. 576.

Table **A-6**	Summary of Normal Urine Lab Values	
Test	**Age**	**Normal Value**
Ammonia	2-12 mo	4-20 μEq/min/m^2
Calcium	1 wk	<2 mg/dl
Chloride	Infant	1.7-8.5 mEq/24 hr
Creatinine	Newborn	7-10 mg/kg/day
Glucose	Preterm	60-130 mg/dl
	Full-term	12-32 mg/dl
Glucose (renal	Preterm	2.21-2.84 mg/ml
threshold)	Full-term	2.20-3.68 mg/ml
Magnesium		180 ± 10 mg/1.73 m^2/dl
Osmolality	Infant	50-600 mOsm/kg
Potassium		26-123 mEq/L
Protein		<100 mg/m^2/dl
Sodium		0.3-3.5 mEq/dl (6-10 mEq/m^2)
Specific gravity	Newborn	1.006-1.008

From Ichikawa I (1990). Pediatric textbook of fluids and electrolytes, Baltimore: Williams & Wilkins.

Table A-7	Electrocardiographic Data in the Neonate*			
	Age			
Parameter	0-24 Hr	1-7 Days	8-30 Days	1-3 Mo
Heart rate (beats/min)	119 (94-145)	133 (100-175)	163 (115-190)	154 (124-190)
PR interval (sec)	0.1 (0.07-0.12)	0.09 (0.07-0/12)	0.09 (0.07-0.11)	0.1 (0.07-0.13)
P wave amplitude II	1.5 (0.8-2.3)	1.6 (0.8-2.5)	1.6 (0.8-2.4)	1.6 (0.8-2.4)
QRS duration (sec)	0.065 (0.05-0.08)	0.06 (0.04-0.08)	0.06 (0.04-0.07)	0.06 (0.05-0.08)
QRS axis (degrees)	135 (60-180)	125 (80-160)	110 (60-160)	80 (40-120)
R amplitude V_m (mm)	8.6 (4-14.2)	—	6.3 (3.3-8.5)	5.1 (1.1-10.1)
R amplitude V_1 (mm)	11.9 (4.3-21)	—	11.1 (3.3-18.7)	11.2 (4.5-18)
R amplitude V_5 (mm)	10.2 (4-18)	10.7 (3.4-19)	11.9 (3.5-27)	13.6 (7.3-20.7)
R amplitude V_6 (mm)	3.3 (2.3-7)	5.1 (2.2-13.1)	6.7 (1.7-20.5)	8.4 (3.6-12.9)
S amplitude V_{18} (mm)	3.8 (0.2-13)	—	1.8 (0.8-4.6)	3.4 (0-9.3)
S amplitude V_1 (mm)	9.7 (1.1-19.1)	—	6.1 (0-15)	7.5 (0.5-17.1)
S amplitude V_5 (mm)	11.9 (0-24)	6.8 (3.6-16.2)	4.8 (2.7-12.3)	4.7 (2-12.7)
S amplitude V_6 (mm)	4.5 (1.6-10.3)	3.3 (0.8-9.9)	2.0 (0.6-9)	2.4 (0.8-5.8)

From Fanaroff A, Martin R (1987). Neonatal-perinatal medicine: diseases of the fetus and infant, ed 4, St Louis: Mosby, p. 1256. As modified from Liebman J, Plonsey R (1977). Electrocardiography. In Moss AJ, Adams FH, Emmanovilldes GC, editors. Heart disease in infants, children and adolescents, ed 2, Baltimore: Williams & Wilkins.

*Mean (5th to 95th percentile).

Table A-8	Time of First Void in 500 Infants								
Hr Since Delivery	395 Full-Term Infants			80 Preterm Infants			25 Postterm Infants		
	No. of Infants	Cumulative (%)		No. of Infants	Cumulative (%)		No. of Infants	Cumulative (%)	
<1	51	12.9		17	21.2		3	12	
1-8	151	51.1		50	83.7		4	38	
9-16	158	91.1		12	98.7		14	84	
17-24	35	100		1	100		4	100	
>24	0	—		0	—		0	—	

From Clark DA (1977). Times of first void and first stool in 500 newborns. Pediatrics, 60, 457-459. Reproduced by permission of Pediatrics.

Table A-9	Time of First Stool in 500 Infants					
Hr Since Delivery	**395 Full-Term Infants**		**80 Preterm Infants**		**25 Postterm Infants**	
	No. of Infants	Cumulative (%)	No. of Infants	Cumulative (%)	No. of Infants	Cumulative (%)
<1	66	16.7	4	5	8	32
1-8	169	59.5	22	32.5	9	68
9-16	125	91.1	25	63.8	5	88
17-24	29	98.5	10	76.3	3	100
24-48	6*	100	18†	98.8	0	—
>48	0	—	1‡	100	0	—

From Clark DA (1977). Times of first void and first stool in 500 newborns. Pediatrics, 60, 457–459. Reproduced by permission of Pediatrics.
*At 25, 26, 27, 28, 33, and 37 hr.
†Five had first stool more than 36 hr after birth, at 38, 39, 40, 42, and 47 hr.
‡At 59 hr.

| Table A-10 | Acid-Base Status |

Determination	Sample Source	Birth	1 Hr	3 Hr	24 Hr	2 Days	3 Days
Vigorous Term Infants (Vaginal Delivery)							
pH	Umbilical artery	7.26					
	Umbilical vein	7.29					
PCO_2 (mm Hg)	Arterial	54.4	38.8	38.3	33.6	34	35
	Venous	42.8					
O_2 saturation	Arterial	19.8	93.8	94.7	93		
	Venous	47.6					
pH	Left atrial		7.30	7.34	7.41	7.39	7.38
CO_2 content			20.6	21.9	21.4	Temporal artery	
Premature Infants (Vaginal Delivery)							
pH (mm Hg)	<1250 g Arterial			7.60	7.35	7.35	
PCO_2 (mm Hg)	Arterial			38	44	37	
pH	>1250 g Arterial			7.39	7.39	7.38	
PCO_2 (mm Hg)	Arterial			38	39	38	

From Schaffer AJ (1971). Diseases of the newborn, ed 3, Philadelphia: WB Saunders.

Table A-11	Selected Chemistry Values in Full-Term and Preterm Infants*			
Constituent	**Preterm**	**Term**	**Reference**
Alkaline phosphatase (U/L) (mean ±SD)	207 ± 60 to 320 ± 142	164 ± 68	8
Ammonia (µg/100 ml)	—	90-150	1
Base, excess (mmol/L)	—	-10 to -2	1
Bicarbonate, standard (mmol/L)	18-26	20-26	2
Bilirubin, total (mg/dl)			
Cord	<2.8	<2.8	2
24 hr	1-6	2-6	
48 hr	6-8	6-7	
3-5 days	10-12	4-6	
≥1 mo	<1.5	<1.5	
Bilirubin, direct (mg/dl)	<0.5	<0.5	2
Calcium, total (mg/dl), wk 1	6.0-10.0	8.4-11.6	3,4
Ceruloplasmin (mg/dl)		1-3 mo: 5-18	1
Cholesterol (mg/dl)			
Cord		45-98	2
3 days–1 yr		65-175	
Creatine phosphokinase (U/L)			
Day 1		44-1150	5
Day 4		14-97	

Continued

Table A-11	Selected Chemistry Values in Full-Term and Preterm Infants*—cont'd			
Constituent	Preterm	Term		Reference
Creatine (mg/dl)	10 days: 1.3 ± 0.07	1-4 days: 0.3-1.0		1
	1 mo: 0.6 ± 0.05	>4 days: 0.2-0.4		
Ferritin (µg/dl)				
Neonate		25-200		
1 mo		200-600		
2-5 mo		50-200		
>6 mo		7-142		
Gamma-glutamyl transferase (GGT) (U/L)	—	14-131		6
Glucose (mg/dl)				
<72 hr	20-125	30-125		7,9
>72 hr	40-125	40-125		
Lactate dehydrogenase (U/L)	—	357-953		6
Magnesium (mg/dl)	—	1.7-2.4		4
Osmolality (mOsm/L)	—	275-295		1
		(may be as low as 266)		
Phosphorus (mg/dl)				
Birth		4.5-8.7		4
Day 5		4.2-7.2		
1 mo		4.5-6.5		
SGOT/AST (aspartate aminotransferase; U/L)		24-81		7
SGPT/ALT (alanine aminotransferase; U/L)		10-33		7
Triglycerides (mg/dl)		10-140		2

Urea nitrogen (mg/dl)	3-25	4-12	1
Uric acid (mg/dl)	—	3.0-7.5	2
Vitamin A (µg/dl) (mean ± SD)	16.0 ± 1.0	23.9 ± 1.8	10
(<10 µg/dl indicates very low hepatic vitamin A stores)			
Vitamin D			
25-hydroxycholecalciferol (ng/ml)*		20-60	11,12
1,25-dihydroxycholecalciferol (pg/ml)*		40-90	11,12

From Fanaroff AA, Martin RJ (2001). *Neonatal-perinatal medicine diseases of the fetus and infant, ed 7, Philadelphia: WB Saunders.*
SD, Standard deviation.
*Serum levels affected by race, age, season, and diet.

References:
[1]Tietz NW, editor (1988). *Textbook of clinical chemistry, Philadelphia: WB Saunders.*
[2]Wallach JB (1983). *Interpretation of pediatric tests, Boston: Little Brown & Co.*
[3]Meites S (1975). Critical reviews of clinical laboratory science, 6, 1.
[4]Nelson N, et al. (1987). Scandinavian journal of clinical laboratory investigations, 47, 111.
[5]Drummond LM (1979). Archives of diseases in children, 54, 362.
[6]Stonestree BS, et al. (1978). Pediatrics, 61, 788.
[7]Statlan BE, et al. (1978). Clinical chemistry, 24, 1010 (abstract).
[8]Cornblath M, Schwartz R, editors. (1976). *Disorders of carbohydrate metabolism, ed 2, Philadelphia: WB Saunders.*
[9]Glass L, et al. (1982). Archives of diseases in children, 57, 373.
[10]Heck LJ, et al. (1987). Pediatric research, 110, 119.
[11]Shenai JP, et al. (1981). Journal of pediatrics, 99, 302.
[12]Hustead VA, et al. (1984). Journal of pediatrics, 108, 610.

| Table **A-12** | Plasma Albumin and Total Protein in Preterm Infants from Birth to 8 Wk |

Gestation (wk)	26	27	28	29	30	31	32	33	34	35	36	37	38	39	40	41	42
Albumin (g/dl)																	
Reference range (95% confidence limits)	—	1.18-3.06	1.09-2.87	1.20-2.74	1.63-2.75	1.08-3.20	1.38-3.14	1.44-3.34	0.53-3.87	1.15-3.87	1.96-3.44	1.50-4.10	1.89-4.15	2.07-4.15	2.07-4.05	2.04-3.90	2.08-3.90
Corrected age																	
26-28 wk gestation		2.13	2.10	2.58	2.29	2.39				2.73							
29-31 wk gestation					2.02	2.14	2.44	2.44	2.54				2.82				
2-34 wk gestation								2.35	2.42	2.46	2.38	2.44				3.35	

Total Protein (g/dl)

	—	1.28-7.94	3.03-5.03	2.18-5.84	2.64-5.80	3.26-5.66	3.63-5.81	3.57-5.87	3.57-6.59	1.52-8.62	3.85-6.91	4.69-6.95	3.32-9.16	4.17-8.25	4.26-8.08	3.73-8.47	3.24-8.76
Reference range (95% confidence limits)																	
Corrected age																	
26-28 wk gestation		4.07	4.45	4.84	4.49	4.45				4.41							
29-31 wk gestation					3.93	4.42	4.70	4.82	4.51				4.55				
32-34 wk gestation								4.54	4.93	4.78	4.86	4.81				4.96	

From Fanaroff A, Martin R (2001). *Neonatal-perinatal medicine: diseases of the fetus and infant*, ed 7, St Louis: Mosby, p. 1654. Modified from Reading RF, et al. (1990). *Early human development*, 22, 81.

| Table **A-13** | | Plasma Immunoglobulin (Ig) Concentrations in Premature Infants (25-28 wk Gestation) | | |

Age (mo)	N	IgG* (mg/dl)[†]	IgM* (mg/dl)[†]	IgA* (mg/dl)[†]
0.25	18	251 (114-552)	7.6 (1.3-43.3)	1.2 (0.07-20.8)
0.5	14	202 (91-446)	14.1 (3.5-56.1)	3.1 (0.09-10.7)
1	10	158 (57-437)	12.7 (3.0-53.3)	4.5 (0.65-30.9)
1.5	14	134 (59-307)	16.2 (4.4-59.2)	4.3 (0.9-20.9)
2	12	89 (58-136)	16 (5.3-48.9)	4.1 (1.5-11.1)
3	13	60 (23-156)	13.8 (5.3-36.1)	3.4 (0.6-15.6)
4	10	82 (32-210)	22.2 (11.2-43.9)	6.8 (1-47.8)
6	11	159 (56-455)	41.3 (8.3-205)	9.7 (3-31.2)
8-10	6	273 (94-794)	41.8 (31.1-56.1)	9.5 (0.9-98.6)

From Ballow M, et al. (1986). Development of the immune system in very low birth weight (less than 1500 g) premature infants: concentrations of plasma immunoglobulins and patterns of infections. Pediatric research, 20, 899-904.
*Geometric mean.
[†]The normal ranges in parentheses were determined by taking the antilog of (mean logarithm ± 2 SD of the logarithms).

| Table **A-14** | | Plasma Immunoglobulin (Ig) Concentrations in Premature Infants (29-32 wk Gestation) | | |

Age (mo)	N	IgG* (mg/dl)[†]	IgM* (mg/dl)[†]	IgA* (mg/dl)[†]
0.25	42	368 (186-728)	9.1 (2.1-39.4)	0.6 (0.04-1)
0.5	35	275 (119-637)	13.9 (4.7-41)	0.9 (0.01-7.5)
1	26	209 (97-452)	14.4 (6.3-33)	1.9 (0.3-12)
1.5	22	156 (69-352)	15.4 (5.5-43.2)	2.2 (0.7-6.5)
2	11	123 (64-237)	15.2 (4.9-46.7)	3.4 (1.1-8.3)
3	14	104 (41-268)	16.3 (7.1-37.2)	3.6 (0.8-15.4)
4	21	128 (39-425)	26.5 (7.7-91.2)	9.8 (2.5-39.3)
6	21	179 (51-634)	29.3 (10.5-81.5)	12.3 (2.7-57.1)
8-10	16	280 (140-561)	34.7 (17-70.8)	20.9 (8.3-53)

From Ballow M, et al. (1986). Development of the immune system in very low birth weight (less than 1500 g) premature infants: concentrations of plasma immunoglobulins and patterns of infections. Pediatric research, 20, 899–904.
*Geometric mean.
[†]The normal ranges in parentheses were determined by taking the antilog of (mean logarithm ± 2 SD of the logarithms).

Table **A-15**	Plasma-Serum Amino Acids in Premature and Term Newborns (µmol/L)		
Amino Acid	**Premature (First Day)**	**Newborn 16 Days–4 Mo (Before First Feeding)**	
Taurine	105-255	101-181	
OH-proline	0-80	0	
Aspartic acid	0-20	4-12	17-21
Threonine	155-275	196-238	141-213
Serine	195-345	129-197	104-158
Aspartic acid + Glutamic acid	655-1155	623-895	
Proline	155-305	155-305	141-245
Glutamic acid	30-100	27-77	
Glycine	185-735	274-412	178-248
Alanine	325-425	274-384	239-345
Valine	80-180	97-175	123-199
Cystine	55-75	49-75	33-51
Methionine	30-40	21-37	31-47
Isoleucine	20-60	31-47	31-47
Leucine	45-95	55-89	56-98
Tyrosine	20-220	53-85	33-75
Phenylalanine	70-110	64-92	45-65
Ornithine	70-110	66-116	37-61
Lysine	130-250	154-246	117-163
Histidine	30-70	61-93	64-92
Arginine	30-70	37-71	53-71
Tryptophan	15-45	15-45	
Citrulline	8.5-23.7	10.8-21.1	
Ethanolamine	13.4-10.5	32.7-72	
Alpha-amino-*n*-butyric acid	0-29	8.7-20.4	
Methylhistidine			

From Klaus MH, Fanaroff AA (2001). *Care of the high-risk neonate*, ed 5, Philadelphia: WB Saunders. Data from Dickinson JC, Rosenblum H, Hamilton PB (1965). Ion exchange chromatography of the free amino acids in the plasma of the newborn infant. *Pediatrics*, 36, 2; Dickinson JC, Rosenblum H, Hamiton PB (1970). Ion exchange chromotography of the free amino acids in the plasma of infants under 2,500 gm at birth. *Pediatrics*, 45, 606. In Behrman RE (1977). *Neonatal-perinatal diseases of the fetus and infant*, ed 2, St Louis: Mosby, Table 20, Appendix.

Table **A-16**	Urine Amino Acids in Normal Newborns (μmol/L)

Amino Acid	mmol/day
Cysteic acid	Tr-3.32
Phosphoethanolamine	Tr-8.86
Taurine	7.59-7.72
OH-proline	0-9.81
Aspartic acid	Tr
Threonine	0.176-7.99
Serine	Tr-20.7
Glutamic acid	0-1.78
Proline	0-5.17
Glycine	0.176-65.3
Alanine	Tr-8.03
Alpha-aminoadipic acid	
Alpha-amino-*n*-butyric acid	0-0.47
Valine	0-7.76
Cystine	0-7.96
Methionine	Tr-0.892
Isoleucine	0-6.11
Tyrosine	0-1.11
Phenylalanine	0-1.66
Beta-aminiosobutyric acid	0.264-7.34
Ethanolamine	Tr-79.9
Ornithine	Tr-0.554
Lysine	0.33-9.79
1-Methylhistidine	Tr-8.64
3-Methylhistidine	0.11-3.32
Carnosine	0.044-4.01
Beta-aminobutyric acid	
Cystanthionine	
Homocitrulline	
Arginine	0.088-0.918
Histidine	Tr-7.04
Sarcosine	
Leucine	Tr-0.918

From Klaus MH, Fanaroff AA (2001). Care of the high-risk neonate, ed 5, Philadelphia: WB Saunders. Modified from Meites S, editor (1997). Pediatric clinical chemistry: a survey of normals, methods, and instruments, Washington, DC: American Association for Clinical Chemistry. In Fanaroff AA, Martin RJ, editors (1997). Neonatal-perinatal medicine: diseases of the fetus and infant, ed 6, St Louis: Mosby, Table B-13. Tr, Trace.

Table **A-17**	Cerebrospinal Fluid Values of Healthy Term Newborns			
	Age			
Component	**0-24 Hr**	**1 Day**	**7 Days**	**Over 7 Days**
Color	Clear or xanthochromic	Clear or xanthochromic	Clear or xanthochromic	Clear or xanthochromic
Red blood cells/mm³	9 (0-1070)	23 (6-630)	3 (0-48)	
Polymorphonuclear	3 (0-70)	7 (0-26)	2 (0-5)	
Leukocytes cells/mm³				
Lymphocytes cells/mm³	2 (0-20)	5 (0-16)	1 (0-4)	
Proteins (mg/dl)	63 (32-240)	73 (40-148)	47 (27-65)	
Glucose (mg/dl)	51 (32-78)	48 (38-64)	55 (48-62)	
Lactate dehydrogenase (IU/L)	22-73	22-73	22-73	0-40

From Fanaroff AA, Martin RJ, editors (1997). Neonatal-perinatal medicine: diseases of the fetus and infant, ed 6, St Louis: Mosby, Table B-16. Data from Naidoo BT (1968). South African medical journal, 42, 933; Neches W, et al. (1968). Pediatrics, 41, 1097.

Table A-18	CSF Values in VLBW Infants by Chronologic Age: Birth Weight ≤1000 g					
	Postnatal Age (days)					
	0-7		**8-28**		**29-84**	
	Mean ± SD	Range	Mean ± SD	Range	Mean ± SD	Range
Birth weight (g)	822 ± 116	630-980	752 ± 112	550-970	750 ± 120	550-907
Gestational age at birth (wk)	26 ± 1.2	24-27	26 ± 1.5	24-28	26 ± 1.0	24-27
Leukocytes/mm^3	335 ± 709	0-1780	1465 ± 4062	0-19,050	808 ± 1843	0-6850
PMNs (%)	11 ± 20	0-50	8 ± 17	0-66	2 ± 9	0-36
Glucose (mg/dl)	70 ± 17	41-89	68 ± 48	33-217	49 ± 22	29-90
Protein (mg/dl)	162 ± 37	115-222	159 ± 77	95-370	137 ± 61	76-260

From Fanaroff AA, Martin RJ (1997). Neonatal-perinatal medicine: diseases of the fetus and infant, ed 6, St Louis: Mosby, Table B-18.
Modified from Rodriguez AF, et al. (1990). Journal of pediatrics, 116, 971.
CSF, Cerebrospinal fluid; VLBW, very low birth weight; SD, standard deviation; PMN, polymorphonuclear neutrophil leukocyte.

Table A-19	CSF Values in VLBW Infants by Chronologic Age: Birth Weight ≥1001-1500 g								
	Postnatal Age (days)								
	0-7			**8-28**			**29-84**		
	Mean ± SD	**Range**		**Mean ± SD**	**Range**		**Mean ± SD**	**Range**	
Birth weight (g)	1428 ± 107	1180-1500		1245 ± 162	1020-1480		1211 ± 86	1080-1300	
Gestational age at birth (wk)	31 ± 1.5	28-33		29 ± 1.2	27-31		29 ± 0.7	27-29	
Leukocytes/mm³	4 ± 4	1-10		7 ± 11	0-44		8 ± 8	0-23	
Erythrocytes/mm³	407 ± 853	0-2450		1101 ± 2643	0-9750		661 ± 1198	0-3800	
PMNs (%)	4 ± 10	0-28		10 ± 19	0-60		11 ± 19	0-48	
Glucose (mg/dl)	74 ± 19	50-96		59 ± 23	39-109		47 ± 13	31-76	
Protein (mg/dl)	136 ± 35	85-176		137 ± 46	54-227		122 ± 47	45-187	

Modified from Rodriguez AF, et al. (1990). Journal of pediatrics, 116, 971.
CSF, Cerebrospinal fluid; VLBW, very low birth weight; SD, standard deviation; PMN, polymorphonuclear neutrophil leukocyte.

| Table A-20 | Thyroid Function in Full-Term and Preterm Infants |

	Serum T4 Concentration in Premature and Term Infants					Serum Free T4 Index in Premature and Term Infants					
	Estimated Gestational Age (wk)										
	30-31	32-33	34-35	36-37	Term	30-31	32-33	34-35	36-37	Term	
Cord											
Mean	6.5*	7.5†	6.7†	7.5	8.2			5.6	5.6	5.9	
SD	1.0	2.1	1.2	2.8	1.8			1.3	2.0	1.1	
N	3	8	18	17	17			12	10	14	
12-72 hr											
Mean	11.5†	12.3†	12.4†	15.5†	19.0	13.1§	12.9§	15.5§	17.1	19.7	
SD	2.1	3.2	3.1	2.6	2.1	2.4	2.7	3.0	3.5	3.5	
N	12	18	17	15	6	12	14	14	14	6	
3-10 days											
Mean	7.7†	8.5†	10.0†	12.7†	15.9	8.3§	9.0§	12.0‖	15.1	16.2	
SD	1.8	1.9	2.4	2.5	3.0	1.9	1.8	2.3	0.7	3.2	
N	7	8	9	9	29	6	9	5	4	11	

11-20 days

Mean	7.5‡	8.3†	10.5	11.2	12.2	8.0¶	9.1#	11.8	11.3	12.1
SD	1.8	1.6	1.8	2.9	2.0	1.6	1.9	2.7	1.9	2.0
N	5	11	9	9	8	5	8	8	5	8

21-45 days

Mean	7.8†	80†	9.3†	11.4	12.1	8.4¶	9.0#	10.9		11.1
SD	1.5	1.7	1.3	4.2	1.5	1.4	1.6	2.8		1.4
N	11	17	13	5	5	11	17	5		5

46-90 days

Mean	9.6			10.2	9.4					9.7
SD	1.7			1.9	1.4					1.5
N	16			17	13					10

From Cuestas RA (1982). Journal of pediatrics, 92, 963. Reprinted with permission.

For comparison of premature vs. term infants (t-test).

T_4, Thyroxine; SD, standard deviation; N, number; P, probability.
*$P < 0.05$.
†$P < .001$.
‡$P < .005$.
§$P = .001$.
‖$P = .025$.
¶$P = .005$.
#$P = .01$.

INTERNATIONAL CONVERSION CHART

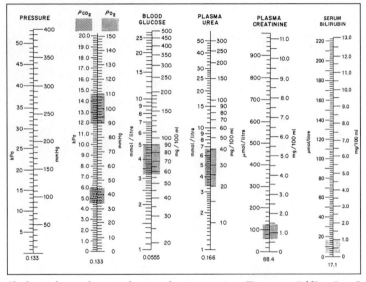

Shading indicates the normal range where appropriate. To convert "old" to "new" units, multiply by the conversion factor at the foot of each column. (Modified from Halliday HL, McClure G, Reid M: Handbook of Neonatal Intensive Care, 2nd ed. Philadelphia: WB Saunders, 1985.)

Table B-1	Conversion Table to Standard International (SI) Units				
Component	**Present Unit**	**×**	**Conversion Factor**	**=**	**SI Unit**
Clinical Hematology					
Erythrocytes	per mm³		1		10^6/L
Hematocrit	%		0.01		(1)vol RBC/vol whole blood
Hemoglobin	g/dL		10		g/L
Leukocytes	per mm³		1		10^6/L
Mean corpuscular hemoglobin concentration (MCHC)	g/dL		10		g/L
Mean corpuscular volume (MCV)	μm³		1		fL
Platelet count	10^3/mm³		1		10^9/L
Reticulocyte count	%		10		10^{-3}
Clinical Chemistry					
Acetone	mg/dL		0.1722		mmol/L
Albumin	g/dL		10		g/L
Aldosterone	ng/dL		27.74		pmol/L
Ammonia (as nitrogen)	μg/dL		0.7139		μmol/L
Bicarbonate	mEq/L		1		mmol/L
Bilirubin	mg/dL		17.1		μmol/L
Calcium	mg/dL		0.2495		mmol/L
Calcium ion	mEq/L		0.50		mmol/L

Continued

Table **B-1**	Conversion Table to Standard International (SI) Units—cont'd			
Component	**Present Unit**	×	**Conversion Factor**	=	**SI Unit**

Component	**Present Unit**	×	**Conversion Factor**	=	**SI Unit**
Clinical Chemistry, cont'd					
Carotenes	μg/dL		0.01836		μmol/L
Ceruloplasmin	mg/dL		10.0		mg/L
Chloride	mEq/L		1		mmol/L
Cholesterol	mg/dL		0.02586		mmol/L
Complement, C_3 or C_4	mg/dL		0.01		g/L
Copper	μg/dL		0.1574		μmol/L
Cortisol	μg/dL		27.59		nmol/L
Creatine	mg/dL		76.25		μmol/L
Creatinine	mg/dL		88.40		μmol/L
Digoxin	ng/mL		1.281		nmol/L
Epinephrine	pg/mL		5.458		pmol/L
Fatty acids	mg/dL		10.0		mg/L
Ferritin	ng/mL		1		μg/L
α-Fetoprotein	ng/mL		1		μg/L
Fibrinogen	mg/dL		0.01		g/L
Folate	ng/mL		2.266		nmol/L
Fructose	mg/dL		0.05551		mmol/L

Galactose	mg/dL	0.05551	mmol/L
Gases			
PO$_2$	mm Hg (= torr)	0.1333	kPa
PCO$_2$	mm Hg (= torr)	0.1333	kPa
Glucagon	pg/ml	1	ng/L
Glucose	mg/dL	0.05551	mmol/L
Glycerol	mg/dL	0.1086	mmol/L
Growth hormone	ng/mL	1	µg/L
Haptoglobin	mg/dL	0.01	g/L

Modified from Young DS: Implementation of SI units for clinical laboratory data. Style specifications and conversion tables. Ann Intern Med 106:114, 1987.

Table B-1 Conversion Table to Standard International (SI) Units—cont'd

Component	Present Unit	×	Conversion Factor	=	SI Unit
Clinical Chemistry, cont'd					
Hemoglobin	g/dL		10		g/L
Insulin	µg/L		172.2		pmol/L
	mU/L		7.175		pmol/L
Iron	µg/dL		0.1791		µmol/L
Iron-binding capacity	µg/dL		0.1791		µmol/L
Lactate	mEq/L		1		mmol/L
Lead	µg/dL		0.04826		µmol/L
Lipoproteins	mg/dL		0.02586		mmol/L
Magnesium	mg/dL		0.4114		mmol/L
	mEq/L		0.50		mmol/L
Osmolality	mOsm/kg H_2O		1		mmol/kg H_2O
Phenobarbital	mg/dL		43.06		µmol/L
Phenytoin	mg/L		3.964		µmol/L
Phosphate	mg/dL		0.3229		mmol/L
Potassium	mEq/L		1		mmol/L
	mg/dL		0.2558		mmol/L
Protein	g/dL		10.0		g/L
Pyruvate	mg/dL		113.6		µmol/L
Sodium ion	mEq/L		1		mmol/L

Steroids			
17-hydroxycorticosteroids	mg/24 h	2.759	μmol/d
17-ketosteroids	mg/24 h	3.467	μmol/d
Testosterone	ng/mL	3.467	nmol/L
Theophylline	mg/L	5.550	μmol/L
Thyroid tests			
Thyroid-stimulating hormone	μU/mL	1	mU/L
Thyroxine (T_4)	μg/dL	12.87	nmol/L
Thyroxine free	ng/dL	12.87	pmol/L
Triiodothyronine (T_3)	ng/dL	0.01536	nmol/L
Transferrin	mg/dL	0.01	g/L
Triglycerides	mg/dL	0.01129	mmol/L
Urea nitrogen	mg/dL	0.3570	mmol/L
Uric acid (urate)	mg/dL	59.48	μmol/L
Vitamin A (retinol)	μg/dL	0.03491	μmol/L
Vitamin B_{12}	pg/mL	0.7378	pmol/L
Vitamin C (ascorbic acid)	mg/dL	56.78	μmol/L
Vitamin D			
Cholecalciferol	μg/mL	2.599	nmol/L
25 OH-cholecalciferol	ng/mL	2.496	nmol/L
Vitamin E (alpha-tocopherol)	mg/dL	23.22	μmol/L
D-xylose	mg/dL	0.06661	mmol/L
Zinc	μg/dL	0.1530	μmol/L
Energy	kcal	4.1868	kJ (kilojoule)
Blood pressure	mm Hg (= torr)	1.333	mbar

TEMPERATURE CONVERSION CHART

To convert from °F to °C:	To convert from °C to °F:
(°F ~ 32) ÷ 1.8 = °C	(°C × 1.8) + 32 = °F

Degrees Fahrenheit	Degrees Celsius	Degrees Fahrenheit	Degrees Celsius
93.2	34.0	101.5	38.6
93.6	34.2	101.8	38.8
93.9	34.4	102.2	39.0
94.3	34.6	102.6	39.2
94.6	34.8	102.9	39.4
95.0	35.0	103.3	39.6
95.4	35.2	103.6	39.8
95.7	35.4	104.0	40.0
96.1	35.6	104.4	40.2
96.4	35.8	104.7	40.4
96.8	36.0	105.2	40.6
97.2	36.2	105.4	40.8
97.5	36.4	105.9	41.0
97.9	36.6	106.1	41.2
98.2	36.8	106.5	41.4
98.6	37.0	106.8	41.6
99.0	37.2	107.2	41.8
99.3	37.4	107.6	42.0
99.7	37.6	108.0	42.2
100.0	37.8	108.3	42.4
100.4	38.0	108.7	42.6
100.8	38.2	109.0	42.8
101.1	38.4	109.4	43.0

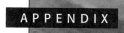

APPENDIX D

NEONATAL WEIGHT CONVERSION FROM POUNDS TO GRAMS

Pounds								Ounces								
	0	**1**	**2**	**3**	**4**	**5**	**6**	**7**	**8**	**9**	**10**	**11**	**12**	**13**	**14**	**15**
0	—	28	57	85	113	142	170	198	227	255	283	312	340	369	397	425
1	454	482	510	539	567	595	624	652	680	709	737	765	794	822	850	879
2	907	936	964	992	1021	1049	1077	1106	1134	1162	1191	1219	1247	1276	1304	1332
3	1361	1389	1417	1446	1474	1502	1531	1559	1588	1616	1644	1673	1701	1729	1758	1786
4	1814	1843	1871	1899	1928	1956	1984	2013	2041	2070	2098	2126	2155	2183	2211	2240
5	2268	2296	2325	2353	2381	2410	2438	2466	2495	2523	2551	2580	2608	2637	2665	2693
6	2722	2750	2778	2807	2835	2863	2892	2920	2948	2977	3005	3033	3062	3090	3118	3147
7	3175	3203	3232	3260	3289	3317	3345	3374	3402	3430	3459	3487	3515	3544	3572	3600
8	3629	3657	3685	3714	3742	3770	3799	3827	3856	3884	3912	3941	3969	3997	4026	4054
9	4082	4111	4139	4167	4196	4224	4252	4281	4309	4337	4366	4394	4423	4451	4479	4508
10	4536	4564	4593	4621	4649	4678	4706	4734	4763	4791	4819	4848	4876	4904	4933	4961
11	4990	5018	5046	5075	5103	5131	5160	5188	5216	5245	5273	5301	5330	5358	5386	5415
12	5443	5471	5500	5528	5557	5585	5613	5642	5670	5698	5727	5755	5783	5812	5840	5868
13	5897	5925	5953	5982	6010	6038	6067	6095	6123	6152	6180	6209	6237	6265	6294	6322
14	6350	6379	6407	6435	6464	6492	6520	6549	6577	6605	6634	6662	6690	6719	6747	6776
15	6804	6832	6860	6889	6917	6945	6973	7002	7030	7059	7087	7115	7144	7172	7201	7228

IMMUNIZATION SCHEDULE

Recommended Childhood Immunization Schedule United States, 2002

Age ▶ Vaccine ▼	Birth	1 mo	2 mos	4 mos	6 mos	12 mos	15 mos	18 mos	24 mos	4 to 6 yrs	11 to 12 yrs	13 to 18 yrs
Hepatitis B[1]	Hep B #1	only if mother HBsAg(−) Hep B #2				Hep B #3					Hep B series	
Diphtheria, Tetanus, Pertussis[2]			DTaP	DTaP	DTaP		DTaP	DTaP		DTaP	Td	
Haemophilus influenzae type b[3]			Hib	Hib	Hib	Hib						
Inactivated Polio[4]			IPVI	PV		IPVI		IPVI		PV		
Measles, Mumps, Rubella[5]						MMR #1				MMR #2	MMR #2	MMR #2
Varicella[6]						Varicella		Varicella		Varicella	Varicella	
Pneumococcal[7]			PCV	PCV	PCV	PCV	PCV		PCV	PPV		
Hepatitis A[8]									Hepatitis A series			
Influenza[9]						Influenza (yearly)						

Vaccines below this line are for selected populations

☐ Range of recommended ages ▢ Catch-up vaccination ▢ Preadolescent assessment

This schedule indicates the recommended ages for routine administration of currently licensed childhood vaccines, as of December 1, 2001, for children through age 18 years. Any dose not given at the recommended age should be given at any subsequent visit when indicated and feasible. ☐ Indicates age groups that warrant special effort to administer those vaccines not previously given. Additional vaccines may be licensed and recommended during the year. Licensed combination vaccines may be used whenever any components of the combination are indicated and the vaccine's other components are not contraindicated. Providers should consult the manufacturer's package inserts for detailed recommendations.

Approved by the Advisory Committee on Immunization Practices (www.cdc.gov/nip/acip), the American Academy of Pediatrics (www.aap.org), and the American Academy of Family Physicians (www.aafp.org).

Drug Guide

Acyclovir

Indications for Use:	Herpes simplex (HSV-I, HSV-2) and varicella-zoster virus infection
Mechanism of Action:	Viral: specified thymidine kinase converts acyclovir to acyclovir monophosphate, which inhibits viral DNA polymerase
Individual Dose:	20 mg/kg
Interval:	Every 8 hr
Route:	Intravenous (IV) over 1 hr
Total Daily Dose:	60 mg/kg
Comments/Cautions:	Little pharmacokinetic data in newborns. $T_{1/2}$: 4 hr. More effective than vidarabine in the treatment of herpetic encephalitis. Side effects uncommon: local phlebitis, transient renal dysfunction, seizures.
Metabolism/Excretion:	Predominantly excreted unchanged in the urine
Stability:	Solution (5 mg/ml) stable for 12 hr–keep at room temperature
Storage:	Below 25° C
Incompatible with:	Unknown
Specific Rx Overdose:	None known
Serum Levels:	Not available

Adrenalin

Indications for Use:	1. Cardiac resuscitation 2. Relief of upper airway obstruction 3. Refractory hypotension
Mechanism of Action:	Potent stimulation of both alpha-and beta-adrenergic receptors
Individual Dose:	For 1. above, 0.1 ml/kg/dose of 1:10,000 solution For 2., 0.5 ml/kg of 1:1000 solution For 3., 0.05-2 ml/kg/min as continuous infusion (protect from light)
Interval:	For 1. above, stat; repeat if necessary For 2., stat; lasts about 40 min For 3., continuous infusion
Route:	For 1. above, IV, endotracheal tube (ETT), intracardiac For 2., nebulized For 3., IV
Comments/Cautions:	May cause dyspnea, hyperglycemia, restlessness, tachycardia, tremor. Large doses may cause cardiac arrhythmias, cerebral hemorrhage, or pulmonary edema. Limited information on continuous infusions in neonates; therefore dopamine,

Comments/ Cautions:	dobutamine, or isoprenaline (isoproterenol) may be a preferred agent. If used as an infusion, intensive peripheral vasoconstriction is a problem, which can be alleviated by the concurrent use of a low-dose dobutamine infusion (2.5 ml/kg/min).
Metabolism/Excretion:	Hepatic metabolism by catecholomethyl transferase and monoamine oxidase enzyme
Supplied as:	1. 1:10,000 Solution (0.1 mg/ml) in 10-ml ampules 2. 1: 1000 Solution (1 mg/ml) in 1-ml ampules
Dilution:	For 1. and 2. above, not required For 3., make (1.5 × wt [kg]) mg of Adrenalin up to 50 ml. 1 ml/hr of this solution = 0.5 mg/kg/min.
Stability:	Discard unused portion after initial use.
Storage:	Store at room temperature; protect ampule from light (not infusion).
Incompatible with:	Total parenteral nutrition (TPN)
Specific Rx Overdose:	Phentolamine followed by beta blocker (e.g., propranolol)

Amikacin

Indications for Use:	Amikacin-sensitive infections, particularly multiply-resistant Enterobacteriaceae
Mechanism of Action:	Inhibits bacterial protein synthesis by interfering with messenger ribonucleic acid (mRNA) at ribosome level
Individual Dose:	1. 7.5 mg/kg: wt <2000 g 2. 10 mg/kg: wt >2000 g
Interval:	1. Age 0-7 days: every 12-24 hr 2. Age >7 days: every 8 hr
Route:	IV over 20 min (preferred); intramuscular (IM)
Total Daily Dose:	1. 15 mg/kg: <2000 g, 0-7 days 2. 20 mg/kg: >2000 g, 0-7 days 3. 30 mg/kg: all infants >7 days
Comments/Cautions:	Relatively resistant to aminoglycoside-inactivating enzymes. Erratic CSF absorption (levels 10%-20% of serum). Nephrotoxic, ototoxic. May potentiate nondepolarizing muscle relaxants.
Metabolism/Excretion:	Excreted almost entirely in urine unchanged
Stability:	Keep open vial 24 hr in refrigerator.
Storage:	Room temperature
Incompatible with:	TPN and most other drugs
Serum Levels:	Trough <5 μg/ml. Peak 20-25 μg/ml.

Aminophylline

Indications for Use:	1. Recurrent apnea or poor respiratory drive in preterm infants 2. To assist weaning from ventilator 3. To reduce airways' resistance in infants with chronic lung disease
Mechanism of Action:	Direct stimulation of respiratory center. Reduces diaphragmatic fatigue. Bronchial smooth muscle cyclic adeosine monophosphate (cAMP) via phosphodiesterase inhibition.
Individual Dose:	1. Loading dose: 10 mg/kg, slowly over 30 min

Individual Dose:	2. Maintenance dose
	   a. 2.5 mg/kg age <2 wk
	   b. 5 mg/kg age >2 wk
	3. Apnea: load with 4-6 mg/kg by mouth (PO) or infused IV over 30 min; then in 8-12 hr begin maintenance of 2 mg/kg/dose IV or PO, given every 6-8 hr. Generally should hold dose if heart rate >180.
	4. Bronchodilation: load with 6 mg/kg IV or PO, then give maintenance of 1 mg/kg/hr

Interval:	Every 12 hr. Begin maintenance dose 12 hr after loading dose.
Route:	IV: loading dose over 30 min; maintenance dose over 15 min
Comments/Cautions:	The maintenance doses are starting doses only and should be adjusted according to serum levels. Theophylline should be omitted if the heart rate is persistently greater than 180/min. If used concurrently with erythromycin, theophylline levels may be increased. A transient diuretic effect is experienced. Theophylline may cause an increase in serum uric acid levels. Complications include gastrointestinal bleeding, hypotension, vomiting, tachycardia, tachypnea, and convulsions. $T_{1/2} \sim 30$ hr (range 15-60 hr).
Metabolism/Excretion:	Hepatic transformation and urinary excretion of metabolites. Caffeine (a metabolite of theophylline) can reach levels 50% those of theophylline and exert a significant stimulatory effect.
Dilution:	Not required
Stability:	Discard unused portion.
Storage:	Room temperature; protect from light
Incompatible with:	Acidic solutions, phenobarbital, phenytoin, morphine, cimetidine, insulin, TPN, furosemide, penicillin
Serum Levels:	Apnea: 5-15 µg/ml Bronchodilation: 15-20 µg/ml

Amoxicillin IV

Indications for Use:	Treating bacterial infections sensitive to amoxicillin
Mechanism of Action:	Inhibits bacterial cell wall synthesis
Individual Dose:	1. Sepsis: 25 mg/kg 2. Meningitis: 50 mg/kg

Interval:	1. <2000 g: age 0-7 days—every 12 hr;
	   >7 days—every 8 hr
	2. >2000 g: age 0-7 days—every 8 hr;
	   >7 days—every 6 hr

Route:	IV, IM
Comments/Cautions:	Amoxicillin has not been used extensively in neonatal practice, and little clinical data exist. However, drug company and in vitro data suggest very little difference compared with ampicillin. The in vitro spectrum of activity is essentially identical to ampicillin, with amoxicillin being more active against Enterobacteriaceae and less active against *Enterobacter* sp. Thrombophlebitis, skin rashes, and transient elevation of liver enzymes may be seen.

| Metabolism/Excretion: | Majority excreted unchanged in urine, with a smaller amount metabolized to the inactive metabolite penicilloic acid. |

Dilution:					
		Vial	Added	Total	
	Route	Strength	Water	Volume	Concentration
	IV	250 mg	4.8 ml	5 ml	50 mg/ml
	IM	250 mg	1.3 ml	1.5 ml	250 mg/1.5 ml
	IV	500 mg	4.6 ml	5 ml	100 mg/ml

Stability:	Use only freshly prepared solutions. Discard unused portion after 30 min.
Storage:	Room temperature
Incompatible with:	Dextrose, TPN, fat or lipid emulsion

Amphotericin

Indications for Use:	Systemic fungal infections—in combination with 5-flurocytosine
Mechanism of Action:	Binds to the sterols of fungal cell membranes, resulting in the loss of intracellular potassium
Individual Dose:	1.0 mg/kg
Interval:	Daily
Route:	IV infusion over 6 hr
Total Daily Dose:	1.0 mg/kg
Comments/Cautions:	Monitor urea, creatinine, and potassium weekly. May cause phlebitis, anemia, hypokalemia, nephrotoxicity. Less frequent but important reactions include cardiovascular toxicity, hypotension/hypertension, convulsions, hemorrhagic gastroenteritis, acute liver failure, anaphylaxis. Cerebrospinal fluid (CSF) concentration, 40%-90% of serum concentration. **Protect from light during administration. (Do not** use with a filter since it is a colloidal dispersion.) 14 days combined treatment (5-Fc + amphotericin) is sufficient for *Candida* sepsis.
Stability:	After reconstitution, room temperature for 24 hr; refrigerate for 1 wk
Storage:	Room temperature for 24 hr or refrigerate. **Protect from light.**
Incompatible with:	Saline, dextrose 10%, penicillin, vitamins, FreAmine, calcium, gentamicin, kanamycin
Specific Overdose Action:	None known
Serum Levels:	As requested; predose level: 0.5-1.5 μg/ml; postdose level: 1.8-3.5 μg/ml

Atracurium

Indications for Use:	Neuromuscular blockage
Mechanism of Action:	Competitive inhibition of neuromuscular transmission
Individual Dose:	0.3-0.5 mg/kg
Interval:	Repeat as necessary.
Route:	IV
Comments/Cautions:	Causes respiratory paralysis; therefore needs ventilation. Causes release of histamine.
Metabolism/Excretion:	Hoffman degradation (nonenzymatic in alkaline environment and not dependent on normal renal or hepatic function)

Dilution:	Not required
Stability:	Discard ampule and unused portion after initial use.
Storage:	Refrigerate; do not freeze.
Incompatible with:	All other drugs
Specific Rx Overdose:	Continued artificial ventilation
Serum Levels:	Not required

Atropine

Indications for Use:	1. Cardiac resuscitation
	2. Premedication
Mechanism of Action:	Competitive antagonist of the action of acetylcholine and other muscarinic agonists
Individual Dose:	For 1. above, 0.02-0.03 mg/kg
	For 2., 0.04 mg/kg
Interval:	For 1. above, 2-3 min as needed (PRN; 2 or 3 doses in 15 min)
	For 2., single dose only
Route:	For 1. above, IV, IM, or subcutaneous (SC)
	For 2., IM
Comments/Cautions:	Cardiac arrhythmia may occur (usually AV dissociation). Abdominal distention, fever, flushing, and pupillary dilation may occur.
Metabolism/Excretion:	Primarily excreted unchanged in urine
Dilution:	IV usage: dilute 1-ml ampule with 5 ml of sterile water
Stability:	Discard unused portion.
Storage:	Room temperature. Protect from light.
Incompatible with:	Alkaline solutions (e.g., $NaHCO_3$)
Specific Rx Overdose:	Physostigmine controls central and peripheral effects. Neostigmine controls peripheral effects only.

Atrovent (Ipratropium Bromide)

Indications for Use:	Chronic lung disease; bronchospasm
Mechanism of Action:	Muscarinic blocker; decreases the level of cyclic guanosine monophosphate (cGMP) in bronchial smooth muscle
Individual Dose:	25 µg/kg (0.1 ml/kg of 0.025% solution)
Interval:	Every 4 hr
Route:	Via nebulizer
Comments/Cautions:	—
Metabolism/Excretion:	Major portion is excreted unchanged in feces. Small amount systemically absorbed and metabolized in liver renal + fecal excretion.
Dilution:	1. <1000 g: dilute to 0.5 ml with 0.9% saline
	2. >1000 g: dilute to 1 ml with 0.9% saline
Stability:	Discard any unused (diluted) solution within 1-2 hr.
Storage:	Room temperature
Incompatible with:	Unknown

Bupivacaine

Indications for Use:	Via interpleural catheter to provide analgesia postoperatively following thoracotomy or upper abdominal procedures

Mechanism of Action:	Bupivacaine is a local anesthetic of the amide group. It interferes with sodium flux across the axonal membrane and thus blocks conduction.
Individual Dose:	Up to 2 mg/kg by bolus injection; 1.25 mg/kg/hr by infusion
Interval:	Every 2 hr
Route:	In this particular technique, the catheter lies between the pleural layers and is directed posteromedially to the paravertebral gutter. The bupivacaine diffuses through the parietal pleura to the intracostal nerves that lie beneath.
Total Daily Dose:	Unknown in the newborn but up to 60 mg/kg/24 hr in children
Comments/Cautions:	Addition of adrenaline 1:200,000 reduces absorption. Plasma levels of bupivacaine are lower, but the duration of blockade is not greatly prolonged.
Metabolism/Excretion:	Hepatic N-dealkylation and hydrolysis
Dilution:	To desired concentration with water for injection or 0.9% saline
Stability:	Solutions are free of preservatives and antibacterials. Opened ampules should not be kept.
Storage:	No special requirements
Incompatible with:	All drugs other than diluents above
Specific Rx Overdose:	1. Convulsions: IV diazepam 2. Hypotension: IV volume expansion +/- inotropes 3. Dysrhythmias: may be extremely refractory to treatment
Serum Levels:	<4 mg/L

Caffeine

Indications for Use:	1. Apnea of prematurity 2. Premedication for infants at risk for postoperative apnea
Mechanism of Action:	CNS stimulant

Individual Dose:	For 1. above
	  a. Loading dose: 12.5 mg/kg
	  b. Maintenance dose: 4.0 mg/kg/day, beginning 24 hr after loading dose
	For 2., loading dose only: 12.5 mg/kg

Interval:	Daily
Route:	For 1.a. above, oral For 1.b., IV
Comments/Cautions:	Stimulates CNS and exerts positive inotropic effect on heart. Stimulates glycogenolysis and lipolysis. Adverse effects include vomiting, gastric irritation, agitation, tachycardia, diuresis, arrhythmia, and seizures. Appears to be less toxic than theophylline. $T_{1/2}$: 80-100 hr depending on gestation.
Metabolism/Excretion:	Excreted unchanged in urine (compare with adults where oxidative metabolism predominates)
Dilution:	None
Stability:	Check that does not precipitate. Shelf life: 7 days.
Storage:	Refrigerate.
Incompatible with:	1. Oral—nil 2. IV—other drugs and blood products
Serum Levels:	Not routinely measured; 25-100 μmol/L

Calcium Chloride

Indications for Use:	1. Hypocalcemia 2. Resuscitation
Mechanism of Action:	Calcium is involved in all membrane stability, neural excitability, and bone formation.

Individual Dose:	1. Hypocalcemia
	  a. Asymptomatic: 1 mmol/kg/day (<1.75 mmol/L) (1.4 ml/kg/day of 10% solution)
	  Note: Calcium gluconate is the preferred agent unless fluid volume critical.
	  b. Symptomatic: 1 ml/kg over 6 hr (0.7 mmol/kg) with ECG monitoring
	  c. Convulsions: 0.15 ml/kg over 1-2 min with electrocardiogram (ECG) monitoring
	2. Resuscitation: 0.15 ml/kg over 1-2 min with ECG monitoring

Interval:	For 1a. above: 4 divided doses, each over 40 min (with ECG monitoring) Stat; repeat if necessary
Route:	IV, umbilical venous catheter (if centrally placed), or oral (maintenance only). Avoid umbilical arterial catheter (UAC) if at all possible.
Comments/Cautions:	May cause bradycardia, hypokalemia, hypotension if IV infusion is administered too rapidly. Skin sloughing may occur if there is extravasation. Chloride combines with citrate; therefore do not give in same line as transfused blood, which would cause coagulation.
Metabolism/Excretion:	Renal excretion
Dilution:	As required
Stability:	Discard ampule and unused portion after initial use.
Storage:	Room temperature
Incompatible with:	Intralipid, sodium bicarbonate, magnesium sulfate, prednisolone, aminoglycosides, TPN, digoxin, transfused blood
Specific Rx Overdose:	Calcitonin, overhydration, diuretics, corticosteroids, IV normal saline

Calcium Gluconate 10%

Indications for Use:	1. Hypocalcemia 2. Resuscitation
Mechanism of Action:	Calcium is involved in all membrane stability, neural excitability, and bone formation.

Individual Dose:	1. Hypocalcemia
	  a. Asymptomatic: 1 mmol/kg/day (<1.75 mmol/L) (4.5 ml/kg/day of 10% solution)
	  b. Symptomatic: 3 ml/kg (i.e., 0.6 mmol/kg) over 6 hr with ECG monitoring
	  c. Convulsions: 0.5 ml/kg over 1-2 min with ECG monitoring
	2. Resuscitation: 0.5 ml/kg over 1-2 min with ECG monitoring

Interval:	For 1.a. above, 4 divided doses, each over 40 min (with ECG monitoring) Stat; repeat if necessary

Route:	IV, umbilical venous catheter (if centrally placed) or PO (maintenance only). Avoid UAC if at all possible.
Comments/Cautions:	May cause bradycardia, hypokalemia, and hypotension if IV infusion is administered too rapidly. Skin sloughing may occur if there is extravasation.
Metabolism/Excretion:	Renal excretion
Dilution:	As required
Stability:	Discard ampule and unused portion after initial use.
Storage:	Room temperature
Incompatible with:	Intralipid, sodium bicarbonate, magnesium sulfate, prednisolone, aminoglycosides, TPN, digoxin
Specific Rx Overdose:	Calcitonin, overhydration, diuretics, corticosteroids, IV normal saline

Cefotaxime

Indications for Use:	Treatment of bacterial sepsis caused by sensitive organisms
Mechanism of Action:	Inhibits bacterial cell wall synthesis
Individual Dose:	50 mg/kg

Interval:	1. Weight <1500 g: every 12 hr
	2. Weight >1500 g
	   a. Every 12 hr at age 0-7 days
	   b. Every 8 hr at age >7 days

Route:	IV over 5 min or IM
Total Daily Dose:	150 mg/kg/day
Comments/Cautions:	Ineffective against *Listeria monocytogenes* and enterococci (e.g., *Streptococcus faecalis*); therefore use in conjunction with amoxicillin. Promotes chromosomally mediated beta-lactamase production, therefore remains a second-choice agent; compare with aminoglycosides (except in renal failure); useful agent in the treatment of meningitis.
Metabolism/Excretion:	30%-50% protein bound, 80% excreted in urine (half as parent compound, half as desacetyl-cefotaxime and inactive metabolites). Hepatic metabolic degradation to desacetyl-cefotaxime and inactive compound. Desacetyl-cefotaxime has significant antibacterial activity itself.

Dilution:

Vial Strength	Added Water	Total Volume
1 g	4.6 ml	5 ml
2 g	9.2. ml	10 ml

Stability:	After reconstituted—24 hr in refrigerator
Storage:	Powder—room temperature; protect from light
Incompatible with:	NaHCO$_3$, aminoglycosides
Specific Rx Overdose:	None known

Ceftazidime

Indications for Use:	Treatment of bacterial sepsis caused by sensitive organisms (especially some *Pseudomonas* species)
Mechanism of Action:	Inhibits bacterial cell wall synthesis
Individual Dose:	25 mg/kg
Interval:	Every 12 hr
Route:	IV (preferred) over 5 min

Total Daily Dose:	50 mg/kg
Comments/Cautions:	Reduce dose in renal failure. Positive Coombs' test may develop. Use in conjunction with an aminoglycoside when treating *Pseudomonas* infections since resistance may develop during treatment. Good CSF penetration. Ineffective against *Listeria monocytogenes* and enterococci (e.g., *S. faecalis*).
Metabolism/Excretion:	Renal excretion via glomerular filtrate

Dilution:

Vial Size	Added Water	Approximate Concentration	IM/IV
1 g	3.0 ml	50 mg/ml	IV
1 g	10.0 ml	90 mg/ml	IM
2 g	10.0 ml	170 mg/ml	IV

Stability:	Discard reconstituted vial after 12 hr.
Storage:	1. Vials: cool, dry place
	2. Reconstituted vial: refrigerator
Incompatible with:	Aminoglycosides
Specific Rx Overdose:	None known

Ceftriaxone

Indications for Use:	Treatment of bacterial sepsis or meningitis caused by sensitive organism
Mechanism of Action:	Inhibits bacterial cell well synthesis
Individual Dose:	1. Septicemia: 50 mg/kg
	2. Meningitis: 100 mg/kg (loading dose), then 50 mg/kg thereafter
Interval:	Once daily
Route:	IV (preferred) over 5 min; IM
Total Daily Dose:	50 mg/kg after loading dose
Comments/Cautions:	Ineffective against *Listeria monocytogenes* and enterococci (e.g., *S. faecalis*). Variable efficacy against *Staphyloccocus epidermidis, Pseudomonas* species, *Bacteroides* species (therefore check sensitivities). May displace bilirubin from albumin.
Metabolism/Excretion:	70% excreted unchanged in urine. Remainder excreted in bile.
Stability:	Replace reconstituted vial every 24 hr.
Storage:	1. Vials: room temperature.
	2. Reconstituted vial: refrigerator
Incompatible with:	None known
Specific Rx Overdose:	None known

Chlorothiazide

Indications for Use:	Diuretic therapy, especially in conjunction with furosemide to prevent the nephrocalcinosis associated with the latter
Mechanism of Action:	Inhibits C1 reabsorption in the distal cortical diluting segment at the top of the ascending loop of Henle
Individual Dose:	20 mg/kg
Interval:	Every 12 hr
Route:	Oral
Comments/Cautions:	Hypokalemia, hyperglycemia, and a deterioration in renal or hepatic function (if already compromised)

Comments/ Cautions:	have been reported in adults. Virtually no data on use in neonates.
Metabolism/Excretion:	Poorly absorbed from gastrointestinal (GI) tract. $T_{1/2}$ ~ 6 hr in newborn infants. Excreted unchanged in urine.
Stability:	Approximately 1 mo. Tendency to settle out; therefore shake well before dispensing.
Storage:	Room temperature
Specific Rx Overdose:	None known

Clonidine

Indications for Use:	1. Opiate withdrawal
	2. Sedation
Contraindications:	Hypotension
Mechanism of Action:	Reduces sympathetic outflow from central nervous system
Individual Dose:	1-4 µg/kg
Interval:	Every 8 hr
Route:	Oral
Comments/Cautions:	Limited experience in newborns. May cause fluid retention. Reduce dose slowly after prolonged use (>1 wk).
Special Observations:	Measure blood pressure before and 1 hr after dose for first 3 doses or after any increase in dose.
Metabolism/Excretion:	Degraded in liver or renally excreted
Storage:	Refrigerator

Dexamethasone

Indications for Use:	1. Treatment of hyaline membrane disease (HMD)
	2. Treatment of chronic lung disease
	3. Pulmonary interstitial emphysema (PIE) (other indications as per consultant)
Mechanism of Action:	Mobilizes pulmonary intestinal edema and suppresses chronic inflammatory response
Individual Dose:	For 1. and 2. above,
	a. Day 1-3: 0.1 mg/kg every 12 hr
	b. Day 4-7: 0.05 mg/kg every 12 hr
	For 3., day 1-6: 0.25 mg/kg every 12 hr
Interval:	See individual dosage.
Total Daily Dosage:	0.2-0.5 mg/kg
Comments/Cautions:	Failure to respond after 5 days of therapy—stop dexamethasone. Deterioration in respiratory status during steroid weaning—return to previous dosage. Repeat courses as necessary. 0.5 mg/kg/day is approximately 70 × the normal glucocorticoid requirement.
Side Effects:	Hyperglycemia, hypertension, GI hemorrhage, electrolyte disturbance, predisposition toward sepsis
Dilution:	Make 0.25 ml up to 1 ml with sterile water (i.e., 1 mg/ml solution).
Stability:	Discard after 24 hr.
Storage:	Room temperature; avoid extreme temperatures
Incompatible with:	Aminoglycosides
Serum Levels:	Not required

40% Dextrose Gel

Indications: Infants with hypoglycemia (i.e., blood sugar level <2.0 mmol/L at age <4 hr or blood sugar level <2.5 mmol/L at age >4 hr)

Method:
1. Draw up 40% dextrose gel, 0.5 ml/kg, into 2-ml syringe (19-gauge needle).
2. Remove needle from syringe.
3. Dry infant's buccal mucosa with gauze swab.
4. Place 40% dextrose gel on your gloved finger, and massage into infant's buccal mucosa.
5. Check blood sugar level 15 min after administration of 40% dextrose gel and feeding.
6. Continue to give feeds as charted, as tolerated.
7. If still hypoglycemic, repeat dose and check blood sugar level further in 15 min. **Do not** give further doses unless instructed by medical staff or neonatal nurse practitioner (NNP).
8. Inform and explain to parents.

Cautions: Infants who are unconscious or experiencing hypoglycemic seizures should receive an urgent bolus of dextrose IV or glucagon IM, as prescribed by medical staff.

40% Dextrose Gel for Analgesia

Indications for Use: Analgesia for mild pain
Contraindications: Birth weight <1000 g
Mechanism of Action: Probably via increased endogenous opioid production, secondary to stimulation of taste cell receptor
Individual Dose: 0.25-1 ml
Interval: Up to 4 times per day
Route:
1. Sublingual: administer 1-2 min before procedure
2. Via pacifier

Total Daily Dose: 4 ml
Comments/Cautions: Limited information available. May be used in conjunction with other analgesics.
Metabolism/Excretion: Metabolized to water and carbon dioxide
Supplied as: 40% dextrose gel
Dilution: None
Storage: Room temperature

Diazepam

Indications for Use: Convulsion control
Mechanism of Action: Enhance gamma-aminobutyric acid (GABA)–mediated presynaptic and postsynaptic inhibitory pathways
Individual Dose:
1. 0.3 mg/kg/hr by continuous infusion
2. 0.3 mg/kg by slow bolus

Interval: For 2., repeat immediately if necessary.
Route: IV only
Comments/Cautions: Respiratory depression and prolonged hypotonia. Hypotension and kernicterus have not been demonstrated in human newborns.
Metabolism/Excretion: Metabolized to N-desmethyldiazepam active CPD, then slowly hydroxylated to other active metabolites
Supplied as: 10 mg/2-ml ampule

Dilution:	1. Continuous infusion: Make 6 mg/kg (body wt) of diazepam up to 10 ml with 0.9% saline or 5% dextrose. Infuse at 0.5 ml/hr = 0.3 mg/kg/hr.
	2. Slow bolus: Dilute to 1 ml with 0.9% saline or 5% dextrose; or administer undiluted.
	Note: Clouding will form on dilution; this represents precipitation of the associated sodium benzoate and does not alter the concentration/effectiveness of the diazepam.
Stability:	Discard ampule and unused portion after initial use. Make fresh infusion every 24 hr.
Storage:	Room temperature; protect from light
Incompatible with:	TPN, other drugs

Digoxin

| Indications for Use: | Supraventricular tachycardia; heart failure |
| Mechanism of Action: | Positive inotropic effect (inhibits Na+/K+ ATPase); depression of conducting tissue; increased vagal activity |

Individual Dose:

	Intravenous Loading doses	Oral
Preterm infants	20 μg/kg	20 μg/kg
Term infants	30 μg/kg	30 μg/kg
	Maintenance doses	
Preterm infants	3.5 μg/kg	5 μg/kg
Term infants	7.5 μg/kg	10 μg/kg

Interval:	1. Loading dose: one-half dose immediately, one-fourth dose 8 hr later, one-fourth dose another 8 hr later
	2. Maintenance dose: daily (beginning 12 hr after completion of loading dose)
Route:	1. IV (over 5 min)
	2. Oral
Comments/Cautions:	Diagnosis of digoxin toxicity in neonates usually rests on ECG abnormalities: first-degree atrioventricular (AV) block is a reliable early sign. Arrhythmias are a late and relatively rare sign. Vomiting and diarrhea are unusual.
Metabolism/Excretion:	Excreted unchanged via kidneys
Dilution:	1. Dilute to 1 ml using normal saline.
	2. Dilute 1 ml of ampule solution to 10 ml with normal saline (i.e., make 25 μg/ml solution).
Stability:	For 1. above, discard used ampule and unused portion
Storage:	Room temperature
Incompatible with:	Calcium
Specific Rx Overdose:	Omit next dose or cease treatment. Correct electrolyte imbalance. Correct arrhythmia. Give phenytoin, 15 mg/kg IV slowly. Digoxin antibodies (Digibind) available through Wellcome (NZ) Ltd.
Serum Levels:	1.1-1.7 ng/ml

Dobutamine

| Indications for Use: | To improve cardiac output |
| Mechanism of Action: | A direct beta$_1$ agonist with minimal beta$_2$ or alpha effects. No dopaminergic action. |

Individual Dose:	2-10 µg/kg/min
Route:	IV, continuous infusion
Comments/Cautions:	Positive inotropic action (similar to dopamine) but lacking any specific vasodilatory action on the splanchnic vasculature. The widespread alpha-mediated vasoconstriction seen with dopamine is not present. Less effective in younger patients. May increase pulmonary wedge pressure; therefore be cautious if pulmonary hypertension. Arrhythmias may be seen at higher doses.
Metabolism/Excretion:	Metabolized (methylation and conjugation) to inactive metabolites, which are excreted in urine and bile; $T_{1/2}$: approximately 2 min
Dilution:	1. Reconstitute vial with 10 ml of diluent (makes solution A, 25 mg/ml). Dilute 1 ml of solution A to 5 ml with 5% dextrose or 0.9% saline to give solution B (5 mg/ml).
	2. For 10-ml syringe: $6 \times$ wt (kg) expressed as mg and made up to 10 ml of solution (0.9% saline, 5% dextrose) = 0.25 ml/hr = 2.5 µg/kg/min
	3. For 20-ml syringe: $6 \times$ wt (kg) expressed as mg and made up to 20 ml of solution (0.9% saline, 5% dextrose) = 0.5 ml/hr = 2.5 µg/kg/min
Stability:	Reconstituted solution
	1. Stable 24 hr at room temperature
	2. Stable 96 hr if refrigerated
Incompatible with:	None known
Specific Rx Overdose:	Discontinue dobutamine infusion.

Dopamine

Indications for Use:	1. Hypotension caused by impaired cardiac output
	2. To improve splanchnic and renal blood flow
Mechanism of Action:	Increases myocordial contractility by direct action on beta-adrenergic receptors, as well as by releasing noradrenaline from myocardial storage sites. Alpha-mediated peripheral vasoconstriction is the predominant mode of action in neonates (compare with adults where this is seen in doses >10 µg/kg/min). Other modes of action
	1. Specific dopaminergic receptors in the renal (and mesenteric) vasculature, which in adults increases renal blood flow, increases glomerular filtration rate (GFR), increases natriuresis (similar responses have not been demonstrated in newborns)
	2. Beta$_1$ effects: increased cardiac output, increased arterial blood pressure (BP)
Individual Dose:	0.5-15 µg/kg/min
Interval:	Continuous infusion
Route:	IV
Comments/Cautions:	Correct hypovolemia before administration. Extravasation may result in tissue necrosis. Doses >10 µg/kg/min have increased pulmonary vascular resistance in newborn lambs; therefore use higher doses cautiously in persistent fetal circulation (PFC).

Metabolism/Excretion:	Biotransformation (via monoamine oxidase and catecholomethyl transferase) to metabolites dihydroxyphenylacetic acid (DOPAC) and homovanillic acid (HVA), which are renally excreted. $T_{1/2}$: 4-5 min.
Dilution:	1. For 50-ml syringe: $15 \times$ wt (kg) expressed as mg and made up to 50 ml of solution (0.9% saline, 5% or 10% dextrose—no heparin) = 0.5 ml/hr = 2.5 μg/kg/min
	2. For 10-ml syringe: $6 \times$ wt (kg) expressed as mg and made up to 10 ml of solution (0.9% saline, 5% or 10% dextrose—no heparin) = 0.25 ml/hr = 2.5 μg/kg/min (250 μL/hr)
Stability:	Discard ampule and unused portion after initial use. Change infusion every 24 hr.
Incompatible with:	NaHCO$_3$ and other alkaline solutions. Use separate route since bolus dose will be administered if flushed through with other drugs.
Specific Rx Overdose:	Cease infusion until patient stabilizes.

Doxapram

Indications for Use:	Apnea of prematurity unresponsive to theophylline
Mechanism of Action:	Increases tidal volume via central stimulation and peripheral carotid chemoreception
Individual Dose:	0.5 mg/kg/hr, increase stepwise to 1.5 mg/kg/hr (as tolerated)
Interval:	Continuous infusion
Route:	IV
Comments/Cautions:	Recognized adverse effects include hypertension, cerebral irritation, convulsions, urinary retention, diarrhea. **Do not** administer to patients who have had convulsions or a recent periventricular hemorrhage. Ampule contains the preservative benzyl alcohol, which is toxic in high doses; at doxapram infusion rate of 1.5 mg/kg/hr approximately 15 mg/kg/day of benzyl alcohol is administered (compare with described toxic symptoms >99 mg/kg/day).
Metabolism/Excretion:	Extensively metabolized in liver with only a small amount of free drug appearing in the urine. Doxapram and metabolites are excreted via bile to feces.
Supplied as:	20 mg/ml; 20-ml vials
Stability:	Stable for 4 yr if stored below 25° C. Make fresh infusion every 48 hr.
Storage:	Room temperature
Incompatible with:	Alkaline solution (e.g., barbiturates, NaHCO$_3$, aminophylline, furosemide, penicillin G)
Specific Rx Overdose:	Stop infusion. Rx anticonvulsants if seizures occur.

Erythromycin (PO and IV) (Lactobionate)
1. IV

Indications for Use:	10 mg/kg
Interval:	Every 12 hr

Route:	IV preferred as an infusion over 30 min
Total Daily Dose:	20 mg/kg/day
Comments/Cautions:	IM injections should be avoided because infants do not have sufficient muscle mass for deep IM injections. Therefore pain is experienced. Interference has been noted with serum transaminase estimations when the patient is receiving erythromycin. Pain and phlebitis at the IV site have been recorded.
Dilution:	IV: Dilute to a 5% solution (i.e., add 6 ml of water for injection). When administering dosage, add 20 ml H_2O; if 1-g vial, further dilute dose $\times$ 4 (i.e., 1% solution).
Stability:	IV 1. 1%: use immediately 2. 5%: suitable for 48 hr in refrigerator
Storage:	Room temperature. After reconstitution, refrigerate for 24 hr.
Incompatible with:	Ampicillin, cephalothin, chloramphenicol, cloxacillin, colistin, heparin, tetracyclines, TPN; inhibits lincomycin
Specific Rx Overdose:	None known
Serum Levels:	When requested: range 1-2 g/ml

2. PO

Indications for Use:	5-10 mg/kg
Interval:	Every 6 hr
Route:	Oral
Total Daily Dose:	20-40 mg/kg
Comments/Cautions:	Should be given 1 hr before feed to ensure maximum absorption. May increase serum theophylline levels. Should not be used with penicillins because they interfere with its action. Shake well before use. May cause cholestatic jaundice. May increase theophylline serum levels.
Stability:	Until expiration date on bottle
Storage:	1. Erythromycin stearate: room temperature 2. Erythromycin ethyl succinate: 10 days refrigerated after reconstitution
Incompatible with:	None known
Specific Rx Overdose:	Aspirate stomach as soon as possible.
Serum Levels:	Not required

Exosurf

Indications for Use:	Respiratory distress syndrome
Mechanism of Action:	Synthetic surfactant, reduces alveolar surface tension
Individual Dose:	5 ml/kg
Interval:	Every 8-12 hr (maximum 4 doses)
Route:	Via endotracheal tube over 20-30 min
Comments/Cautions:	Desaturation may accompany administration. Pulmonary hemorrhage has been observed to occur more frequently in those <750 g.
Metabolism/Excretion:	Locally degraded
Supplied as:	Sterile, lyophilized powder
Dilution:	Dissolve dry powder in 8 ml of sterile water.
Stability:	Reconstituted solution is stable for 12 hr.
Storage:	Room temperature

Fentanyl

Indications for Use:	Sedation while ventilated
Mechanism of Action:	Binds to the opioid receptor
Individual Dose:	1. 2-5 µg/kg
	2. 2-5 µg/kg/hr
Interval:	For 1. above, as needed (PRN), every 2-4 hr; if receiving muscle relaxants give every 4 hr
	For 2., continuous IV infusion
Route:	For 1. above, IV, over 2-3 min
	For 2., continuous IV infusion
Comments/Cautions:	Rapid onset of action (few minutes). Significant respiratory depression can occur. Muscle rigidity has been described if the IV push is administered too quickly or if 25 µg/kg is administered. Cardiovascular effects are negligible in these doses.
Metabolism/Excretion:	Hepatic metabolism
Dilution:	For 1. above, dilute with 0.9% NaCl up to 5 or 10 ml (depending on infant's wt). Dilution to 5 ml gives 20 µg/ml; dilution to 10 ml gives 10 µg/ml.
	For 2., make fentanyl, 100 µg/kg, up to 10 ml with 0.9% saline = 0.5 ml/hr = 5 µg/kg/hr
Stability:	Discard unused portion once ampule opened. Make fresh infusion every 12 hr.
Storage:	Room temperature; protect ampule from light (not infusion)
Incompatible with:	TPN, phenobarbital
Specific Rx Overdose:	Naloxone

Flucloxacillin (Floxacillin)

Indications for Use:	Staphylococcal infections (*S. aureus, S. epidermidis*) if organism sensitive
Mechanism of Action:	Inhibits bacterial cell wall synthesis
Individual Dose:	25-50 mg/kg
Interval:	Body weight
	1. <2000 g
	a. Age 0-7 days : every 12 hr
	b. Age >7 days : every 8 hr
	2. >2000 g
	a. Age 0-7 days: every 8 hr
	b. Age >7 days: every 6 hr
Route:	IV (over 3-4 min), IM, oral
Total Daily Dose:	Not to exceed 150 mg/kg
Comments/Cautions:	Eosinophilia and neutropenia have been reported in 5% of treated patients. May displace bilirubin from albumin. If administered orally, give 30-60 min before feed.
Metabolism/Excretion:	Most of the drug is excreted unchanged in the urine.
Supplied as:	1. 250-mg vials (500-mg and 1-g vials also available)
	2. 125 mg/5 ml powder for reconstitution
Dilution:	For 1. above, IV/IM: dilute 250-mg vial with 1.9 ml of water for injection. This makes a solution of 125 mg/ml.
	For 2., oral: reconstitute syrup by adding 60 ml of sterile water (125 mg/5 ml)

Stability:	For 1. above, powder: 3 yr from date of manufacture, reconstituted; use freshly prepared solution only
	For 2., powder: 2 yr from date of manufacture, reconstituted, after 7 days
Storage:	1. Powder—room temperature
	2. Syrup—refrigerate (8° C)
Incompatible with:	Gentamicin, kanamycin, blood products, TPN

Fluconazole

Indications for Use:	Treatment of serious fungal infection
Mechanism of Action:	Inhibits cytochrome P-450 in susceptible fungi, leading to decreased concentrations of ergosterol and hence increased cell membrane permeability
Individual Dose:	1. Mucosal infection: 3 mg/kg
	2. Systemic infection: 6 mg/kg
	3. Severe, life-threatening infection: 12 mg/kg
Interval:	1. <2 wk old—single dose every third day
	2. 2-4 wk old—single dose every second day
	3. >4 wk old—single dose every day
Route:	PO or IV (over 30 min)
Comments/Cautions:	Limited data on use in newborn. In adults, pharmacokinetics are similar following IV or PO administration. Rapidly absorbed from GI tract with no first-pass metabolism. Distributed widely throughout body tissues (CSF levels 50%-90% of plasma levels) following IV or PO administration. Transient increase in transaminase may be seen (especially if phenytoin used concomitantly).
Metabolism/Excretion:	Predominantly excreted unchanged in urine—increase dose interval if renal impairment. $T_{1/2}$: 50-90 hr; decreases with increasing postnatal age as GFR increases.
Dilution:	None required
Storage:	Room temperature
Incompatible with:	Amphotericin B, ampicillin, calcium, cefotaxime, furosemide

5-Flucytosine

Indications for Use:	Systemic fungal infections
Mechanism of Action:	Fungal cells convert flucytosine to fluorouracil, which is metabolized to 5-fluorodeoxyuridylic acid, an inhibitor of thymidylate synthetase.
Individual Dose:	1. IV: 25 mg/kg every 12 hr administered over 20 min
	2. PO: 25 mg/kg every 6 hr
Comments/Cautions:	Bone marrow suppression, especially if serum levels >750 μmol/L or with concurrent amphotericin B usage. Despite the possible potentiation of side effects it is recommended that systemic candidiasis treatment begin with combination of 5-FC plus amphotericin B since there is evidence of synergy.
Metabolism/Excretion:	Well absorbed from the GI tract; minimally bound plasma proteins. CSF levels 65%-90% of plasma levels. 80% is excreted unchanged in urine.
Dilution:	May dilute with 0.9% saline or 5% dextrose

Stability:	Stable for 3 yr from the date of manufacture
Storage:	Room temperature; protect from light
Incompatible with:	All but 5% dextrose or 0.9% saline
Specific Rx Overdose:	None known
Serum Levels:	Trough >80 μmol/L. Peak 250-400 μmol/L.

Furosemide

Indications for Use:	Fluid overload; poor urine output in presence of adequate renal perfusion; chronic lung disease
Mechanism of Action:	Inhibits electrolyte reabsorption in the ascending limb of the loop of Henle
Individual Dose:	1. IV: 1 mg/kg 2. PO: 1-2 mg/kg

Interval:	1. IV
	  a. <30 wk postconceptual age—once daily
	  b. >30 wk postconceptual age—once daily initially, may increase to every 12 hr
	2. PO
	  a. <30 wk postconceptual age—alternate day
	  b. >30 wk postconceptual age—alternate day, may increase to every 12 hr on alternate days

Route:	IV or PO
Comments/Cautions:	Usually used in conjunction with chlorothiazide to prevent hypercalciuria. Displaces bilirubin from albumin; therefore avoid in hyperbilirubinemia. Ototoxic in higher doses or presence of renal failure.
Metabolism/Excretion:	Excreted unchanged in urine
Dilution:	None required
Stability:	1. IV: discard ampule and unused portion 2. PO: until 3 wk after opening.
Storage:	1. IV: room temperature; protect from light 2. PO: refrigerate; protect from light
Incompatible with:	TPN

Fusidic Acid

Indications for Use:	Treatment of *Staphylococcus aureus* and *Staphylococcus epidermidis* infections. Penicillinase-producing and methicillin-resistant forms are usually sensitive to fusidic acid.
Mechanism of Action:	Inhibits bacterial protein synthesis by interfering with protein G
Individual Dose:	1. IV: 20 mg/kg 2. PO: 6.5 mg/kg
Interval:	For 1. above: >37 wk, every 12 hr; 30-37 wk, every 18 hr; <30 wk, every 24 hr For 2., every 8 hr
Route:	1. IV over 2 hr 2. PO **Do not give IM or SC.**
Total Daily Dose:	40 mg/kg/day
Comments/Cautions:	No pharmacokinetic data available for neonates. Limited reports on clinical usage. In adults, causes impairment of liver functions when given IM;

Comments/ Cautions:	therefore monitor LFTs (liver function tests). Displaces bilirubin from albumin.
Metabolsim/Excretion:	Metabolized in liver. Degradation products primarily excreted in bile. Little renal excretion.
Dilution:	Dissolve dry powder in vial with supplied diluent (i.e., 500 mg in 50 ml or 100 mg/ml solution). Dilute required dose a further 10 times ($\times$10) with normal saline or 5% dextrose.
Stability:	Infusion stable for 24 hr once reconstituted
Storage:	Cool place. Do not freeze.
Incompatible with:	Parenteral nutrition, gentamicin, whole blood
Specific Rx Overdose:	None known

Gentamicin

Indications for Use:	Gentamicin-sensitive infections
Mechanism of Action:	Inhibits bacterial protein synthesis by interfering with mRNA at ribosome level
Individual Dose:	1. Loading dose: 5 mg/kg (made up to 1 ml if <1500 g or 2 ml if >1500 g)
	2. Maintenance dose: 2.5 mg/kg (see below for interval)

Interval:	Initial Maintenance Dose (following loading dose) (hr)	Subsequent Doses (hr)
<1000 g	30	24
1000-1500 g	24	18
>1500 g, age 0-7 days	18	12
>1500 g, age >7 days	12	8

Route:	For 1. above, infuse IV over 1 hr (by pump)
	For 2., IV over 20 min (preferred), IM
Comments/Cautions:	Ototoxicity, nephrotoxicity. Variable CSF penetration. $T_{1/2}$: 4-14 hr depending on postnatal age and gestation.
Metabolism/Excretion:	Excreted unchanged in urine
Stability:	Open vial—24 hr in refrigerator
Storage:	Room temperature
Incompatible with:	TPN, calcium gluconate, penicillins, cephalosporins, heparin, chloramphenicol, amphotericin
Serum Levels:	Check on second dose or on next dose following a prescription change; if stable, check weekly. Trough: <2 μg/ml. Peak: 8-12 μg/ml.

Glucagon

Indications for Use:	Hypoglycemia
Mechanism of Action:	Activates glycogen phosphorylase via cAMP. Opposes action of insulin and hence promotes hyperglycemia.
Individual Dose:	1. Bolus: 200 μg/kg
	2. Infusion: 5-10 μg/kg/hr
Interval:	For 1. above, stat; repeat every 4-6 hr as required
	For 2., loading dose 200 μg/kg; thereafter continuous infusion
Route:	For 1. above, SC, IM, or IV
	For 2., IV
Comments/Cautions:	If no response to infusion rate of 2 mg/day, a further dosage increase is unlikely to be of value. Vomiting may occur.

Metabolism/Excretion:	Extensively degraded in liver, in kidney, and at tissue receptor sites.
	Plasma $T_{1/2}$~ 3-6 mmol (adults).
Dilution:	Add (300 × birth wt [kg]) micrograms of glucagon to 30 ml of normal saline. 1 ml/hr of this solution = 10 μg/kg/hr.
Stability:	Discard reconstituted vial after initial use. Remake IV infusion every 24 hr.
Storage:	Room temperature
Incompatible with:	Chloride-containing solutions

Heparin

Indications for Use:	1. To heparinize IV and intraarterial (IA) infusions
	2. Anticoagulation
Mechanism of Action:	Inhibits thrombin formation by the activity of antithrombin III and heparin co-factor II that in turn form complexes with thrombin
Individual Dose:	For 1. above, IV: 1 unit per 1 ml of solution; IA: 2 units per 1 ml of solution
	For 2., 50 units/kg bolus followed by 20 units/kg/hr (preterm) or 25 units/kg/hr (term). Increase by 5 units/kg/hr if antiprothrombin time (APTT) less than 2 × normal.
Route:	IV or IA
Total Daily Dose:	For 1. above, 30 units/kg/day
	For 2., determined by APTT
Comments/Cautions:	Monitor APTT every 4 hr during infusion.
Metabolism/Excretion:	Metabolized in liver and inactive compounds appear in the urine
Stability:	Discard after 24 hr.
Storage:	Refrigerate.
Incompatible with:	All other drugs
Specific Rx Overdose:	Stop giving heparin. Treat hypovolemia. Give protamine sulfate, 1 mg/kg, or calculate how much heparin remains (assume a heparin $T_{1/2}$ of 2 hr and give 1 mg of protamine to reverse each 100 units of heparin).
Serum Levels:	Not required

Hyaluronidase

Indications for Use:	Prevention of tissue injury following IV extravasation
Mechanism of Action:	Hyaluronidase is a mucolytic enzyme that disrupts the normal intercellular barrier and allows rapid dispersion of extravasated fluids through the tissues.
Individual Dose:	15 units
Interval:	Single dose only
Route:	SC or intradermal: inject 3 units in five separate sites around the periphery of the extravasation site
Comments/Cautions:	**Do not** use for the treatment of extravasation of vasoconstrictive agents (e.g., dopamine, adrenaline). Allergic reactions have been encountered (rarely).
Metabolism/Excretion:	Not known

Dilution:	Dilute powder (1500 units) with 10 ml of normal saline, making solution A (150 units/ml). Further dilute 1 ml of solution A with 9 ml normal saline, making solution B (15 units/ml).
Stability:	Reconstituted powder is stable for 2 wk at room temperature.
Storage:	Room temperature
Incompatible with:	None known
Specific Rx Overdose:	Inotropes, corticosteroids, antihistamine

Hydralazine

Indications for Use:	1. Persistent systemic hypertension 2. Pulmonary hypertension related to chronic lung disease
Mechanism of Action:	Direct action on vascular smooth muscle, arterioles more than venules
Individual Dose:	First dose: 0.1 mg/kg over 5 min; repeat until desired fall in arterial pressure is seen. Subsequent doses: 0.15-0.3 mg/kg.
Interval:	Every 4 hr once desired effect seen
Route:	IV/IM (IV preferred)
Total Daily Dose:	1-9 mg/kg/24 hr
Comments/Cautions:	In ventilated infants, consider increasing sedation first. Profound hypotension may follow initial dose especially if there is unrecognized hypovolemia. Hydralazine causes tachycardia mediated partly via aortic baroreceptor reflex.
Metabolism/Excretion:	Acetylated. Very variable half-life time depending on acetylator status (2-8 hr in adults and probably longer in newborns).
Dilution:	Add 2 ml water for injection to give 10 mg/ml solution. May be further diluted in water or saline, **not** 5% glucose. **Use a plastic cannula.**
Stability:	Diluted solution can be kept at **room temperature** for up to 12 hr (if the solution is in contact with steel [e.g., a syringe needle], then a purple-colored but inactive product is formed by oxidation).
Storage:	Protect ampules and solution from heat/light.
Incompatible with:	Glucose-containing solutions
Specific Rx Overdose:	Correct hypotension by volume replacement initially. Vasoconstrictors are a logical second line; the more direct-acting drugs (e.g., methoxamine, metaraminol) by choice. Adrenaline should be avoided since it exacerbates tachycardia.

Hydrocortisone

Indications for Use:	1. Replacement therapy in adrenal insufficiency 2. Intractable hypoglycemia 3. Severe bronchospasm
Mechanism of Action:	Steroids control intracellular protein synthesis by binding to cytoplasmic steroid receptors. Affect lipid, protein, CHO metabolism; water and electrolyte balance; immune response.

Individual Dose:	For 1. above, 12.5 mg/meter squared To calculate: surface area (meters squared) = $0.05 \times$ wt (kg) + 0.05 For 2., 2.5 mg/kg increasing to 7.5 mg/kg For 3., 5-10 mg/kg
Interval:	For 1. above, daily, in four divided doses For 2. and 3., every 6 hr
Route:	IM or IV

Comments/Cautions:	Cushingoid, hyperglycemia, protein catabolism,
	    increased bleeding tendency, decreased growth,
	    increased infection

Metabolism/Excretion:	Metabolized in liver and excreted by kidneys
Stability:	Discard after 24 hr.
Storage:	Room temperature
Incompatible with:	Adrenaline, chloramphenicol, heparin, isoproterenol, phenobarbital, TPN

Indomethacin

Indications for Use:	Medical closure of patent ductus arteriosus (PDA)
Mechanism of Action:	Inhibition of prostaglandin synthesis
Individual Dose:	1. Treatment: 0.2 mg/kg (initial dose) 2. Prophylactic: 0.1 mg/kg

Interval:	For 1., either
	    a. 0.2 mg/kg every 24 hr for a total of 3 doses if the
	       PDA remains patent, *or*
	    b. 0.1 mg/kg daily for a further 5 doses if PDA
	       closed
	For 2., 3 doses at 24-hr intervals. Initial dose at age <6
	    hr (following stabilization and cerebral ultrasound).

Route:	IV (not arterial)—**slowly over 30 min**

Comments/Cautions:	Transient renal dysfunction occurs in the majority of
	    infants—oliguria. Hypoglycemia, hyponatremia,
	    decreased platelet aggregation, GI bleeding, and
	    convulsions may be seen. To avoid oliguria
	    immediately follow each dose of indomethacin with
	    furosemide, 1 mg/kg IV.

Contraindications:	1. Serum creatinine >0.13 mmol/L 2. Urine output <0.5 ml/kg/hr for preceding 8 hr 3. Platelets <50,000/mm^3 4. Clinical bleeding or necrotizing enterocolitis (NEC)

Metabolism/Excretion:	Elimination $T_{1/2}$ shows great variability (especially in
	    very low–birth weight [VLBW] infants): 5-90 hr. Renal
	    excretion and biliary excretion (following hepatic
	    metabolism). Significant enterohepatic circulation.

Dilution:	Dilute with 2 ml of water for injection. This makes a solution of 0.5 mg/ml.
Stability:	Discard unused portion immediately.
Storage:	Room temperature; protect from light

Incompatible with:	Any solution with pH <6.0. Therefore avoid mixing
	    with TPN or other drugs. Flush line before and after
	    administration with 5% or 10% dextrose.

Insulin

Indications for Use:	1. Hyperglycemia 2. Hyperkalemia

Mechanism of Action:	Binds to cell membrane insulin receptors and promotes protein, lipid, and glycogen synthesis. Promotes peripheral glucose uptake. Insulin is a major fetal growth factor and the improved weight gain seen in preterm infants given insulin may reflect this as well as the improved CHO intolerance.
Individual Dose:	For 1. above, 0.05-0.2 units/kg/hr For 2., 0.1 unit/kg of Actrapid HM insulin plus 50% dextrose, 2 ml/kg
Interval:	For 1. above, infusion For 2., PRN as indicated
Route:	IV
Comments/Cautions:	Initially check blood sugar every 30 min, thereafter hourly, or as per unit protocol.
Metabolism/Excretion:	10% appears unchanged in urine. Remainder metabolized in the liver.
Supplied as:	Actrapid HM insulin (100 units/ml)
Dilution:	For 1. above, 20-ml and 50-ml syringe Take 0.1 ml insulin and make up to 10 ml total volume with 9.9 ml of 0.9% saline (this gives 1 unit/ml = solution A). Then make a 20-ml solution (B) containing ($4 \times$ body wt [kg]) ml of solution A and the remainder 0.9% saline. 0.5 ml/hr of this final solution (B) = 0.1 unit/kg/hr. For 2., 10-ml syringe (via pump) Take 0.1 ml insulin and make up to 10 ml total volume with 9.9 ml of 0.9% saline (this gives 1 unit/ml = solution A). Then make a 10-ml solution (B) containing ($4 \times$ body wt [kg]) ml solution A and the remainder 0.9% saline. 0.25 ml/hr of this final solution (B) = 0.1 unit/kg/hr. **Note:** At initiation of infusion, flush 2 ml of the insulin infusion through the giving set and tubing to saturate the plastic binding capacity (before connecting to baby).
Stability:	Infusion: 24 hr
Storage:	Refrigerate.
Incompatible with:	Chlorothiazide, phenobarbital, phenytoin, $NaHCO_3$, thiopental

Isoprenaline

Indications for Use:	Hypotension caused by impaired cardiac output
Mechanism of Action:	Beta$_1$- and beta$_2$-adrenergic agonist. It increases cardiac contractility and heart rate, with little increase in systemic vascular resistance. May reduce pulmonary vascular resistance (beta$_2$ effect).
Individual Dose:	0.05-0.5 µg/kg/min
Interval:	Continuous infusion
Route:	IV
Comments/Cautions:	May cause tachycardia, arrhythmias, hypotension, cardiac enlargement, and rarely, pulmonary edema
Metabolism/Excretion:	Metabolized in liver by catecholomethyl transferase

Dilution:	$(0.3 \times$ body wt [kg]) mg and make up to 25 ml with 0.9% saline, 5% or 10% dextrose. 0.5 ml/hr = 0.1 μg/kg/min.
Stability:	Discard ampule and unused portion after initial use. Change IV solution every 24 hr.
Storage:	Room temperature; protect from light
Incompatible with:	**Any other drug in solution.** Use with extreme caution if patient has high serum digoxin levels. Separate line preferable to avoid the hazard of bolus dose with injection of other drugs or volume.
Specific Rx Overdose:	Support patient.

Ketoconazole

Indications for Use:	*Candida* infections (excluding meningitis)
Mechanism of Action:	Inhibits synthesis of ergosterol in fungi
Individual Dose:	5 mg/kg
Interval:	Daily
Route:	Oral
Total Daily Dose:	5 mg/ml
Comments/Cautions:	Interferes with cytochrome P-450 enzyme system in gonads, adrenals, kidneys, and liver, which in higher dose leads to reduced cortisol and testerone production (long-term effects?). Displaces estradiol and dihydrotestosterone from sex-hormone binding globulin. Mild GI upsets, rarely hepatitis. Avoid co-administration with cimetidine or antacids.
Metabolism/Excretion:	Mostly metabolized in liver to inactive substance. Small amount appears in the urine.
Storage:	Room temperature

Magnesium Sulfate

Indications for Use:	Hypomagnesemia
Mechanism of Action:	An essential activator for approximately 300 enzymes and a necessary co-factor for APTase. Involved in oxidative phosphorylation, neuromuscular excitability, and muscular contraction. Slows SA nodal impulse formation and prolongs conduction time.
Individual Dose:	0.1 ml/kg of 50% solution (i.e., 50 mg/kg)
Interval:	Every 6 hr for 4 doses (check serum Mg++ between doses)
Route:	IV (over 10-15 min) or IM (preferred)
Comments/Cautions:	Hypotension, CNS, and respiratory depression may all occur. Contraindicated in renal failure.
Metabolism/Excretion:	Renal excretion
Dilution:	1. IM: no dilution necessary 2. IV: dilute dose to 1 ml with normal saline
Stability:	Discard ampule and unused portion after initial use.
Storage:	Room temperature
Incompatible with:	TPN, NaHCO$_3$, calcium solutions, hydrocortisone
Specific Rx Overdose:	Calcium gluconate

Midazolam

Indications for Use:	Sedation
Mechanism of Action:	Binds to CNS benzodiazepine receptors
Individual Dose:	1. Infusion
	a. Loading dose: 0.2 mg/kg over 5 min
	b. Maintenance: 0.4-2 µg/kg/min
	2. Stat dose: 0.2 mg/kg over 5 min
Interval:	For 1. above, continuous infusion
	For 2., every 4 hr; continuous infusion preferred
Route:	IV
Comments/Cautions:	There is very little information relating to the use of midazolam in newborn infants. Causes respiratory depression and hypotension (less commonly). These effects may be potentiated by concomitant use of opioids or barbiturates.
Metabolism/Excretion:	Extensively metabolized by the liver. Metabolism decreased by concomitant use of cimetidine or ranitidine. Principal metabolite alpha-hydroxymidazolam has weaker hypnotic effects than midazolam itself.
Dilution:	1. Loading dose/stat dose: make up required dose to 1 ml with 5% dextrose
	2. Infusion: make midazolam, 2.4 mg/kg, up to 25 ml with 5% dextrose/normal saline: 0.25 ml/hr = 0.4 µg/kg/min
Stability:	Reconstitute infusion every 24 hr.
Storage:	Room temperature
Incompatible with:	Henobarbitone, ranitidine
Specific Rx Overdose:	Flumazenil (Anexate)

Morphine

Indications for Use:	Pain relief
Mechanism of Action:	Binds to opioid receptors in CNS (especially beta receptor). Releases histamine—vasodilation and decreased BP.
Individual Dose:	1. Bolus: 0.1 mg/kg
	2. Infusion
Interval:	For 1. above,
	a. Term infant: every 4-6 hr
	b. 31-37 wk: every 6 hr
	c. 28-31 wk: every 8 hr
	d. <29 wk: every 10 hr
	For 2., continuous infusion
	a. Term infant: maximum 15 µg/kg/hr
	b. Preterm infant: maximum 10 µg/kg/hr
Route:	For 1. above, IM or IV (over 5 min)
	For 2., IV
Comments/Cautions:	Bolus may cause hypotension. All routes will depress respiration and decrease bowel mobility.
Metabolism/Excretion:	Very little excreted unchanged in urine. Hepatic conjugation.
Dilution:	IV: dilute to 1 ml with sterile water
Storage:	Room temperature; protect ampule from light (not infusion). Locked in dangerous-drug cupboard. Make fresh solution after 24 hr.

Incompatible with:	Sodium bicarbonate, iodides, sulfas, thiopental, sodium, phenytoin, aminophylline, phenobarbital, heparin, methicillin, Pethidine
Specific Rx Overdose:	Naloxone: 0.01 mg/kg IV or IM. Assisted ventilation if required.

Naloxone

Indications for Use:	1. Opiate drug depression 2. Refractory apnea of prematurity 3. Refractory hypotension in septicemia
Mechanism of Action:	Competitive antagonist at opioid receptors
Individual Dose:	For 1. above, 0.1 mg/kg For 2. and 3., 0.1-0.5 mg/kg/hr (begin at lowest dose)
Interval:	For 1. above, stat: repeat $\times$ 3 if necessary For 2. and 3., continuous infusion
Route:	For 1. above, SC, IM, IV For 2. and 3., IV
Comments/Cautions:	Exercise caution when administering drug to infants of known or suspected drug addicts: precipitates withdrawal syndrome. Ensure adequate therapeutic theophylline level before beginning infusion for apnea (synergistic action).
Metabolism/Excretion:	Conjugated in liver
Stability:	Discard ampule and unused portion after initial use. Infusion stable for 24 hr.
Storage:	Room temperature

Neostigmine

Indications for Use:	1. Reversal of nondepolarizing neuromuscular blockers 2. Treatment of myasthenia gravis
Mechanism of Action:	Cholinesterase antagonist leads to acetylcholine accumulation at cholinergic receptor sites; therefore the effects are prolonged or exaggerated.

Individual Dose:	For 1. above, 0.05 mg/kg (mixed in same syringe with atropine, 0.025 mg/kg)
	For 2., initial dose 0.1 mg IM 30 min prefeed, then:
	  a. 0.05-0.25 mg IV every 4 hr 30 min prefeed, *or*
	  b. 1 mg PO 2 hr prefeed
	Maintenance doses may need to be increased.

Interval:	For 1. above, may need repeating after 12-24 hr if neuromuscular blockade recurs For 2., see individual dosage
Route:	For 1. above, IV or IM For 2., see individual dosage
Comments/Cautions:	May cause bradycardia, hypotension, salivation, bronchorrhea, increased bowel activity. Overdose causes nondepolarizing neuromuscular blockade (i.e., paralysis).
Metabolism/Excretion:	Degraded by plasma esterases. Degradation products and parent compound both excreted in urine.
Dilution:	Not required
Stability:	Discard unused portion.
Storage:	Room temperature; protect from light

Incompatible with:	Suxamethonium, $NaHCO_3$
Specific Rx Overdose:	Ventilation, atropine, anticonvulsants (if seizures occur)

Netilmicin

Indications for Use:	Suspected/proven sepsis after the first week of life
Contraindications:	Renal failure or a history of adverse reaction to aminoglycosides
Mechanism of Action:	Inhibits bacterial protein synthesis at the ribosome
Individual Dose:	1. Loading dose: 5 mg/kg (made up to 1 ml if 1500 g, or 2 ml if >1500 g) 2. Maintenance dose: 4 mg/kg

Interval:	Corrected Gestation (wk)	Initial Maintenance (following load)	Subsequent Doses
	<32	36 hr	Every 36 hr
	>31	36 hr	Every 24 hr

(**Note:** This dose regimen is for infants >7 days of age.)

Route:	For 1. above, infuse IV over 1 hr (Graseby Pump) For 2., IV over 20 min (preferred), IM
Comments/Cautions:	Ototoxicity, nephrotoxicity. Variable CSF penetration.
Metabolism/Excretion:	Excreted unchanged in the urine
Dilution:	Make up to 1-2 ml with normal saline or 10% dextrose.
Stability:	Open vial: 24 hr in refrigerator
Storage:	Room temperature; store below 25°C. **Do not freeze.**
Incompatible with:	TPN, most other drugs
Serum Levels:	Check on third dose (or on second dose if suspected renal impairment). Trough <3 μg/ml. Peak 6-10 μg/ml.

Nitroglycerin

Indications for Use:	Hypertension. To improve peripheral perfusion in the presence of an adequate circulating volume and cardiac output.
Mechanism of Action:	Vasodilator, which is dependent on protein kinase in vascular smooth muscle. In the vascular system it acts largely on the systemic veins and coronary arteries.
Individual Dose:	1-10 μg/kg/min
Interval:	Continuous infusion
Route:	IV
Comments/Cautions:	Limited experience in newborn infants. Hypotension uncommon. Methemaglobinemia is a potential problem. **Use polyethylene-lined syringe and tubing (not PVC).**
Metabolism/Excretion:	Hydrolyzed in liver to less active metabolites
Stability:	Infusion stable for 48 hr at room temperature
Storage:	Room temperature
Incompatible with:	None known

Nitroprusside

Indications for Use:	Hypertension, congestive heart failure (decreased after load) to improve peripheral perfusion (in presence of adequate BP)

Mechanism of Action:	Directly relaxes arteriolar and venous smooth muscles
Individual Dose:	0.5 µg/kg/min, increasing to 5 µg/kg/min
Route:	IV infusion (protect from light)
Comments/Cautions:	Slight tachycardia is common. Hypotension, restlessness, twitching may be seen. Prolonged use leads to cyanide poisoning (see below). Limit continuous infusion period to 3 days.
Metabolism/Excretion:	Metabolized by rapid uptake into red blood cells and release of cyanide (converted in liver to thiocyanate)
Stability:	A fresh solution should be made every 24 hr. Protect infusion from light.
Storage:	Room temperature
Incompatible with:	Most other drugs
Specific Rx Overdose:	Stop infusion. Cyanide intoxication: Rx sodium nitrate.

Norepinephrine

Indications for Use:	Refractory hypotension
Mechanism of Action:	$Beta_1$ stimulant (similar to adrenaline), $alpha_1$ stimulant (less than adrenaline). Weak $beta_2$ action.
Individual Dose:	0.05-0.5 µg/kg/min
Interval:	Continuous infusion
Route:	IV (preferably central venous line [CVL])
Comments/Cautions:	Increases coronary blood flow. Reduces splanchnic and hepatic blood flow. May cause arrhythmias and hyperglycemia (less so than adrenaline).
Metabolism/Excretion:	Metabolized by catecholomethyl transferase and monoamine oxidase
Stability:	Discard unused portion. Reconstitute solution every 24 hr.
Storage:	Room temperature
Incompatible with:	Alkali, barbiturates, phenytoin
Specific Rx Overdose:	Treat cardiac arrhythmias

Pancuronium

Indications for Use:	Skeletal muscle paralysis (usually to assist ventilation)
Mechanism of Action:	Competitive neuromuscular blockade. Binds to cholinergic receptor site at the postjunctional membrane and thereby blocks competitively the transmitter action of acetylcholine.
Individual Dose:	0.1 mg/kg
Interval:	Repeat as necessary every 1-4 hr
Route:	IV
Comments/Cautions:	Causes respiratory paralysis, therefore needs ventilation. Vagolytic effect causes tachycardia and elevation in blood pressure. Does not release histamine.
Metabolism/Excretion:	Partially hydroxylated by liver; 40% excreted unchanged in urine
Dilution:	None required
Stability:	Discard ampule and unused portion after initial use.
Storage:	Refrigerate; **do not freeze.**
Incompatible with:	All other drugs
Specific Rx Overdose:	Ventilation. Reversed by neostigmine and atropine (combination).

Paracetamol Acetaminophen

Indications for Use:	Analgesia
Mechanism of Action:	Uncertain; may inhibit local prostaglandin production
Individual Dose:	1. 10-15 mg/kg 2. 20-25 mg/kg
Interval:	Every 6-8 hr
Route:	For 1. above, PO For 2., rectal
Comments/Cautions:	Limited data available for neonates. Hepatic necrosis (excessive doses), bone marrow depression, rash, fever.
Metabolism/Excretion:	Variable rectal absorption. $T_{1/2}$: 2-5 hr (prolonged in rectal failure). Metabolized in liver, primarily sulfation (little glucuronidation), and then renally excreted.
Stability:	Months
Storage:	Room temperature
Incompatible with:	Unknown
Specific Rx Overdose:	Acetylcysteine (Parvolex)
Serum Levels:	Toxic levels in newborn—unknown

Paraldehyde

Indications for Use:	Convulsions
Mechanism of Action:	Generalized CNS depression: hypnotic, anticonvulsant

Individual Dose:	1. IV infusion: loading dose: 200 mg/kg (4 ml/kg of 5% solution); maintenance dose: 16 mg/kg/hr (0.3 ml/kg/hr of 5% solution)
	  a. Add 1 ml of paraldehyde to 19 ml of 5% dextrose (i.e., make a 5% solution) (200 mg/kg)
	  b. Give 4 ml/kg over 1 hr (5% solution)
	  c. Continue to infuse 0.3 ml/kg/hr (5% solution)
	  d. If seizures continue after 1-hr continuous infusion, repeat loading dose of 4 ml/kg over 1 hr, then continue infusion at 0.3 ml/kg/hr
	2. IM: 0.2 ml/kg
	3. Rectal: 0.2 ml/kg

Interval:	For 1. above, continuous infusion For 2., every 6 hr For 3., every 2 hr
Comments/Cautions:	Plastic syringe and tubing can be used. Protect from light during infusion. May cause prolonged unconsciousness, respiratory depression, pulmonary edema, impaired renal function, skin rashes.
Metabolism/Excretion:	70%-80% metabolized in liver, 20% exhaled. Small amount appears in urine.
Stability:	Use immediately after opening. Discard ampule and unused portion after initial use. Make fresh solution (infusion) after 24 hr.
Storage:	Cool place; protect from light
Incompatible with:	Do not mix with other drugs.
Specific Rx Overdose:	Correct acidosis; support cardiorespiratory function; hydrocortisone

Penicillin (Benzyl)

Indications for Use:	Treatment of infection caused by penicillin-sensitive organisms
Mechanism of Action:	Inhibits bacterial cell wall synthesis through interaction with penicillin-binding proteins
Individual Dose:	1. 15 mg/kg: local infection or colonization 2. 45 mg/kg: septicemia 3. 60 mg/kg: meningitis

Interval:	1. Infants <2000 g
	   a. Every 12 hr for days 0-7
	   b. Every 8 hr for days >7
	2. Infants >2000 g
	   a. Every 8 hr for days 0-7
	   b. Every 6 hr for days >7

Route:	IV (preferred), IM
Comments/Cautions:	Larger dosages recommended for treatment of group B streptococcal meningitis than for pneumococcal meningitis; excessive dosage (150 mg/kg/day) should be avoided because of possible CNS toxicity.
Metabolism/Excretion:	Renal excretion; small amount via bile
Stability:	Discard 30 min after reconstitution.
Storage:	Refrigerate.
Incompatible with:	TPN, phenytoin, sodium, adrenaline, methylprednisolone. Incompatible in solution with aminoglycoside antibodies, heparin, cephalothin, amphotericin.
Serum Levels:	Not required 15 mg = 25,000 units. This is the direct conversion from units to milligrams for penicillin; it is just useful information.

Phenobarbitone Sodium (Phenobarbital)

Indications for Use:	1. Convulsions 2. Sedation
Mechanism of Action:	Depression of reticular activating system and enhancement of gamma-aminobutyric acid binding to neuroinhibitory receptors

Individual Dose:	For 1. above,
	   a. Loading dose: 30 mg/kg (term), 20 mg/kg (preterm)
	   b. Then maintenance dose of 5 mg/kg (starting 24 hr after loading dose) *or* 2.5 mg/kg in the presence of significant asphyxia or renal failure
	For 2.,
	   a. 5-10 mg/kg initially
	   b. Then maintenance dose as above (if required)

Interval:	Daily beginning 24 hr after loading dose
Route:	IV slowly over 20 min IM, PO
Comments/Cautions:	Overdose may cause hypoventilation, hypotension, hypothermia, renal failure, decreased clotting factors. Withdrawal symptoms after prolonged use.
Metabolism/Excretion:	25% excreted unchanged in urine. Remainder metabolized to inactive metabolites in liver and

Metabolism/ Excretion:	excreted in urine. $T_{1/2}$: varies with duration of treatment (and maturity); initially 100-150 hr falling to 30-60 hr by 4 wk of therapy.
Dilution:	IV: dilute to desired volume with 0.9% saline
Stability:	Discard ampule and unused portion after initial use.
Storage:	Room temperature
Incompatible with:	Phenytoin, erythromycin, hydrocortisone
Specific Rx Overdose:	Maintain respirations; treat shock; eliminate drug (diuretics and dialysis).
Serum Levels:	Measure at 48 hr and at 5-7 days or earlier if indicated. Therapeutic range: 65-130 μmol/L

Phenytoin

Indications for Use:	Convulsions
Mechanism of Action:	Stabilizes neuronal membranes
Individual Dose:	1. Loading dose: 15 mg/kg
	2. Maintenance dose: 5 mg/kg (beginning 24 hr after loading dose)
Interval:	Daily
Route:	IV over 5 min; IM and PO routes ineffective in newborn infants
Comments/Cautions:	Thrombophlebitis, bone marrow depression, hypotension
Metabolism/Excretion:	5% excreted unchanged in urine. Remainder metabolized in liver to inactive metabolites and excreted in bile and urine. $T_{1/2}$: 80-120 hr during first postnatal week.
Stability:	Discard ampule and unused portion after initial use.
Storage:	Room temperature
Incompatible with:	Most medications. Flush line before and after administration with normal saline.
Specific Rx Overdose:	Ventilation, exchange transfusion
Serum Levels:	48 hr after loading dose, then weekly thereafter. Therapeutic levels: 40-80 μmol/L.

Piperacillin

Indications for Use:	Infections caused by organisms sensitive to piperacillin, especially *Klebsiella* species and *Pseudomonas* species
Mechanism of Action:	Inhibits bacterial cell wall synthesis through interaction with penicillin-binding proteins
Individual Dose:	1. Sepsis: 100 mg/kg
	2. Meningitis: 150 mg/kg
Interval:	Every 12 hr
Route:	IV or IM (painful)
Total Daily Dose:	<300 mg/kg/day
Comments/Cautions:	Can be inactivated by beta lactamases. Effective synergism when combined with aminoglycoside. Low sodium content (1.98 mmol/g). Diarrhea, skin rash, transient leukopenia, and transient increase in alanine aminotransferase (ALT), aspartate aminotransferase (AST).
Metabolism/Excretion:	Predominantly excreted unchanged in urine. Remainder excreted in bile.

Dilution:	Reconstitute dry powder with 8.6 ml sterile water for injection, making a concentration in vial of 200 mg/ml. Dilute further with sterile water for injection if necessary.
Stability:	24 hr after reconstitution
Storage:	Below 25° C
Incompatible with:	Do not mix with other drugs in solution.
Serum Levels:	Not routinely measured

Potassium Chloride

Indications for Use:	1. Daily maintenance 2. Hypokalemia
Mechanism of Action:	Involved in membrane stability and neural excitability

Individual Dose:	1. Maintenance: 3 mmol/kg/day
	2. Hypokalemia
	   a. 2.5-3.0 mmol/L: double maintenance amount and check serum potassium in 6 hr
	   b. <2.5 mmol/L (or symptomatic hypokalemia): 1 mmol/kg over 6 hr; ECG monitoring

Interval:	1. Maintenance: daily 2. Hypokalemia: check serum K+ every 6 hr and review
Route:	1. Maintenance or asymptomatic hypokalemia: PO or IV 2. Symptomatic hypokalemia or serum K+ <2.5 mmol/L: IV
Comments/Cautions:	Potassium is renally excreted; therefore administer with caution in the presence of renal impairment or following birth asphyxia.
Metabolism/Excretion:	Renal excretion
Dilution:	As required
Stability:	Discard unused portion of ampule immediately.
Storage:	Room temperature
Incompatible with:	Amphotericin
Specific Rx Overdose:	CPR, $CaCl_2$, $NaHCO_3$
Serum Levels:	3-5 mmol/L

Prostacyclin

Indications for Use:	Persistent pulmonary hypertension of newborn (PPHN)
Mechanism of Action:	Vasodilation of pulmonary system more than systemic (especially in presence of hypoxia). Inhibits platelet aggregation by elevating platelet cAMP.
Individual Dose:	1-30 ng/kg/min
Interval:	Continuous infusion
Route:	IV
Comments/Cautions:	Limited experience in newborn. Bleeding and hypotension may occur—both are reversible and disappear within 30 min of ceasing infusion.
Metabolism/Excretion:	Not fully understood. Majority hydrolyzed and excreted in urine. $T_{1/2}$: 2-3 min.
Stability:	Make fresh solution every 12 hr.
Storage:	2°-8° C. Protect from light.
Incompatible with:	All fluids, except 0.9% normal saline
Specific Rx Overdose:	Hypotension: reduce or discontinue infusion and expand plasma volume

Prostaglandin E$_1$

Indications for Use:	Patent ductus arteriosus (PDA)–dependent congenital heart disease
Mechanism of Action:	Relaxes ductus arteriosus via unknown mechanism
Individual Dose:	0.01 µg/kg/min initially, then increase stepwise up to 0.05 µg/kg/min (if inadequate response)
Interval:	Continuous infusion
Route:	IV
Comments/Cautions:	Apnea occurs in 10%-20% of neonates, usually in those weighing <2 kg and during the first hour of the infusion. Fever, diarrhea, seizures, hypotension have all been noted. High doses cause medial edema of the ductus and make surgery more difficult.
Metabolism/Excretion:	Metabolized (oxidation) in the lungs and metabolites excreted in the urine. No active drug in urine.
Stability:	Change infusion every 24 hr.
Storage:	Up to 2 yr in refrigerator (2°-8° C)

Pyridoxine (Vitamin B$_6$)

Indications for Use:	Treatment of pyridoxine-dependent seizures
Mechanism of Action:	Pyridoxine is essential in the synthesis of gamma-aminobutyric acid (GABA), an inhibitory neurotransmitter in the CNS. GABA increases the seizure threshold.
Individual Dose:	1. Diagnostic dose: 100 mg 2. Maintenance dose: 100 mg
Interval:	For 1. above, single dose with electroencephalogram (EEG) monitoring For 2., daily
Route:	For 1. above, IV over 5 min For 2., IV, IM, or PO
Comments/Cautions:	May cause respiratory depression
Metabolism/Excretion:	Metabolized in liver to 4-pyridoxic acid
Dilution:	Not required
Stability:	Discard ampule and unused portion after initial dose.
Storage:	Room temperature; protect from light

Racemic Adrenaline

Dose:	0.05 ml/kg
Interval:	Every 4-6 hr
Comments/Cautions:	Use to prevent laryngeal edema after long-term ventilation; may be used concurrently with dexamethasone or prednisolone. May cause tachycardia, arrhythmias, poor peripheral circulation, and sweating although blood pressure is normal or elevated. Cease Rx if tachycardia becomes too great. Gastric distention, bleeding, or paralytic ileus may occur. Hyperglycemia and hypokalemia have also been reported.
Dilution:	Dilute in 2 ml of inhalation diluent.
Storage:	Protect from light.
Specific Rx Overdose:	Cease treatment; support patient.
Indications for Use:	Bronchitis, croup, epiglottal edema reduction and upper airway resistance following intubation then

Indications for Use:	used to prevent edema post long-term ventilation. This medication may be used concurrently with dexamethasone and/or prednisolone.
Onset of Action:	Within 5 min
Duration of Action:	1 to 3 hr

Ranitidine

Indications for Use:	Acute upper GI tract hemorrhage
Mechanism of Action:	Competitive antagonist of histamine on H_2 receptor. Inhibits gastric acid secretion. No effect on H_1 receptor.
Individual Dose:	1. 0.5 mg/kg (gestation <37 wk)
	2. 1.5 mg/kg (gestation >37 wk)
Interval:	For 1. above, every 12 hr
	For 2., every 8 hr
Route:	IV slowly over 45 min
Total Daily Dose:	4.5 mg/kg
Comments/Cautions:	Limited data on use in neonates. Diarrhea, constipation, somnolence, granulocytopenia, and impaired liver function have been reported in adults. Does not reverse the effects of tolazoline.
Metabolism/Excretion:	Primarily excreted unchanged in the urine. Some hepatic excretion.
Stability:	Stable for 24 hr following dilution
Storage:	Below 25°C. Protect from light.
Incompatible with:	None known
Specific Rx Overdose:	None known
Serum Levels:	Not available

Salbutamol

Indications for Use:	1. Bronchospasm, chronic lung disease (nebulizer)
	2. Hyperkalemia (IV)
Mechanism of Action:	$Beta_2$ sympathomimetic, relaxes bronchial musculature
Individual Dose:	For 1. above, 0.5 mg (i.e., 0.5 ml made up to 2 ml with 0.9% saline). Nebulize until chamber empty.
	For 2., 4 µg/kg diluted to 2 ml with water
Interval:	For 1. above, PRN up to every 4 hr
	For 2., every 2 hr up to 2 doses
Route:	For 1. above, via nebulizer running air/oxygen mixture at 8-10 L/min
	For 2., IV over 20 min
Comments/Cautions:	Tachycardia, hypertension, tremor may be seen at higher dosage.
Metabolism/Excretion:	Metabolized in liver via monoamine oxidase and catecholomethyl transferase enzyme systems.
Dilution:	For 1. above, 0.9% normal saline
	For 2., water for injection
Stability:	Discard unused portion.
Storage:	Room temperature
Incompatible with:	TPN

Sodium Bicarbonate

Indications for Use:	1. Cardiac resuscitation
	2. Correction of metabolic acidosis
	3. Induction of metabolic alkalosis in PPHN

Mechanism of Action:	HCO_3^- binds to H^+ $\rightarrow H_2O + CO_2$
Individual Dose:	For 1. above, 1-3 mmol/kg For 2., if base excess -5 to -8, give 1 mmol/kg; if -8 to -12, give 2 mmol/kg; if >-12, give 3 mmol/kg For 3., 6-12 mmol/kg/day
Interval:	For 1. above, stat; repeat every 10 min if necessary For 2., according to blood gases For 3., daily infusion
Route:	For 1. and 2. above, IV for 20-30 min For 3., IV infusion

Comments/Cautions:	Rapid administration may cause intraventricular
	  hemorrhage (IVH). Hyperosmolar
	  (1680 mOsmol/L); therefore dilute twofold to
	  fourfold with sterile water for injection. May
	  temporarily increase $PaCO_2$ and therefore reduce
	  pulmonary artery blood flow; increases sodium
	  load.

Metabolism/Excretion:	Converted to H_2O and CO_2
Supplied as:	Sodium bicarbonate 8.4% solution

Dilution:	For 1. and 2. above, 1 part sodium bicarbonate to 2-4
	  parts water for injection
	For 3., dilute with sterile H_2O, 5%-10% dextrose as
	  indicated

Stability:	Discard unused portion after initial use.
Storage:	Room temperature
Incompatible with:	TPN, calcium, neostigmine

Sodium Chloride

Indications for Use:	1. Daily maintenance 2. Hyponatremia
Mechanism of Action:	Major extracellular cation involved in membrane stability, neural excitability, and fluid distribution

Individual Dose:	1. Maintenance: 3 mmol/kg/day (may be considerably
	  more in preterm infants, i.e., 4-10 mmol/kg/day)
	2. Hyponatremia
	  a. [Na] 130-135 mmol/L: double maintenance and
	    check in 6-8 hr
	  b. [Na] <130 mmol/L: correct IV over 6 hr
	Formula for Correction:
	Sodium deficit (mmol/L) = (135 − SNa) × total
	  body weight (0.6 × wt in kg) in which SNa represents
	  the measured serum sodium concentration.

Interval:	1. Maintenance: daily 2. Hyponatremia: check serum Na^+ every 6 hr and review
Route:	1. Maintenance or mild hyponatremia (Na >130 mmol/L): PO or IV 2. Hyponatremia (Na <130 mmol/L): IV over 6 hr

Comments/Cautions:	Changes in the serum Na levels are accompanied by
	  similar changes in osmolarity; which may affect
	  cerebral water content. Prolonged hyponatremia
	  (>24 hr) requires more cautious correction of
	  serum Na.

Metabolism/Excretion:	Renal excretion

Stability:	Discard unused portion of vial immediately.
Storage:	Room temperature
Incompatible with:	None known

Spironolactone

Indications for Use:	Secondary hyperaldosteronism as seen in syndrome of inappropriate antidiuretic hormone secretion (SIADH) or ascites
Mechanism of Action:	Competitive inhibition of aldosterone in distal tubules and collecting system
Individual Dose:	1 mg/kg
Interval:	Every 12 hr
Route:	PO
Comments/Cautions:	Do not use in presence of renal failure or hyperkalemia.
Metabolism/Excretion:	70% of oral dose absorbed. Hepatic metabolism to canrenone and canrenoate, the former being an aldosterone antagonist.
Stability:	1 mo
Storage:	Refrigerate.

Survanta

Indications for Use:	Respiratory distress syndrome
Mechanism of Action:	Modified bovine surfactant. Reduces alveolar surface tension.
Individual Dose:	4 ml/kg
Interval:	Every 8-12 hr (maximum 4 doses)
Route:	Via endotracheal tube as rapidly as tolerated
Comments/Cautions:	Desaturation may accompany administration. Rapid change in oxygenation and compliance may follow administration. Should be warmed for 20 min at room temperature before use.
Metabolism/Excretion:	Local degradation
Supplied as:	8-ml vial (contains 200 mg phospholipid)
Dilution:	None
Stability:	Unopened vials should be returned to refrigerator within 8 hr of warming. Discard unused portion of vial.
Storage:	Refrigerate at 2°-8° C.

Suxamethonium

Indications for Use:	Skeletal muscle paralysis (to assist intubation)
Mechanism of Action:	Depolarizing agent. Sustained depolarization at neuromuscular junction resulting in a brief period of repetitive excitation (fasciculation may be seen), followed by flaccid paralysis.
Individual Dose:	3 mg/kg
Interval:	May be repeated but beware that repeated doses increase the risk of severe bradycardia
Route:	IV, IM, umbilical arterial catheter
Comments/Cautions:	Precede IV suxamethonium with atropine (to avoid bradycardia). May elevate potassium in patients with already raised [K+]. Known to cause malignant

Comments/ Cautions:	hyperthermia in susceptible patients and chest wall rigidity in patients with myotonia. Bradycardia caused by vagal ganglia stimulation.
Metabolism/Excretion:	Rapidly hydrolyzed by pseudocholinesterase in plasma
Dilution:	Sterile water or saline if necessary
Stability:	Discard ampule and unused portion after initial use.
Storage:	Refrigerate; **do not freeze**.
Incompatible with:	Other drugs
Specific Rx Overdose:	Mechanical ventilation. Atropine for bradycardia. Do not give neostigmine; this may potentiate the paralysis.

Theophylline

Indications for Use:	1. Recurrent apnea or poor respiratory drive in preterm infants 2. To assist weaning from ventilator 3. To reduce airways' resistance in infants with chronic lung disease
Mechanism of Action:	Direct stimulation of respiratory center. Reduces diaphragmatic fatigue, increasing bronchial smooth muscle cAMP via phosphodiesterase inhibition.
Individual Dose:	1. Loading dose: 8 mg/kg followed 12 hr later by maintenance dose 2. Maintenance dose: 2 mg/kg in first 2 wk of life; 4 mg/kg for age >2 wk
Interval:	Every 12 hr
Route:	PO
Comments/Cautions:	The maintenance doses are starting doses only and should be adjusted according to serum levels. When changing from aminophylline to theophylline (with serum levels satisfactory) Rx the same dose of theophylline as was prescribed for aminophylline. Should be omitted if the heart rate is persistently greater than 180/min. If used concurrently with erythromycin, theophylline levels may be increased. A transient diuretic effect is experienced. Theophylline may cause an increase in serum uric acid levels. Complications include GI bleeding, hypotension, vomiting, tachycardia, tachypnea, and convulsions. $T_{1/2} \sim 30$ hr (range 15-60 hr).
Metabolism/Excretion:	Hepatic transformation and urinary excretion of metabolites. Caffeine (a metabolite of theophylline) can reach levels 50% those of theophylline and exert a significant stimulatory effect.
Stability:	Until expiration date
Storage:	Room temperature; **do not refrigerate.**
Incompatible with:	Acidic solutions, phenobarbital, phenytoin, penicillins, vitamins
Serum Levels:	40-90 μmol/L

Thiopental

Indications for Use:	Convulsions uncontrolled by conventional anticonvulsant agents

Mechanism of Action:	General CNS depressant. Facilitates GABA-ergic inhibition.
Individual Dose:	1. Loading dose: 10 mg/kg over 30 min 2. Maintenance dose: 1-2 mg/kg/hr as continuous infusion
Interval:	Continuous infusion
Route:	IV
Comments/Cautions:	Depresses ventilation (ensure patient intubated before initiation). Hypotension may occur. Increases the rate of metabolism of hepatic cytochrome P-450 metabolized drugs and steroids (vitamin D).
Metabolism/Excretion:	Highly lipid soluble—rapid brain uptake. No correlation between duration of action and elimination half-life. Biotransformation (oxidation) primarily in the liver. Small amount of renal excretion.
Stability:	Make fresh solution every 24 hr.
Storage:	Room temperature
Incompatible with:	TPN
Serum Levels:	150-200 μmol/L

Tobramycin

Indications for Use:	Treatment of infections caused by tobramycin-sensitive organisms, especially *Pseudomonas* species
Mechanism of Action:	Inhibits bacterial protein synthesis by interfering with mRNA at ribosomal level
Individual Dose:	2 mg/kg

Interval:	1. Age 0-7 days: every 12 hr
	2. Age >7 days
	   a. <2000 g: every 12 hr
	   b. >2000 g: every 8 hr

Route:	IV/IM
Total Daily Dose:	1. 4 mg/kg for infants 0-7 days 2. 6 mg/kg for infants >7 days and >2000 g
Comments/Cautions:	Potential ototoxicity and nephrotoxicity. Superior activity against *Pseudomonas* sepsis (compare with gentamicin). Poor synergy with penicillin against enterococci (compare with gentamicin).
Metabolism/Excretion:	Excreted unchanged in urine
Dilution:	1. IM: no dilution 2. IV: dilute requested dose with 1.2 ml water for injection
Stability:	Discard after 24 hr.
Storage:	Room temperature
Incompatible with:	TPN. Do not mix with other drugs in solution.
Serum Levels:	Trough <2 μg/ml. Peak 5-8 μg/ml.

Tolazoline

Indications for Use:	1. Persistent pulmonary hypertension of newborn 2. Lower limb ischemia secondary to umbilical arterial catheter (UAC)

Mechanism of Action:	Alpha-adrenergic blocker; direct effect on vascular smooth muscle $\rightarrow$ vasodilation. Histamine-like effects.
Individual Dose:	0.25-0.5 mg/kg/hr
Interval:	Continuous infusion
Route:	1. IV for PPHN
	2. Intraaortic for UAC complications
Comments/Cautions:	Clinical response unpredictable: nonselective effects on both pulmonary and systemic circulation (approximately 50% of infants with PPHN may derive benefit). Hypotension and diminished cardiac output (direct depressant effect on myocardium) may be seen. Loss of hypoxic vasoconstriction reflex (pulmonary) and worsening of V/Q matching. GI bleeding and thrombocytopenia.
Metabolism/Excretion:	Median $T_{1/2}$ ~ 5 hr. Largely excreted unchanged in urine; therefore use with caution in presence of oliguria.
Stability:	Discard unused portion in ampule immediately after initial use. Change infusions every 24 hr.
Storage:	Room temperature; protect ampule from light (not infusion)
Incompatible with:	No specific interaction known
Specific Rx Overdose:	Volume, inotropes. Cease infusion of tolazoline.

Tromethamine (THAM)

Indications for Use:	Metabolic acidosis, when $NaHCO_3$ is contraindicated because of elevated serum sodium or $PaCO_2$
Mechanism of Action:	Tromethamine acts as a proton acceptor actively binding H+. Binds to the cations not only of fixed and metabolic acids but also of carbonic acid, increasing HCO_3 (thus lowering $PaCO_2$). $H_2O + CO_2 = H_2CO_3 = H+ + HCO_3$
Individual Dose:	3-5 ml/kg
Interval:	Repeat after 15 min.
Route:	IV over 20 min
Comments/Cautions:	Hepatic necrosis if administered via malplaced umbili venous catheter (UVC) Hyperkalemia, hypoglycemia, and respiratory depression ($PaCO_2$). Extravasation may cause skin sloughing (infiltrate skin with hyaluronidase if this occurs). Do not use if patient in renal failure.
Metabolism/Excretion:	Renally excreted
Dilution:	Not necessary
Stability:	Single-use bottle only (contains no bacteriostatic agent); therefore discard after use
Storage:	Room temperature
Incompatible with:	TPN

Vancomycin

Indications for Use:	Methicillin-resistant staphylococcal infections
Mechanism of Action:	Inhibits cell wall synthesis by binding to cell wall precursors

Individual Dose:	15 mg/kg			
Interval:	Gestation (wk)	<27	27-31	32-37	>37
	Interval (hr)	36	24	18	12
Route:	IV slowly over 30 min			
Comments/Cautions:	Thrombophlebitis, necrosis of tissues if extravasates. Convulsions, eosinophilia, and anaphylaxis have been reported. Nephrotoxicity and ototoxicity (especially with concomitant use of aminoglycosides).			
Metabolism/Excretion:	Not metabolized, excreted unchanged in urine			
Storage:	Room temperature			
Incompatible with:	Other drugs and TPN, heparin. Flush IV Luer with nonheparinized saline before and after vancomycin dose, then final flush with heparinized saline.			
Specific Rx Overdose:	Peak: 30 mg/L (must be monitored; contact microbiology). Trough: 6 mg/L.			

Vasopressin (8-Arginine Vasopressin)

Indications for Use:	Refractory hypotension
Contraindications:	None known
Mechanism of Action:	Increases systemic vascular resistance
Individual Dose:	0.0005–0.001 unit/kg/min
Interval:	Continuous infusion only
Route:	Central line/UVC
Comments/Cautions:	Cutaneous vasoconstriction, skin necrosis, and GI upset may occur. Hyponatremia (through binding to V_2 receptor) may occur. *Do not use Pitressin Tannate (oil-based).*
Special Observations:	Monitor renal output and serum sodium every 6 hr initially.
Metabolism/Excretion:	Minimal renal excretion. Predominantly cleared to inactive form in liver and kidney.
Supplied As:	20 units/ml, 1-ml ampules
Trade Name:	Pitressin (Parke-Davis)
Dilution:	Make 1.5 unit/kg up to 25 ml with 5%-10% dextrose or saline (0.5 ml/hr = 0.0005 unit/kg/min).
Stability:	Discard unused portion of vial.
Storage:	Room temperature
Incompatible with:	None known
Specific Rx Overdose:	Stop infusion.

Vecuronium

Indications for Use:	Neuromuscular blockage
Mechanism of Action:	Competitive inhibition of neuromuscular transmission
Individual Dose:	0.1 mg/kg
Interval:	Repeat as necessary.
Route:	IV
Comments/Cautions:	Causes respiratory paralysis, therefore needs ventilation. No release of histamine.
Metabolism/Excretion:	50% excreted unchanged in bile, 25% excreted unchanged in urine, and 25% metabolized in liver.
Stability:	Discard remainder of ampule.
Storage:	Stable at room temperature in powder form

Incompatible with:	Most other drugs
Specific Rx Overdose:	Continued artificial ventilation
Serum Levels:	Not necessary

Vitamin K1 (Phytonadione)

Indications for Use:	Prevention and treatment of hemorrhagic disease of the newborn. Vitamin K deficiency.
Mechanism of Action:	An essential co-factor in the synthesis of the vitamin K–dependent clotting factors (II, VII, IX, X)

Individual Dose:	1. Prophylaxis in well, term babies: 2 mg
	2. Prophylaxis in at-risk babies
	  a. >1500 g: 1 mg
	  b. <1500 g: 0.5 mg
	3. Treatment: 1 mg

Interval:	For 1. above, first dose with the first feed. If breast-fed, then second dose at 5 days, third dose at 6 wk of age. If formula fed, then follow-up doses not required. For 2., single dose only For 3., according to coagulation profile
Route:	For 1. above, PO For 2., IM For 3., IV slowly over 5 min
Comments/Cautions:	IV administration may be associated with hypotension.
Metabolism/Excretion:	Hepatic metabolism. Excreted in bile and urine.
Dilution:	For 1. above, none necessary For 2., none necessary For 3., dilute to 2 ml with 5% dextrose
Stability:	Discard ampule and unused portion after initial use.
Storage:	Room temperature; protect from light
Incompatible with:	Phenytoin, ascorbic acid, dextran, vitamin B_{12}
Serum Levels:	Not required

CRITICAL PATHWAYS

HISTORY:
Age:_____G_____P_____AB_____
NSVD_____C/S_____
GA:_____APGARS_____/_____
B/W_____
Special Family Needs/Requests:

CONSULTS

SKIN / WOUND CARE / SPECIAL NEEDS

MISC
Neomap Review Date:_____ / SHIFT_____
Isolette Change Date: _____
Phototherapy:
Spot _____   K-PAD _____
Bank _____
Wallaby _____

Tour SCN with family_____
MD/ARNP _____
1st Feed _____

RESPIRATORY
Vent: _____ FiO$_2$:_____PIP/PEEP_____
CPAP:_____ FiO$_2$:_____PEEP_____
NC:_____ FiO$_2$:_____LPM_____
Hood_____ FiO$_2$:_____Weaning Orders:_

Surfactant Doses:_____
Aerosol:_____ CPT: _____
ABG:_____ CBG:_____

VS / BLD GLUCOSE
TPR:_____ BP: _____
Bld Gluc._____

FLUIDS   **TOTAL FLUIDS:**
CVC_____ @ _____
PICC_____ @ _____
PAL_____ @ _____
UAC_____ @ _____
PIV _____ @ _____
Additional Fluids
_____ @ _____
_____ @ _____
_____ @ _____
_____ @ _____
_____ @ _____
UAC Level _____UVC Level___
CVL Drsg. Change:_____
NUTRITION   NPO_____
TPR_____ Nutrition: ___
COG _____ _____
OG/NG_____
PO_____ Amt/Freq: ___
LABS PENDING   **RADIOLOGY**

CULTURES

DIAGNOSTIC STUDIES

NEOMAP

Aspect of Care	DAY 1 Date:	Init.	DAY 2 Date:	Init.	DAY 3 Date:	Init.
RESPIRATORY - Optimal gas exchange and perfusion at minimal settings.	Respiratory support as needed. CXR. Surfactant per protocol. Suction PRN. Continuous pulse oximeter, monitor blood gases.		Respiratory support as needed. Suction PRN. Continuous pulse oximeter, monitor blood gases.		⟶	
CARDIAC - Optimal perfusion without pressor agents. Heart rate within normal limits.	Assess perfusion (capillary refill, pulses, BP x4 extremities.) Vital signs per protocol.		Assess perfusion (capillary refill, pulses). Vital signs per protocol.		Assess perfusion (capillary refill, pulses) Vital signs per protocol. Assess for PDA. ECHO?	
NUTRITION / FLUIDS - Adequate fluid/electrolyte and hydration status. Progress toward all nipple feeds.	NPO. Establish IV access, provide fluid needs. Blood glucose per protocol. Initial weight/head circumference.		Maintain IV access. Consider PICC. Consider feeds. Blood glucose per protocol. Daily weights and head circumference.		Maintain IV access. Consider feeds. Blood glucose per protocol. Daily weights and head circumference. Assess feeding tolerance. Offer pacifier.	
ELIMINATION - cc/kg output within acceptable range while on continuous fluids. No less then 6 wet diapers in 24 hours when off IVF.	I&O, calculate urine output every day and PRN. Utilize appropriate diapers per developmental / clinical needs.		⟶		⟶	
THERMAL REGULATION - Temperature maintained within normal limits.	Radiant warmer on ISC and K-pad, if necessary. Shield with plastic and use humidity as indicated.		Consider double-wall isolette on ISC. K-pad as necessary.		⟶	
NEURODEVELOPMENT - Progress toward oral-motor readiness with subsystem stability.	Cluster care/minimal handling. Narcotics prior to painful procedures. Offer pacifier for consoling and during procedures. Maintain flexion using developmental supports. Minimize sensory stimulation by decreasing exposure to light and noise.		⟶			
SKIN INTEGRITY - Minimal skin irritation. Integrity of epidermal barrier maintained.	Assess skin integrity. Bathe when stable. Minimal tape usage. Tegaderm under adhesives as needed. Cord care per protocol.		Minimal tape usage. Tegaderm under adhesive as needed. Cord care per protocol. Bathe with warm sterile water prn. Eucerin/Aquaphor pm.		⟶	
INFECTION - No signs nor symptoms of infection.	Admission labs as ordered. Antibiotics as ordered. Hand washing per protocol, always before and after patient contact.		Check Gentamycin level. Hand washing per protocol. Monitor results of cultures.		Monitor results of cultures. Hand washing per protocol.	
FAMILY SUPPORT - Optimal family involvement and knowledge.	Admission packet given. Discuss breast feeding. Explain equipment / unit routines including hand washing protocol. Provide support for initial contact.		Encourage and facilitate communication with MD/ ARNP. Introduce concept of Kangaroo Care. Reinforce unit routine information. If breast feeding, arrange to introduce parents to a Lactation Consultant. Discuss collection and storage of breask milk.		Discuss signs of stress and soothing techniques. Encourage involvement in care as appropriate. Reinforce information regarding collection and storage of breast milk.	
DISCHARGE PLANNING - Family will demonstrate ability to perform basic skills needed post discharge.	Initial assessment of family needs/referrals as needed. Family supports identified.		Assessment of family needs. Family supports identified. Interdisciplinary Assessment tool completed by Clinical Care Coordinator.		Assessment of family needs. Family supports identified. Teach as appropriate: Take a temperature_____ Diaper change_____ Cord care_____ Skin care_____ Use of bulb syringe_____	

Before performing these routines, a physician's order must be received for those activities requiring an order.

SIGNATURE	INITIALS	SIGNATURE	INITIALS

CODE - VARIANCE SOURCE:	A. Patient/Family	B. Caregiver / Clinician	C. Hospital	D. Community
1. Event not applicable	3. Patient condition	10. Physician's order	20. Information/Data availability	30. Placement delay
2. Unpredicted event	4. Patient/family decision	11. Caregivers decision	21. Supplies/Equipment availability	31. Transportation delay
	5. Patient/family availability	12. Caregiver action	22. Department overbooked/closed	32. Community-other
	6. Patient/family cognition		23. Delayed/incorrect medication/fluids	33. Home Healthcare delay
	7. Mother's condition		24. Bed Availability	

DAY 4 Date:	Init.	DAY 5 Date:	Init.	DAY 6 Date:	Init.	DAY 7 Date:	Init.
⟶		⟶		⟶		⟶	
Assess perfusion (capillary refill, pulses). Vital signs per protocol.		⟶		⟶		⟶	
Maintain IV access. Blood glucose per protocol. Daily weights & head circumference. Assess feeding tolerance. Offer pacifier.		⟶		⟶		⟶ Florida Infant Screen Weekly length assessment	
⟶		⟶		⟶		⟶	
⟶		Double-wall isolette with ISC & K-pad if necessary.		⟶		Double-wall isolette as necessary. D/C K-pad if temperature stable.	
⟶		⟶		⟶		⟶	
⟶		⟶		⟶		⟶	
⟶		⟶		⟶		⟶	
Discuss signs of stress and soothing techniques. Encourage involvement in care as appropriate.		⟶		⟶		⟶	
Teach as appropriate: Take a temperature_____ Diaper change_____ Cord care_____ Skin care_____ Use of bulb syringe_____		⟶		⟶		⟶	

DATE	CODE	VARIANCE	CAUSE	ACTION	DATE RESOLVED

PAGE 3 of 4

Aspect of Care	DAY 14 Date: Gestational Age:	Init.	Date: Gestational Age: 30 weeks	Init.	Date: Gestational Age: 32 weeks	Init.
RESPIRATORY - Optimal perfusion and gas exchange at minimal settings.	Respiratory support as needed. Monitor blood gases as needed. Continuous pulse oximeter.		➝		➝	
CARDIAC - Optimal perfusion without pressor agents. Heart rate within normal limits.	Assess perfusion (capillary refill, pulses). Vital signs per protocol.		➝		➝	
NUTRITION / FLUIDS - Adequate fluid/electrolyte and hydration status. Progress toward all nipple feeds.	Maintain IV access. Advance feeds as tolerated. Offer pacifier with gavage feeds. Blood glucose per protocol. Daily weights and head circumference. Weekly length assessment.		➝		➝ Assess po readiness.	
ELIMINATION - cc/kg output within acceptable range while on continuous fluids. No less than 6 wet diapers in 24 hours when off IVF.	I&O. Calculate urine output daily and PRN. Utilize appropriate diapers per developmental / clinical needs.		➝		➝	
THERMAL REGULATION - Temperature maintained within normal limits.	Double-walled isolette with ISC as needed. Change isolette weekly.		➝		DWI. D/c ISC if > 15000 gms. Change isolette weekly.	
NEURODEVELOPMENT - Progress toward oral-motor readiness with subsystem stability.	Cluster care/minimal handling. Narcotics prior to painful procedures. Offer pacifier for consoling and during procedures. Maintain flexion using developmental supports. Minimize sensory stimulation by decreasing exposure to light and noise.		➝		➝	
SKIN INTEGRITY - Minimal skin irritation. Integrity of epidermal barrier maintained.	Minimal tape usage. Tegaderm under adhesives as needed. Bathe with mild soap prn. Eucerin prn.		➝		➝	
INFECTION - No signs nor symptoms of infection.	Hand washing per protocol, always before and after patient contact.		➝		➝	
FAMILY SUPPORT - Optimal family involvement and knowledge.	Reinforce signs of stress and soothing techniques. Encourage involvement in care as appropriate. Consider Kangaroo Care.		Encourage involvement in care as appropriate. Kangaroo Care.		➝	
DISCHARGE PLANNING - Family will demonstrate ability to perform basic skills needed post discharge.	Teach as appropriate: Taking a temperature _____ Diaper change_____ Skin care_____ Use of bulb syringe_____		Return demonstration of: Taking a temperature _____ Diaper change _____ Skin care _____ Use of bulb syringe _____		Discuss clothing needs.	

Before performing these routines, a physician's order must be received for those activities requiring an order.

SIGNATURE	INITIALS	SIGNATURE	INITIALS

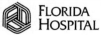

FLORIDA HOSPITAL

NEONATAL CARE MAP

665-NNCM (12/01)

Date:	Init.	Date:	Init.	Date:	Init.	Date:	Init.
Gestational Age: 33 weeks		Gestational Age: 34 weeks		Gestational Age: 36 weeks		Gestational Age: 37-40 weeks	
———→		———→		Consider d/c pulse oximeter.		———→	
———→		———→		———→		———→	
Maintain IV access. Assess po readiness. Full feeds. Offer pacifier with gavage feeds. Daily weights and head circumference. Weekly length assessment.		Assess readiness for increased frequency of po feeds. Maintain IV access. Full feeds. Offer pacifier with gavage feeds. Daily weights and head circumference. Weekly length.		Assess fluid needs. Full feeds. Consider gavage prn/po with cues. Daily weights and head circumference. Weekly length.		PO all feeds. Daily weights and head circumference. Weekly length.	
Diaper checks if no IV.		———→		———→		———→	
DWI. Change isolette weekly. Dress in light clothing.		———→		Assess readiness for open crib. Provide containment by swaddling.		Open crib. Dress in appropriate clothing.	
Cluster care. Offer pacifier for consoling. Maintain flexion using developmental supports. Minimize sensory stimulation by decreasing exposure to light and noise.		———→		Cluster care. Place in supine position. Provide containment by swaddling.		Cluster care. Place in supine position.	
Bathe prn. Eucerin prn. Minimal tape usage. Protective barriers for diaper area.		———→		———→		———→	
———→		———→		———→		———→	
Encourage involvement in care as appropriate. Kangaroo care.		———→		———→		———→	
Bath demonstration. Discuss feeding techniques with family. Encourage family to schedule CPR training.		Family doing baby care / feeding. Demonstration of medication administration and return demonstration by family.		Family doing baby care / feeding. Teach as appropriate: Formula preparation_____ Adequate I&O_____ Circumcision care_____ Signs&symptoms of illness_____ Car seat instruction_____ Prescriptions to family.		Teach as appropriate: Formula preparation_____ Adequate I&O_____ Circumcision care_____ Signs&symptoms of illness_____ Car seat instruction_____	

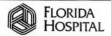

FLORIDA
HOSPITAL

NEONATAL CARE MAP

665-NNCM (12/01)

Index